Clinical Dermatology

a LANGE medical book

Clinical Dermatology
Diagnosis and Management of Common Disorders

Second Edition

Carol Soutor, MD
Adjunct Professor
Department of Dermatology
University of Minnesota Medical School
Minneapolis, Minnesota

Maria K. Hordinsky, MD
Professor and Chair
Department of Dermatology
University of Minnesota Medical School
Minneapolis, Minnesota

New York Chicago San Francisco Lisbon London Madrid Mexico City
Milan New Delhi San Juan Seoul Singapore Sydney Toronto

Clinical Dermatology: Diagnosis and Management of Common Disorders, Second Edition

Copyright © 2022, 2013 by McGraw Hill, LLC. All rights reserved. Printed in China. Except as permitted under the United States Copyright Act of 1976, no part of this publication may be reproduced or distributed in any form or by any means, or stored in a data base or retrieval system, without the prior written permission of the publisher.

1 2 3 4 5 6 7 8 9   DSS   27 26 25 24 23 22

ISBN 978-1-264-25737-9
MHID 1-264-25737-6

This book was set in Minion by Thomson Digital.
The editors were Leah Carton and Christina M. Thomas.
The production supervisor was Catherine Saggese.
Project management was provided by Dr. Sudhi Singh, Thomson Digital.

Library of Congress Control Number: 2021947609

McGraw Hill books are available at special quantity discounts to use as premiums and sales promotions, or for use in corporate training programs. To contact a representative please visit the Contact Us pages at www.mhprofessional.com.

Contents

List of Videos

Videos are accessible via mhprofessional.com/clinicaldermatology

Contributors

Rehana Ahmed, MD, PhD
Assistant Professor
Department of Dermatology
University of Minnesota Medical School
Minneapolis, Minnesota

Gretchen Bellefeuille, BS
Clinical Research Intern
Department of Dermatology
University of Minnesota Medical School
Minneapolis, Minnesota

Andrea Bershow, MD
Assistant Professor
Department of Dermatology
University of Minnesota Medical School
Veterans Affairs Healthcare System
Minneapolis, Minnesota

Paul L. Bigliardi, MD
Professor
Department of Dermatology
University of Minnesota Medical School
Minneapolis, Minnesota

Kimberly Bohjanen, MD
Professor
Department of Dermatology
University of Minnesota Medical School
Minneapolis, Minnesota

Christina L. Boull, MD
Assistant Professor
Department of Dermatology
University of Minnesota Medical School
Minneapolis, Minnesota

Caleb Creswell, MD
Adjunct Assistant Professor
Department of Dermatology
University of Minnesota Medical School
Minneapolis, Minnesota

Nada Elbuluk, MD, MSc
Associate Professor
Director, Skin of Color & Pigmentary Disorders Program
Director, Dermatology Diversity & Inclusion Program
Department of Dermatology
Keck School of Medicine of USC
Los Angles, California

Ronda Farah, MD
Assistant Professor
Department of Dermatology
University of Minnesota Medical School
Minneapolis, Minnesota

Lori A. Fiessinger, MD
Assistant Professor
Department of Dermatology
University of Minnesota Medical School
Minneapolis, Minnesota

Neal Foman, MD, MS
Professor
Department of Dermatology
University of Minnesota Medical School
Minneapolis, Minnesota

Kevin Gaddis, MD
Assistant Professor
Department of Dermatology
University of Minnesota Medical School
Minneapolis, Minnesota

Yi Gao, MD
Resident
Department of Dermatology
University of Minnesota Medical School
Minneapolis, Minnesota

Noah Goldfarb, MD
Assistant Professor
Department of Dermatology
Department of Medicine
University of Minnesota Medical School
Veterans Affairs Healthcare System
Minneapolis, Minnesota

Amrita Goyal, MD
Adjunct Assistant Professor
Department of Dermatology
University of Minnesota Medical School
Minneapolis, Minnesota

Sara Hylwa, MD
Assistant Professor
Department of Dermatology
University of Minnesota Medical School
Hennepin Healthcare
Minneapolis, Minnesota

Kristen Hook, MD
Associate Professor
Department of Dermatology
University of Minnesota Medical School
Minneapolis, Minnesota

Maria K. Hordinsky, MD
Professor and Chair
Department of Dermatology
University of Minnesota Medical School
Minneapolis, Minnesota

Juan Jaimes, MD
Adjunct Associate Professor
Department of Dermatology
University of Minnesota Medical School
Minneapolis, Minnesota

Hadley Johnson, BS
Medical Student
University of Minnesota Medical School
Minneapolis, Minnesota

Tiana Kazemi, MD
Resident
Department of Dermatology
University of Minnesota Medical School
Minneapolis, Minnesota

Daniel Knabel, MD
Assistant Professor
Department of Dermatology
University of Minnesota Medical School
Veterans Affairs Healthcare System
Minneapolis, Minnesota

Nikifor K. Konstantinov, MD
Assistant Professor
Department of Dermatology
University of New Mexico School of Medicine
Albuquerque, New Mexico

Ioannis G. Koutlas, DDS, MS
Associate Professor
Division of Oral and Maxillofacial Pathology
Director
University of Minnesota Oral Pathology Laboratories
Minneapolis, Minnesota

Jing Liu, MD
Assistant Professor
Department of Dermatology
University of Minnesota Medical School
Hennepin Healthcare
Minneapolis, Minnesota

Erin Luxenberg, MD
Assistant Professor
Department of Dermatology
University of Minnesota Medical School
Hennepin Healthcare
Minneapolis, Minnesota

Sheilagh Maguiness, MD
Associate Professor
Department of Dermatology
University of Minnesota Medical School
Minneapolis, Minnesota

Adam Mattox, DO
Assistant Professor
Department of Dermatology
University of Minnesota Medical School
Minneapolis, Minnesota

David R. Pearson, MD
Assistant Professor
Department of Dermatology
University of Minnesota Medical School
Minneapolis, Minnesota

Ingrid C. Polcari, MD
Associate Professor
Department of Dermatology
University of Minnesota Medical School
Minneapolis, Minnesota

Daniel Miller, MD
Associate Professor
Department of Dermatology
University of Minnesota Medical School
Minneapolis, Minnesota

Nora K. Shumway, MD
Assistant Professor
Department of Dermatology
University of Minnesota Medical School
Veterans Affairs Healthcare System
Minneapolis, Minnesota

Autumn L. Saizan, BS
Student Research Fellow
School of Medicine and Dentistry
University of Rochester
Rochester, New York

Brittney Schultz, MD
Assistant Professor
Department of Dermatology
University of Minnesota Medical School
Minneapolis, Minnesota

Carol Soutor, MD
Adjunct Professor
Department of Dermatology
University of Minnesota Medical School
Minneapolis, Minnesota

Allison Smith, MD
Staff Hospitalist
Department of Internal Medicine
Hennepin Healthcare
Minneapolis, Minnesota

Cindy Firkins Smith, MD
Adjunct Professor
Department of Dermatology
University of Minnesota Medical School
Minneapolis, Minnesota

Lindsey M. Voller, MD
Intern
Santa Clara Medical Center
San Jose, California

Ryan M. Wells, MD, PhD, Pharm D
Staff Dermatologist
Dermatology Clinic of Idaho
Boise, Idaho

Barbara D. Wilson, MD
Professor
Department of Dermatology
Medical College of Wisconsin
Milwaukee, Wisconsin

Christopher B. Zachary, MBBS, FRCP
Professor, Chair Emeritus
Department of Dermatology
University of California
Irvine, California

Preface

Clinical Dermatology: Diagnosis and Management of Common Disorders is the product of decades of interaction with our primary care colleagues and residents. It features concise and practical information on the diagnosis and management of common skin disorders. Diagnostic features, cost-effective management, evidence-based medicine, and patient-centered care are emphasized.

▼ INTENDED AUDIENCE

Clinicians, residents, and medical students will find this textbook helpful in their understanding and management of skin disorders. Our advisory group, consisting of primary care physicians, residents, nurse practitioners, physician assistants, and medical students was instrumental in the design and review of this textbook.

▼ ORGANIZATION AND CONTENT

Clinical Dermatology is divided into three sections.

- **Section One** covers the principles of diagnosis, management of common skin disorders, diagnostic and surgical procedures.

- **Section Two** covers common skin disorders and selected less common disorders with high morbidity. The information on each disease is formatted into 11 sections: introduction, pathogenesis, history, physical examination, laboratory findings, diagnosis, differential diagnosis, management, clinical course and prognosis, indications for consultation, and patient information. Evidence-based reviews and national and international guidelines are used when available in the management sections.

- **Section Three** focuses on the differential diagnosis of diseases in specific body regions based on history and physical examination. This section also includes the differential diagnosis of purpura, fever and rash, hospital-acquired rashes, pruritus, and skin ulcers.

▼ ONLINE LEARNING CENTER

The online learning center for this textbook at mhprofessional.com/clinicaldermatology has videos with detailed demonstrations of common cutaneous diagnostic and surgical procedures.

Clinical unknown cases with self-assessment questions and PowerPoint presentations that cover the diagnosis, evaluation, and management of common skin disorders are available at AccessDermatologyDxRx, dermatology. mhmedical.com, which is available at many institutions or as a paid subscription.

▼ ACKNOWLEDGMENTS

The editors would like to thank our McGraw Hill editors: Leah Carton, Associate Editor and Christina Thomas, Senior Project Development Editor for all their assistance in the development and publication of this textbook and Dr. Sudhi Singh, Thomson Digital Project Manager. We thank our reviewers Jamie Santilli, MD, Cynthia Olson, MD, Dori Henderson, PhD, Elizabeth Norheim NP, Brittney Busse PA, Deana Gruenhagen PA, and our medical student reviewers Carissa Klarisch and Brett Macleod.

We are grateful for contributions of photographs from Doctors Whitney Tope, Spencer Holmes, and Charles Crutchfield III.

We want to especially acknowledge Robert W. Goltz, MD, who was our mentor and chairman of the Department of Dermatology at the University of Minnesota (1971–1985). His mastery of the art, science, and practice of medicine influenced all who were privileged to train with him.

We are especially grateful for our husbands' support and patience during this project.

Structure and Function of the Skin

Amrita Goyal

Kimberly Bohjanen

INTRODUCTION TO CHAPTER

Human skin is the site of many complex structures and dynamic processes as demonstrated in Figure 1-1 and Table 1-1. These processes include barrier and immunologic functions, sensation, vitamin D synthesis, thermoregulation, and protection from ultraviolet (UV) light and trauma.

BARRIER FUNCTION

One of the most important function of human skin is to act as a barrier between us and the external environment.[1] It protects against a variety of forms of physical damage, ranging from desiccation to infection, heat loss, and UV damage.[2] The skin is a multilayered stalwart against these insults. First, the stratum corneum, with its corneocytes wrapped in cornified cell envelopes, water-impenetrable lipid lamellae, and filaggrin, forms a barrier that protects us from infectious organisms and water loss. Tight junctions help seal the spaces between neighboring cells in the stratum granulosum. Langerhans cells in the epidermis project their dendrites beyond this barrier to capture foreign antigens and act as antigen-presenting cells, alerting the immune cells in the epidermis and dermis to potential

foreign insults.[3] The skin helps to provide protection against infections from bacteria, yeasts, fungi, and viruses via daily desquamation, antimicrobial peptides, and the overall acidic pH of the corneum. The epidermis also contains epidermal nerve fibers and numerous molecules including urocanic acid, DNA, and melanin that protect us from UV damage by absorbing UV rays.[4] Eccrine glands and smooth muscle cells that control blood flow help to regulate body temperature. Subcutaneous fat offers cushioning, energy storage, and hormonal synthesis.

An understanding of the epidermal barrier is particularly important for the study of dermatology. The epidermal barrier is created by the differentiation and keratinization of epidermal cells as they move from the basal cell layer to the stratum corneum. The keratinocytes of the epidermis are produced and renewed by stem cells in the basal layer resulting in replacement of the epidermis approximately every 28 days. It takes 14 days for these cells to reach the stratum corneum and another 14 days for the cells to desquamate.[5]

Keratinocytes produce keratins, structural proteins that form filaments which are part of the keratinocyte cytoskeleton. In the stratum spinosum, keratin filaments radiate outwards from the nucleus and connect with desmosomes which are prominent under the microscope giving a

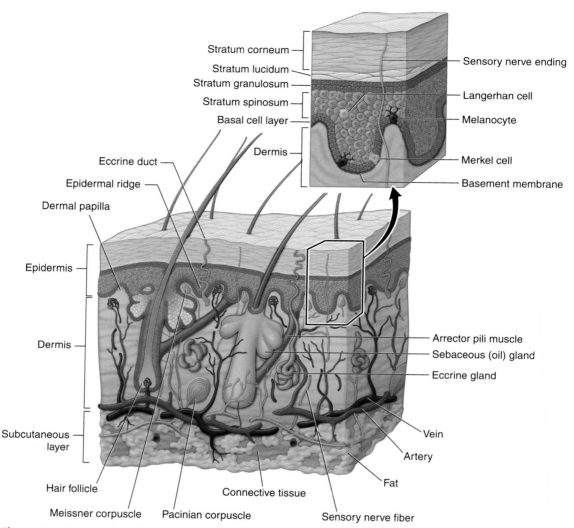

Figure 1-1. Cross-section of skin. Diagram showing layers of the skin, appendages, blood vessels, sensory nerve fibers, and sensory receptors.

"spiny" appearance to cells. As cells move into the stratum granulosum, keratohyalin granules composed of keratin and profilaggrin are formed. Profilaggrin is converted into filaggrin (filament aggregation protein) which aggregates and aligns keratin filaments into tightly compressed parallel bundles that form the matrix for the cells of the stratum corneum.[6] Filaggrin gene mutations are associated with ichthyosis vulgaris[7] and atopic dermatitis.[8] As keratinocytes move into the stratum corneum, they lose their nuclei and organelles and develop a flat hexagon shape. These cells are stacked into a "bricks and mortar" like pattern with 15–25 layers of cells (bricks) surrounded by lipids (mortar). The lipids consist of ceramides, free fatty acids, and cholesterol. The lipid "mortar" plays a critical role in preventing transepidermal water loss.

IMMUNOLOGIC FUNCTION

Epithelial cells at the interface between the skin and the environment provide the first line of defense via the innate immune system.[9] Epithelial cells are equipped to respond to the environment through a variety of structures including toll-like receptors (TLRs) of which there are at least 10, nucleotide-binding oligomerization

Table 1-1. Structure and Function of the Skin

Component	Structure and Function
Stratum corneum	Semipermeable barrier with "bricks" (stacked cornified cells) and "mortar" (ceramides, cholesterol, and fatty acids) like construction.
Stratum granulosum	Cells contains keratohyalin granules which are primarily composed of profilaggrin.
Stratum spinosum	Contains desmosomes for intercellular adhesion.
Langerhans cells	Dendritic cell important in the modulation of the adaptive immune response.
Merkel cells	Specialized cell with neuroendocrine function.
Melanocytes	Dendritic cells that produce melanin for ultraviolet light protection.
Basal cell layer	Contains the stem cells that divide and produce the rest of the keratinocytes in the epidermis.
Basement membrane	Interface between the epidermis and dermis.
Ground substance	Amorphous gel of mucopolysaccharides that is the substrate for the dermis.
Collagen	Network of fibrous proteins for skin tensile strength.
Elastic fibers	Fibrous proteins responsible for skin elasticity.
Fibroblasts	Cells that produce ground substance, collagen, and elastic fibers.
Mast cells	Leukocytes that release histamine and heparin.
Histiocytes/macrophages	Leukocytes which phagocytize and present antigen.
Eccrine glands	Sweat glands which help in temperature regulation.
Apocrine glands	Axillary and anogenital glands responsible for body odor.
Sebaceous glands	Component of pilosebaceous unit which produces sebum.
Hair follicle	Component of pilosebaceous unit that produces the hair fiber.
Somatic sensory and sympathetic autonomic nerves	Supply blood vessels, glands, and hair follicles.
Meissner's corpuscles	Specialized nerve receptor for light touch.
Pacinian corpuscles	Specialized nerve receptor for pressure and vibration.
Blood vessels	Two horizontal plexuses in the dermis which are connected and can shunt blood flow.
Lymphatics	Parallel to blood vessels with two plexuses for flow of plasma.
Fat	Provides protection from cold and trauma. Essential for storage of energy and metabolism of sex hormones and glucocorticoids.
Fascia	Connective tissue layer overlying the muscle beneath the fat.

domain-like receptors, C-type lectins, and peptidogly-can-recognition proteins.[10] TLR-mediated activation of epithelial cells is also associated with the production of defensins and cathelicidins, families of antimicrobial peptides.[11]

Dendritic cells bridge the gap between the innate and adaptive immune systems. Dermal dendritic cells can induce autoproliferation of T cells, production of cytokines, and nitric oxide synthase. The exact function of epidermal Langerhans cells is an area of rapidly evolving research suggesting that these cells are very important to the modulation of the adaptive immune response.[12]

MELANIN PRODUCTION AND PROTECTION FROM ULTRAVIOLET LIGHT DAMAGE

Melanocytes comprise 10% of the cells in the basal cell layer. There is another population of melanocytes in the hair follicle which is responsible for hair color and replacing epidermal melanocytes as needed (Figure 1-2). Melanocytes produce melanin, a pigmented polymer that absorbs UV light. Melanin is synthesized from tyrosine in several steps that require the enzyme tyrosinase. As melanin is produced, it is then packaged into melanosomes, a specialized organelle. Melanosomes are phagocytosed by

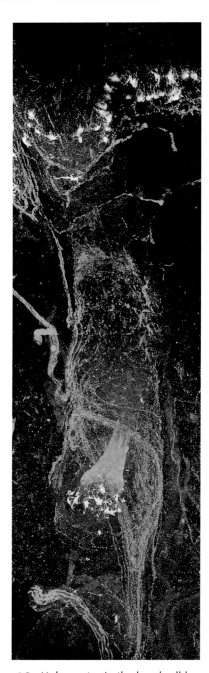

▲ **Figure 1-2.** Melanocytes in the basal cell layer and in the hair bulb region. Confocal image of nerves *(aqua)* and melanocytes *(yellow)* in the epidermis and the hair bulb region of a human anagen scalp hair follicle. Montage of three fields of view. Sample was immunostained with antibodies to a pan-neuronal marker PGP9.5 *(aqua)* and melanocytes (MEL5) *(yellow)*. Reproduced with permission from Marna Ericson, PhD.

keratinocytes and moved to an area above the keratinocyte's nucleus acting as a protective shield from UV light. One melanocyte provides melanosomes for as many as 30–40 keratinocytes. All humans have the same number of melanocytes. The variation in the degree of skin color is due to variations in melanosomes. Individuals with darker brown skin tones have more abundant, larger, and more dispersed melanosomes. Exposure to UV light stimulates the production of melanin within melanosomes producing a "tan." Tryosinase deficiency is associated with albinism and vitiligo is associated with absence of melanocytes.

SYNTHESIS OF VITAMIN D

The main sources for vitamin D are dietary intake and production of vitamin D precursors by the skin. With exposure to UV light provitamin D3 (7-dehydrocholesterol) in the epidermis is converted into previtamin D that converts into vitamin D3. Vitamin D3 is converted to its metabolically active form in the liver and kidneys.

SENSATION

The skin is one of the principal sites of interaction with the environment and many types of stimuli can be processed by the peripheral and central nervous systems. Initially, cutaneous nerves were classified as being either "afferent" controlling sweat gland function and blood flow, or "efferent" transmitting sensory signals to the central nervous system, but after the discovery of the neuropeptide substance P (SP) and other neuropeptides in sensory nerves, many trophic properties of nerve fibers and neuropeptides have been reported.

There are three major nerve types in the skin:

- Aβ fibers—large, heavily myelinated nerve fibers which transmit tactile sensation.
- Aδ fibers—thinly myelinated nerve fibers involved in the transmission of short and fast painful stimuli.
- C-fibers—unmyelinated nerves which transmit pain and itch sensations.

Mixed nerve fiber bundles form a plexus from which individual nerve fibers extend toward their specific targets. The first tier is underneath the epidermis and innervates the epidermis and cutaneous mechanoreceptors or the upper dermis (Figure 1-3).

The second and third tiers are located between the dermis and subcutis or in the deep subcutis and innervate hair follicles, the arrector pili muscles, and sweat glands as well as the lower dermis and subcutis. All three plexi innervate blood vessels, smooth muscle cells, and are closely aligned with mast cells thereby connecting different skin cell populations with the brain.

TEMPERATURE REGULATION

The skin helps to regulate and maintain core body temperature through regulation of sweating and varying the blood flow in the skin. Evaporation of sweat contributes to

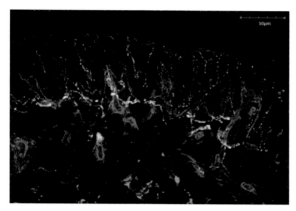

Figure 1-3. Epidermal nerve fibers and blood vessels. Confocal image of epidermal nerve fibers *(green)*, blood vessels *(red)* and the neuropeptide calcitonin gene related peptide (CGRP) *(blue)* in human scalp skin. The dermal/epidermal boundary is delineated by Collagen Type IV. Sample was immunostained with antibodies to protein gene product (PGP) 9.5 *(green)*, Collagen Type IV *(red)*, and CGRP *(blue)*. Reproduced with permission from Marna Ericson, PhD.

temperature control of the body. Under normal conditions 900 mL of sweat is produced daily. With increased physical activity or increased environmental temperature, 1.4–3 L of sweat per hour can be produced.

The regulation of blood flow in the capillaries in the dermal papillae and other cutaneous vessels plays an important role in convective heat loss and heat conservation. Normally, the blood flow in the skin is approximately 5% of the cardiac output, but in extremely cold temperatures it can drop to almost zero and in severe heat stress it can be as high as 60%. Dysfunction of thermoregulation can lead to hyper- and hypothermia which is more common in older adults and diabetic patients.

PROTECTION FROM TRAUMA

The dermis varies in thickness from 1 to 4 mm. It protects and cushions underlying structures from injury and provides support for blood vessels, nerves, and adnexal structures. It is separated from the epidermis by the basement membrane, which is created by the basal layer of the epidermis. Collagen is responsible for the tensile strength of the skin and comprises 75% of the dry weight of the dermis. Defects in collagen synthesis are associated with diseases such as Ehlers–Danlos syndrome (hyperextensible joints and skin). Elastic fibers are responsible for the elasticity and resilience of the skin and are 2%–3% of the dry weight of the skin. Defects in elastic fibrils can be associated with cutis laxa and Marfan syndrome.

STRUCTURAL INTEGRITY OF THE SKIN AND THE BASEMENT MEMBRANE

The basement membrane is the adhesive layer between the epidermis and dermis, and is composed of a vast array of proteins which bind and interact with one another in a carefully orchestrated pattern. Critical structures include desmosomes, focal adhesions, hemidesmosomes, the basement membrane itself, and dermal fibrils including collagen VII. Desmosomes permit adhesion of keratinocytes to one another and are composed of desmosomal cadherins (desmogleins and desmocollins), plakins (desmoplakin, envoplakin, and periplakin), as well as armadillo family proteins (plakoglobin and plakophilin). Hemidesmosomes allow adhesion of basal layer keratinocytes to the basement membrane, which itself is composed of collagen IV. Hemidesmosomes are composed of plakins, integrins, and collagens. The dermal–epidermal junction is anchored to the papillary dermis by interactions between anchoring filaments and type VII collagen in the dermis. These components are not only structural but also play an active role in cellular signaling.

SKIN MICROBIOME

One of the most important components of human skin is not produced by ourselves at all, but rather our symbionts, the microbes that live in and on our skin. They are myriad, including bacteria, fungi, and viruses. They range from colonizers to commensals, pathogens, and perform a variety of functions.[13–15]

The human microbiome is defined as all the microorganisms, genomes, and surrounding environmental conditions in the ecosystem of our skin. Studies of the microbiome must thus not include single organisms, but rather the cutaneous microbial communities. It is important to recognize that the skin is not one monolithic environment; rather, the microbial communities on our skin are incredibly diverse and can vary from location to location, for example, from the seborrheic areas of the face to the axillae, palms, and soles. Even different skin structures (e.g., hair follicles vs. eccrine glands) can contain different types of microorganisms even at the same locations.

Different pathologic conditions may be associated with their own changes in the microbiome. For example, acne is characterized by the proliferation of *Cutibacterium acnes* (previously *Propionobacterium acnes*).[16] Atopic dermatitis demonstrates an increased abundance of *Staphylococcus aureus* and *S. epidermidis* in the flaring skin, as well as higher fungal diversity.[17] Diabetic ulcers are associated with staphylococcal species and fungi, while primary immunodeficiency syndromes are associated with *Aspergillus* and *Candida*. Finally, psoriasis may be associated with decreased bacterial diversity but higher fungal diversity; this may be a function of increased production of antibacterial peptides in psoriatic skin.[18]

IDENTITY AND ESTHETICS

The perception of an individual's ethnicity, age, state of health, and attractiveness is affected by the appearance of their skin and hair. Sun damaged skin, rashes, hair disorders, pigment disorders, and acne can have a profound effect on how individuals perceive themselves and others.

REFERENCES

1. Dąbrowska AK, Spano F, Derler S, Adlhart C, Spencer ND, Rossi RM. The relationship between skin function, barrier properties, and body-dependent factors. *Ski Res Technol.* 2018;24(2):165–174.
2. Burke KE. Mechanisms of aging and development—A new understanding of environmental damage to the skin and prevention with topical antioxidants. *Mech Ageing Dev.* 2018;172:123–130.
3. Jakob T. The changing faces of Langerhans cells. *J Eur Acad Dermatology Venereol.* 2017;31(11):1773–1773.
4. Hart PH, Norval M. The multiple roles of urocanic acid in health and disease. *J Invest Dermatol.* 2021;141(3):496–502.
5. Has C. Peeling skin disorders: A paradigm for skin desquamation. *J Invest Dermatol.* 2018;138(8):1689–1691.
6. Sandilands A, Sutherland C, Irvine AD, McLean WHI. Filaggrin in the frontline: role in skin barrier function and disease. *J Cell Sci.* 2009;122(9):1285–1294.
7. Thyssen JP, Godoy-Gijon E, Elias PM. Ichthyosis vulgaris: the filaggrin mutation disease. *Br J Dermatol.* 2013;168(6):1155–1166.
8. Liang Y, Chang C, Lu Q. The genetics and epigenetics of atopic dermatitis—Filaggrin and other polymorphisms. *Clin Rev Allergy Immunol.* 2016;51(3):315–328.
9. Coates M, Blanchard S, MacLeod AS. Innate antimicrobial immunity in the skin: A protective barrier against bacteria, viruses, and fungi. Hogan DA, ed. *PLOS Pathog.* 2018;14(12):e1007353.
10. Gallo RL. Human skin is the largest epithelial surface for interaction with microbes. *J Invest Dermatol.* 2017;137(6):1213–1214.
11. Weinberg A, Krisanaprakornkit S, Dale BA. Epithelial antimicrobial peptides: Review and significance for oral applications. *Crit Rev Oral Biol Med.* 1998;9(4):399–414.
12. Kaplan DH. In vivo function of Langerhans cells and dermal dendritic cells. *Trends Immunol.* 2010;31(12):446–451
13. Byrd AL, Belkaid Y, Segre JA. The human skin microbiome. *Nat Rev Microbiol.* 2018;16(3):143–155.
14. Dréno B, Araviiskaia E, Berardesca E, et al. Microbiome in healthy skin, update for dermatologists. *J Eur Acad Dermatology Venereol.* 2016;30(12):2038–2047.
15. Lunjani N, Hlela C, O'Mahony L. Microbiome and skin biology. *Curr Opin Allergy Clin Immunol.* 2019;19(4):328–333.
16. Xu H, Li H. Acne, the skin microbiome, and antibiotic treatment. *Am J Clin Dermatol.* 2019;20(3):335–344.
17. Lee S-Y, Lee E, Park YM, Hong S-J. Microbiome in the gut-skin axis in atopic dermatitis. *Allergy Asthma Immunol Res.* 2018;10(4):354.
18. Lewis DJ, Chan WH, Hinojosa T, Hsu S, Feldman SR. Mechanisms of microbial pathogenesis and the role of the skin microbiome in psoriasis: A review. *Clin Dermatol.* 2019;37(2):160–166.

Morphology and Terminology of Skin Lesions

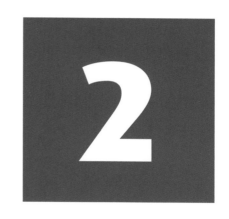

Carol Soutor

INTRODUCTION TO CHAPTER

Identification and classification of a patient's skin lesions are important steps in the diagnosis of any skin disorder.[1] The numerous descriptive terms used in dermatology can be overwhelming and at times confusing as there are some variations in the use and meaning of these words in the literature.[2] The International League of Dermatology Societies developed a glossary for the description of cutaneous lesions which has helped to standardize terminology for skin findings.[3] A few simple terms can be used to describe the cutaneous findings in most skin diseases. Using proper terminology to describe skin findings is essential for both documentation and communication with other clinicians. The effort to use precise descriptive terms also encourages a clinician to look with more care and more closely at a patient's skin lesions. Key terms used in the description of lesions are (1) type of primary lesion, (2) secondary features, (3) color of lesion, (4) shape of the lesion, and (5) arrangement and distribution of the lesions.

TYPES OF PRIMARY SKIN LESIONS

It is important to identify and categorize the primary skin lesion(s). This may be difficult if the lesions are excoriated or if the examination takes place late in the disease process. The lesion may need to be lightly touched or deeply palpated to accurately assess its features. Most diagnostic algorithms for skin disease start with the primary lesion. See Chapter 5 for lists of diseases and their primary skin lesions.

Table 2-1 lists the 10 most common morphological terms for types of skin lesions. These are based on:

- Diameter of the lesion.

Table 2-1. Primary lesions and their morphology.

Terminology	Diameter	Morphology	Example
Macule Patch	< 1 cm >1 cm	Flat, level with surface of skin and differs in color from surrounding skin.	Vitiligo (Figure 2-1)
Papule Plaque	< 1 cm > 1 cm	Solid, elevated lesion.	Chronic allergic contact dermatitis (Figure 2-2)
Wheal	Any size	White to pink edematous, smooth, papule, or plaque that lasts less than 24 hours.	Urticaria (Figure 2-3)
Nodule	> 1 cm	Dermal or subcutaneous solid elevated lesion.	Amelanotic melanoma (Figure 2-4)
Vesicle Bulla	< 1 cm > 1 cm	Blister containing fluid or blood.	Bullous pemphigoid (Figure 2-5)
Pustule	< 1cm	Cavity filled with pus, may be sterile.	Pustular psoriasis (Figure 2-6)
Cyst	> 1 cm	Cavity filled with pus or keratin.	Boil (Figure 2-7)

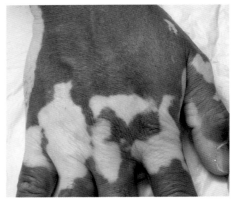

Figure 2-1. Macules and patches. Vitiligo on dorsum of hand.

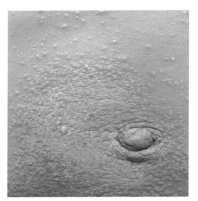

Figure 2-2. Papules and a plaque. Chronic allergic contact dermatitis to metal button.

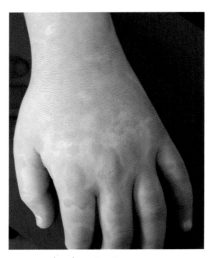

Figure 2-3. Wheal. Urticaria.

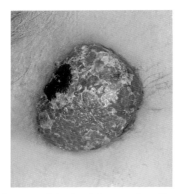

Figure 2-4. Nodule. Nodular amelanotic melanoma.

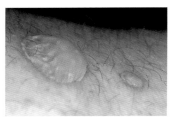

Figure 2-5. Vesicle and bulla. Pemphigus.

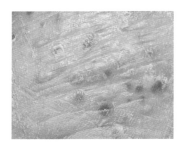

Figure 2-6. Pustules. Pustular psoriasis.

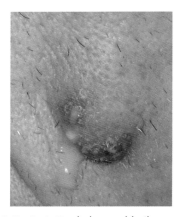

Figure 2-7. Cyst. Staphylococcal boil.

Table 2-2. Examples of secondary changes in skin lesions.

Terminology	Secondary Surface Changes in Lesions	Example
Scale	Loose or adherent flakes composed of stratum corneum cells.	Psoriasis (Figure 2-8)
Crust	Deposits of serum, pus and/ or blood, may be yellow, brown, black, or green.	Pemphigus (Figure 2-9)
Lichenification	Thickening of the epidermis with accentuation of skin markings.	Atopic Dermatitis (Figure 2-10)
Fissure	Linear, sharply defined, deep crack in the skin.	Callous (Figure 2-11)
Erosion	Localized loss of part or all of the epidermis.	Drug rash (Figure 2-12)
Excoriation	Linear or punctate, superficial, erosions in the epidermis caused by fingernails and sharp objects. It may extend into the dermis.	
Ulcer	Loss of the entire epidermis and a portion of the dermis. May extend into subcutaneous tissue.	Venous ulcer. (Figure 2-13)
Eschar	Black, hard crust resulting from tissue necrosis of the epidermis and/or dermis.	Heparin necrosis. (Figure 2-14)
Atrophy	Depression and/or surface change in skin as the result of diminution of a component(s) of the epidermis, dermis or fat.	Lichen sclerosus (Figure 2-15)
Scar	Depressed or elevated proliferation of connective tissue that has replaced inflamed or traumatized skin.	Depressed scar (Figure 2-16) Hypertrophic scar (Figure 2-17)

- Relationship of the lesion to the surface of the skin— is the lesion flat or elevated above the surface of the skin?
- Composition of the lesion—is it solid or fluid filled?

Most textbooks use a lesion diameter of 1 cm to distinguish between various lesion types. It is not uncommon for a skin disease to have multiple types of lesions. Therefore, terms such as maculopapular and vesiculobullous are commonly used.

SECONDARY FEATURES

Some lesions have a smooth surface such as urticarial wheals, but most skin diseases have some secondary changes to the surface of the lesions (Table 2-2). These surface changes may often quickly develop during the course of a skin disease. For example, vesicles, bullae, and pustules often collapse leaving crusts or erosions. Some infectious and inflammatory diseases will result in skin atrophy or scarring. Papulosquamous is a term used to describe diseases that have papules or plaques with scale as in psoriasis and lichen planus.

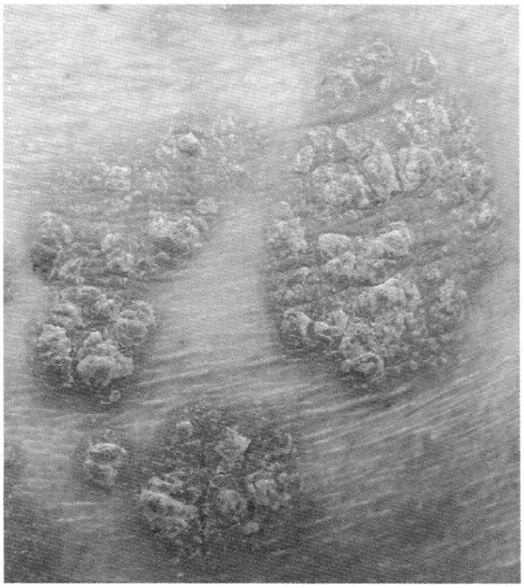

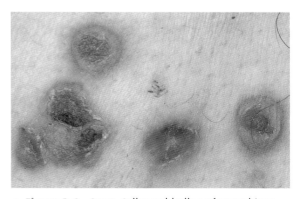

Figure 2-8. Scale. Psoriasis.

Figure 2-9. Crust. Collapsed bullae of pemphigus.

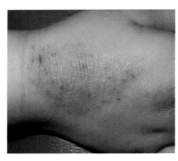

▲ **Figure 2-10.** Lichenification. Atopic dermatitis on dorsal hand.

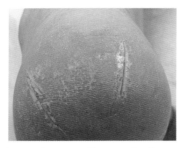

▲ **Figure 2-11.** Fissure. Callous on heel.

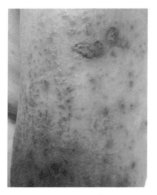

▲ **Figure 2-12.** Excoriations and erosions. Lichenoid drug rash.

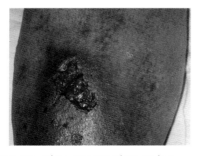

▲ **Figure 2-13.** Ulcer. Venous ulcer on leg.

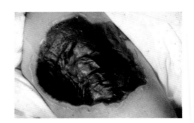

▲ **Figure 2-14.** Eschar. Heparin necrosis.

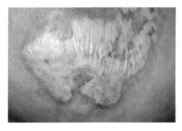

▲ **Figure 2-15.** Atrophy. Lichen sclerosis, extragenital.

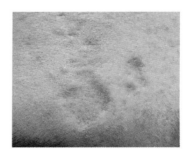

▲ **Figure 2-16.** Depressed scar. Scar after herpes zoster.

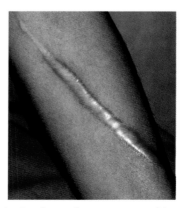

▲ **Figure 2-17.** Elevated scar. Hypertrophic scar after laceration.

Table 2-3. Selected colors of lesions and their causes.

Color	Examples of Causes of Color Change	Example
Pale pink	Edema or dilated blood vessels.	Urticaria
Pink	Dilated blood vessels	Dermatitis
Red	Dilated blood vessels or extravasated blood.[5]	Angiomas
Purple	Dilated blood vessels or extravasated blood.	Vasculitis
Yellow	Carotenemia, bilirubinemia.	Xanthoma
Brown	Increased melanin or dermal hemosiderin.	Melasma, nevi
Black	Increased melanin, necrotic skin.[6]	Nevus, eschar
Blue	Melanin deep in dermis, cyanosis.	Blue nevus
White	Decreased or absent melanin or melanocytes, vasoconstriction.[7]	Vitiligo

COLOR

The color of the lesion often correlates with underlying pathophysiologic changes (Table 2-3). Terms such as hyperpigmented and hypopigmented are often used to describe lesions that are darker or lighter than the patient's overall skin color. Erythema or erythematous are terms used for red hues of lesions that are due to dilated blood vessels in the dermis. It is important to note that in individuals with darker tones erythematous skin rashes may appear purple or hyperpigmented.[4] Also postinflammatory hypopigmentation and postinflammatory hyperpigmentation of lesions may result in color changes in lesions ranging from white to black.

SHAPE

The shape of the lesion may also aid in diagnosis (Table 2-4). Some common skin disorders such as tinea corporis, which typically presents with annular lesions, are characterized by the shape of the lesion.

ARRANGEMENT AND DISTRIBUTION

The lesions of many skin disorders often have characteristic arrangements and distributions (Table 2-5). For instance, the lesions in viral exanthems and drug rashes are typically symmetrical and herpes simplex vesicles are usually grouped.

DOCUMENTATION

The most important features when documenting or describing a *skin rash* are:

- Type of primary skin lesion(s).
- Secondary surface changes if present.
- Color.
- Location of lesions.
- The percentage of affected body surface should be documented in cases of extensive rashes.
- The arrangement/distribution and shapes of lesions may be helpful in some cases.

Table 2-4. Shapes of individual lesions.

Terminology	Shapes of Lesions	Example
Discoid/round	Circular or coin shaped.	Nummular dermatitis (Figure 2-18)
Oval	Round with elliptical shape.	Pityriasis rosea (Figure 2-19)
Annular	Ring shaped with variation in appearance between center and periphery.[8]	Tinea corporis (Figure 2-20)
Arcuate	Arc shaped, may be a portion of an annular lesion.[9]	Erythema multiforme (Figure 2-21)
Targetoid	Target like with distinct zones.	Erythema multiforme (Figure 2-22)

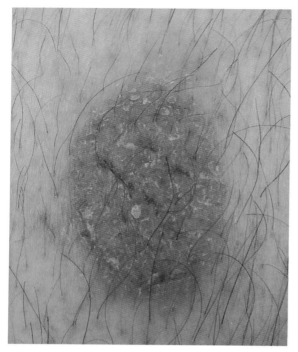

▲ **Figure 2-18.** Discoid/round. Nummular dermatitis.

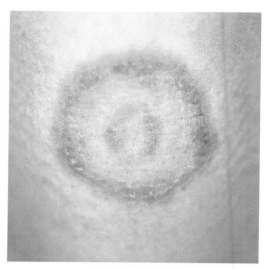

▲ **Figure 2-20.** Annular lesion. Tinea corporis.

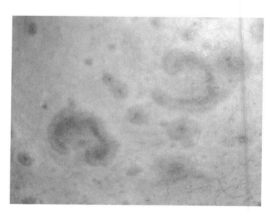

▲ **Figure 2-21.** Arcuate lesion. Erythema multiforme.

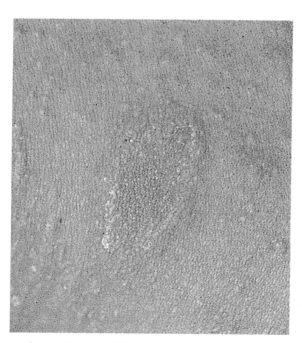

▲ **Figure 2-19.** Oval. Pityriasis rosea.

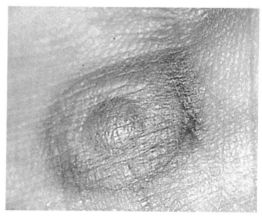

▲ **Figure 2-22.** Targetoid lesion. Erythema multiforme.

Table 2-5 Arrangement and distribution of lesions.

Terminology	Arrangement and Distribution of Lesions	Example
Grouped	Clustered next to each other.	Herpes simplex (Figure 2-23)
Discrete/Isolated	Separated from one another.	Miliaria (Figure 2-24)
Linear/Streak	Thin straight line of lesions.	Poison ivy dermatitis (Figure 2-25)
Dermatomal	Distributed along a dermatome.	Herpes zoster (Figure 2-26)
Serpiginous	Wave or snake-like streak.	Larva migrans (Figure 2-27)
Reticular	Lace or net like.	Livedo reticularis (Figure 2-28)
Symmetrical	Uniform distribution on an axis of the body such as the midline.	Drug rash (Figure 2-29)
Generalized/Disseminated	Spread over wide areas of the body.	
Photodistributed	Located In areas of sunlight exposure.[10]	Phototoxic drug rash (Figure 2-30)

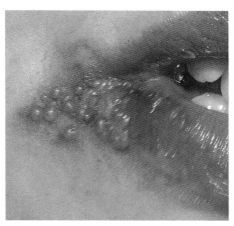

▲ **Figure 2-23.** Grouped lesions. Vesicles of herpes simplex.

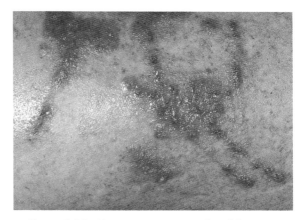

▲ **Figure 2-25.** Linear arrangement of vesicles. Allergic contact dermatitis due to poison ivy.

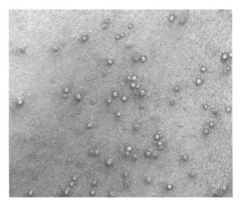

▲ **Figure 2-24.** Discrete lesions. Pustules of miliaria pustulosa.

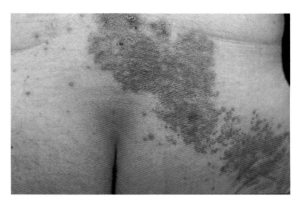

▲ **Figure 2-26.** Dermatomal distribution of hemorrhagic vesicles. Herpes zoster.

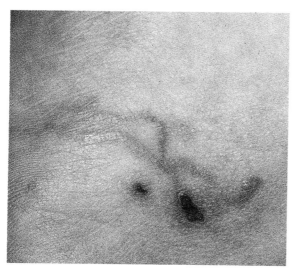

▲ **Figure 2-27.** Serpiginous lesions. Cutaneous lava migrans.

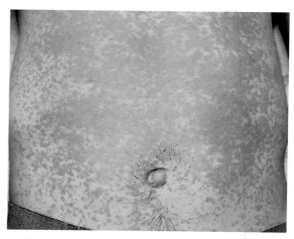

▲ **Figure 2-29.** Symmetrical and generalized distribution of macules. Drug rash.

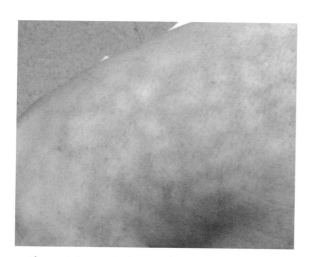

▲ **Figure 2-28.** Reticular. Livedo reticularis.

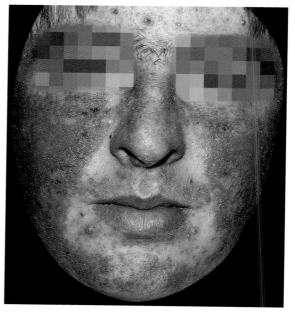

▲ **Figure 2-30.** Photodistribution of crusted plaques. Phototoxic drug rash. Note sparing of periorbital and perioral areas, and nasolabial folds.

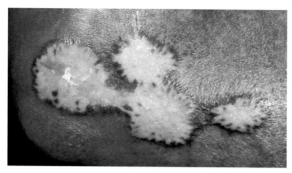

▲ **Figure 2-31.** Discoid lupus erythematosus. Multiple round, pink plaques with scale on the elbow. Dark brown hyperpigmentation and white scarring are seen on the edge of the plaques

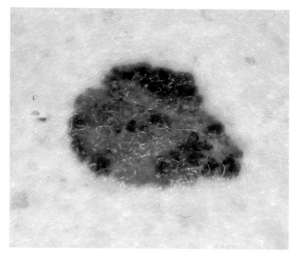

▲ **Figure 2-32.** Melanoma. Plaque with an irregular border and variations in color including black, brown, red, and blue.

Utilizing these various terminologies, the lesions of discoid lupus erythematosus in Figure 2-31 could be described as "multiple round, pink plaques with scale on the elbow. Dark brown hyperpigmentation and white scarring are seen on the edge of the plaques."

The most important features when documenting or describing a *skin tumor (growth)* are:

- Type of primary lesion.
- Surface changes if present, especially any erosions or ulceration.
- Color(s).
- Diameter of lesion.
- Precise location of lesion especially if malignancy is suspected.

For example, the melanoma in Figure 2-32 could be described as "2 cm plaque with an irregular border and variations in color including black, brown, red, and blue. No ulcerations are seen."

REFERENCES

1. Rimoin L, Altieri L, Craft N, Krasne S, Kellman PJ. Training pattern recognition of skin lesion morphology, configuration, and distribution. *J Am Acad Dermatol.* 2015;72(3):489–495.

2. Cardili RN, Roselino AM. Elementary lesions in dermatological semiology: literature review. *An Bras Dermatol.* 2016;91(5):629–633.
3. Nast A, Griffiths CEM, Hay R, Sterry W, Bolognia JL. The 2016 International League of Dermatological Societies' revised glossary for the description of cutaneous lesions. *Br J Dermatol.* 2016;174(6):1351–1358.
4. Kelly A, Taylor SC, Lim HW, Serrano A. eds. *Taylor and Kelly's Dermatology for Skin of Color,* Second edition. McGraw-Hill Education; 2016.
5. Elias M, Patel S, Schwartz RA, Lambert WC. The color of skin: red diseases of the skin, nails, and mucosa. *Clin Dermatol.* 2019;37(5):548–560.
6. Qiu CC, Brown AE, Lobitz GR, Shanker A, Hsu S. The color of skin: black diseases of the skin, nails, and mucosa. *Clin Dermatol.* 2019;37(5):447–467.
7. Brown AE, Qiu CC, Drozd B, Sklover LR, Vickers CM, Hsu S. The color of skin: white diseases of the skin, nails, and mucosa. *Clin Dermatol.* 2019;37(5):561–579.
8. Trayes KP, Savage K, Studdiford JS. Annular Lesions: Diagnosis and Treatment. *Am Fam Physician.* 2018;98(5):283–291.
9. Sharma, A, Lambert, P J, Maghari, A, et al. Arcuate, annular, and polycyclic inflammatory and infectious lesions. *Clin Dermatol.* 2011; 29(2):140–150.
10. Choi D, Kannan S, Lim HW. Evaluation of patients with photodermatoses. *Dermatol Clin.* 2014;32(3):267–275.

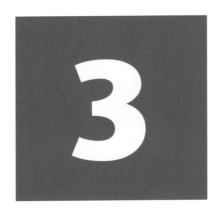

History and Physical Examination of the Skin, Hair, and Nails

Carol Soutor

INTRODUCTION TO CHAPTER

There is no more difficult art to acquire than the art of observation, and for some it is quite as difficult to record an observation in brief and plain language.
—Sir William Osler, 1903

The physical examination was a primary tool in the diagnosis of most diseases prior to the widespread availability of diagnostic laboratory tests and imaging.[1] Many skin diseases are currently diagnosed on the basis of a short history and physical examination.

Typically, the history and physical examination for skin problems are done in the same sequence and manner as with any other organ system. However, in some cases, it is helpful to examine the patient after taking only a brief history, so that the questions for the patient can be more focused.

The history and physical examination play an important part in establishing rapport, confidence, and trust in the patient–clinician relationship. In this chapter, information on the challenges and opportunities in the care of select populations will be covered.

SELECTED KEY POINTS FOR HISTORY OF CUTANEOUS DISORDERS

A problem-focused history is sufficient for most common skin disorders. If the patient has systemic complaints, or if diseases such as lupus erythematosus or vasculitis are suspected, a detailed or comprehensive history may be needed.

History of Present Illness (HPI)

- Initial and subsequent morphology of the lesions.
- Location of lesion(s).
- Symptoms (e.g., itch, pain, tenderness, burning).
- Date of onset/duration.
- Severity-current and in the past.
- Factors causing flares.
- Use of medications, including over-the-counter products.
- Response to prior treatment.
- History of previous similar outbreaks.

If the patient's main complaint is a *skin tumor or growth*, the following additional questions should be added.

- What changes have occurred in size and appearance of the lesion?
- Is there a history of spontaneous or trauma-induced bleeding of the lesion?
- Is there a history of sunburns or tanning bed use?
- What is the history of use of sunscreens?

It is also important to determine the patient's Fitzpatrick skin type, as this helps to identify patients at risk for skin cancer. The patient should be asked if they burn easily or tan after initial exposure to approximately 45–60 minutes of sunlight in early summer.[2] The patient's response determines the Fitzpatrick skin type.

- Skin type I: Always burns, never tans.
- Skin type II: Usually burns, tans with difficulty.
- Skin type III: Sometimes burns, tans normally.
- Skin type IV: Rarely burns, tans easily.
- Skin type V: Very rarely burns, tans easily.
- Skin type VI: Never burns, tans darkly.

Typically, there is some correlation between a patient's Fitzpatrick skin type and skin color. However, there are patients with darker skin tones who do experience sunburns and sun damage.

If indicated, the patient should also be asked about the effect of their skin condition on work, social, and home life. Patients with the following chronic skin disorders often report quality of life concerns:

- Acne
- Atopic dermatitis
- Chronic bullous diseases
- Chronic pruritus
- Hair disorders
- Hidradenitis suppurativa
- Melanoma
- Nail disorders
- Pigment disorders
- Psoriasis
- Rosacea
- Scars/keloids

The Dermatology Life Quality Index, at www.dermatology.org.uk, has a 10-point questionnaire that can be used to more accurately assess a patient's quality of life concerns. Skindex is another widely used instrument for quality of life evaluations.[3]

Past Medical History

Past and current diseases, personal history of skin cancer, and other skin disorders.

Medications

All systemic and topical medications, including over-the-counter medications and supplements.

Allergies and Medication Intolerances

Medications, foods, pollens, chemicals.

Family History

Skin cancer, atopy (atopic dermatitis, allergic rhinitis, and asthma), psoriasis, autoimmune diseases, or any disorder similar to the patient's current skin problem.

Social History

Occupation(s), hobbies, travel history, marital status, housing status.

Review of Systems (ROS)

High-yield questions for cutaneous disorders include fever, chills, fatigue, weight changes, lymphadenopathy, joint pain/stiffness, wheezing, rhinitis, menstrual history, birth control history, photosensitivity, depression, and anxiety.

PHYSICAL EXAMINATION OF THE SKIN, HAIR, AND NAILS

Introduction

A careful, systematic examination of the skin, hair, and nails is an essential and cost-effective method for evaluation and diagnosis of skin disorders. It is important to examine the skin for lesions that are directly related to the chief complaint, and also for incidental findings, especially lesions that may be skin cancer. A study done in a dermatology clinic in Florida found that 56.3% of the melanomas that were found during a full body skin examination were not mentioned in the patient's presenting complaint.[4] A full body skin examination can easily be incorporated into routine physical examinations of other areas of the body.

A limited problem-focused exam may be all that is needed for some chief complaints, such as warts or acne in a child or young adult. However, there are several indications for a total body skin exam. These include:

- Personal history or family history of skin cancer, and presence of risk factors for skin cancer (e.g., history of severe sunburns, immunocompromised status).
- Presence of a generalized skin rash, such as atopic dermatitis or psoriasis.
- An ill patient.
- Diagnosis is unknown or in doubt.

Some clinicians may be hesitant to perform a full body skin examination because of concerns that a patient will be reluctant to agree to it. However, a study of female veterans showed that most patients prefer a full body skin examination.[5] As with any examination, the clinician should explain which areas of the body are to be examined and the reasons for the examination and ask for permission/consent to proceed. Also, the patient should be asked if they would like to have a room attendant/chaperone present during the examination. Be especially sensitive to cultural concerns of the patient regarding examination of the skin.

The Exam Room and Equipment

It is important to create a comfortable setting for the patient. The exam room should be warm, with the door and window shades closed. The patient should remove all clothing from the area(s) to be examined and should be given an examination gown of adequate size, and a sheet. Wigs, eyeglasses, bandages, and makeup should be removed as needed. Hearing aids and dentures should be removed at the time of the ear and mouth examination.

The following equipment should be available: additional lighting for the exam (e.g., penlight, otoscope, or ophthalmoscope), magnifying lens, examination gloves, tongue blade, gauze pad, and a centimeter ruler. Other equipment that may be needed includes a Wood's lamp (black light), a dermatoscope, bacterial and viral transport media, a #15 scalpel blade, microscope slides, and/or a sterile collection jar for skin scrapings, and a camera, to document findings. It is also helpful to have a body diagram available, for documentation of skin findings.

If the patient cannot get onto the exam table because of issues with limited mobility, the upper body and the anterior surface of the legs can be examined while the patient is seated, and the lower body skin exam of the buttocks and posterior legs can be done with the patient standing, with appropriate support. In a hospital setting, a patient may be unconscious or have limited ability to turn over. In such circumstances, it may be necessary to have the nurses turn the patient, so that the posterior trunk and extremities can be seen. Many common skin conditions, such as drug rashes and vasculitis, are more prominent in dependent areas of the body.

Examination of Suspected Skin Cancers and Rashes

A full body examination should include a systematic examination of the entire surface of the skin, hair, and nails. Many skin diseases and skin cancers present in areas that are not normally examined or are not easily seen by the patient. For example, a melanoma in a toe web (Figure 3-1), or a basal cell carcinoma on the posterior surface of the ear (Figure 3-2).

When examining and screening patients for **skin cancer** and **precancerous lesions**, give close attention to the following areas:

- Any areas of chronic sun exposure, such as the scalp, face, ears, neck, extensor forearms, dorsal hands, and upper trunk, with special attention to:
  - The head and neck, which are the most common sites of basal and squamous cell carcinomas.

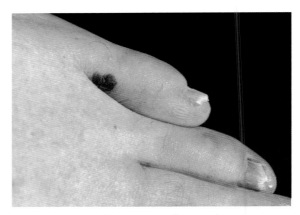

▲ **Figure 3-1.** Melanoma in web space between fourth and fifth toes.

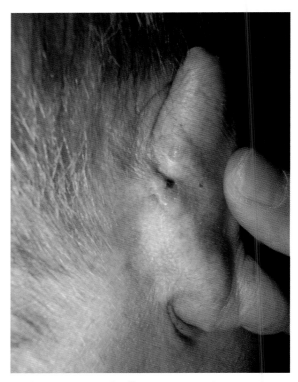

▲ **Figure 3-2.** Basal cell carcinoma on the posterior aspect of the helix of the ear.

- The back, which is the site of almost 40% of melanomas in men.[6]
- The legs, which are the site of over 40% of melanomas in females.[6]

When performing skin examinations for **dermatoses (rashes):**

- Carefully and systematically examine all skin surfaces. Refer to Chapters 30–42 for common skin diseases that occur in specific body regions.
- Pay close attention to areas that are difficult for patients to see, such as the scalp, back, buttocks, and posterior legs.
- Examine the eyes, ears, nose, and oral cavity. These areas are of particular importance in exanthems, bullous diseases, and connective tissue disorders.

▼ STEPS IN THE PHYSICAL EXAMINATION

Overall Assessment of the Skin

- Begin the examination with the patient seated and facing you.
- Scan the skin for variations in skin tone, looking for features, such as pigment variations, erythema, flushing, jaundice, pallor, or cyanosis.
- Touch the skin lightly, to check for abnormal variations in skin temperature and for increased sweating.
- Check the turgor and elasticity of the skin, by pinching the skin over the dorsal hand or forearm and quickly releasing it. The skin should quickly return to its normal shape.

Scalp and Hair

- Evaluate the hair for any abnormal changes of texture, fractured hair fibers, and patterned hair loss.
- Palpate the scalp for tumors, cysts, papules, plaques, or scale.
- Visually inspect the scalp by parting the hair at regularly spaced intervals.
- Lightly palpate any balding or areas with hair thinning for the presence of gritty, rough, keratotic areas that could indicate the presence of actinic keratoses.

Head, Face, and Neck

- The face is the most common area for basal and squamous cell carcinomas, so careful inspection is important.
- Lightly palpate the face for the presence of gritty, rough keratotic areas that could indicate the presence of actinic keratoses.
- Carefully examine all areas of the face, especially the central portions, for any evidence of skin cancer.
- Inspect the neck for evidence of sun damage or tumors and palpate the lymph nodes. Metastatic head and neck

carcinomas may involve the anterior and/or posterior cervical lymph nodes.

Eyes, Ears, Nose, and Throat

- Eyes: Check sclerae for evidence of injection of blood vessels or jaundice. Evert the eyelids to examine the palpebral conjunctivae.
- Nose: Examine the nostrils for tumors or erosions.
- Oral cavity: Using a tongue blade and a light source, examine all surfaces of the mucosa, looking for erosions, vesicles, or white, red, or brown macules or plaques. Gently grasp the tongue with a gauze pad, so that all surfaces can be examined. Examine the teeth and gums for abnormal dentition, cavities, abscesses, or periodontal disease.
- Ears: Lightly palpate the ears for the presence of rough, gritty keratotic areas. Examine all aspects of the ears for tumors, with special attention to the postauricular areas, where tumors may go undetected.

Arms

- Examine all surfaces, with close attention to the elbows and antecubital fossae, as these are common sites for psoriasis and atopic dermatitis, respectively.
- The flexor wrists are common sites for atopic dermatitis, scabies, and lichen planus.

Hands

- Examine all surfaces of the hands, including the web spaces. The hands are the site of involvement for many common skin disorders, such as irritant and allergic contact dermatitis, and less common disorders, such as connective tissue diseases.
- The dorsal hands are common sites for sunlight-related disorders, such as actinic keratoses and photodermatoses.

Fingernails

- Examine the nail plates for any abnormalities, such as thickening, onycholysis (distal nail plate detachment from the nail bed), horizontal or vertical defects, and for evidence of clubbing.
- Examine the nail beds for pigment or color changes or splinter hemorrhages.
- Use a dermatoscope or ophthalmoscope, at a setting of +12 to +20, to examine the nail bed capillaries, which should look like a picket fence. Look for evidence of capillary dilation or any irregularities in pattern, as these findings may indicate the presence of a connective tissue disorder.

Trunk

The trunk examination in males can be done with the patient remaining in the seated position. Many clinicians perform the trunk examination in females with the patient lying down, to allow for appropriate draping.

- Begin with the examination of chest, paying special attention to the central upper chest, which is an area of frequent sun exposure and sunburns.
- In females, lift the breasts, if needed, to examine the inframammary areas, to check for candida infections or intertrigo.
- Examine the axillae for the presence or absence of hair and any skin lesions. Check for lymphadenopathy, if indicated.
- Carefully examine the back, 40% of melanomas in men are located on the back, especially the upper central back.

Abdomen

The patient should be asked to lie down for the rest of the examination, if they have been in the seated position.

- Lift and spread the skin as needed, to examine body fold areas in obese patients, to check for any evidence of a candida infection or intertrigo.
- Check the inguinal area for lymphadenopathy and signs of a fungal infection.

Genitals

- As covered in the introduction, the patient should be informed of the extent of the examination of the genital area and consent to the examination.
- In males, examine the surface of the scrotum and penis for skin lesions. If the patient is uncircumcised, the foreskin should be retracted.
- In females, examine the entire vulva. The vagina should be examined if there are any signs of warts or malignancy on the vulva.

Legs

- Examine the anterior and medial surfaces of the legs. Over 40% of melanomas in women are on the legs, so it is important that any pigmented or other suspicious lesions are noted.
- The knees and popliteal surfaces are common areas of involvement in psoriasis and atopic dermatitis, respectively.
- The lower legs should be evaluated for signs of edema, stasis dermatitis, and ulcers.

Feet

- Check the feet for pallor and decreased temperature, as this may indicate vascular disease.
- Check the dorsalis pedis and posterior tibial pulses, if indicated.
- Carefully examine the feet, especially the plantar surfaces in diabetic patients, for evidence of neuropathic diabetic ulcers.
- Check all toe webs for presence of scaling or fissures, which could indicate a fungal infection.

Toenails

- As with the fingernails, examine the nail plates for any abnormalities, such as thickening, onycholysis, horizontal or vertical defects, and ingrowing of the nail plate into the cuticle folds.

Buttocks and Posterior Legs

At this point in the examination, the patient should be asked to turn, lying face down on the examination table, so that the buttock area and posterior surfaces of the legs can be examined. If this is difficult or uncomfortable for the patient, complete the examination with the patient lying on his/her side.

- Examine the gluteal cleft and perianal area. These sites are often affected in inflammatory diseases, such as psoriasis and lichen sclerosus, respectively. The perianal area is also a potential site for warts.

Lastly, help patients step off of the examination table, if needed.

TELEDERMATOLOGY AND THE PHYSICAL EXAMINATION

Introduction

Dermatology was one of the first medical specialties to utilize telemedicine and telehealth.[7] The growth of teledermatology was initially slow in the United States and was mostly limited to the academic centers and Veterans Administration Health Centers. However, the COVID-19 pandemic resulted in a rapid surge in the use of teledermatology by all types of dermatology and primary care practices.[8]

Teledermatology is useful to follow up patients with known diagnoses. However, there are issues involved in using it for the diagnosis of new skin rashes and in the performance of total body examinations in patients with suspicious tumors.

Teledermatology can be done in a store-and-forward manner, in which a healthcare professional takes photographs of the rash or tumor and forwards them to the consulting clinician, with a brief history. More commonly, the patient takes photographs of the rash or tumor, and schedules a video or telephone appointment with a clinician.

Challenges in Teledermatology

The challenges in the teledermatology physical examination include:

- Picture may be out of focus or have other quality issues, such as poor lighting.
- Picture may not be taken at a proper distance.
- Picture may not represent the most typical and diagnostic portion of the rash or tumor.
- It may be difficult to determine the morphology of the primary lesion, for example, vesicles may appear to be papules, or macules may appear to be papules.
- It is difficult to photograph the extent of widespread rashes or do a total body skin exam in patients with suspicious tumors or confirmed melanoma.
- It is impossible to determine the consistency or depth of a tumor.
- Examination with a dermatoscope is usually not possible.

Asking additional questions of the patient may help to clarify the true presentation of the rash or tumor. These could include:

- Are your spots or the growth level with the skin, or are they elevated?
- Are your spots rough or smooth?
- How large is your growth—the size of a pea, a grape, or larger?
- What color are your spots—red, pink, blue, gray, purple, white, tan, brown, or black?
- Are your spots or the growth soft like a balloon, firm like rubber, or hard like a rock?

Tips on Photography in Teledermatology

High-quality photographs are needed to reliably diagnose most skin conditions. Unfortunately, many telemedicine photographs are out of focus or have other quality issues.

The following instructions can be given to a patient to improve the quality of their photographs:

- Use good lighting, preferably natural lighting, such as sunlight. However, bright, direct sunlight may result in an overexposed photograph.
- Hold the phone or camera steady, with both hands.

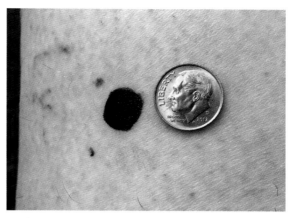

▲ **Figure 3-3.** Picture taken with smart phone to demonstrate use of a coin to focus and estimate the size of a 1 cm lesion.

- Hold the phone or camera parallel to the skin's surface.
- Get a close-up picture of the skin condition and also some pictures of the entire rash.
- On a smartphone, touch the screen and pinch the fingers together to get a close-up photograph of the skin condition.
- On a camera, use the flower icon or macro setting to get a close up. The flower icon or the macro setting should be used for most pictures.
- Place a coin adjacent to the skin rash or tumor, to help sharpen the focus and to clarify the size of the spots (Figure 3-3).
- If you are concerned about a single spot, circle it with a pen or marker.
- If you cannot photograph areas of your body, such as your back, ask another person to take photographs, if possible.
- Make sure you are in a quiet, private place for your visit. You may be asked confidential questions, and/or be asked to take additional pictures.
- When possible, submit your photographs in advance of your visit.

THE HISTORY AND PHYSICAL EXAMINATION IN SELECTED POPULATIONS

Introduction

The clinical setting should be welcoming to patients of all socioeconomic, gender, racial, ethnic, and cultural populations. Patient literature, posters, and pictures in the office should reflect the community and the people who are served in the clinic. Several studies have shown that cultural competency is essential for patient communication, trust, compliance, and optimal outcomes.[9]

A culturally competent clinician:

- Keeps an open and flexible mind.
- Asks patients about their cultural values and health beliefs, as they relate to the patient's understanding of their disease and treatment options.
- Is aware of their explicit and implicit bias tendencies toward certain populations.
- Provides individualized patient care.

Clinicians may need to expand and modify certain elements of the history and physical examination in selected populations. It is important to note that an individual patient may belong to several populations, such as a black, elderly immigrant. Often the history will need to include more specific details of the demographic and social history. Medical terms and the patient's responses to questions may need to be clarified. A simple question such as "What do you think caused your skin problem?" may reveal much about the patient's belief system regarding his/her disease.

In some situations, the physical examination may need to be modified based on age, mobility, or cultural and religious preferences. The principle of "talk before you touch" is even more important in some of the selected populations listed below.[10] Appropriate draping of the skin is important, even if permission has been given for the examination.

Pediatric Population

Office visits may be stressful for children.[11] Creating a safe and child-friendly setting, with children's books and toys, can help relax a child. Document the relationship of the child with the accompanying adult(s) and whether or not that person is the child's legal guardian. When appropriate, ask the child to confirm elements of their history, using age-appropriate language. If the child's parent or parents are not present, call them, if needed, for additional information.

The physical examination in younger children can be done in the caregiver's lap. If an infant or young child is placed on an exam table, take care that the child does not roll off of the table. Start with examining the hands and feet, which is less fearful for a child. When possible, clothing can be lifted, rather than removed. At or after puberty, a patient may prefer to have the parent leave the room for the physical examination. In that case, a room attendant should be present.

Geriatric Population

People over 85 years are the fastest growing segment of the United States population. Elderly patients disproportionally account for visits related to cutaneous problems, as for other organ systems. The presence of hearing loss and dementia may complicate obtaining a good history. The prevalence of dementia between ages 71 and 79 is 5.0% but rises to 37.4% in those over 90 years of age. [12] Hearing impairment is present in 39.3% of the population between 60 and 69 years, is more prevalent in males, and continues to worsen with age.[13]

Speaking more slowly and more distinctly is beneficial in communicating with the older patients.

As with the pediatric population, the clinician should document the relationships of any person(s) who accompany the patient, especially if they are providing some of the patient's history. The application of topical medications and dressings may be difficult in older patients who have limited range of motion. Therefore, it is helpful to know who is living in the patient's household, and what, if any, support system the patient has, in terms of care of their skin.

If an elderly patient has difficulty getting onto an examination table, the physical examination of the skin can be done with the patient seated in an office chair. The patient can be asked to stand, with support, for examination of the lower back, buttocks, and posterior portions of the legs.

Many people over 60 years of age have multiple benign tumors, including seborrheic keratoses, solar lentigines, cherry angiomas, and skin tags. These tumors may distract a clinician from detecting a malignant tumor. Therefore, special attention should be given to any atypical growths.

Skin of Color Population

Skin of color populations include a diverse group of individuals with skin tones that are darker than those of the White population such as Black, Asian, and Native American individuals.[14] In the last United States census, the skin of color population comprises almost a quarter of the total population.[15]

One of the common concerns in skin color of patients are pigment disorders, such as vitiligo, melasma, and post inflammatory hyper- and hypopigmentation. The history should include documentation of sun exposure and use of sunscreens. It is a common misconception that darker pigmented individuals do not need to use sunscreens. Another misconception is that more darkly pigmented individuals do not get skin cancer.[16] The incidence of skin cancer, including melanoma, is lower in darker-pigmented individuals but the diagnosis is frequently delayed, resulting in an increase in morbidity and mortality. It is important to examine the skin in areas of relatively less pigment, such as the palms, soles, and nail beds.

Black individuals have a greater risk for several cutaneous disorders, including keloids, pseudofolliculitis barbae (razor bumps), atopic dermatitis, sarcoidosis, traction alopecia, and other hair disorders such as central centrifugal scarring alopecia. Healthcare disparities in the African American populations can result in the patient presenting with more advanced skin disease.[9]

Various ethnic and cultural practices may affect the skin and hair, such as cupping, coining, acupuncture, tribal tattoos or scarification, use of various skin-lightening agents, hair braiding or twisting (dreadlocks), and hair straightening.[17]

LGBT Population

The lesbian, gay, bisexual, transgender (LGBT) self-identified population in the United States is over 10 million, with females, millennials, and city dwellers predominant.[18] Bias and a clinician's lack of knowledge can negatively impact healthcare in this population. This often begins with the medical history. It is important that LBGT patients have the opportunity to document their preferred name, sex (male, female, intersex), their sexual orientation (e.g., heterosexual, gay, lesbian, bisexual) and their gender identity, expression, and transgender status. If the patient identifies a preference in personal pronouns, use these in conversation and in documentation. When indicated, a sexual behavior history should be included.

For various reasons, some segments of the LGBT population are at higher risk for certain conditions that may have cutaneous manifestations. These include sexually transmitted diseases (genital warts, molluscum, genital herpes, syphilis, and hepatitis B and C), cutaneous signs of HIV, and signs of substance abuse or self-harming.[18] Transgender patients may have cutaneous signs related to the use of systemic testosterone or estrogen therapy, such as androgenetic alopecia, hirsutism, and acne. These patients may also have signs of gender-affirming procedures.

Homeless Population

Over 500,000 adults and children in the United States are homeless.[19] Being homeless can cause and exacerbate many skin problems, due to exposure to the elements, overcrowding in shelters, inadequate nutrition, and poor hygiene. Patients who are homeless face multiple challenges in accessing and utilizing healthcare. The patient's housing status should be documented in the social history section, to clarify what, if any, shelter they have. It is important to ask the patient about access to a mobile phone, bathing and laundry facilities, transportation, food, and a place to store medications. Most homeless patients qualify for Medicaid, and should be assisted in enrollment, if they are not already enrolled. Medicaid covers a wide range of over-the-counter and prescription medications used to treat skin disorders.

The physical examination should include surveillance for cutaneous disorders that are common in the homeless population, such as bacterial and fungal infections, chronic wounds, cold injuries, trauma, ectoparasites/infestations, malnutrition, and signs of intravenous drug use.[20]

Immigrant Population

The immigrant population represents a diverse group that may have various issues with the healthcare system. Most prominently, language barriers, or even illiteracy, may be a factor in obtaining a good health history. Interpreters vary in their skill level and availability. Translation apps or telephone interpretation services can be used if a qualified interpreter cannot be present.[21]

Recent immigrants from some countries may have cutaneous signs of certain infections, infestations, and ectoparasites that occur primarily outside of the United States, Canada, and Europe. The patient's history should include questions regarding diseases specific to the patient's country of origin.

Diverse Ethnic and Religious Populations

When pertinent, it is helpful to know if patients have specific concerns with healthcare visits relating to their ethnic or religious traditions. In some situations, direct eye contact, shaking hands, or communication and examination by a clinician of the opposite gender is not preferred by some patients.[21]

The physical examination may need to be modified, especially in females. It is important to clarify exactly which parts of the body need to be examined, the reasons for the examination, and what modifications can be made. Consent to proceed with the examination is important and cannot be assumed. The patient should be carefully draped, with only the site of examination exposed.

Websites for Additional Information on Selected Populations

- U.S Department of Health and Human Services, A Physician's Practical Guide to Culturally Competent Care. https://cccm.thinkculturalhealth.hhs.gov/default.asp
- National Center for Cultural Competence. https://nccc.georgetown.edu
- AAMC Tool for Assessing Cultural Competency. https://www.aamc.org/what-we-do/mission-areas/diversity-inclusion/tool-for-assessing-cultural-competence-training
- Howard University College of Medicine. National Multicultural Center. https://www.aetcnmc.org/translate.php
- National Health Care of the Homeless Council. https://nhttps://www.hudexchange.info/resource/5639/2017-ahar-part-1-pit-estimates-of-homelessness-in-the-us/hchc.org
- Health Professionals Advancing LFBTQ Equality. http://www.glma.org

REFERENCES

1. Verghese A, Brady E, Kapur CC, Horwitz RI. The bedside evaluation: Ritual and reason. *Ann Int Med.*2011; 155:550–553.
2. Kelly AP, Jamoussi M, Skin of color: A historical perspective. In: Kelly AP, Taylor SC, Lim HW, Serrano AMA, eds. Taylor

and Kelly's Dermatology for Skin of Color. 2nd ed. McGraw-Hill Education; 2016.

3. Chren M. The Skindex instruments to measure the effects of skin disease on quality of life. *Dermatol Clin.* 2012;30(2):231–236.

4. Kantor J, Kantor DE. Routine dermatologist-performed full-body skin examination and early melanoma detection. *Arch Dermatol.* 2009;145(8):873–876.

5. Federman DG, Kravetz JD, Haskell SG, Ma F, Kirsner RS. Full-body skin examinations and the female veteran: prevalence and perspective. *Arch Dermatol.* 2006;142(3):312–316.

6. Garbe C, Leiter U. Melanoma epidemiology and trends. *Clin Dermatol.* 2009;27(1):3–9.

7. Weinstein RS, Krupinski EA, Doarn CR. Clinical examination component of telemedicine, telehealth, mHealth, and connected health medical practices. *Med Clin N America.* 2018;102(3):533–544.

8. Perkins S, Cohen JM, Nelson CA, Bunick CG. Teledermatology in the era of COVID-19: Experience of an academic department of dermatology. *J Am Acad Dermatol.* 2020;83(1):e43–e44.

9. McKesey J, Berger TG, Lim HW, McMichael AJ, Torres A, Pandya AG. Cultural competence for the 21st century dermatologist practicing in the United States. *J Am Acad Dermatol.* 2017;77(6):1159–1169.

10. Hussain A. Recommendations for culturally competent dermatology care of muslim patients. *J Am Acad Dermatol.* 2017;77(2):388–389

11. LaRosa C, Makkar H, Grant-Kels JM. Approach to the total body skin examination in adults and children: Kids are not just little people. *Clin Dermatol.* 2017;35(6):500–503.

12. Plassman BL, Langa KM, Fisher GG, et al. Prevalence of dementia in the United States: The aging, demographics, and memory study. *Neuroepidemiology.* 2007;29(1-2):125–132.

13. Hoffman HJ, Dobie RA, Losonczy KG, Themann CL, Flamme GA. Declining prevalence of hearing loss in US adults aged 20 to 69 years. *JAMA Otolaryngol Head Neck Surg.* 2017;143(3):274.

14. Taylor SC, Kyei A. Defining skin of color. In: Kelly A, Taylor SC, Lim HW, Serrano A, eds. *Taylor and Kelly's Dermatology for Skin of Color,* New York, New York: McGraw-Hill; 2016.

15. United States Census Bureau. Accessed July 1, 2020. https://www.census.gov/topics/population/race/data.html

16. Hu S, Parmet Y, Allen G, et al. Disparity in melanoma: A trend analysis of melanoma incidence and stage at diagnosis among whites, Hispanics, and blacks in Florida. *Arch Dermatol.* 2009;145(12):1369–1374.

17. Vashi NA, Patzelt N, Wirya S, Maymone MBC, Zancanaro P, Kundu RV. Dermatoses caused by cultural practices. *J Am Acad Dermatol.* 2018;79(1):1–16.

18. Yeung H, Luk KM, Chen SC, Ginsberg BA, Katz KA. Dermatologic care for lesbian, gay, bisexual, and transgender persons. *J Am Acad Dermatol.* 2019;80(3):581–589.

19. HUD Exchange. Accessed July 1, 2020. https://www.hudexchange.info/resource/5639/2017-ahar-part-1-pit-estimates-of-homelessness-in-the-us

20. Coates SJ, Amerson EH, Chang AY. Dermatologic care of persons experiencing homelessness: Key concepts in an era of housing instability. *JAMA Dermatol.* May 13, 2020.

21. Attum B, Shamoon Z. Cultural competence in the care of Muslim patients and their families. In: *StatPearls.* StatPearls Publishing; 2020.

Diagnostic Procedures and Dermoscopy

Lori A. Fiessinger
Juan Jaimes
Carol Soutor

INTRODUCTION TO CHAPTER

This chapter covers selected diagnostic tools that a clinician can use in the office to confirm their diagnoses including laboratory tests, patch testing, and dermoscopy.

A few simple diagnostic tests such as potassium hydroxide (KOH) examinations, Tzanck smears, and scrapings for scabies can be helpful to confirm a clinical diagnosis. However, these tests can have false positive and false negative results which are typically due to the following problems most of which are operator dependant.[1]

- Improper site or lesion selection
- Faulty collection technique
- Failure to systematically scan entire specimen
- Artifacts in the specimen

Polymerase chain reaction (PCR) tests for herpes and fungal infections are replacing some of the diagnostic tests used in dermatology, but they are not yet widely available in all clinical settings.[2,3]

The use of a dermatoscope to visualize structures that are beneath the surface of the skin has become a major diagnostic tool in dermatology. This chapter will focus on dermoscopy of skin tumors. However, dermoscopy is useful in the diagnosis of many other disorders such as hair diseases and dermatoses.[4]

POTASSIUM HYDROXIDE (KOH) EXAMINATIONS AND FUNGAL CULTURES

KOH examinations (Table 4-1) are a cost effective method for the detection of superficial fungal skin infections. In the hands of an experienced clinician, this test has a high level of specificity and sensitivity. However, cotton or nylon fibers from clothing and socks can mimic fungal hyphae and a mosaic artifact created by cell membranes can also mimic fungal hyphae and air bubbles can mimic spores. Some of these false positives can be reduced by the use of special stains such as Chicago Sky Blue or Chlorazol Black E.[5] Fungal cultures are another option for detection of fungal infections. Dermatophyte Test Media (DTM) media, a modified Sabouraud's agar contains an indicator dye that turns red within 7–14 days in the presence of viable dermatophytes (Figure 4-3).

Table 4-1. Potassium hydroxide (KOH) examination for superficial fungal infections.

Equipment needed
- # 15 scalpel blade (for skin and nails), small curette (for nails), tweezers or needle holder, swab or gauze (for scalp and hair).
- Microscope, glass slides, cover slip, 20% potassium hydroxide solution (plain or with dimethyl sulfoxide (DMSO) or with dyes such as Chlorazol Black E or Chicago Sky Blue).
- If specimens are submitted for culture, a sterile urine container or petri dish is needed for transport of the specimens to the laboratory. Modified Sabouraud's agar, such as Dermatophyte Test Medium (DTM) or Mycosel ™ or Mycobiotic™ should be available if specimens will be directly placed onto the fungal media.

Techniques for specimen collection
- **Skin:** Select an area of scale from the edge of the lesion. Clean the area with an alcohol pad. Gently scrape off the scale using a #15 scalpel blade onto a glass slide or sterile urine container. If the lesions are vesicular (e.g., vesicular tinea pedis), trim off the roof of a vesicle with iris scissors and submit that as a specimen.
- **Nails:** Scrape out subungual debris using a small metal skin or ear curette or a #15 scalpel blade.
- **Scalp:** Pluck involved hairs with a needle holder or tweezers, cut the hair saving the proximal 1 to 2 cm of the hair fiber and bulb. Scalp scales can be collected for culture using a bacterial culturette swab that has been pre-moistened by the transport media or sterile gauze or a sterile toothbrush. The involved areas of the scalp should be vigorously rubbed with these devices.

Examination of specimens
- Place the skin scales or proximal hair fibers on a glass slide and cover the specimen with 2–4 drops of 20% KOH solution (plain or with DMSO) to partially dissolve keratin. Apply a coverslip.
- Let the slide sit for 20 minutes.
- Lower the condenser on the microscope and decrease the intensity of the light.
- Scan the entire preparation at low power (10 X) magnification looking for branching septate hyphae (Figure 4-1) which are seen in dermatophyte infections or pseudohyphae and spores (Figure 4-2) which are seen in yeast infections. These may be slightly refractile. Switch to high power (40 X magnification) to confirm findings.
- Be aware of the many causes of false positive examinations, such as clothing fibers, hair fibers, and the cell walls of keratinocytes, which can look like hyphae. Also, air bubbles and oil droplets can look spores.

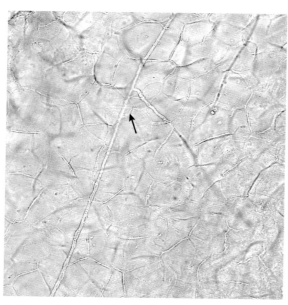

Figure 4-1. Potassium hydroxide (KOH) preparation. Fungal hyphae with branches.

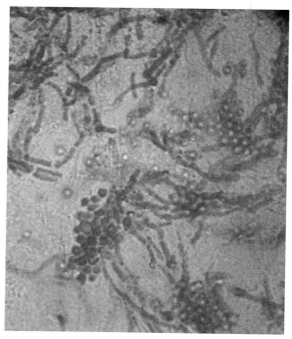

Figure 4-2. Chicago Sky Blue and potassium hydroxide (KOH) preparation. Pseudohyphae and spores in tinea versicolor infection.

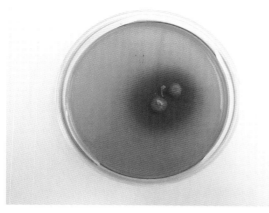

△ **Figure 4-3.** Dermatophyte Test Media (DTM). Change in color of medium from yellow to red indicating the presence of a dermatophyte fungus.

Indications for a KOH examination or fungal culture include the presence of scaly annular plaques, areas of scale and/or alopecia on the scalp (primarily in preadolescents), vesicular lesions on the feet and thickened nail plates.

Fungal cultures of toenail subungual debris can identify the specific species of fungus which may be helpful in choosing the proper oral medication; however, these cultures have a low level of sensitivity. Sending a nail clipping for PAS staining to pathology for detection of fungal hyphae has a high level of specificity and results are usually available in a few days while fungal cultures may take 2 weeks.[5]

A video demonstrating specimen collection techniques and preparation of the specimen for KOH examination is available at mhprofessional.com/clinicaldermatology.

▼ TZANCK TEST

The Tzanck test (Table 4-2) is a cost-effective method for the detection of cutaneous herpes simplex and herpes zoster infections[1]; however, there can be significant rates of false positives and false negatives. Therefore, it is being replaced in many clinics and hospitals by polymerase chain reaction (PCR) tests which have higher rates of sensitivity and specificity.[2]

Indications for a Tzanck test include vesicles on an erythematous base, primarily on the central face, genitals, or in a unilateral dermatome.

A video demonstrating specimen collection techniques and preparation of the Tzanck smear is available at mhprofessional.com/clinicaldermatology.

▼ SCABIES SCRAPING

A scabies scraping (Table 4-3) can be used to confirm the presence of the scabies mite, which is less than 0. 5 mm and invisible to the naked eye.[6] The specimens are examined for

Table 4-2. Tzanck test for herpes simplex and zoster.

Equipment needed
- # 15 scalpel blade, alcohol pad
- Microscope, glass slide, coverslip
- Stain for specimen (Giemsa, Wright, toluidine blue, or methylene blue)

Technique for specimen collection
- Select an intact vesicle(s) and swab with an alcohol pad.
- If there are no intact blisters a crusted lesion or an erosion could be sampled.
- Remove the roof of the blister or the crust with a #15 blade.
- Gently scrape the base of the blister with the #15 blade.
- Smear a thin film of the collected contents onto a microscope slide.
- Let the slide air dry.

Examination of specimen
- Apply 2-4 drops of one of the above stains and leave the stain on for the amount of time recommended by the manufacturer.
- Rinse the slide with water and allow it to dry completely.
- Scan the entire specimen first at low power (10 X magnification) looking for cells (keratinocytes) with large nuclei.
- Switch to high power (40 X magnification) or oil immersion to confirm the presence of multinucleated giant cells (Figure 4-4) which represent infected keratinocytes

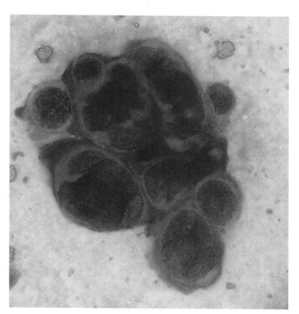

△ **Figure 4-4.** Positive Tzanck smear. Giant, multinucleated keratinocytes in herpes simplex infection.

the mites (Figure 4-6), eggs, and or fecal material (scybala). If these are present in the preparation, they can be easily detected, but false negatives can occur because there are typically few mites present in scabies infestations and the chance of finding them in any one lesion is low, with the

Table 4-3. Scabies skin scraping.

Equipment needed
- #15 scalpel blade, alcohol pad, mineral oil
- Microscope, glass slide, cover slip

Technique for specimen collection
- Select a burrow (Figure 4-5) or papule(s) that have not been excoriated and swab the lesion(s) with an alcohol pad.
- Apply a small amount of mineral oil on the scalpel blade or on the lesion(s).
- Using firm pressure scrape the burrow or papules with a #15 scalpel blade and smear the contents on a glass slide.

Examination of specimens
- Cover the contents with 2-4 drops of mineral oil and apply a cover slip. Do not use KOH as this may dissolve the mite's fecal material.
- Scan the entire specimen at low power (10 X) for the presence of mites, eggs, and or fecal material (Figure 4-6).

Table 4-4. Wood's light findings in selected skin disorders.

Disease	Color with Wood's Light Examination
Vitiligo, post-inflammatory depigmentation, halo nevus, tuberous sclerosis (ash leaf macules).	Bright white to off white.
Melasma (melanin in *epidermis*), lentigo, freckles, café au lait spots.	Darker than surrounding skin.
Melasma (melanin in *dermis*), Mongolian spot.	No change from surrounding skin.
Tinea capitis due to *Microsporum* species.	Blue-green.
Tinea/pityriasis versicolor due to *Malassezia sp.*	Yellow-white or copper-orange.
Pityrosporum/Malassezia folliculitis.	Blue-white around hair follicles.
Erythrasma (coproporphyrins produced by *Corynebacterium minutissimum*).	Coral red. (Figure 4-7)
Pseudomonas due to pyocyanin.	Green.
Porphyrins in urine, blood and teeth.	Red-pink.

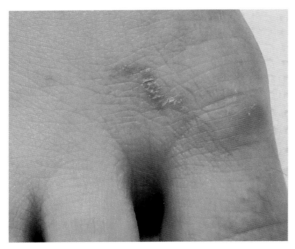

▲ **Figure 4-5.** Scabies burrow. Thin white line above the toe web.

exception of burrows (Figure 4-5) which are short, wavy lines typically seen on the wrists, finger webs, feet, and penis.[6]

The indications for scabies scraping include intensely pruritic papules in patients of any age on the hands, feet, extensor extremities, or genitals.

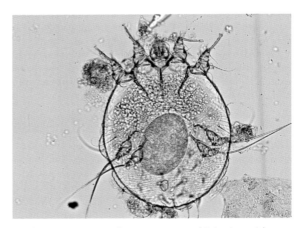

▲ **Figure 4-6.** Female *Sarcoptes scabiei* mite with egg.

WOOD'S LIGHT EXAMINATION (BLACK LIGHT)

A Wood's light is a handheld mercury vapor bulb (ultraviolet light 360 nm) that is helpful in the diagnosis in several conditions (Table 4-4).[7] The examination should take place in a dark room with the Wood's light held about 10 cm from the skin. Patients should not look directly into the light during the examination. A Wood's light examination is most helpful in pigment disorders and certain infections. Lesions with increased melanin in the epidermis appear darker than surrounding skin. In contrast, lesions with increased melanin confined to the dermis do not appear darker than the surrounding skin. There are also some fungal and bacterial infections that produce compounds that can be detected with a Wood's light.

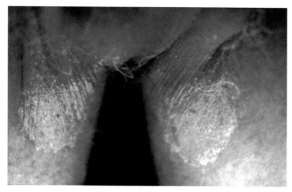

▲ **Figure 4-7.** Erythrasma in medial and anterior thighs. Coral red fluorescence with Wood's light examination due to porphyrins produced by *Corynebacterium minutissimum*.

▼ PATCH TESTING

Skin patch testing is used to detect allergens responsible for allergic contact dermatitis which is a type IV delayed hypersensitivity reaction.[8,9] The Thin-layer Rapid Use Epicutaneous Patch Test (T.R.U.E.) is a commercially available patch test kit which is Food and Drug Administration (FDA) approved. It consists of 35 common allergens and allergen mixes in a gel coating on polyester sheeting. There are also other companies that supply standardized allergens for skin patch testing that can be placed in small aluminum discs (Finn chambers) (Figure 4-8). The tests are placed on the patient's back and taped in place and left on for 48 hours. The results are read at 48 hours, 72 hours, and 96 hours after application. The presence of erythema, papules, and/or vesicles indicates a positive test (Figure 4-9). However, clinical correlation is needed to confirm that positive reactions are indeed the cause of the patient's dermatitis.[8,9]

▼ INTRODUCTION TO DERMOSCOPY

Dermoscopy can benefit any clinician who routinely evaluates skin lesions. Dermatoscopes are relatively affordable, easy to use, and noninvasive. The earliest studies showed that dermoscopy improved diagnostic accuracy compared to naked eye evaluation of pigmented skin lesions, which has since been confirmed in meta-analyses.[10] Dermoscopy improves sensitivity of diagnosis of pigmented lesions without reducing specificity.[11] Dermoscopy allows for diagnosis of melanoma at earlier stages which results in more treatable melanomas. Use of dermoscopy reduces the number of benign lesions biopsied or excised.[10] Dermoscopy can also be useful in nonpigmented skin tumors by aiding in visualization of blood vessels and other structures.[12] While outside the scope of this chapter, it should be noted that

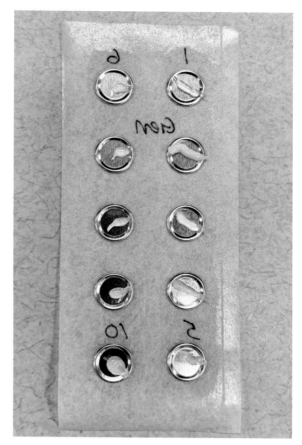

▲ **Figure 4-8.** Allergens diluted in petroleum jelly on aluminum discs (Finn chambers) which are taped to patient's back.

dermoscopy can be useful in evaluation of nonpigmented lesions, rashes, alopecia, and nail changes.[13]

Use of dermoscopy is steadily increasing among dermatologists, but adaptation by nondermatologist physicians in the United States has been slower. Because many patients with skin cancer will present to their primary care provider first, it is important to encourage use of dermoscopy in the primary care setting in particular. A recent survey targeting primary care physicians in the United States found that only 15% had ever used a dermatoscope and only 6% are currently using a dermatoscope in their practice.[14] Studies have identified that barriers to using dermoscopy include the cost of equipment, insufficient reimbursement for use in practice, and need for training.[15]

The benefit of dermoscopy does depend on user expertise and experience. One study showed that without formal training, diagnostic accuracy actually decreased when dermatologists were presented with a dermoscopy photograph compared to when they were shown a clinical photograph.[16]

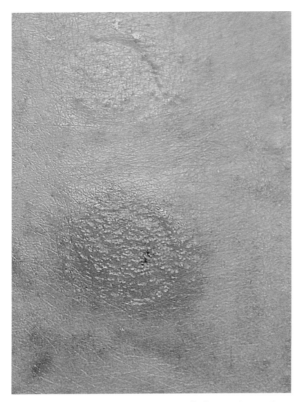

Figure 4-9. Positive reaction to balsam of Peru in patch test. Erythema and papules present at 48 hours after application of patch tests.

A similarly structured study found that diagnostic accuracy improved significantly with just 9 hours of training.[17] There is no one best way to learn dermoscopy. Training in dermoscopy could include reading textbooks, examining patients, attending conferences, and using online learning resources (see end of chapter for our recommendations). For less expert users, use of algorithms may be particularly helpful.[18]

The purpose of this chapter is to give the reader the background knowledge necessary to understand dermoscopy while providing a foundation for evaluation of potential skin malignancies. This chapter is particularly designed for those who are new to dermoscopy. The information provided here will provide a basic knowledge level of dermoscopy of pigmented lesions on the body in particular.

DERMOSCOPY DEVICES

A dermatoscope is a handheld microscope with a light source that has a magnification of 10x. While this seems simple, dermatoscopes are not mere magnifiers. Dermoscopy adapts light to allow the user to see past the surface of the skin.

When light hits the skin normally, the majority of the light is then reflected off the stratum corneum due to its high refractive index. The reflected light goes to the retina, resulting in what we see. Very little light penetrates the stratum corneum and is then reflected back to the retina. The retina is overwhelmed by the much higher amounts of light reflected off the stratum corneum, so we only see the surface or stratum corneum changes with our naked eyes.

Non-polarized dermoscopy uses a liquid interface and direct contact of the dermatoscope's glass plate with skin to decrease reflection of light off the stratum corneum. More light then penetrates beneath the stratum corneum before being reflected back to the retina. This mode allows us to see deeper into the skin and visualize structures that are not seen on naked eye examination. Typical liquid interfaces include mineral oil, ultrasound gel, and alcohol. Nonpolarized dermoscopy allows us to see into the superficial epidermis.

Polarized dermatoscopes use cross polarization to allow us to see past the stratum corneum. Light passes through a polarizer as it exits the device to make it unidirectional. Light reflected off of the stratum corneum maintains this polarization and is then filtered out by a cross-polarized filter before it can reach our retina. Only light that has penetrated beneath the stratum corneum and superficial layers of the epidermis will have a change in polarization and be able to pass through the cross-polarized filter and to the retina. Polarized dermoscopy allows us to see into the deep epidermis or superficial dermis.

Since they work in different ways, there are differences between nonpolarized and polarized dermoscopy. As opposed to nonpolarized dermoscopy, polarized dermoscopy does not require contact with the skin or a liquid interface. Nonpolarized dermoscopy shows surface changes and superficial epidermal findings better than polarized dermoscopy. This is best displayed in examining seborrheic keratoses. The milia-like cysts and comedone-like openings are much more apparent on nonpolarized dermoscopy (Figure 4-10A) than on polarized dermoscopy (Figure 4-10B). Polarized dermoscopy allows the user to see changes in the deep epidermis or superficial dermis. Fibrosis or alteration in collagen in the dermis is visible as white shiny structures on polarized dermoscopy only (Figure 4-11A). Polarized dermoscopy is often better to see vessels (Figure 4-11A). This is because vessels are deeper in the skin and polarized dermoscopy does not require skin contact. Contact of the dermatoscopes with the skin puts pressure on the skin that can cause the vessels to blanch and thus not be visible (Figure 4-11B). The differences between nonpolarized and polarized dermoscopy are summarized in Table 4-5.

DERMOSCOPY TERMINOLOGY

The language of dermoscopy, or terminology, can seem complex to new learners. Once dermoscopy was recognized as a useful tool in diagnosing skin disease, publications

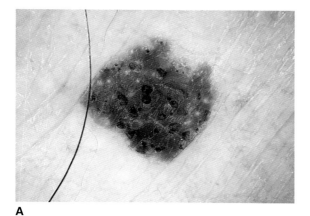

A

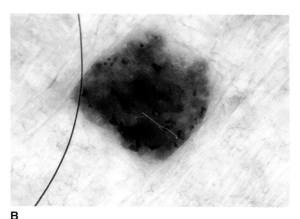

B

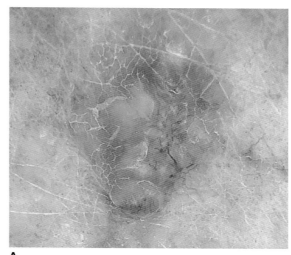

A

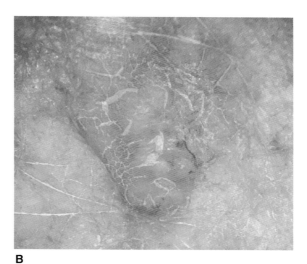

B

▲ **Figure 4-10.** A, B. Nonpolarized versus polarized dermoscopy of a seborrheic keratosis. **A**. Nonpolarized mode. The surface invaginations (called comedone-like openings) and white circular milia are much more visible on this nonpolarized image than on image **B**. Polarized image.*

▲ **Figure 4-11** A, B. Polarized versus nonpolarized dermoscopy of a basal cell carcinoma. **A**. Polarized mode. White shiny circular areas are visible only on the polarized image as these represent changes to collagen at the superficial dermal level. Note that there are more blood vessels visible on this polarized image than in **B**. Nonpolarized image.*

describing dermoscopic findings rapidly grew, but there was often poor consistency and heterogeneity in terminology. The International Dermoscopy Society has made efforts to make dermoscopy language more standardized.[19]

There are two different systems of terminology in dermoscopy. *Metaphoric terminology* draws on comparisons to other things. One example of metaphoric terminology is the description of arborizing vessels in basal cell carcinomas (BCCs). Arborizing vessels have many branches, making them appear tree like. While use of metaphors can make quick and lasting memories in some learners, metaphoric terminology relies on the user being familiar with the metaphor that is drawn upon. Metaphoric terminology can be less precise, more subjective, harder to define, and more difficult to communicate to others. This was the driving force in creating descriptive terminology.

Descriptive terminology describes all features as one of six categories: lines, dots (object too small to have a discernable shape), clods or globules (solid object bigger than a dot), circles, pseudopods (line with a bulbous end), and structureless areas. It follows a simple and logical structure, making it more reproducible. However, for complex structures, descriptive terminology can become quite long and cumbersome. For example, the arborizing vessels described

Table 4-5. Nonpolarized vs polarized dermoscopy.

Feature	Nonpolarized dermoscopy	Polarized dermoscopy
Contact with skin surface	Required.	Not required.
Liquid interface	Required.	Not required.
Better for	Surface changes (stratum corneum to superficial epidermis).	Deeper changes (deep epidermis to superficial epidermis).
Visualization of vessels	Impaired as contact pressure causing vessel blanching.	Improved as contact is not required.

in metaphoric terminology would be described as linear, serpentine, branched vessels in descriptive terminology. A criticism of metaphorical terminology is that it may not be reproducible between different dermoscopists. As an example, sometimes a term is only used after the diagnosis has been determined. For instance, you may call a structure a maple leaf after you have made the diagnosis of BCC; however, if the lesion came back as a melanoma then you would call the same structure a radial streak or radial streaming (Figure 4-12). Terminology should exist to help you arrive at the correct diagnosis. Thus, we recommend the reader uses terminology to describe a lesion before reaching a diagnosis. The terminology that you choose should be that which can be reproducible to others. If others cannot see what you are describing, then it will be difficult to understand and communicate your knowledge; and gaps will be created. The majority of dermoscopy experts use a

combination of metaphoric and descriptive terminology, so familiarity with both systems is needed to build a foundation of the dermoscopy knowledge.

To introduce the basic terminology, we will go through some of the most commonly used metaphoric terminology, the corresponding descriptive terminology, the most common diagnoses associated, and an example image of the feature in Table 4-6.

BEGINNER'S APPROACH TO DERMOSCOPY

There are many different ways to approach dermoscopy. We find that starting with a simplified algorithm approach is best for beginners. Algorithms are particularly useful when one is not yet familiar with dermoscopic structures. The goal of most algorithms is not to reach a diagnosis at the end, but rather to decide if the lesion is concerning enough to warrant biopsy/referral. There have been many different algorithms developed. Some of the more commonly cited ones include the three-point checklist, the ABCD (asymmetry, border, color, and dermoscopic structures) rule, the seven-point checklist, Menzies' method, the CASH (color, architecture, symmetry, and homogeneity) algorithm, the two-step algorithm, chaos and clues, and TADA (Triage Amalgamated Dermoscopic Algorithm).[20] Each of these has their own strengths and weaknesses. For beginners, the three-point checklist is a good starting point as it has a relatively high sensitivity and is easy to implement. The three-point checklist algorithm is discussed in detail in the following section.

After mastering an algorithm, the next step in learning dermoscopy is to identify specific dermoscopic criteria associated with a diagnosis. By learning features common in a diagnosis, you will be able to better triage lesions. For example, a pigmented BCC on the face does not require urgent referral but a suspected melanoma on the face does. Learning diagnosis-specific dermoscopic criteria does require familiarity with the terminology and experience.

Many expert dermoscopists most often use pattern analysis rather than algorithms to examine lesions. Pattern analysis requires the user to recognize a number of dermoscopic structures that when found together result in a reproducible diagnosis. It is a powerful and flexible method that is more involved than the simple scoring algorithms. Unlike some of the algorithms, the end goal is to reach a

▲ **Figure 4-12.** This image demonstrates that metaphoric language is not always reproducible. If a clinician thinks the diagnosis is a BCC or a melanoma, they may be influenced to describe the pigmentation within the white square as a maple leaf in a BCC or as radial streaks or streaming in a melanoma. Terminology should be used to communicate dermoscopy findings and not be influenced by the diagnosis. In this case the diagnosis was an invasive melanoma.**

Table 4-6. Commonly used metaphoric and descriptive terminology with associated diagnoses and example images.

Metaphoric terminology	Descriptive terminology	Most commonly found in	Example see later in this chapter in Figure(s)
Pigment network	Reticular lines	Nevi, melanoma, solar lentigines, dermatofibromas	4-13A, 4-13C
Atypical pigment network	Thick or variable in color reticular lines	Melanoma	4-13B, 4-13C, 4-21
Cobblestone pattern	Large brown or skin colored polygonal clods	Dermal nevus, congenital nevus	4-17, 4-19
Negative network	White reticular lines	Melanoma, spitz nevus	4-21
Shiny white streaks (AKA chrysalis, chrysalids, crystalline structures)	Polarizing-specific white lines or clods	Melanoma, spitz nevus, BCC, dermatofibroma	4-11A, 4-22
Radial streaming	Peripheral radial lines	Melanoma, recurrent nevi after biopsy	4-22
Blue-whiteish veil	Blue structureless zone	Melanoma	4-13C
Scar like depigmentation	White structureless zone	Melanoma	4-23
Peppering	Gray dots	AK, melanoma, lichen planus like keratosis	4-22
Leaf like areas	Radial lines converging on a common base	BCC	4-25C
Spoke wheel areas	Radial lines converging on a central base or clod within a clod	BCC	4-25B
Arborizing vessels	Serpentine lines, arranged in branching pattern	BCC	4-25B
Blue gray ovoid nests	Blue or gray clods	BCC	4-25C
Cerebriform pattern	Curved, thick lines	SK	4-27A
Comedo-like openings	Brown, orange, yellow, or black clods	SK	4-10A, 4-27B
Milia-like cysts	White or yellow clods	SK	4-10A, 4-27B

AK, Actinic keratosis; BCC, Basal Cell Carcinoma; SK, Seborrheic Keratosis.

diagnosis. Teaching pattern analysis is more difficult than teaching an algorithm. With experience, experts often identify a diagnosis without being able to clearly articulate how they arrived at the diagnosis, as their thought process does not follow steps rather it is the sum of past experiences. Work has been done on standardizing the orders and rules of pattern analysis that is outside the scope of this beginner's chapter. For the interested readers and budding expert dermoscopists, we recommend Harald Kittler's *Dermatoscopy: Pattern analysis of pigmented and non-pigmented lesions*[21] for further reading.

THE THREE-POINT CHECKLIST

Dermoscopists can start using the three-point checklist with little training. It was designed for the evaluation of pigmented lesions on the body, but not on the face or acral surfaces. The goal of the algorithm is not to miss a melanoma, so high sensitivity is needed. It takes into account only three criteria: asymmetry, atypical network, and blue-white structures.

- Asymmetry can be in either color or structure of the lesion.
- Atypical network refers to a pigment network without a uniform honeycomb pattern, with either irregular holes or thickened lines.
- Blue-white structures include any type of blue or white coloration.

If two out of three criteria are present, the lesion should be biopsied. If only one out of three criteria is present but that criterion is blue-white structures, biopsy should be considered. Studies have found good interobserver reproducibility for these criteria. With a short training period,

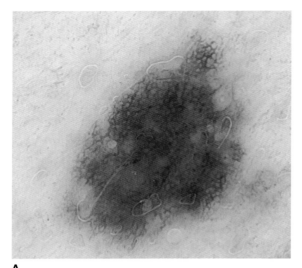

A

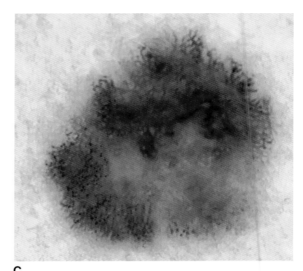

C

B

Figure 4-13 A, B, C. Examples of 3-point checklist criteria. **A.** 0/3 criteria. This image shows a pigment network and pigmented globules centrally. It is overall symmetric, does not have an atypical network, and lacks blue-white structures. No biopsy needed. This lesion shows loss of pigment network around hair follicles, which is normal; globules are distributed fairly uniformly in the center of the lesion. **B**. 2/3 criteria. This image shows a pigmented lesion with asymmetry of patterns and atypical network (thickened reticular network) on the left. No blue white structures. Biopsy needed. The biopsy showed a severely dysplastic nevus.* **C**. 3/3 criteria. Pigmented lesion with asymmetry (loss of pigment in bottom right quarter, darker pigment in top half), atypical network (thickened in top half), and subtle blue structures (top half). Irregularly distributed globules from 6 o'clock to 9 o'clock are present. Biopsy needed. Biopsy showed melanoma, superficial spreading subtype with a Breslow depth of 0.3mm.*

non-experts in dermoscopy improved their sensitivity from 69.7% to 96.3% using the three-point checklist.[22]

In Figures 14-13 A–C, we go through some examples of how to use the three-point checklist to examine lesions and determine if biopsy is needed.

The three-point checklist gives a framework to start evaluating dermoscopic lesions. Take time when you are learning to look at several lesions on a patient, including some that you are sure of the diagnosis based on the naked eye examination. After you become familiar with practicing the three-point checklist, you will find that the end point is a decision, to biopsy or refer; and it is a major downside of this technique. To achieve high sensitivity, specificity is sacrificed. The technique does not get you to a final diagnosis. The algorithm was designed to detect melanomas but it could miss other skin cancers.

▼ DERMOSCOPIC FEATURES BY DIAGNOSIS

After getting more familiar with dermoscopy by mastering the three-point checklist, the next step is learning about specific features that are commonly found in other diagnostic categories. While these features are not always specific for a single diagnosis, they provide clues to the diagnosis, especially when multiple features of a diagnosis are present.

Pigment patterns tend to be more specific than vascular patterns for a diagnosis. For this reason, it is helpful to start by analyzing pigment first when looking at lesions by dermoscopy. We will focus on pigmented lesions by going through features seen in benign nevi, melanoma, Bowen's disease (squamous cell carcinoma in situ), BCC, seborrheic keratoses, and dermatofibromas.

Benign Nevi

Benign nevi can have a number of different patterns on dermoscopy. The most common patterns include the following:

1. The diffuse reticular network pattern shows hyperpigmented thin lines with hypopigmented holes (Figure 4-14). The lines should be of same color and size throughout. The holes are larger in size than the lines. The brown lines correspond to melanin in the rete ridges and the hypopigmented holes correspond to the dermal papilla. In descriptive terminology, this would be made up of reticular lines.

2. The patchy reticular network pattern has islands made up of reticular network divided evenly throughout the lesion (Figure 4-15).

3. Benign nevi can show peripheral reticular network with central hypopigmentation or hyperpigmentation (Figure 4-16), or central globules (Figure 4-17). Note all of these are still symmetric despite having two different components.

4. Homogeneous pattern shows only one color that is uniform throughout the lesion (Figure 4-18). In descriptive terminology, these are termed as structureless.

5. Globular pattern shows uniformly distributed globules (metaphoric language) or clods (descriptive terminology) of similar size, shape, and color (Figure 4-19).

6. Centrally, a peripheral network with uniform globules on the outside of the lesion (Figure 4-20) is indicative of a growing nevus. This is normal in children, but it would be abnormal for adults over the age of 40 years to have growing nevi. Care must be taken to observe the peripheral globules and ensure that they are uniformly distributed as well, as asymmetric peripheral globules can be a concerning finding on dermoscopy.

Melanoma

In contrast to benign nevi, melanoma also has a wide array of dermoscopic features to be familiar with. Here, we will focus on features found in the pigmented melanomas on the body. Features to diagnose melanoma on the face, acral, or mucosal surfaces requires more advanced dermoscopy skill and is beyond the scope of this chapter. The most common features concerning for melanoma are listed below and highlighted in the mentioned figures:

1. An atypical network shows irregular size and color of the hyperpigmented lines and hypopigmented holes (Figure 4-21 & 4-13C). Often, the hyperpigmented lines appear larger than the hypopigmented holes.

2. Irregularly distributed or different sized globules/clods within a lesion (Figure 4-13C).

3. Irregular streaks are straight lines radiating outward from a center point that do not involve the entire lesion (Figure 4- 22). Pseudopods are similar to streaks but have a bulbous head. When distributed irregularly, both are concerning for melanoma.

4. Regression structures can be seen as pepper-like blue-gray granules (metaphoric) or dots (descriptive) (Figure 4- 22) or scar-like areas within a lesion (Figure 4-23).

5. Blue structures are blue-gray-white areas that appear somewhat out of focus or smudged. A blue-white veil (Figure 4-13C) is particularly concerning for melanoma and is thought to represent either deeply invasive melanoma or regression of melanoma, depending on if palpable or not.

6. A negative network shows the inverse of the normal reticular network (Figure 4-21). Instead of hyperpigmented lines, the lines are hypopigmented compared to the holes which are hyperpigmented.

7. An atypical blotch is a pink, black, brown, or gray off-center structureless area (Figure 4-13C).

8. Polymorphic vessels within a lesion are the presence of two or more types of blood vessels. Vessels can be described as dotted, glomeruloid/clods/lacunae, or linear (straight, curved, serpentine, looped, coiled). Polymorphic vessels can be one of only a few clues to melanoma diagnosis in amelanotic melanoma (Figure 4-24).

9. White shiny lines are perpendicular white lines that do not intersect (Figure 4-22). These are only visualized on polarized dermoscopy and are thought to represent changes to the collagen-like fibrosis. White shiny lines can be seen in a number of benign diagnoses, including scars, dermatofibromas, and spitz nevi. They can also

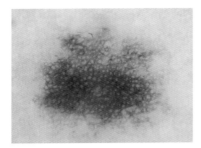

Figure 4-14. Benign nevus with diffuse reticular pattern.**

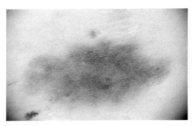

Figure 4-15. Benign nevus with islands of patchy reticular network.*

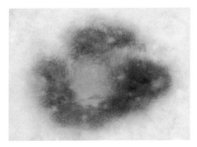

Figure 4-16. Mildly atypical nevus with reticular network peripherally and central hypopigmented structureless zone. Note the overall symmetry of the lesion.*

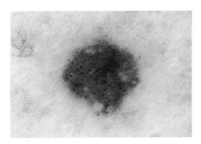

Figure 4-17. Benign nevus with reticular network peripherally and central globules. Note the overall symmetry of the lesion.*

Figure 4-18. Benign blue nevus with homogeneous or structureless pattern.**

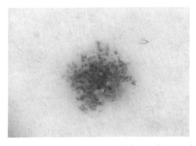

Figure 4-19. Benign nevus with uniform globules/clods.*

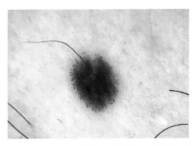

Figure 4-20. Nevus with peripheral globules and central reticular network. This pattern is indicative of a growing nevus. This is normal in children, but abnormal in adults. This lesion was in an adult and showed dysplastic nevus with moderate to severe atypia.*

be seen in malignant diagnoses like BCC and melanoma.

Basal Cell Carcinoma

BCCs can be both pigmented and nonpigmented. The majority of BCCs are nonpigmented. The most common features of *nonpigmented BCCs* include:

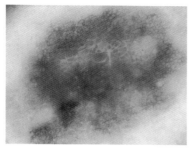

▲ **Figure 4-21.** Melanoma. This melanoma shows a negative network centrally and atypical network (notice the thickening of the network on the left lower side of the image).✲✲

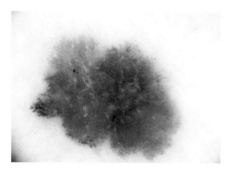

▲ **Figure 4-22.** Melanoma. This melanoma shows regression structures with peppered pigment dots centrally, white shiny lines, irregular streaks (9 o'clock).✲✲

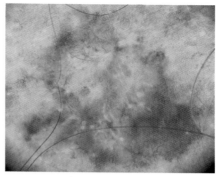

▲ **Figure 4-23.** Melanoma with white scar like areas. Note the pink-white structureless areas scattered throughout.✲✲

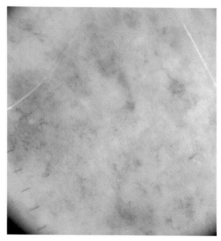

▲ **Figure 4-24.** Melanoma in situ showing polymorphic vessels. Note dotted vessels at 9 o'clock, short linear or serpentine vessels throughout the lesion, and coiled, almost corkscrew like vessel at 3 o'clock.✲✲

1. Erosion or ulceration or structureless (Figure 4-25A). These often appear as homogeneous or structureless yellow or orange areas. Because serum crust can be sticky, there are sometimes adherent fibers in the area. Erosions and ulcerations can have overlying hemorrhagic crust as well.

2. Arborizing vessels (linear vessels, serpentine) (Figure 4-25B). These vessels are branching vessels that often have a tree-like pattern. They are sharply in focus on dermoscopy, unlike the background blood vessels of the adjacent normal skin.

When *pigment is present* in BCCs, it has unique patterns compared to nevi. Pigment can be:

1. Leaf-like structures (Figure 4-25C). Linear to oval-shaped pigment coming together to at a common, off-center base to form patterns that look like leaves.

2. Spoke wheel-like structures (clods in clods) (Figure 4-25B). Radial projects coming together at a common central point to give the appearance of a wheel with spokes.

3. Blue-gray ovoid nests (clods) (Figure 4-25C). Round- or oval-shaped blue, black, or gray collections of pigment.

4. Blue-gray dots and globules (dots and clods) (Figure 4-25B). Small blue or gray dots or globules scattered throughout a lesion or collected in one area in a lesion.

Squamous Cell Carcinoma

The dermoscopy of squamous cell carcinoma is different for invasive disease compared to in situ disease. The majority of invasive squamous cell carcinomas are not pigmented. Bowen's disease (squamous cell carcinoma in situ)

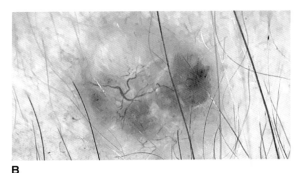

B

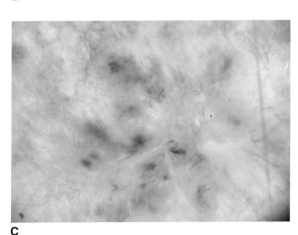

C

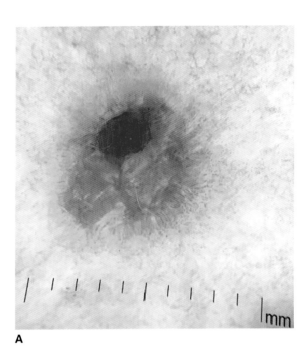

A

△ **Figure 4-25** A, B, C. Basal cell carcinoma (BCC). **A.** Non-pigmented BCC showing erosion (superior half of lesion with bright red appearance) and white shiny lines/strands* **B.** Pigmented BCC. Arborizing vessels, spoke wheel pigmentation (best seen near 3 o'clock), and blue gray dots of pigment (around 9 o'clock).* **C.** Pigmented BCC. Arborizing vessels and blue gray ovoid pigment clods. Notice the leaf like pigmentation toward the bottom of the image at approximate 5 o'clock.**

can occasionally be pigmented. When pigment is present, it will be arranged as brown or gray dots in linear arrays, most commonly at the periphery of a lesion (Figure 4-26). Bowen's disease often has dotted or coiled blood vessels that line up and sometimes they are linearly arranged (Figure 4-26).

Seborrheic Keratoses

Seborrheic keratoses (SKs) can be difficult to differentiate from melanocytic lesions by naked eye examination but show very different features on dermoscopy. Pigment is arranged in thick curved lines that can resemble the sulci and gyri of the brain (Figure 4-27A) rather than in a reticular network. The borders of SKs are sharply defined and often have a scalloped edge to them. SKs have both milia-like cysts and comedo-like openings visible on the surface (Figure 4-27B). When vessels are visible in less pigmented

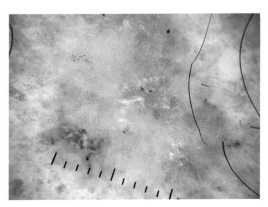

△ **Figure 4-26.** Squamous cell carcinoma in situ with dotted vessels in linear arrays and dotted brown pigment toward the periphery (best seen around 9 o'clock).*

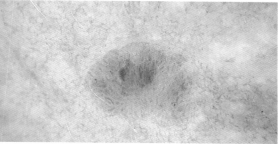

A

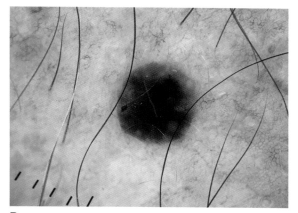

B

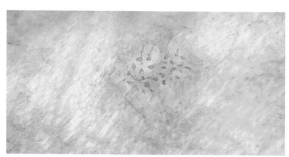

C

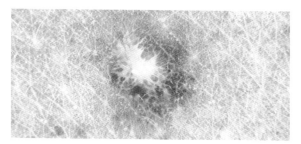

▲ **Figure 4-28.** Dermatofibroma with central scar like area and peripheral reticular network.*

Diagnoses by dermoscopy requires time and training. Skills are gained by looking at examples in textbooks or online resources and by practicing on patients. If possible, taking dermoscopic photographs of lesions that are biopsied is very helpful in enforcing learning further.

▼ **TOTAL BODY PHOTOGRAPHY AND SEQUENTIAL DIGITAL DERMOSCOPY**

In high-risk patients, total body photography with sequential dermoscopy imaging can be very helpful in diagnosing melanomas early. Baseline total body photography, also referred to as mole mapping helps to identify if moles are new and clinical changes are occurring. It is often difficult for patients with a large number of nevi to determine if moles are new or changing on their own. Sequential digital dermoscopy imaging or serial dermoscopy photos of moles, provides even further baseline data to determine if nevi are changing and need to be biopsied. Studies have shown that the combination of both these techniques allows for earlier diagnosis of melanoma (most are diagnosed at less than 1 mm in depth) and allows for diagnosis of melanoma in lesions that show no dermoscopic or clinical features of melanoma by identifying changing lesions.[23] This technology is not yet widely available in the United States.

▼ **ONLINE RESOURCES FOR DERMOSCOPY EDUCATION**

• Dermoscopedia. https://dermoscopedia.org
• Dermoscopy made simple blog. http://dermoscopymadesimple.blogspot.com/
• DermNet NZ. https://dermnetnz.org/topics/dermoscopy/

*Reproduced with permission from Lori A. Fiessinger, MD
**Reproduced with permission from Juan Jaimes, MD, MS

▲ **Figure 4-27** A, B, C. Seborrheic keratosis.
A. Cerebriform pattern of curved thick brown lines.
B. Scalloped edge, sharply defined borders, milia like cysts, and comedo-like openings in the surface.
C. Looped vessels with no pigmentation.*

seborrheic keratoses, they are looped or coiled in curved lines that resemble a hairpin (Figure 4-27C).

Dermatofibroma

Dermatofibromas most commonly have a center scar-like area and peripheral reticular network (Figure 4-28).

▼ **REFERENCES**

1. Ruocco E, Baroni A, Donnarumma G, Ruocco V. Diagnostic procedures in dermatology. *Clin Dermatol.* 2011;29(5): 548-556.

2. Dominguez SR, Pretty K, Hengartner R, Robinson CC. Comparison of herpes simplex virus PCR with culture for virus detection in multisource surface swab specimens from neonates. *J Clin Microbiol.* 2018;56(10).

3. Petrucelli MF, Abreu MH de, Cantelli BAM, et al. Epidemiology and diagnostic perspectives of dermatophytoses. *J Fungi (Basel).* 2020;6(4):310–325.

4. Micali G, Verzì AE, Lacarrubba F. Alternative uses of dermoscopy in daily clinical practice: An update. *J Am Acad Dermatol.* 2018;79(6):1117–1132.

5. Pihet M, Le Govic Y. Reappraisal of conventional diagnosis for dermatophytes. *Mycopathologia.* 2017;182(1–2):169–180.

6. Chandler D, Fuller L. A review of scabies: An infestation more than skin deep. *Dermatology* 2019;235(2):79–90.

7. Klatte JL, van der Beek N, Kemperman PMJH. 100 years of Wood's lamp revised. *J Eur Acad Dermatol Venereol.* 2015;29(5):842–847.

8. Uyesugi BA, Sheehan MP. Patch testing pearls. *Clin Rev Allergy Immunol.* 2019;56(1):110–118.

9. Johansen JD, Aalto-Korte K, Agner T, et al. European Society of Contact Dermatitis guideline for diagnostic patch testing - recommendations on best practice: ESCD PATCH TEST GUIDELINE. *Contact Dermatitis.* 2015;73(4):195–221.

10. Mayer JE, Swetter SM, Fu T, Geller AC. Screening, early detection, education, and trends for melanoma: current status (2007-2013) and future directions: Part I. Epidemiology, high-risk groups, clinical strategies, and diagnostic technology. *J Am Acad Dermatol.* 2014;71(4):599.e1–e12.

11. Usatine RP, Shama LK, Marghoob AA, Jaimes N. Dermoscopy in family medicine: A primer. *J Fam Pract.* 2018;67(12):e1–e11.

12. Zalaudek I, Kreusch J, Giacomel J, Ferrara G, Catricalà C, Argenziano G. How to diagnose nonpigmented skin tumors: a review of vascular structures seen with dermoscopy: part I. Melanocytic skin tumors. *J Am Acad Dermatol.* 2010;63(3):361–374.

13. Micali G, Verzì AE, Lacarrubba F. Alternative uses of dermoscopy in daily clinical practice: An update. *J Am Acad Dermatol.* 2018;79(6):1117–1132.

14. Morris JB, Alfonso SV, Hernandez N, Fernández MI. Use of and intentions to use dermoscopy among physicians in the United States. *Dermatol Pract Concept.* 2017;7(2):7–16.

15. Fee JA, McGrady FP, Rosendahl C, Hart ND. Dermoscopy use in primary care: A scoping review. *Dermatol Pract Concept.* 2019;9(2):98–104.

16. Binder M, Schwarz M, Winkler A, et al. Epiluminescence microscopy. A useful tool for the diagnosis of pigmented skin lesions for formally trained dermatologists. *Arch Dermatol.* 1995;131(3):286–291.

17. Binder M, Puespoeck-Schwarz M, Steiner A, et al. Epiluminescence microscopy of small pigmented skin lesions: short-term formal training improves the diagnostic performance of dermatologists. *J Am Acad Dermatol.* 1997;36(2 Pt 1): 197–202.

18. Dinnes J, Deeks JJ, Chuchu N, et al. Dermoscopy, with and without visual inspection, for diagnosing melanoma in adults. *Cochrane Database Syst Rev.* Dec 4 2018;12(12):Cd011902.

19. Kittler H, Marghoob AA, Argenziano G, et al. Standardization of terminology in dermoscopy/dermatoscopy: Results of the third consensus conference of the International Society of Dermoscopy. *J Am Acad Dermatol.* 2016;74(6):1093–1106.

20. Carrera C, Marchetti MA, Dusza SW, et al. Validity and reliability of dermoscopic criteria used to differentiate nevi from melanoma: A Web-Based International Dermoscopy Society Study. *JAMA Dermatol.* 2016;152(7):798–806.

21. Harald Kittler CR, Alan Cameron, Philipp Tschandl. *Dermatoscopy: Pattern analysis of pigmented and non-pigmented lesions.* 2nd ed. Facultas Verlags; 2016.

22. Soyer HP, Argenziano G, Zalaudek I, et al. Three-point checklist of dermoscopy. A new screening method for early detection of melanoma. *Dermatology.* 2004;208(1):27–31.

23. Guitera P, Menzies SW, Coates E, et al. Efficiency of detecting new primary melanoma among individuals treated in a high-risk clinic for skin surveillance. *JAMA Dermatol.* 2021;157: e1–e11.

Principles of Diagnosis

Carol Soutor

INTRODUCTION TO CHAPTER

Diagnosing a cutaneous problem can be challenging compared to other organ systems. Blood studies, imaging, and other standardized testing are usually not that helpful in diagnosing dermatologic diseases as they may be for example in endocrinology, cardiology, or orthopedics.

Fortunately, the skin can be easily examined directly without using special technologies or invasive procedures. Some of the common skin diseases were accurately described and categorized in great detail over 2000 years ago.[1]

Diagnosis of cutaneous disorders can be done using two different systems, *system 1*, a rapid, intuitive, non-analytical method primarily based on visual pattern recognition, or *system 2,* an analytic method using algorithms and decision trees.[2–4] In general, more experienced clinicians use system 1 and novices use system 2 for diagnosis.[2]

PATTERN RECOGNITION FOR DIAGNOSIS

Clinicians utilizing pattern recognition rapidly identify the cutaneous findings and compare them to a set of images stored in their long-term memory (sometimes called the "blink" diagnosis).[2,3] These images are typically from clinical findings seen earlier in patients or from pictures in textbooks and other sources. Pattern recognition is more effective in common disorders with typical presentations and in the hands of more experienced clinicians. However, studies have shown that in electrocardiogram (ECG) interpretation[5] and in dermoscopy,[6] pattern recognition can be an effective diagnostic strategy even for less-experienced clinicians.

Human beings and all animals are hardwired for visual pattern recognition. Otherwise, we could not easily and quickly identify each other, objects, or predators. We know that pattern recognition can be learned, but can it be taught? One of the problems is that much of visual pattern recognition occurs subconsciously.[2] An experienced clinician can usually tell a student what cutaneous findings led to their diagnosis, but there may be other subtle, important factors, not easily elucidated that also contributed to the diagnosis.

The most common features of skin disorders used in pattern recognition include the following:

- The morphology of the primary lesion, its surface changes, color, and size.
- Location of lesions.
- Configuration of lesions.

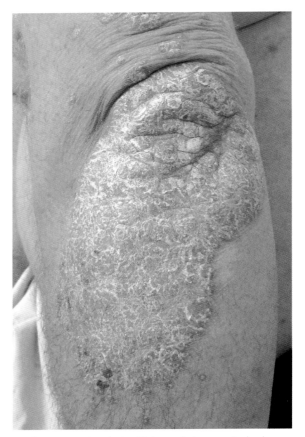

▲ **Figure 5-1** Psoriasis. Pink, well demarcated, plaque with silvery scale on elbow is a characteristic finding.

Many common skin disorders have characteristic features. For example, pink plaques with silvery scale on knees and elbows are characteristic for psoriasis (Figure 5-1). These patterns are covered in more detail in individual diseases in Section II.

ANALYTIC METHOD FOR DIAGNOSIS

An analytic method for diagnosis is slower and more methodical. It utilizes a step-by-step evaluation of the patient's history, the physical examination findings, and results of diagnostic tests (e.g., potassium hydroxide (KOH) examination and skin biopsies).[2,3] These are used as the basis for searches in differential diagnoses lists or decision tree algorithms. An analytic method is helpful in complex cases with atypical or numerous cutaneous findings and systemic complaints. Section III of this book contains lists of differential diagnoses of skin diseases in various body regions based on the patient's history, lesion morphology, and laboratory results. It also contains differential diagnosis lists for purpura, pruritus, rash and fever, and leg ulcers.

THE PRIMARY LESION

Both strategies for diagnosis rely heavily on identification and classification of the primary lesion(s).[4] Table 5-1 lists the various forms of primary lesions and the disorders commonly associated with them.[7] Many common skin diseases can present with more than one type of primary lesion.

Pitfalls in Identifying the Primary Lesion

There are several pitfalls in the identification and classification of primary lesions. These include:

- Excoriations may alter or partially damage the primary lesions (Figure 5-2).

Table 5-1. Primary skin lesions and common skin diseases.

Primary Lesion	Skin disease
Macule/patch	• Vitiligo, melasma, guttate hypomelanosis. • Pityriasis versicolor, erythrasma. • Drug rash, purpura, lupus erythematosus. • Viral exanthem.
Papule	• Dermatitis (atopic, dyshidrotic), keratosis pilaris, prurigo nodularis, guttate psoriasis, secondary syphilis, lichen planus, granuloma annulare. • Acne, rosacea, perioral dermatitis, folliculitis. • Warts (verrucae), molluscum, scabies, arthropod bites. • Urticaria, drug rash, vasculitis.
Plaque	• Dermatitis (atopic, contact, nummular, dyshidrotic, stasis, seborrheic), psoriasis, pityriasis rosea, lichen planus, lichen sclerosus, granuloma annulare. • Tinea(corporis, capitis, manuum, cruris, pedis), candidiasis, cellulitis, erythrasma, secondary syphilis. • Urticaria, drug rash, erythema migrans, vasculitis, erythema multiforme, erythema nodosum, discoid lupus.
Pustule/cyst	• Acne, rosácea, perioral dermatitis, boil/furuncle, folliculitis, hidradenitis supurativa. • Impetigo, boils, candida, herpes simplex/zoster. • Pustular psoriasis, keratosis pilaris, drug rash.
Vesicle/bullae	• Dermatitis (atopic, contact, dyshidrotic). • Herpes simplex/zoster, varicella, bullous impetigo. • Arthropod bites, scabies. • Bullous pemphigoid, pemphigus, dermatitis herpetiformis.
Wheal	• Urticaria, angioedema, dermatographism, mastocytosis. • Urticarial phase of bullous pemphigoid.

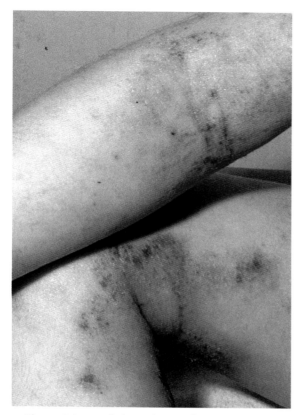

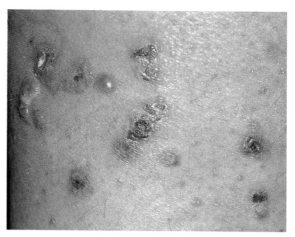

▲ **Figure 5-3** Bullous pemphigoid. An example of vesicles breaking to form crusts and erosions.

▲ **Figure 5-2** Excoriations altering the appearance of plaques in a child with atopic dermatitis.

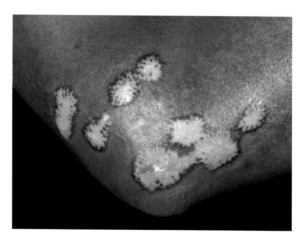

▲ **Figure 5-4** Post inflammatory hyper and hypopigmentation partially obscuring the erythematous plaques of discoid lupus erythematosus.

- Vesicles, bullae, and pustules may easily break leaving only erosions or erythema (Figure 5-3). Also, vesicles may develop into pustules as in some case of herpes simplex and zoster.

- Post inflammatory hyper- and hypopigmentation may obscure the primary lesion especially individuals with darker skin tones (Figure 5-4).

- The examination may take place too early or too late in an evolving skin disease. For instance, many skin rashes present with pink macules in the first 1 to 2 days and then evolve into their more characteristic findings. As an example, herpes zoster could evolve from a pink macule/patch → pink plaque → plaque with vesicles → bullae → crusts → erosions → scars (Figure 5-5) .

- Treatment may alter the skin findings, for example, the use of a topical antifungal cream for tinea corporis may remove the characteristic scale or make it difficult to find fungal hyphae on a KOH examination.

- Lastly, many common diseases present with multiple types of primary lesions. For example, atopic dermatitis may present with macules, patches, papules, plaques,

vesicles, and pustules and with surface changes that may include scale, crust, lichenification, fissures, erosions, and excoriations (Figure 5-6).

Location(s) of Primary Lesions and Diagnosis

The location(s) of the primary lesions are a helpful clue to the diagnosis. Many common skin rashes occur in specific areas of the body.[7] Section III of this book covers skin diseases in each area of the body. A summary of the sites of the most common rashes is as follows:

- **Scalp**: Dermatitis (atopic, allergic contact, seborrheic), psoriasis, folliculitis, tinea capitis, herpes zoster, head lice, cicatricial alopecias.

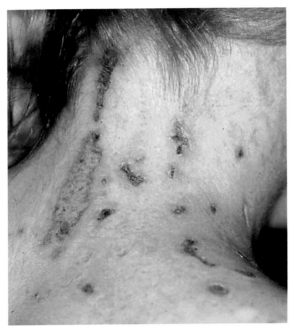

▲ **Figure 5-5** Herpes zoster. Crust, erosions, and scars on neck representing evolution of the lesions.

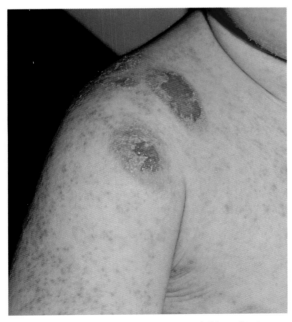

▲ **Figure 5-6** Atopic dermatitis in a child. Multiple types of primary lesions are present, for example, papules, plaques, and vesicles.

- **Face:** Acne, rosacea, dermatitis (atopic, contact, seborrheic, perioral), herpes simplex/zoster, impetigo, melasma, vitiligo.
- **Arms:** Atopic dermatitis, keratosis pilaris, lichen simplex chronicus, allergic contact dermatitis, psoriasis, lichen planus, tinea corporis.
- **Hands:** Dermatitis (atopic, contact, dyshidrotic), psoriasis, lichen planus, tinea manuum.
- **Legs:** Dermatitis (atopic, contact, nummular, stasis), psoriasis, cellulitis, erythema nodosum, vasculitis.
- **Feet:** Dermatitis (atopic, contact, dyshidrotic), psoriasis, tinea pedis, cellulitis.
- **Trunk:** Dermatitis (atopic, contact, seborrheic, nummular), psoriasis, pityriasis rosea, tinea versicolor, tinea corporis, candidiasis, acne, folliculitis, hidradenitis suppurativa, herpes zoster, viral exanthems, drug rash, urticaria.
- **Genitals:** Herpes simplex, human papillomavirus infection (HPV), molluscum contagiosum, tinea cruris, candidiasis, erythrasma, folliculitis, hidradenitis, contact dermatitis, lichen simplex chronicus, psoriasis, lichen sclerosus.
- **Oral cavity:** Candidiasis, herpes simplex, viral enanthems, aphthous ulcers, geographic tongue, lichen planus, leukoplakia.
- **Multiple sites:** Dermatitis (atopic, contact, nummular), psoriasis, lichen planus, herpes simplex/zoster, tinea corporis, urticaria, drug rash, viral exanthem, bug bites, scabies, vitiligo.

BROAD DIAGNOSTIC CATEGORIES

Once the primary lesion(s) and their locations have been identified. It is important to consider the broad categories of disease in the differential diagnosis before making a specific diagnosis. The common skin diseases covered in this textbook fall into 9 broad categories.

- Dermatitis
- Psoriasis and other papulosquamous diseases
- Urticaria and drug rashes
- Infections (fungal, bacterial, viral)
- Acne and other pilosebaceous diseases
- Infestations and bites
- Hair and nail disorders
- Pigment disorders
- Benign and malignant tumors

LABORATORY CONFIRMATION OF DIAGNOSIS

A study of primary care physicians' errors found that 68% of misdiagnoses could be eliminated by three simple diagnostic tests: (1) KOH examination of scale for fungus (2) Tzanck smear or viral culture for herpes, and (3) skin scraping for scabies.[8] There are several other laboratory and diagnostic studies such as bacterial cultures and skin biopsies that can be done to confirm diagnoses. However, false positive and negative results can occur due to errors in collection of specimens and in the interpretation of microscopic findings. Therefore, clinical correlation is important. The following are examples of laboratory tests that can be used to confirm diagnoses in various clinical findings:[7]

- Potassium hydroxide (KOH) examination and/or fungal cultures: Scaling with or without alopecia in preadolescent children, annular scaly plaques at any age, scaling or vesicles on feet, hands or groin area or body folds and dystrophy of nails.
- Tzanck smear, polymerase chain reaction (PCR), or viral culture for herpes simplex or varicella zoster virus: Vesicles on an erythematous base especially on face, genitals, or a unilateral dermatome.
- Scabies scraping: Intensely pruritic papules or vesicles and/or burrows in patients of any age especially on the hands, feet, extensor extremities, or genitals.
- Bacterial cultures: Cysts or nodules with purulent drainage, crusted plaques surrounded by erythema.
- Skin biopsies: Histopathologic examination of skin biopsy specimens preserved in formalin is useful in the diagnosis of benign and malignant tumors. It is also helpful in the diagnosis of psoriasis, lichen planus, pemphigoid, pemphigus, vasculitis, connective tissue disorders, and many scalp disorders. It is also is useful in the diagnosis of fungal infections, but special stains such as the periodic acid Schiff stain (PAS) need to be done to visualize the fungal elements. Skin biopsies are generally not useful in differentiating between various forms of dermatitis. The diagnostic accuracy of pathology reports is enhanced by the inclusion of detailed history and clinical findings on the biopsy requisition form.

Skin biopsies for direct immunofluorescence are diagnostic in pemphigoid, pemphigus, dermatitis herpetiformis, and cutaneous lupus erythematosus.

There can be differences in the interpretation between some pathologists, so as with any laboratory test; clinical correlation is needed.[9] Chapter 7 has more details on skin biopsy procedures.

- Blood studies: These are generally not helpful in the diagnosis of common skin disorders but are helpful in connective tissue disorders.

DIAGNOSTIC ERROR

Most errors in the diagnosis of rashes are made between inflammatory diseases and diseases associated with microbes (Table 5-2), for example, misdiagnosing dermatitis as a fungal infection.[8] Misdiagnosis is especially problematic in these cases, because the diseases in these two categories have different treatments. However, it is

Table 5-2. Common inflammatory diseases and diseases associated with microbes.

INFLAMMATORY DISEASES
Dermatitis • Allergic and irritant contact dermatitis • Atopic dermatitis • Lichen simplex chronicus • Nummular dermatitis • Stasis dermatitis • Dyshidrotic dermatitis
Papulosquamous • Psoriasis • Seborrheic dermatitis • Pityriasis rosea • Lichen planus
Urticaria and drug rashes • Acute and chronic urticaria • Morbilliform drug rash
DISEASES ASSOCIATED WITH MICROBES
Bacterial • Boils • Impetigo • Cellulitis • Pilosebaceous diseases (acne, rosacea, perioral dermatitis, hidradenitis)
Viral • Herpes simplex • Herpes zoster • Human papillomavirus • Molluscum contagiosum
Fungal • Tineas (capitis,corporis,manuum, pedis,cruris) • Tinea versicolor • Candidiasis

important to note that there are some clinical cases in which an inflammatory disease and an infectious process coexist. The following are some examples:

- Atopic dermatitis and staphylococcal skin infection or herpes simplex (Figure 5-7).
- Contact dermatitis and bacterial infection (Figure 5-8).
- Stasis dermatitis and cellulitis.
- Dermatitis and molluscum contagiosum.
- Dyshidrotic dermatitis and tinea pedis.

Cutaneous Mimics

Many common skin diseases that are in different broad diagnostic categories not only mimic each other but may also closely resemble skin findings in systemic diseases and diseases with high morbidity (Table 5-3). Drug rashes and syphilis are well known imitators of many other diseases. Drug rashes can present with cutaneous findings that are

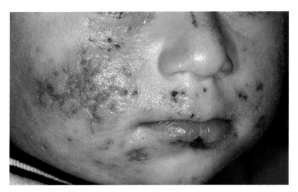

▲ **Figure 5-7** Atopic dermatitis with secondary herpes simplex and *Staphylococcal aureus* infection. Eczema herpeticum with erythema, deep erosions, vesicles, and crusts.

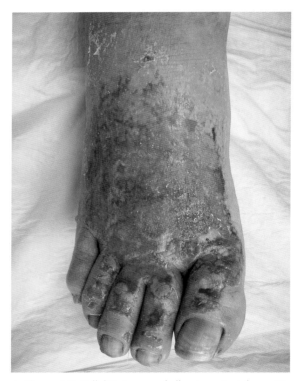

▲ **Figure 5-8** Cellulitis in area of allergic contact dermatitis on dorsal foot. Erythematous, edematous plaque with vesicles, crusts, erosions and purulent drainage.

similar to many common skin diseases including papules, plaques, blisters, pustules, ulcers, skin necrosis, nail dystrophy, and alopecia (Figure 5-9). Syphilis can mimic many of the common papulosquamous diseases such as pityriasis rosea and guttate psoriasis.

Table 5-3. Common dermatoses which mimic each other and their systemic mimics.

Location	Common Dermatoses Which Mimic each Other	High Morbidity Mimics
Scalp	Tinea capitis Seborrheic dermatitis Contact dermatitis	Dermatomyositis.
Face	Acne Rosacea Dermatitis (perioral, seborrheic)	Malar rash (butterfly) of systemic lupus erythematosus.
Oral cavity	Aphthous ulcers Herpes simplex	Bechet disease. Erythema multiforme, Steven-Johnson syndrome /toxic epidermal necrolysis.
Hands	Contact dermatitis Tinea manuum	Dermatomyositis, Systemic lupus erythematosus, Porphyria cutanea tarda.
Feet	Tinea pedis Allergic contact dermatitis	Cellulitis.
Nails	Fungal infection Psoriasis Trauma	Nail changes due to systemic diseases.
Genitals	Herpes simplex	Chancre (lesion of primary syphilis) Behcet's disease.
Multiple locations	Drug rash Viral exanthem	Early stages of Steven's Johnson syndrome/toxic epidermal necrolysis, Staphylococcal scalded skin syndrome, Toxic shock syndrome.
	Tinea corporis Nummular dermatitis Granuloma annulare	Subacute cutaneous lupus erythematosus.
	Dermatitis Psoriasis	Cutaneous T-cell Lymphoma.
	Pityriasis rosea Guttate psoriasis Lichen planus	Secondary syphilis.
	Urticaria Dermatitis	Prebullous phase of bullous pemphigoid.
	Acute allergic contact dermatitis	Bullous Pemphigoid, Pemphigus.
	Dermatitis Scabies	Dermatitis herpetiformis.

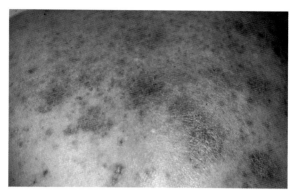

▲ **Figure 5-9** Drug rash due to hydrochlorothiazide mimicking a dermatitis or papulosquamous disease. Hyperpigmented, erythematous, scaly, papules, and plaques on back.

Table 5-4. Benign tumors and dermatoses and their malignant mimics.

Benign tumors and dermatoses which can mimic malignant neoplasms	Malignant mimics
Seborrheic keratosis Benign nevus Atypical nevus	Melanoma. Pigmented basal cell carcinoma.
Dermatitis. Psoriasis.	In situ basal cell carcinoma. Bowen's disease. Squamous cell carcinoma in situ. Paget's disease of the nipple or extramammary Paget's disease. Cutaneous T cell lymphoma
Viral wart. Seborrheic keratosis.	Squamous cell carcinoma.
Genital lichen sclerosus Lichen planus Dermatitis	Vulvar squamous intraepithelial neoplasias. Erythroplasia of Queyrat (in situ squamous cell carcinoma).
Oral candidiasis Lichen planus	Oral squamous cell carcinoma.

There are also several skin cancers that are very similar in appearance to benign skin diseases (Table 5-4). Superficial forms of basal carcinoma and in-situ squamous cell carcinoma are often misdiagnosed initially as being a rash, for example, psoriasis and dermatitis (Figure 5-10 A, B). On genital skin and oral mucosa all forms of squamous cell carcinoma, especially those in the premalignant and in situ stage can resemble benign inflammatory dermatoses and candida infections (Figure 5-10 C).

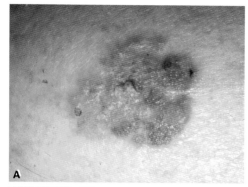

A

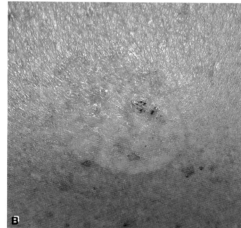

B

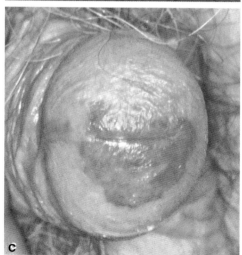

C

▲ **Figure 5-10 A, B, C** Skin cancers that are often misdiagnosed as a rash. A. In situ basal cell carcinoma. Well demarcated, erythematous, crusted plaque. B. In situ squamous cell carcinoma on arm. Subtle pink, thin plaque. C. In situ squamous cell carcinoma on head of penis (Bowen's disease). Well demarcated erythematous plaque.

Table 5-5. Clinical presentations of diseases with high potential morbidity.

Clinical presentations	Diseases with high potential morbidity
Multiple persistent, red plaques that only partially respond to steroids.	Cutaneous T-cell lymphoma, connective tissue disorders.
Red plaques primarily in sun exposed areas in patients with systemic complaints.	Lupus erythematosus, dermatomyositis (see chapter 15).
Urticaria like lesions that last longer than 24 hours.	Urticarial vasculitis, prebullous phase of pemphigoid.
Urticaria and/ or angioedema in a patient with acute breathing difficulty (stridor).	Laryngeal edema, anaphylaxis (see chapter 16).
Widespread vesicles or bullae, especially if mucosa is involved.	Pemphigoid, pemphigus, Stevens Johnson syndrome/ Toxic epidermal necrolysis (see chapter 18).
Widespread areas of red painful skin.	Stevens Johnson/Toxic epidermal necrolysis, staphylococcal scalded skin syndrome (see chapter 18).
Widespread areas of peeling (desquamation) leaving areas of denuded skin.	Stevens Johnson syndrome/toxic epidermal necrolysis, staphylococcal scalded skin syndrome, toxic shock syndrome, exfoliative erythroderma (see chapter 18).
Localized area of red, tender, warm skin.	Cellulitis, erysipelas (see chapter 11).
Dusky, red to blue, painful, edematous area. May have hemorrhagic bullae or crepitus.	Necrotizing fasciitis.
Necrosis of the skin with ulceration and/or eschar.	Occlusion or inflammation of blood vessels from arteriosclerosis, localized infection, emboli, sepsis, clotting disorders, vasculitis, paraproteinemia, calciphylaxis.
Red or purple papules or macules that don't blanch.	Purpura, (see chapter 24 Purpura for differential diagnosis).
Purple or red papules primarily in children with fever and neurological symptoms.	Rocky Mountain Spotted Fever, other rickettsial diseases, meningococcemia.
Rash and fever with multiple systemic complaints and findings.	Exanthems due to certain infections, such as measles, varicella, parvovirus B19, meningococcemia, scarlet fever, mononucleosis, covid-19, zika, rickettsioses, west Nile virus, Kawasaki disease, connective tissue diseases, Still's disease, vasculitis. (See chapter 26 Fever and Rash for differential diagnosis).
Widespread persistent pruritus in patient with no primary skin disease.	Liver, kidney and myeloproliferative disease. (See chapter 25 Pruritus for differential diagnosis).

Misdiagnosis of Cutaneous Diseases with High Morbidity

"Could this be a serious disease?" is a common concern in medicine. Most skin disorders that have high morbidity or are associated with systemic disease have features that should alert a clinician that they may be dealing with a serious disorder. Table 5-5 lists some of the clinical findings that could indicate a serious disease.

Cognitive Errors

Flaws in clinicians thinking/cognitive processes account for more than 75% of diagnostic errors.[10] These cognitive errors are well studied and are predictable, some of the more common are listed below.[3,11,12]

- Anchoring and premature closure of diagnosis: Sticking with your initial diagnosis and closing your mind to other possible diagnoses before all the information is known.
- Confirmation bias: Looking only at evidence that confirms your diagnosis and ignoring evidence that refutes it.
- Availability bias: Choosing a diagnosis you are most familiar with.
- Bandwagon effect/diagnostic momentum: Colleagues' opinions overly influence diagnosis.
- Racial, ethnic, gender bias: Patient's demographics lead to underestimating or overestimating likelihood of diagnosis.[13]

REFERENCES

1. Santoro R Skin over the centuries. A short history of dermatology: physiology, pathology and cosmetics. *Medicina Historica*. 2017. 1(2):94–102.
2. Croskerry P. A universal model of diagnostic reasoning. *Acad Med*. 2009;84(8):1022–1028.
3. Norman GR, Monteiro SD, Sherbino J, Ilgen JS, Schmidt HG, Mamede S. The causes of errors in clinical reasoning: cognitive biases, knowledge deficits, and dual process thinking. *Academic Medicine*. 2017;92(1):23–30.
4 Ko CJ, Braverman I, Sidlow R, Lowenstein EJ. Visual perception, cognition, and error in dermatologic diagnosis: Key cognitive principles. *J Am Acad Dermatol*. 2019;81(6):1227–1234.
5. Ark TK, Brooks LR, Eva KW. Giving learners the best of both worlds: do clinical teachers need to guard against teaching pattern recognition to novices? *Acad Med*. 2006;81(4):405–409.
6. Carli P, Quercioli E, Sestini S, et al . Pattern analysis, not simplified algorithms, is the most reliable method for teaching dermoscopy for melanoma diagnosis to residents in dermatology. *Br J Dermatol*. 2003;148(5):981–984.
7 Kang S, Amagai M, Bruckner AL, Enk AH, Margolis DJ, McMichael AJ, Orringer JS. eds. *Fitzpatrick›s Dermatology,* 9th ed. McGraw-Hill; 2019.
8. Pariser RJ, Pariser DM. Primary care physicians' errors in handling cutaneous disorders. *J Am Acad Dermatol*. 1987;17(2):239–245.
9. Aslan C, Gktay F, Mansur A T, Aydıngöz I E, Güneş P, Ekmekçi T R. Clinicopathological consistency in skin disorders: A retrospective study of 3949 pathological reports. *J Am Acad Dermatol*. 2012;66(3):393–400.
10. O'Sullivan E, Schofield S. Cognitive bias in clinical medicine. *J R Coll Physicians Edinb*. 2018;48(3):225–232.
11. Cohen JM, Burgin S. Cognitive biases in clinical decision making: a primer for the practicing dermatologist. *JAMA Dermatol*. 2016;152(3):253.
12. Lowenstein EJ, Sidlow R, Ko CJ. Visual perception, cognition, and error in dermatologic diagnosis: Diagnosis and error. *J Am Acad Dermatol*. 2019;81(6):1237–1245.
13. Hall WJ, Chapman MV, Lee KM, et al. Implicit racial/ethnic bias among health care professionals and its influence on health care outcomes: a systematic review. *Am J Public Health*. 2015;105(12):60–76.

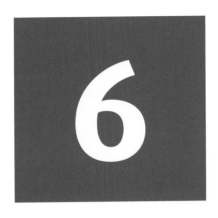

Principles of Management

Lindsey M. Voller
Ingrid C. Polcari
Carol Soutor

INTRODUCTION TO CHAPTER

Most of the common skin disorders can be treated with a formulary of generic, widely available topical and oral medications. Several medicinal products are over the counter including those used for fungal and bacterial infections, acne, urticaria, pruritus, and head lice. Topical medications are effective for most common skin disorders and they have fewer serious adverse side effects when compared to their oral counterparts. Oral medications may be needed if a skin disease is widespread or more severe.

There are several things to consider before prescribing a topical product such as the vehicle, quantity to dispense, and cost.

VEHICLE SELECTION

The vehicle of a topical product may be as important as the active ingredient. Table 6-1 lists commonly used vehicles. "If it's dry, wet it and if it's wet, dry it" is still a good general guideline for the treatment of common dermatoses. Most skin disorders, especially the chronic dermatoses (e.g.,

psoriasis, chronic contact dermatitis) are "dry"; therefore, ointments are preferred as they are more moisturizing. Also, ointments do not contain preservatives which can cause stinging and burning. The main problem with ointments, especially in adults, is that they are greasy and can stain clothing and bedding. Creams are a good option for the "wet" dermatoses, such as acute contact dermatitis, and other blistering or exudative dermatoses. They are also a good option for adults who don't want to use an ointment. However, some cream preparations are slightly drying and preservatives and other ingredients may sting or burn.

QUANTITY TO DISPENSE

The quantity of medication to be dispensed and the amount of medication that is needed per application are important considerations in prescribing medications, especially topical steroids and calcineurin inhibitors.

There are a few general rules that can be used to estimate the quantity of topical medication that a patient will need; however, the required amount may vary a great deal

Table 6-1 Vehicles for topical products.

Vehicle	Formulation	Indications
Ointment	80% oil and 20% or less water, petroleum jelly base, greasy, no preservatives, effective at moisturizing skin. May stain paper, clothing, and bedding.	Best choice for most "dry," thick, lichenified, or fissured dermatoses (e.g., atopic dermatitis and psoriasis), doesn't sting.
Cream	Oil and 20%–80% water emulsion, moderate moisturizing effects, some residue, contains preservatives.	Acute dermatitis and cases in which ointments are not tolerated (e.g., hot, humid climate, intertriginous skin, and cosmetic concerns).
Lotion	Similar to cream with more water and lower viscosity, spreads easily, minimal residue, and contains preservatives.	Used in many moisturizers and sunscreens, cosmetically acceptable.
Gel	Transparent base that liquefies on contact with skin, residue minimal, but may be shiny, drying.	Best choice for hair bearing areas, cosmetically acceptable. Often used for acne and rosacea medications.
Solution	Low viscosity, transparent, base of water and or alcohol, very drying, evaporates quickly leaving no residue.	Best for use in scalp dermatoses, too drying and irritating for use on other body areas.
Foam	Leaves minimal residue, may be drying.	Usually used in hair bearing areas.
Powder	Talc-based, drying, decreases frictional forces in intertriginous areas.	Good choice for body fold areas and feet.

depending on the age of the patient, body size, type of vehicle, and how thickly the product is applied. In general:

- Approximately 30 grams of cream will cover the entire adult body for 1 application.
- As an approximation, infants will need 1/5 of the adult quantity, children 2/5 of the adult quantity, and adolescents 2/3 of the adult quantity.[1]

It is also important to give instructions to patients on what quantity of medication they need to apply per application. The fingertip unit (FTU) is a commonly used measurement.[2] A FTU is the amount of medication dispensed (squeezed) from a tube with a 5 mm nozzle that covers the skin of the index finger from the tip to the distal crease (Figure 6-1). One FTU is equal to approximately 0.5 gram. One FTU will cover an area of skin equivalent to the area covered by 2 hands. Another option for estimating larger quantities is the use of a standardized kitchen tablespoon. One tablespoon holds slightly less than 15 grams of a cream or ointment which will cover approximately half of an adult body.

Topical medications are usually packaged in increments of 15 grams, most commonly in tubes and bottle sizes of 15, 30, 45, and 60 grams. Many generic topical steroid medications can be dispensed in jars of larger sizes, typically at a lower cost per gram.

COST CONSIDERATIONS

The cost of medications is an increasingly important issue and may affect a patient's decision about the purchase and use of a prescription medication. There are generic forms of most of the commonly used topical medications and in general they are cheaper than their branded counterparts.

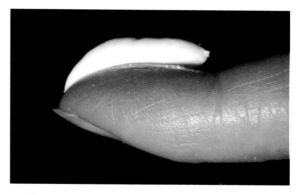

▲ **Figure 6-1.** Fingertip unit. Amount of medication dispensed from tube from the tip of the index finger to the distal crease is 0.5 g.

However, even the price of generic topicals has been increasing.[3]

There were concerns about the quality of topical generic medications several years ago, but recent studies on selected products have shown that they are equivalent in efficacy to brand name medications.[4] There are, however, some products such as augmented steroids, combination medications, and certain vehicle preparations that are available only as a branded product.

Some large retailers (e.g., Kroger, Target, Walgreens, Walmart) have a few selected medications that they offer at a low price ($4 for 30 day supply). These medications typically include a choice of low, medium, and high potency topical steroids, and some oral antibiotics.

ANTI-INFLAMMATORY MEDICATIONS

Introduction

Many common diseases fall into the inflammatory category (e.g., dermatitis and papulosquamous) and respond to topical and systemic medications that reduce inflammation. For many years, topical and oral corticosteroids were the main treatment options for these diseases. But clinicians now have many more options, including topical calcineurin inhibitors, biologic agents, and Janus kinase (JAK) inhibitors.

Topical Steroids

Since the 1950s, topical steroids have been used for a wide range of inflammatory skin disorders such as dermatitis and papulosquamous diseases. They have anti-inflammatory, anti-proliferative, and immunosuppressive effects on the skin. In the United States, topical steroids are ranked from class 1 to 7 with superpotent steroids in class 1 and the least potent steroids in class 7. The steroids in any one class have equivalent potency, so a limited formulary of topical steroids is sufficient in most cases (Table 6-2).[5]

There are many factors to consider when prescribing a topical steroid, including the nature of the disease to be treated, the location of the rash, the amount of steroid needed, duration and frequency of treatment, and the age of the patient (Table 6-3).[6]

The risks of topical steroids are less severe than those associated with the use of oral corticosteroids; however, in certain situations the topical adverse effects can be cosmetically distressing to the patient and damaging to the skin. Some of the most common adverse effects including striae, atrophy, and purpura (Figures 6-2, 6-3) are listed in Table 6-4.[6,7] Systemic adverse reactions, similar to those seen with systemic steroids, can occur with the use of more potent topical steroids, especially in children.

Systemic Steroids

Most common inflammatory dermatoses can be managed without systemic steroids. However, there are a few indications for their *short-term use*, such as widespread severe allergic contact dermatitis (e.g., dermatitis due to poison ivy) and in some cases of atopic dermatitis that are unresponsive to other therapies. The risks of long-term use of systemic corticosteroids limit their use for chronic dermatoses; however, there are risks to even brief use (< 14 days), including gastrointestinal bleeding, sepsis, heart failure, and hyperglycemia.[8]

Topical Calcineurin Inhibitors

Topical calcineurin inhibitors (tacrolimus and pimecrolimus) are nonsteroidal, immunosuppressant medications that are Food and Drug Administration (FDA) approved for short-term use as a *second-line therapy* in moderate to severe atopic dermatitis. Stinging and burning are common side effects of these medications. Pimecrolimus 1% cream and tacrolimus 0.03% ointment are approved for children 2 years and older and tacrolimus 0.1% ointment is approved for adults.

Several studies have been conducted on the off-label use of tacrolimus and pipecuroniums in cases in which

Table 6-2. Potency ranking of selected topical steroid medications.[a]

Class and Potency	Generic Name	Formulations
1 Ultra high potency	Clobetasol propionate	Cream, ointment, gel, solution, foam, shampoo 0.05%
	Halobetasol propionate	Cream, ointment 0.05%
2 High potency	Desoximetasone	Cream, ointment, 0.25% Gel 0.05%
	Fluocinonide	Cream, ointment, gel, solution 0.05%
	Halcinonide	Cream, ointment 0.1%
3,4,5 Mid potency	Betamethasone valerate	Cream, ointment, lotion 0.1%, and foam 0.12%
	Fluocinolone acetonide	Cream, ointment, 0.025% and oil, shampoo 0.01%
	Hydrocortisone valerate	Cream, ointment 0. 2%
	Triamcinolone acetonide	Cream, ointment, gel, lotion 0.1%
6 Low potency	Desonide	Cream, ointment 0.05%
	Fluocinolone acetonide	Cream, solution 0.01 %
7 Least potent	Hydrocortisone acetate	Cream, ointment, gel, lotion 0.5% 1% and 2.5%

[a]This table does not include all the available topical steroids.

Table 6-3. Factors in the usage and selection of topical steroids.

Disease and Lesion Category
- Acute inflammatory diseases such as contact dermatitis and atopic dermatitis usually respond to medium to low potency topical steroids. However, short-term use of more potent steroids may be needed for initial treatment.
- Chronic localized dermatoses with thick lesions such as psoriasis may require high potency steroids.

Location of Lesions
- Areas of thin skin such as the face, axilla, groin, diaper areas, and other intertriginous areas should be treated with low potency steroids. The use of steroids in these locations should be limited in quantity and duration.
- Dermatoses on the palms and soles may require high potency steroids.

Extent of Area to be Treated
- Medium to low potency steroids should be used if large areas are to be treated.

Quantity of Steroid
- A thin layer of steroid is sufficient for treatment.
- Package insert for clobetasol indicates that no more than 50 g should be used in 1 week.

Duration of Treatment
- The package insert on superpotent topical steroids such as clobetasol recommends use of no more than 2 consecutive weeks.
- Topical steroids should be discontinued when the rash has resolved.

Frequency of Application
- Once to twice a day application is the usual recommendation.

Age of Patient
- Children have a higher ratio of total body surface to body weight and are more likely to have systemic adverse effects from topical steroids. Low potency steroids are recommended.
- Low to mid potency steroids are recommended in elderly adults with thin and/or fragile skin as they may more easily develop adverse cutaneous problems with high potency steroids.

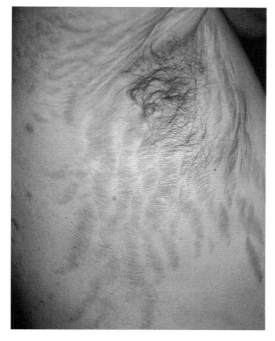

▲ **Figure 6-2.** Striae in axillae caused by chronic use of high potency steroid ointment for psoriasis.

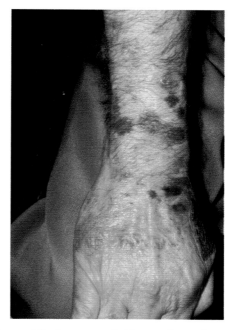

▲ **Figure 6-3.** Purpura and skin atrophy on forearm and dorsal hand due to use of high potency steroid ointment.

Table 6-4. Selected potential adverse effects of topical steroids.

Adverse Effects	Notes
Atrophy	More common in children and the elderly, intertriginous areas, and face. Risk increases with strength of steroid.
Telangiectasia	Most commonly occurs on the face.
Striae	Most common in intertriginous and flexural areas.
Purpura and ulcerations	More common in the elderly due to dermal atrophy.
Delayed wound healing	May occur in ulcers and surgical sites.
Hypopigmentation	More prominent in darker skin.
Increased incidence of infections (bacterial, fungal, and viral)	May mask clinical features of fungal infections.
Flares of acne, rosacea perioral dermatitis	May occur with mid to high potency steroids.
Allergic or irritant contact dermatitis	Most commonly caused by a chemical in the vehicle or to the steroid itself.
Glaucoma	Uncommon, occurs with use near or on periorbital skin.
Systemic adverse effects	More common in children or with use of high potency steroids in any age group.
Osteoporosis and osteoporotic bone fractures.	In adults using high potency topical steroids.

the long-term use of topical steroids is contraindicated such as in dermatoses on the face (especially the periorbital region), intertriginous areas and other areas of thin skin. These studies have shown that calcineurin inhibitors are effective in seborrheic dermatitis, perioral dermatitis, intertriginous psoriasis, oral lichen planus, lichen sclerosus, and vitiligo.[9]

Tacrolimus and pimecrolimus have black box warnings that warn about the potential for an increased risk of skin and other cancers. However, a prospective 10-year study on the safety of tacrolimus ointment in children found no evidence of an increased incidence of cancer in the study group.[10]

MOISTURIZERS

The barrier function of the skin is impaired in many of the common dermatoses, especially in atopic dermatitis. It is essential that the skin's barrier function be restored and maintained with the use of moisturizers.[11] Moisturizers should be applied liberally at least twice a day including immediately after bathing. The use of a low detergent bar or liquid soap is also important in the maintenance of the barrier. Examples of moisturizers and cleansers that can be used in patients with dermatitis and other inflammatory skin disorders are listed in Chapter 8.

Creams or lotions with ceramides, colloidal oatmeal, lactic acid, or urea may be helpful in some conditions, such as dry skin or dermatitis. At lower concentrations, lactic acid and urea act as moisturizers (humectants) and at higher concentrations, they act as keratolytic agents, which are especially helpful in thick, fissured skin. Generic versions of the products are available; the following are some examples of branded options:

- Ceramides: CeraVe Moisturizing Cream, Cetaphil Restoraderm Eczema Soothing moisturizer
- Colloidal Oatmeal: Aveeno Active Naturals Skin Relief Moisture Repair Cream
- Lactic acid: AmLactin Moisturizing Lotion, Lac-Hydrin Lotion
- Urea: Eucerin Roughness Relief Cream

THERAPEUTIC BATHS

Tub baths with emollients added to the water are an efficient method of moisturizing the entire skin's surface. Bath products that contain detergents should not be used on skin that is inflamed or dry. Aveeno Soothing Bath Treatment (colloidal oatmeal powder) and RoBathol Bath Oil (cotton seed oil) are examples of such products, as are several generic options. Bath products with emollients may make the tub slippery, so caution is needed when entering or exiting the bathtub.

WET DRESSINGS

Wet dressings are a safe and cost effective treatment for dermatoses that are vesicular or have crusts or exudate such as acute contact dermatitis, atopic dermatitis, bullous diseases, and impetigo.[12] Topical emollients or topical steroid creams can be applied before or after the wet dressings. Table 6-5 covers the materials and procedure for wet dressings.

Table 6-5. Wet dressings materials and procedure.

Materials needed
- For Burrow's solution 1:40, mix one tablet or one powder packet of aluminum sulfate (generic or Domeboro Medicated Soak Rash Relief) in one pint (16 oz. /473 cc) of water.
- For 1% acetic acid solution mix 1/2 cup (2 oz.) of white household vinegar (5% acetic acid) in one pint of water.
- Cotton material for dressings, for example, 4" gauze (e.g., Kerlix) or bed sheets, pillowcases, or T-shirts.

Procedure
- Apply a bland emollient or the appropriate steroid cream to the affected area.
- Fold the cotton material to produce 4-8 layers of sufficient size to cover the affected area.
- Drip the material into the solution and wring it out slightly so it is not dripping wet.
- Apply the wet dressings to the affected area(s) and keep them in place for 15–30 minutes. Reapply 2-4 times a day until crusts and inflammation have resolved which typically takes 2-5 days
- Discontinue wet dressings if skin becomes fissured or dry.
- If a large area is treated, cover wet dressings with a blanket or dry clothing to prevent hypothermia.

TOPICAL ANTIPRURITIC MEDICATIONS

Over the counter lotions containing calamine, camphor, menthol, or pramoxine are commonly used to reduce the symptoms of pruritus. Many of the these are available as generic products; some of the widely available branded products and their active ingredients are as follows:

- Benadryl Gel (diphenhydramine)
- Prax Lotion (pramoxine)
- Sarna Original Anti-Itch Moisturizing Lotion (camphor and menthol)
- Sarna sensitive Anti-Itch Lotion (pramoxine)

ORAL ANTIHISTAMINES

Oral antihistamines for urticaria are listed in in Chapter 14. They are also commonly used for treatment of pruritus due to other etiologies. However, in conditions such as atopic dermatitis, it may be the soporific effect of the sedating antihistamines that is responsible for their efficacy in the treatment of pruritus.

ANTIFUNGAL MEDICATIONS

Superficial dermatophyte infections such as tinea pedis, tinea cruris, and tinea corporis will usually respond to non prescription topical antifungal agents, such as clotrimazole, miconazole, terbinafine, and tolnaftate. However, prescription medications may be needed in cases that do not respond to these products. Table 6-6 lists some common antifungal products.[6]

Table 6-6. Selected topical medications for superficial fungal infections.

Medication	Formulations	Dosing	Nonprescription
Allylamines			
Naftifine	Cream, gel 2%.	Once a day.	No
Terbinafine	Cream, spray 1%.	Twice a day.	Yes
Imidazoles			
Clotrimazole	Cream, lotion, solution 1%.	Twice a day.	Yes
Econazole	Cream 1%.	Once a day.	No
Ketoconazole	Cream, gel, foam 2%.	Twice a day.	
Miconazole	Cream, ointment, lotion, spray Solution, powder 2%.	Twice a day.	Yes
Oxiconazole	Cream, lotion 2%.	Twice a day.	No
Sulconazole	Cream, solution 1%.	Once a day to twice a day.	No
Miscellaneous			
Butenafine	Cream 1%.	Once a day.	Yes
Ciclopirox	Cream, 0.77%, gel 3%, lotion 0.77%.	Twice a day.	No
Tolnaftate	Cream, lotion, solution, spray, powder 1%.	Twice a day.	Yes

Oral antifungal medications are used for treatment of fungal infections in the scalp and nails and in some cases of fungal infections of the skin that do not respond to topical agents. These are covered in Chapter 12.

ANTIVIRAL MEDICATIONS

Oral antiviral medications are effective treatments for herpes zoster and herpes simplex. In general, they have a good safety profile. The antiviral medications and dosing for herpes simplex infection in immunocompetent adults are listed in Table 6-7. The dosing for oral antiviral medications for herpes zoster in immunocompetent adults is as follows:

- Acyclovir 800 mg every 4 hours, 5 times a day for 7–10 days.
- Famciclovir 500 mg every 8 hours for 7 days.
- Valacyclovir 1000 mg three times a day for 7 days.

MEDICATIONS FOR SCABIES AND LICE

Topical and oral medications for the treatment of scabies and lice are covered in Chapter 14.

Table 6-7. Oral medications for initial genital herpes and recurrent orolabial and genital herpes infections in immunocompetent adults.

Medication	Selected dosing options for herpes simplex infections.	Duration
Acyclovir	Initial genital: 200 mg every 4 hours, 5 times a day.	10 days
	Recurrent genital: 200 mg every 4 hours, 5 times a day.	5 days
Famciclovir	Initial orolabial: 250 mg every 8 hours.	7-10 days
	Recurrent orolabial: 1500 mg one dose.	1 day
	Recurrent genital: 1000 mg twice a day.	1 day
Valacyclovir	Initial genital: 1 gram twice a day.	10 days
	Recurrent genital: 500 mg twice a day.	3 days
	Recurrent orolabial: 2 g every 12 hours.	1 day

ACNE AND ROSACEA MEDICATIONS

Topical and oral medications for the treatment of acne and rosacea are covered in Chapter 10.

ANTIBIOTICS

Topical antibiotics are useful for the treatment of localized areas of impetigo and superficial bacterial skin infection.[6] Mupirocin ointment and cream 2% and retapamulin ointment 1% are examples of prescription topical antibiotics. Over the counter topical antibiotics can also be used, but they have a higher rate of risk for allergic contact dermatitis. These include bacitracin, neomycin, and triple antibiotic (polymyxin, neomycin, and bacitracin) ointments.

Oral antibiotics for skin infections are covered in Chapter 11 and for acne and rosacea in Chapter 10.

SUNSCREENS AND SUN SAFETY

Importance of Sun Protection

Sunlight emits a wide range of radiation energy along the electromagnetic spectrum, including visible light and ultraviolet (UV) light. UV radiation can be subdivided into three main categories based on its wavelengths:[13]

- UVC: 200–290 nm
- UVB: 290–315 nm
- UVA: 315–400 nm

Of these, UVB and UVA possess the greatest potential to cause skin damage; UVB is primarily absorbed in the epidermis, while UVA's longer wavelength facilitates deeper penetration into the dermis.[13] Cumulative exposure to UV radiation in the form of direct sunlight and/or tanning beds is a well-described risk factor in the development of skin cancer. Keratinocyte skin cancer (e.g., basal cell carcinoma (BCC) and squamous cell carcinoma (SCC)) is the most common form of malignancy in the United States, and its incidence continues to rise.[14] Melanoma—the deadliest type of skin cancer, causing more than 9,000 US deaths per year—has also demonstrated a steady increase in incidence over the past few decades.[15] Fortunately, many of these cases are preventable. The primary prevention of skin cancer therefore remains a worthwhile public health endeavor, beginning with an emphasis on proper education and the incorporation of sun safety routines from an early age.

Sun Safety Recommendations

Adequate photoprotection is most effectively accomplished through a combination of strategies, including seeking shade, wearing sun-protective clothing, and regularly applying sunscreen to exposed areas not covered by clothing (Table 6-8). For all patients, particularly adolescents, strict avoidance of tanning beds is strongly advised.

Seeking shade

Whenever possible, outdoor activities should be scheduled before 10 am and after 4 pm to avoid the peak intensity of the sun's strongest rays. Activities can be adjusted to take advantage of the shade; examples include choosing playgrounds with shade structures or nearby trees, as well as bringing umbrellas, canopies, or tents to create makeshift shade. The "shadow rule" serves as a general rule of thumb in estimating the intensity of UV radiation; shadows which are shorter than the height of an individual indicate increased sunburn risk ("Short shadow? Seek shade!").[16] A more specific measurement is the UV index, which provides a calculated forecast of the strength of

Table 6-8. Summary of sun safety recommendations.

Category	Recommendation
Shade	• Schedule outdoor activities before 10 a.m. and after 4 p.m. • Seek shade whenever possible.
Clothing	• UPF 50+ clothing (or dark, tightly woven clothing). • Wide-brimmed hats (2″ brim). • Sunglasses (oversized or wrap-around style preferred).
Sunscreen	• Apply to all skin not covered by clothing. • SPF 30+, broad-spectrum, water-resistant sunscreen. • Apply 1 oz, at least 15 minutes prior to outdoor activities. • Reapply every 2 hours, and after swimming/sweating.

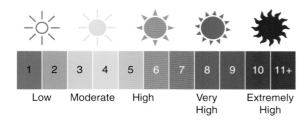

1	2	3	4	5	6	7	8	9	10	11+

Low　　Moderate　　High　　Very　　Extremely
　　　　　　　　　　　　　　High　　　High

▲ **Figure 6-4.** Depiction of the ultraviolet light (UV) index, a linear scale describing sunburn risk for the average individual.

sunburn-inducing UV radiation at a particular place and time.[17] The UV index is displayed as an open-ended linear scale (Figure 6-4), which is directly proportional to the intensity of UV radiation. The average individual requires sun protection at a level ≥ 3. Importantly, clouds do not confer photoprotection; an overcast day can still emit high levels of UV radiation.

Sun-protective clothing

Even while seeking shade, UV light can be reflected off environmental surfaces such as sand, water, and grass; sun-protective clothing is thus an important addition to routine sun safety practices. Photoprotective clothing is often labeled with an ultraviolet protection factor (UPF), which indicates the fabric's ability to confer protection from UVA and UVB radiation. The Skin Cancer Foundation promotes a Seal of Recommendation for approved UPF clothing, with UPF levels of 30–49 rated as "very good" protection and UPF 50+ rated as "excellent."[18] The following are examples of UPF-clothing brands which offer a variety of photoprotective options for individuals of all age groups:

• Coolibar: coolibar.com
• L.L. Bean: llbean.com

• Lands' End: landsend.com
• Solbari: solbari.com
• Solumbra: sunprecautions.com
• UV Skinz: uvskinz.com

If UPF clothing is deemed cost-prohibitive, certain regular clothing items may be used as an alternative. In general, patients should be counseled to wear clothing that provides full coverage (e.g., long sleeves and pants) and is darker, densely woven, loosely fitting, and composed of unbleached cotton or polyester. Practically, holding the fabric against a light source to determine whether light shines through can help estimate the quality of photoprotection.

In addition to clothing, wearing wide-brimmed hats (≥ 2-inch brim) and sunglasses that provide up to 400 nm of UV absorption (e.g., 100% UVA and UVB protection) is advised. These measures are not only important in preventing skin cancer of the face, ears, neck, and scalp, but also in reducing the risk of ocular complications such as cataracts and macular degeneration.[19]

Avoidance of tanning beds

Similar to cigarette smoking and ionizing radiation, tanning beds are considered a group 1 carcinogen; associations have been demonstrated with indoor tanning and the subsequent development of SCC, BCC, and most concerningly, melanoma.[20] Indoor tanning is particularly common among adolescents and young adults, leading to the introduction of legislation to restrict access to tanning beds by minors across many states. However, adherence to these restrictions has been substandard, highlighting the need for increased education efforts in this population.[21] Younger patients should be counseled that a tan indicates skin damage, and that the concept of "preventive tanning" to decrease future sunburn risk is both damaging and strongly discouraged. Individuals desiring a tanned appearance should instead be directed to sunless tanning products.

Sunscreens

Sunscreen basics

While avoidance of UV exposure is the most effective means of skin cancer prevention, consistent sunscreen use is also important. Sunscreens are topically applied agents designed to protect the skin from the adverse effects of UV light, including sunburn, photoaging (e.g., wrinkles), photosensitivity, and skin cancer. Prospective studies have largely demonstrated that sunscreen is effective in reducing the risk of actinic keratoses, SCCs, and melanoma, and may be effective in preventing BCCs.[22,23] The American Academy of Dermatology (AAD) specifically recommends the use of broad-spectrum, water-resistant sunscreen with a sun protection factor (SPF) of 30 or greater (Figure 6-5).[24] Higher SPF values may be utilized to compensate for underapplication, but minimal additional benefit is offered for SPF

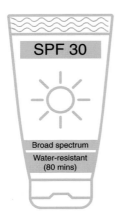

▲ Figure 6-5. Basic labeling guidelines for selecting a sunscreen.

values >50. Definitions of the SPF, broad-spectrum, and water-resistant designations can be found in Table 6-9.[25]

Sunscreen should be applied to all exposed skin not covered by clothing (including the ears, eyelids, and lips) approximately 15 minutes prior to outdoor activities, and reapplied every 2 hours while outdoors. Adults require approximately one ounce of sunscreen (roughly the size of a shot glass) to cover their entire body in a swimsuit. Sunscreens should be stored at room temperature, and not used past their expiration date. As the best sunscreen is the one used most consistently, the optimal vehicle (e.g., lotion, stick, or spray) primarily depends on consumer preference, although sprays and sticks may pose difficulties with quantifying the appropriate amount to use for adequate coverage. In addition, the U.S. Food & Drug Administration (FDA) has expressed concern regarding particles in spray sunscreens, which may be inhaled during application and

Table 6-9. Common sunscreen labeling terms[24,25]

Sunscreen Label	Typical Definition
FDA-regulated terms	
Broad-spectrum	• Indicates UVA and UVB protection.
Extended protection	• Provides protection >typical 2-hour reapplication period. • Requires reapplication at stated time intervals.
Instant protection	• Provides protection immediately after application.

Sun protection factor (SPF)	• Primarily specifies UVB protection/attenuation of sunburn.
	  • SPF 15: 93% of UVB filtered.
	  • SPF 30: 97% of UVB filtered.

Water resistant	• Maintains protection while swimming and sweating. • Label must report how long the sunscreen will confer SPF protection. • Maximum effectiveness: 80 minutes.
FDA-unregulated terms	
Baby/safe for children	• No standard meaning. • Misleading label as strict sun avoidance is generally. recommended in infants <6 mos. • Does not necessarily indicate gentle or hypoallergenic.
Dermatologist recommended/ clinically proven	• Product may have undergone clinical testing. • Not endorsed by the American Academy of Dermatology.
Hypoallergenic	• Notoriously misused claim in cosmetic products. • Does not necessarily indicate absence of common allergens.
Contains insect repellent	• Not Recommended; insect repellent and sunscreen should be applied as separate products.
Natural/organic	• Often used if certain inactive ingredients meet the criteria. of "organic" (e.g., contain carbon.) • Organic sunscreens typically contain chemical active ingredients.
Non-comedogenic	• Typically avoids use of common irritants (e.g., fragrance) and comedogenic ingredients.
Sensitive skin	• Typically avoids use of common irritants (e.g., fragrance).
Sport	• Maintains protection while swimming and sweating.
Tanning/instant bronzing	• Often combined with sunless tanning products. • May have lower than recommended SPF values.

Table 6-10. Types of sunscreens.[27]

Sunscreen Type	Physical Sunscreens	Chemical Sunscreens
Synonyms	Inorganic, mineral.	Organic.
Mechanism of Action	Blocks and scatters UV and visible light.	Absorbs light and re-emits energy as insignificant quantities of heat.
Active Ingredients	Titanium dioxide. Zinc oxide.	Benzophenones (oxybenzone). Cinnamates (octinoxate). Para-aminobenzoic acid (PABA). Salicylates (octisalate). Avobenzone, octocrylene, others.
Advantages	Less irritating to sensitive skin, immediately effective, protects against visible light.	Not as messy, easier to apply, less apparent white sheen.
Disadvantages	Inferior UVB protection, can be difficult to rub in, may leave a white sheen.	Requires approximately 15 min to start working, may be irritating to sensitive skin.

cause damage to small airways.[26] This risk can be mitigated by avoiding spraying near the face and mouth, and choosing a different vehicle for use in children.

Sunscreen basics

There are two main categories of sunscreens: physical (also termed mineral or inorganic) and chemical (organic). Physical sunscreens, formulated with the active ingredients titanium dioxide and/or zinc oxide, provide protection by absorbing, reflecting, and scattering UV and visible light. Organic filters, of which there are many, consist of aromatic rings which allow for absorption of UV light and re-emission of that energy as insignificant quantities of heat.[27] Given the various advantages and disadvantages of the two types of sunscreens (Table 6-10), many sunscreens include a combination of both physical and chemical blockers. In addition, tinted sunscreens containing iron oxides and pigmentary titanium dioxide have emerged for photoprotection against visible light; these sunscreens may be particularly suitable for patients with darker skin types, visible light-induced photodermatoses, and/or hyperpigmentation disorders.[28]

Sunscreen labeling

Despite previous regulations by the FDA to standardize sunscreen labeling practices, studies have demonstrated sunscreen labels to be poorly understood by the general public.[29,30] In addition to basic features meeting American Academy of Dermatology guidelines (e.g., water-resistance, broad spectrum, and SPF value $\geq$ 30), many supplementary claims are marketed by companies, such as "sport," "hypoallergenic," and "safe for children" (Table 6-9). Though many of these claims are unregulated, they have nonetheless been shown to influence purchasing behaviors.[31] In February 2019, the FDA issued a proposed rule as part of the Sunscreen Innovation Act to update

the regulatory requirements for sunscreen products. The rule would institute regulations for over-the-counter sunscreen products, establishing specific guidelines for evaluating the safety and efficacy of sunscreens. Once finalized, it also aims to improve labeling requirements to help consumers more easily interpret specific statements found on many sunscreens.[26] In addition to these national regulations, clinicians are encouraged to provide routine counseling to their patients on selecting sunscreens and overall sun safety behaviors. Prior sunscreen counseling by any healthcare provider has been shown to significantly improve sunscreen knowledge, underscoring the importance of these continued education efforts.[32]

Sunscreen safety

While the safety of physical sunscreens has been relatively established, questions have arisen regarding the active ingredients used in certain chemical sunscreens. Oxybenzone (benzophenone-3), a well-known contact allergen, has previously been shown to influence the endocrinologic function of rats and fish with chronic exposure; however, these results have not been replicated in human studies.[33] In vitro studies have also demonstrated a correlation between oxybenzone and bleaching of coral reefs, and some states have banned the use of oxybenzone and octinoxate from their sunscreens owing to these concerns.[33] The effects of coral reef bleaching in reality are likely multifactorial, occurring in conjunction with other pollutants and rising ocean temperatures.

The systemic absorption of chemical sunscreens has also become a point of discussion. A 2019 randomized controlled trial published in the Journal of the American Medical Association requested men and women to apply commercially available sunscreens to 75% of their body surface area four times a day for 4 days, and found serologically detectable levels of four chemicals (e.g., avobenzone, oxybenzone, octocrylene, and ecamsule) exceeding the FDA's limit of >0.5 ng/mL, or the cutoff requiring safety studies.[34] The study required an amount of sunscreen significantly higher than typical use, and did not provide evidence of linking the systemic absorption of sunscreen ingredients to adverse health effects. Nonetheless, the demonstration of systemic absorption affirms the FDA's request for further studies on the safety and efficacy of 12 chemical sunscreen ingredients before considering them to be generally recognized as safe and effective.[26] It should be noted that these ingredients are not considered unsafe by the FDA; rather, further safety data is requested regarding their potential for irritation/allergy, safety/efficacy in children, and the extent of absorption.[35] Ultimately, the known benefits of sunscreen in preventing skin cancer and photoaging are thought to outweigh the uncertain implications of systemic absorption.

▶ Sun Protection in Infants

Approximately 25–50% of the total erythema dose that an individual is exposed to prior to the age of 60 is received in childhood.[36] Infants and children are particularly susceptible to the damaging effects of the sun, due in part to their underdeveloped skin barrier function, as well as an increased total body surface area to volume ratio as compared to adults.[37] It is therefore critical to practice strict sun safety with infants and children, and to incorporate these routines early on. For infants less than 6 months old, sun avoidance is recommended (e.g., seeking shade and dressing in sun-protective clothing, as discussed previously).[37] If sun avoidance is not possible and the infant has exposed skin, a small amount of physical blocking sunscreen may be applied to exposed areas, as these sunscreens are generally less irritating to sensitive skin. Sunscreens which are labeled as "baby" or "safe for children" typically have no actual standard criteria for their labeling, and do not necessarily indicate the inclusion of gentle or hypoallergenic ingredients. Importantly, infants overheat easily, so caution should be exercised during any activities taking place in warm temperatures. After 6 months, sunscreen can be applied as usual.

ADHERENCE ISSUES

Patient adherence to medication usage is not often optimal, but in the case of topical products, it is even more challenging. Studies show that many patients do not actually purchase their prescriptions, or they use the medications less frequently or in smaller quantities than recommended.[38] Adherence is particularly low in chronic conditions such as atopic dermatitis, psoriasis, and acne. Some of these adherence challenges can be addressed by clinicians with the following measures:

- Ask patients and/or parents about their preferences for various treatment regimens.

- Utilize shared decision-making tools which are currently available for such conditions as psoriasis, systemic lupus erythematosus, and melanoma.[39]
- Set realistic treatment goals and expectations for the patient's specific circumstances.
- Limit the frequency and complexity of treatment schedules for medications that are used in a school, assisted living or nursing home setting.
- Give clear written instructions about the importance and proper use of medications. Instructions should be translated into the appropriate language, as needed.
- Discuss concerns about side effects, risks, and cost of medications.
- If non-adherence is a recurrent issue, clarify, and when possible, address the underlying problems.
- If a patient has a preference for complementary and integrative medicine, explore those options or refer to an appropriate provider.
- Encourage use of medication reminder cell phone apps and a follow up visit to assess the patient's response and adherence with the treatment plan.

BARRIERS TO MANAGEMENT

Many of the patient adherence issues are related to various barriers patients face in accessing medications and dermatologic therapies. Many of these barriers are related to socioeconomic disparities. Tens of millions of Americans remain uninsured or underinsured or live in healthcare or pharmacy deserts even in urban areas.[40] Healthcare racial disparities also create barriers. For example, studies have shown that Black patients on Medicare with moderate to severe psoriasis were 70% less likely to receive biologic medications than white Medicare patients independent of pertinent variables.[41] It is important for clinicians to be aware of these barriers and assist patients in overcoming them.

QUALITY OF LIFE AND MENTAL HEALTH ISSUES

Patients with chronic skin disorders (e.g., psoriasis, atopic dermatitis, chronic pruritus) have higher rates of anxiety and depression than healthy controls.[42] These negative emotional states can trigger or worsen their skin disease, setting off a vicious cycle. Patients with skin disorders and psychiatric comorbidities are best managed by a team approach, including clinicians in primary care, mental health, and dermatology.[42] These patients can be treated with standard psychotropic medications commonly used for anxiety and depression. Nonpharmacologic management such as psychotherapy, hypnosis, biofeedback, support groups, meditation, and other stress reduction techniques are also beneficial.[43]

There are several free websites that have more detailed information about prescription and nonprescription products. The following is a list of selected sites.

- Dailymed.com has the most recent FDA labels (package inserts) for many commonly used prescription medications. It is a free website of the US National Library of Medicine.

- Drugstore.com lists the ingredients in many common topical nonprescription products.

- Drugs.com contains a drug interaction checker and pill identifier.

- GoodRx lists prices of medications at various pharmacies in most cities in the United States. It also offers coupons for discounts on medications.

- Medlineplus.gov/druginformation.html has patient information for prescription products and herbs and supplements

- The American Academy of Dermatology has information on sun protection at www.aad.org/public/every-day-care/sun-protection

REFERENCES

1. Nelson AA, Miller AD, Fleischer AB, et al. How much of a topical agent should be prescribed for children of different sizes? *J Dermatolog Treat.* 2006;17(4):224–228.
2. Long CC, Finlay AY, Averill RW. The rule of hand: 4 hand areas = 2 FTU = 1 g. *Arch Dermatol.* 1992;128(8):1129–1130.
3. Bhatt MD, Bhatt BD, Dorrian JT, et al. Increased topical generic prices by manufacturers. *J Am Acad Dermatol.* 2019;80(5):1353–1357.
4. Payette M, Grant-Kels JM. Generic drugs in dermatology: part I. *J Am Acad Dermatol.* 2012;66(3):343.e1-8; quiz 351–352.
5. Sewell M, Burkhart C, Morrell D. Dermatological Pharmacology. In: Brunton L, Hilal-Dandan R, Knollmann B, eds. *Goodman & Gilman's: The Pharmacological Basis of Therapeutic.* 13th ed. New York: McGraw-Hill Education; 2017.
6. Drake LA, Dinehart SM, Farmer ER, et al. Guidelines of care for the use of topical glucocorticosteroids. American Academy of Dermatology. *J Am Acad Dermatol.* 1996;35(4): 615–619.
7. Egeberg A, Schwarz P, Harsløf T, et al. Association of potent and very potent topical corticosteroids and the risk of osteoporosis and major osteoporotic fractures. *JAMA Dermatol.* January 2021.
8. Yao T-C, Huang Y-W, Chang S-M, et al. Association between oral corticosteroid bursts and severe adverse events: A nationwide population-based cohort study. *Ann Intern Med.* 2020;173(5):325–330.
9. Guenther L, Lynde C, Poulin Y. Off-label use of topical Calcineurin inhibitors in dermatologic disorders. *J Cutan Med Surg.* 2019;23(4suppl):27S–34S.
10. Paller AS, Fölster-Holst R, Chen SC, et al. No evidence of increased cancer incidence in children using topical tacrolimus for atopic dermatitis. *J Am Acad Dermatol.* 2020;83(2): 375–381.
11. Purnamawati S, Indrastuti N, Danarti R, et al. The role of moisturizers in addressing various kinds of dermatitis: A review. *Clin Med Res.* 2017;15(3–4):75–87.
12. Dabade TS, Davis DMR, Wetter DA, et al. Wet dressing therapy in conjunction with topical corticosteroids is effective for rapid control of severe pediatric atopic dermatitis: experience with 218 patients over 30 years at Mayo Clinic. *J Am Acad Dermatol.* 2012;67(1):100–106.
13. Rünger TM. Ultraviolet radiation. In: Bolognia J, Schaffer J, Cerroni L, eds. *Dermatology.* Fourth. Philadelphia, PA: Elsevier; 2018:1536–1547.
14. Rogers HW, Weinstock MA, Feldman SR, et al. Incidence estimate of nonmelanoma skin cancer (keratinocyte carcinomas) in the US Population, 2012. *JAMA Dermatol.* 2015;151(10):1081–1086.
15. Paulson KG, Gupta D, Kim TS, et al. Age-specific incidence of melanoma in the United States. *JAMA Dermatol.* 2020;156(1):57–64.
16. Carter OBJ, Mills BW, Mazzucchelli GN, et al. Testing children's ability to correctly use the "Shadow Rule" for sun protection. *Int J Environ Health Res.* 2016;26(3):317–325.
17. United States Environmental Protection Agency. UV Index. https://www.epa.gov/sunsafety/uv-index-1. Accessed August 11, 2020.
18. Skin Cancer Foundation. Sun-Protective Clothing. https://www.skincancer.org/skin-cancer-prevention/sun-protection/sun-protective-clothing/. Accessed August 11, 2020.
19. Li H, Colantonio S, Dawson A, et al. Sunscreen application, safety, and sun protection: The evidence. *J Cutan Med Surg.* 2019;23(4):357–369.
20. Madigan LM, Lim HW. Tanning beds: Impact on health, and recent regulations. *Clin Dermatol.* 2016;34(5):640–648.
21. Williams MS, Buhalog B, Blumenthal L, et al. Tanning salon compliance rates in states with legislation to protect youth access to UV tanning. *JAMA Dermatol.* 2018;154(1):67–72.
22. Watts CG, Drummond M, Goumas C, et al. Sunscreen use and melanoma risk among young Australian adults. *JAMA Dermatol.* 2018;154(9):1001–1009.
23. Waldman RA, Grant-Kels JM. The role of sunscreen in the prevention of cutaneous melanoma and nonmelanoma skin cancer. *J Am Acad Dermatol.* 2019;80(2):574–576.e1.
24. American Academy of Dermatology. How to select a sunscreen. https://www.aad.org/public/everyday-care/sun-protection/sunscreen/how-to-select-sunscreen. Accessed August 11, 2020.
25. Yang EJ, Beck KM, Maarouf M, et al. Truths and myths in sunscreen labeling. *J Cosmet Dermatol.* 2018;17(6): 1288–1292.
26. U.S. Food and Drug Administration - Department of Health and Human Services. Sunscreen drug products for over-the-counter human use. *Fed Regist.* 2019;84(38):6204–6275. https://www.govinfo.gov/content/pkg/FR-2019-02-26/pdf/2019-03019.pdf.
27. Mancuso JB, Maruthi R, Wang SQ, et al. Sunscreens: An update. *Am J Clin Dermatol.* 2017;18(5):643–650.
28. Lyons AB, Trullas C, Kohli I, et al. Photoprotection beyond ultraviolet radiation: A review of tinted sunscreens. *J Am Acad Dermatol.* 2020; In press.
29. Chao LX, Sheu SL, Kong BY, et al. Identifying gaps in consumer knowledge about sunscreen. *J Am Acad Dermatol.* 2017;77(6):1172–1173.e2.

30. Kong BY, Sheu SL, Kundu R V. Assessment of consumer knowledge of new sunscreen Labels. *JAMA Dermatol.* 2015;151(9):1028.

31. Xu S, Kwa M, Agarwal A, et al. Sunscreen product performance and other determinants of consumer preferences. *JAMA Dermatol.* 2016;152(8):920–927.

32. Voller LM, Polcari IC. Public misperceptions of common sunscreen labeling claims: A survey study from the Minnesota State Fair. *J Am Acad Dermatol.* 2020;83(3):908–910.

33. Yeager DG, Lim HW. What's new in photoprotection - a review of new concepts and controversies. *Dermatol Clin.* 2019;37(2):149–157.

34. Matta MK, Zusterzeel R, Pilli NR, et al. Effect of sunscreen application under maximal use conditions on plasma concentration of sunscreen active ingredients. *JAMA.* 2019;321(21):2082–2091.

35. Adamson AS, Shinkai K. Systemic absorption of sunscreen - balancing benefits with unknown harms. *JAMA.* 2020;323(3):223–224.

36. Gilaberte Y, Carrascosa JM. Sun protection in children: realities and challenges. *Actas Dermo-Sifiliográficas (English Ed.)* 2014;105(3):253–262.

37. Julian E, Palestro AM, Thomas JA. Pediatric sunscreen and sun safety guidelines. *Clin Pediatr (Phila).* 2015;54(12):1133–1140.

38. Ahn CS, Culp L, Huang WW, et al. Adherence in dermatology. *J Dermatolog Treat.* 2017;28(2):94–103.

39. Morrison T, Johnson J, Baghoomian W, et al. Shared decision-making in dermatology: A scoping review. *JAMA Dermatol.* 2021;157(3):330–337.

40. Pednekar P, Peterson A. Mapping pharmacy deserts and determining accessibility to community pharmacy services for elderly enrolled in a State Pharmaceutical Assistance Program. *PLoS One.* 2018;13(6):e0198173.

41. Takeshita J, Gelfand JM, Li P, et al. Psoriasis in the US Medicare Population: Prevalence, treatment, and factors associated with biologic use. *J Invest Dermatol.* 2015;135(12):2955–2963.

42. Balieva FN, Finlay AY, Kupfer J, et al. The role of therapy in impairing quality of life in dermatological patients: A multinational study. *Acta Derm Venereol.* 2018;98(6):563–569.

43. Shenefelt PD. Complementary psychocutaneous therapies in dermatology. *Dermatol Clin.* 2005;23(4):723–734.

Dermatologic Procedures

Daniel Knabel
Adam Mattox

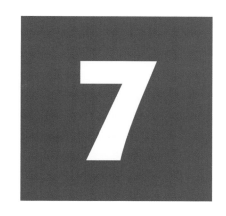

▼ INTRODUCTION TO CHAPTER

This chapter focuses on the most common procedures in dermatology that include biopsy techniques as well surgical procedures for removal of benign and malignant tumors. Videos of these procedures on simulated skin, pig's feet, and in a clinical setting are available. The reader should seek hands-on supervised training to supplement the content in this section.

▼ SKIN BIOPSY

Introduction

A skin biopsy is a diagnostic test done to gather more information than is available from the patient's history and physical examination. This information can be used to establish or confirm a diagnosis of a rash or tumor. Often clinicians hesitate to perform a biopsy. There may be concerns about the cosmetic impact on the patient, the risks associated with the procedure, or the technical aspects involved. Some disease processes are prone to sampling error and may require multiple skin biopsies for diagnosis. This is classically the case with cutaneous T-cell lymphoma or diseases with lesions of various stages or morphology.

Types of Biopsy Techniques

It is important to select the appropriate site, lesion, and technique for a biopsy to obtain an adequate sample. Having an understanding of the location of the pathology within the skin is important, for example, the epidermis, the dermal epidermal junction, deeper dermal structures, or subcutaneous dermal fat or muscle. The suspected location of the pathology will determine if a shave, punch, or an excisional biopsy is most appropriate (Table 7-1).[1–4] A biopsy should not be done on lesions that are excoriated or eroded.

- **Shave biopsy:** This is the most commonly used biopsy technique. It has the advantage of being less time consuming, yielding a good cosmetic result, and having a limited downtime for the patient. It is typically limited to processes occurring to the depth of the mid dermis. A saucerization biopsy is similar to a shave biopsy, but usually extends to the mid to lower dermis.[2,3,5,6] If done too deeply, in certain locations the biopsy site may heal slowly (e.g., on the lower leg) or leave a scar (e.g., on the nose).
- **Punch biopsy:** This has the advantage of providing a sample of full thickness skin, rapid healing, and uniform control. It is limited by the diameter of the punch tool

Table 7-1. Lesion, site, and biopsy selection for skin disorders.

Disorder	Procedures for Biopsy	Lesion or Site Selection
Dermatoses (rash) in epidermis or superficial dermis (lesions are not indurated, sclerotic or deep).	Punch or shave.	Select lesions that are characteristic or typical of the rash. Avoid old resolving lesions and excoriated lesions. If possible avoid cosmetically sensitive areas, such as the central face.
Dermatoses in deep dermis or fat (lesions are indurated, sclerotic or deep).	Punch, incision or excision.	
Vesiculobullous diseases for routine histology.	Punch or shave.	Biopsy new lesions 2–7 days old with bullae intact. Include the edge of blister and perilesional normal skin.
Vesiculobullous diseases for immunofluorescence studies.	Punch or shave.	For suspected vasculitis, biopsy lesional skin (the area of purpura). For suspected pemphigoid and pemphigus, biopsy perilesional skin. For suspected dermatitis herpetiformis, biopsy perilesional or normal skin.
Ulcers.	Punch or incision.	Biopsy edge of ulcer, not the necrotic center.
Tumors that are not suspected to be of melanocytic origin.	Deep shave, punch, incision or excision.	Biopsy the thickest or elevated area.
Tumors that are suspected to be of melanocytic origin (e.g., lentigo, nevus, atypical nevus, or melanoma).	Deep shave, saucerization biopsy, excision or punch biopsy (for small lesions.)[5,7]	Remove entire lesion for biopsy, ensure adequate depth.

and may not be adequate for processes in the subcutaneous tissue. Many dermatopathologists prefer a punch biopsy for adequate histologic assessment of a rash.[2,3]

- **Excision and incision/wedge biopsy:** These are more advanced procedures which are done using a sterile technique. Advantages include an adequate sample down to the subcutaneous tissues. Margins can also be controlled and adjusted as needed. Limitations include the increased duration of the procedure and a longer healing time with a greater potential for scarring.

EQUIPMENT FOR PROCEDURES

The following is a list of standard equipment that is essential for most dermatologic procedures. For each type of procedure discussed, additions to the standard tray are listed within the associated section. When surgical trays are being prepared, it is important to decide if the procedure will be clean or sterile. Shave biopsy and punch biopsy are performed with a clean technique. Deeper procedures like excisions require a full sterile technique including a sterile tray, gloves, and disposables (e.g., gauze sponges).

Dermatology Standard Equipment Tray

- 70% isopropyl alcohol pads/swabs, surgical marking pen, cotton-tipped applicators and 4"× 4" gauze sponges.
- Sterile pack containing no. 3 scalpel handle, Iris scissors and Adson or Bishop forceps with small teeth.

- Dressing including bandage and sterile petroleum jelly.
- Pathology materials including a biopsy bottle (with 10% formalin for routine biopsies) labeled with the patient's name, identification number, birthdate, and the biopsy site. A pathology requisition slip and a biohazard bag are also needed.

Electrosurgery Devices

The terms electrosurgery and electrocautery are often applied incorrectly. Electrosurgery involves the passage of electrical current through patient's tissue to achieve coagulation or cutting.[8] This method relies on high frequency, alternating electrical current passed from one unheated electrode through human tissue, to a dispersive electrode. Resistance encountered by tissue results in the conversion of electrical energy to heat. When a grounding electrode is utilized, this is *biterminal electrosurgery*. Electrocoagulation and electrosection are examples of biterminal electrosurgery. When a grounding electrode is absent, this is *monoterminal electrosugery*. Electrodessication and electrofulguration are examples of monoterminal electrosurgery.[9] While the specific differences between these methods of electrosurgery are beyond the scope of this text, it is important to note that *electrodessication* is the primary method utilized in the office to destroy tissue in superficial benign or malignant tumors and to control bleeding following biopsies. This is performed using a device with a single electrode tip (monoterminal) and use

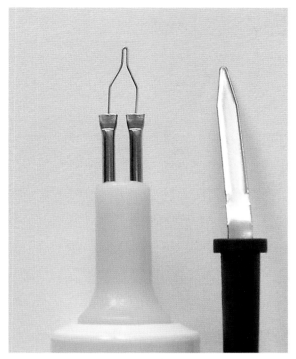

▲ **Figure 7-1.** Electrocautery (left) employs a thermal mechanism; no electric current is transferred to tissue (safe around implanted electric devices). In the battery-operated device shown, the current passes through the wire generating heat. Electrodessication and electrofulgaration (right) are done with a single electrode tip (monoterminal).

of high voltage and low amperage (Figure 7-1) that directly contacts the skin. The electrical spark generated by this device causes desiccation (dehydration) of the treated tissue. Electrodesiccation should not be used in any patient with a pacemaker or implantable cardiac defibrillator as it can interfere with their function. The difference between electrodessication and electrofulguration, is that the former involves direct contact with the tissue and the latter does not.

Electrocautery involves the use of a heated object that is applied to tissue to control bleeding. A classic example would be that of a hot iron. Battery-operated, disposable electrocautery devices are more commonly employed (Figure 7-1) and utilize direct current passed through the device's tip to generate heat which is applied directly to the tissue. Advantages of electrocautery include their portability, effectiveness in a wet field and ability to be safely used in patients with implantable cardiac devices.[8,9]

Care must be taken to properly inform the patient of the risks of any dermatologic procedure. Setting clear expectations is critical. The patient may have unrealistic expectations for scarring (or the expected lack thereof), or the anticipated duration of healing. This leads to frustration on the part of the patient and may lead to a negative impression of an otherwise normal outcome. Discussing these aspects clearly with the patient prior to the biopsy is critical, as is a review of post procedure care. Current guidelines recommend patients undergoing cutaneous surgery continue prescription anticoagulation, as the risks associated with thrombosis outweigh the risks of post-operative bleeding.[10]

After the risks, benefits, and alternatives of the procedure have been discussed, informed consent should be obtained and documented in the chart. Once the equipment is prepared, attention should turn to preparing the patient. Patient care should focus on limiting the physical and emotional discomfort that may be associated with the procedure. The patient should be in a reclined and comfortable position that they can maintain during the entire procedure.

Injectable local anesthetics are commonly used for skin biopsies. 1% lidocaine with epinephrine added at 1:100,000 is generally standard for most dermatologic procedures. Epinephrine decreases bleeding and increases the duration of the anesthetic effect. Onset of anesthesia after injection is very rapid with lidocaine. If epinephrine is used as part of the injection, a decrease in bleeding due to vasoconstriction is expected but may be delayed by 5–15 minute. In sites with a high vascular network, like the scalp, waiting 5–15 minute postinjection will allow for vasoconstriction onset and greatly reduce bleeding during the procedure.

The maximum dose of lidocaine varies with the weight of the patient. The package insert recommendations for adult patients are 4.5 mg/kg (not to exceed 300 mg) for plain lidocaine and 7 mg/kg (not to exceed 500 mg) for lidocaine with epinephrine. Some patients metabolize lidocaine at a much higher rate and will require a larger dose. Other amide anesthetics vary in timing of onset and duration; further discussion of these is beyond the scope of this text.

Lidocaine toxicity may initially present with tinnitus, lightheadedness, circumoral numbness, diplopia, or a metallic taste in the mouth. Nystagmus, slurred speech, localized muscle twitching, or fine tremors may occur with more profound toxicity. Epinephrine can lead to tachycardia and a feeling of uneasiness

A syringe is selected to match the anticipated volume of lidocaine, typically 1–3 mL for shave or punch biopsies and small excisions. Needle sizes of 26, 30, or 33 gauge are preferred for patient comfort but require increased pressure on the plunger and a slower rate of injection. Multiple syringes may be more appropriate for a large site as the needle will dull with repeated injections.

There are several things that can be done to minimize the pain and stinging associated with anesthetic injection.[6]

- 8.4% sodium bicarbonate added to the anesthetic at 10:1 ratio to lower the pH.[6]
- The use of a smaller gauge needle.[11]
- Slowing the rate of injection to reduce injection pressure.
- Vibratory distraction with use of battery-operated vibratory device.[12]
- Pinching/other distraction.[13]

Topical anesthetics have a limited role in skin biopsy procedures due to the limited depth of penetration and the duration of application required to get an adequate effect. Generally, they do not penetrate past the dermal epidermal junction. For younger or more apprehensive patients, a topical anesthetic can be applied to the site prior to injectable anesthesia for procedures extending into the dermis. Options include EMLA (lidocaine 2.5% and prilocaine 2.5%) cream or topical lidocaine. Absorption is slow and takes upward of 20–30 minute for onset and 1 h for maximum effect. The topical anesthesia must be applied to a sufficient thickness with the recommended number of grams as per the package insert and covered with an occlusive dressing. Peak anesthesia is achieved only after 1 hour or longer. If the need for anesthesia is anticipated, the anesthetic could be applied at home 1 hour before the procedure.

SHAVE BIOPSY

A shave technique is appropriate for removal of benign superficial lesions and the biopsy of lesions that extend into the mid to lower dermis. Lesions appropriate for a shave biopsy include the following.

- Seborrheic keratoses and skin tags.
- Suspected squamous and basal cell carcinomas.
- Nevi (when melanoma is not a concern).
- A controlled deep dermal shave biopsy (saucerization biopsy) can be appropriate for a lesion considered for melanoma if adequate depth is obtained. However, consider a punch biopsy for smaller lesions or an excisional biopsy for larger lesions.
- Dermatoses may be sampled with a shave biopsy; however, a punch biopsy is preferred if possible.

In addition to the standard tray, the following items are added.

- Occupational Safety and Health Administration (OSHA) approved safety blade (e.g., DermaBlade or a no. 15 blade on a scalpel handle.
- 20% aluminum chloride solution (e.g., Drysol) for hemostasis with cotton-tipped applicators.

Table 7-2. Shave biopsy procedure.

- Clean the biopsy site with 70% isopropyl alcohol pads.
- Mark the borders of the lesion with the surgical marking pen.
- Inject 1% lidocaine with epinephrine 1:100,000 subcutaneously at the margin of the biopsy site, followed by intradermal infiltration creating a slightly elevated wheal above the plane of the skin.
- For a superficial shave biopsy with a safety blade or scalpel, enter the skin parallel or at an angle of approximately 10^0 to the plane of the skin and at a steeper angle for deeper shave biopsies. For a saucerization biopsy, enter the skin at an angle of approximately 45^0.
- Use a smooth, short, back and forth motion of the blade to allow the cutting edge to slide through the tissue. (Figure 7-2A)
- Diminish the angle to maintain depth within the dermal plane.
- If a safety blade (DermaBlade®) is being used, control the depth of the biopsy by adjusting the curvature of the blade (Figure 7-2B).
- Use pressure with the tip of a cotton applicator to minimize tissue movement during the shave biopsy.
- Exit the biopsy with a more acute angle.
- Place the sample in the previously labeled specimen container.
- Wipe the biopsy site with a gauze pad and press a cotton tipped applicator soaked in aluminum chloride on the site to control bleeding.
- Use electrodessication if the biopsy site continues to bleed. Remember to ask patients about implanted cardiac devices *before* using electrodessication and to rinse any aluminum chloride solution from the field (flammable). *If the patient has a cardiac device use electrocautery if needed.*
- After hemostasis is obtained, cover the biopsy site with sterile petroleum jelly and a bandage with adhesion on all sides sufficient to cover the biopsy site.
- Instruct the patient to remove the bandage in 24 hours and wash the area with soap and water and apply petroleum jelly for 14 days or until the wound is healed.

The steps for a shave biopsy are presented in Table 7-2.[5,6]

Video demonstrations of shave biopsy procedures on simulated skin, pig's feet, and in a clinical setting are available at mhprofessional.com/clinicaldermatology.

PUNCH BIOPSY

A punch biopsy can be used as a diagnostic tool for lesions or dermatoses that extend into the deeper dermis or for removal of small- to medium-sized lesions such as compound/dermal nevi. Punch biopsy tools are typically available in increments of 1 mm and range in size from 1 to 10 mm in diameter. The most commonly used sizes for diagnostic biopsies are 3–4 mm.

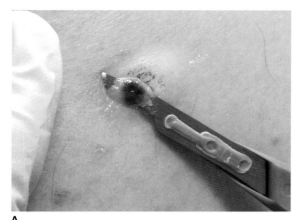

A

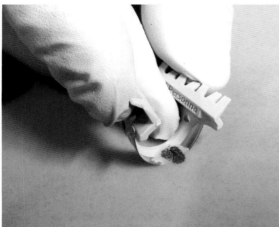

B

⬛ **Figure 7-2** A, B. Shave biopsy. A. Scalpel blade held parallel to plane of the skin cutting through the dermis below the lesion. B. Bendable blade used to scoop under the lesion.

In addition to the standard tray, the following items are needed for a punch biopsy:

- A punch tool of the appropriate size.
- 20% aluminum chloride solution for hemostasis with cotton-tipped applicators.
- A needle holder.
- Suture, typically 4.0 or 5.0 polypropylene, nylon, chromic gut or fast absorbing gut on a P-3 needle.

The steps for a punch biopsy are presented in Table 7-3.[5,6]

Video demonstrations of shave biopsy procedures on simulated skin, pig's feet and in a clinical setting are available at mhprofessional.com/clinicaldermatology.

Table 7-3. Punch biopsy procedure.

- Cleanse, mark and inject the biopsy site with lidocaine as in the shave biopsy procedure in Table 7-2.
- Stretch the skin with the nondominant hand perpendicular to the relaxed tension lines (e.g., wrinkle or Langer's lines) of the skin so that an oval rather than round defect will be created.
- Place the punch tool vertically over the lesion and twist and push down with increasing pressure. (Figure 7-3A)
- When the punch tool reaches the depth of the subcutaneous fat, there will be a decrease in tissue tension and the surrounding tissue will reach the level of the punch bezel.
- Remove the core of tissue by very gently grasping the edge with forceps, taking care to not squeeze or crush the tissue. If the tissue is still attached to the skin, use scissors to snip the base of the specimen. (Figure 7-3B)
- Place the biopsy specimen directly into the appropriate specimen bottle.
- Control bleeding by wiping the biopsy site with a gauze pad and pressing a cotton tipped applicator soaked in aluminum chloride over the site. Electrocautery is generally not necessary.
- Small ≤ 4 mm punch biopsies can be left open to heal by secondary intention.[5]
- If the biopsy is > 4 mm or continues to bleed, the site can be closed with one or several simple interrupted sutures.
- Use 4.0 polypropylene, 4.0 nylon or 4-0 Chromic gut sutures on a P-3 needle for the trunk and extremities. Use 5-0 polypropylene or 5-0 fast absorbing gut sutures on a P-3 needle for the face. The number of sutures is determined by the diameter of the defect. Alternatively, a figure of 8 suture technique can be used.
- Place sterile petroleum jelly over the site and apply a bandage.
- Instruct the patient to come back for suture removal in approximately 7 days for the face and in 14 days for the trunk and extremities.

▼ EXCISION

Excisions are used for biopsy lesions (e.g., when suspecting melanoma) or inflammatory processes (e.g., panniculitis) that are in the deep dermis or subcuticular fat. They also can be used for removal of large benign lesions or malignant tumors such as basal or squamous cell carcinomas. These procedures are performed under sterile technique.

In addition to the standard tray, the following items are needed for an excision:

- Sterile drapes, gloves, and bandages.
- Povidone–iodine solution or chlorhexidine scrub.
- A number 15-scalpel blade and tissue scissors.
- A needle holder.
- 3-0 or 4-0 absorbable sutures (e.g., Vicryl, Monocryl) on a PS-2 or P-3 needle and non-absorbable 4-0 or 5-0

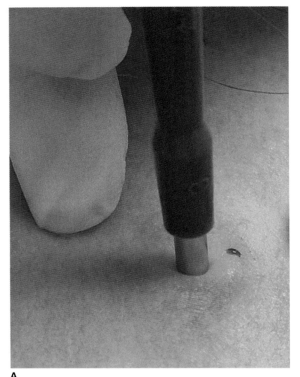

A

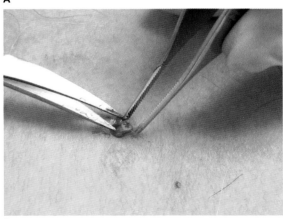

B

▲ **Figure 7-3** A, B. Punch biopsy. A, Punch biopsy tool held perpendicular to the skin and pressed halfway into the dermis. B. Tissue sample is gently grasped with forceps and the subcutaneous tissue is cut with scissors. An assistant may control bleeding with a cotton-tipped applicator.

sutures (e.g., Prolene) on a P-3 needle. Alternative suture and needle sizes may be needed depending on the location and degree of wound tension (Table 7-4).

The steps for an excision are presented in Table 7-5.[14–16]

Table 7-4. Selection of suture size and timing of suture removal.

Location	Deep absorbable sutures (e.g., Vicryl, Monocryl)	Non-absorbable sutures for closure of Epidermis (e.g., Prolene, nylon)	Timing of suture removal in days*
Face and Neck	5.0 to 6.0	5.0 to 6.0	Face-5-7 Neck-7-10
Back, Scalp	3.0 to 4.0	3.0 to 4.0	14–21
Trunk and Extremities	4.0	4.0	10–14

*Longer duration decreases risk of dehiscence, but may increase scarring.

Video demonstrations of suturing techniques and excisions on simulated skin, pig's feet, and in a clinical setting are available at mhprofessional.com/clinicaldermatology.

DESTRUCTIVE TECHNIQUES

Cryotherapy

Cryotherapy is a common office procedure and is the mainstay for the treatment of many benign and precancerous lesions. Liquid nitrogen, which has a boiling point of −196°C (−321°F) is the coldest and most commonly used cryogen. A 30 s spray of liquid nitrogen will result in tissue temperatures of −25°C to −50°C (−13°F to −58°F). Most benign lesions will be destroyed at a tissue temperature of −20°C to 30°C.[17]

The use of cryosurgical devices (e.g., CRY-AC, CryoPro, FrigiSpray) with a spray tip and fingertip trigger is a safe and accurate way to use liquid nitrogen. Lesions commonly treated with cryotherapy include actinic keratosis, viral warts (human papillomavirus and molluscum contagiosum), seborrheic keratosis, and skin tags.

The patient should be informed that cryotherapy is painful during and sometimes for several minutes after the procedure. Erythema, bullae, and sometimes hemorrhagic bullae may develop. Hypo- and/or hyperpigmentation may also occur in darker-skinned individuals. Scarring can occur if the freezing extends into the dermis.

Procedure

- Position the nozzle of the spray tip 1–1.5 cm from the lesion to be treated.
- Spray the lesion until a 2 mm rim of frost develops around the lesion and then continue spraying for 5–30 seconds depending on the thickness, diameter, and location of the lesions (Figure 7-5). For larger lesions

Table 7-5. Excision procedure.

- Mark the planned surgical margins using a surgical marking pen. The width of the fusiform excision should include 2 mm margins for benign lesions and 4–6 mm for basal or squamous cell carcinomas. The length of the excision should be three times greater than the width and the angle at the corner of the excision should be 30° or less. The long axis of the excision should be along the relaxed skin tension lines or at a cosmetic junction. (Figure 7-4).
- Cleanse the skin with 70% isopropyl alcohol pads.
- Inject 1% lidocaine with epinephrine 1:100,000 subcutaneously around the margin of the planned excision, carefully placing the needle into the edge of area that has already been anesthetized. Then inject the lidocaine intradermally until there is a slight swelling of the tissue.
- Cleanse the skin with povidone-iodine solution and allow to dry or scrub the surgical site with chlorhexidine (avoid using near the eyes/ears) and place sterile drapes around the surgical site.
- Apply tension to the surgical site with the surgeon (non-dominant hand) and assistant pulling the skin in opposite directions.
- To begin the excision, insert the tip of the scalpel blade at the distal apex of the incision perpendicular and at 90° angle to the plane of the skin.
- Lower the blade to a 45° angle and use the belly of the blade to cut the tissue rather than the tip, as the belly of the blade is the sharpest part of the blade.
- Continue with increased pressure and a smooth steady motion perpendicular to the surface of the skin to the depth of the subcutaneous fat. At that point the tissue relaxes around the excision. It may take two passes to extend through the dermis depending on the site.
- As the proximal apex of the excision is reached, increase the angle of the blade back to a 90° to generate a clean excision with the tip of the blade.
- Repeat the previous 4 steps on the other side of the excision.
- Lift the skin specimen with forceps and separate the tissue specimen from the base of the excision at the level of the subcutaneous fat with the scalpel blade held parallel to the skin or with iris scissors. The thickness of the specimen should be uniform.
- Place the sample in the previously labeled specimen container.
- Use electrosurgery or electrocautery to achieve hemostasis. Limit thermal damage to the epidermis. Larger caliber arterioles or named vessels would benefit from ligature with braided absorbable suture (i.e., 4/5-0 Vicryl) in a figure-of-eight technique to prevent hematoma.
- Narrowly undermine (0.5 to 1.0 cm) the skin at the level of the subcutaneous fat with rounded tip Mayo, Metzenbaum curved iris or Gradle scissors.
- Use absorbable sutures placed in buried vertical mattress fashion to approximate the deep dermis. Place each suture deep to superficial on one wound edge and superficial to deep on the other wound edge, creating a "heart-shaped" path to improve eversion. This technique buries the knot deep in the wound. Sutures can be placed from either the center to each apex for wounds of low tension ("rule of halves" technique), or from the apex to the center for high tension wounds.
- Close the epidermis with either interrupted sutures or a running suture. Wound margins should be carefully approximated without tension to achieve a satisfactory cosmetic result.
- Place sterile petroleum jelly is placed over the excision site and cover with an adhesive bandage.

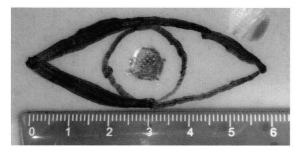

▲ **Figure 7-4.** Elliptical excision. The margins of the excision are marked (inner inked circle) and an ellipse is drawn with a 3:1 length to width ratio and less than 30 degree terminal angles.

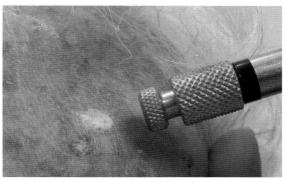

▲ **Figure 7-5.** Cryotherapy. The tip of the cryosurgical unit is held 1 cm from an actinic keratosis creating a 2 mm freeze margin.

this can be done in spiral or paintbrush pattern. Approximate freeze times vary.

- Actinic keratosis: 5–20 seconds freeze cycle, depending on the location and size of the lesion. [18]
- Seborrheic keratosis: 5–10 seconds for thin, flat lesions.[17]
- Warts: 10 seconds. Plantar warts may require a second freeze cycle.[19]
- Skin tags: 5 seconds.[17]
- Cover the eyes, nostrils, and external auditory canal with gauze or cotton, if cryosurgery is done near those sites. Care should also be taken not to deeply freeze the skin near the digital nerves on the medial and lateral aspects of the fingers and toes.

Video demonstrations of cryotherapy are available at mhprofessional.com/clinicaldermatology.

Curettage and Electrodesiccation

Curettage and electrodesiccation is a commonly used procedure for the treatment of seborrheic keratosis, certain types of viral warts, pyogenic granulomas, as well as low risk basal and squamous cell carcinomas.[20,21] Electrodesiccation without cautery can be used on small skin tags and cherry angiomas. *Electrodesiccation should not be used on any patient with an implantable cardiac device.* If needed, a battery operated, disposable heat cautery device could be used in these patients.

The patients should be informed of the risks of the procedure that include bleeding, infection, scars, and hyper- or hypopigmentation.

Equipment needed in addition to the standard tray is as follows:

- Fox round or oval curette, sizes 3–5 mm are most commonly used.
- Monoterminal electrodesiccation unit.

The steps for curettage and electrodesiccation are presented in Table 7-6.[22]

Wound Care and Follow-Up

Wound care and follow-up are dictated by the type of procedure that was performed. Many patients have the false notion that air drying the wound will promote a more rapid healing response. In general, a clean wound will heal more rapidly and with less scarring if a good moisture barrier is maintained throughout the healing process. A firm pressure dressing is helpful for any full thickness procedure and should be left in place for 24–48 hour.

SURGICAL COMPLICATIONS

Bleeding

Excessive bleeding during a procedure is disconcerting both to the clinician and the patient. Firm application

Table 7-6. Curettage and electrodesiccation procedure.

- Cleanse and anesthetize the skin as for shave and punch biopsies.
- Let the alcohol dry completely before proceeding to prevent possible fire.
- Hold the curette in the dominant hand at a 45° angle and with firm pressure scrape the curette across the lesion with one or more smooth strokes. The non-dominant hand can be used to provide counter traction. (Figure 7-6 A,B)
- Repeat the procedure by scraping perpendicular to the original direction of curettage until a firm base is obtained.
- Electrodesiccate the treated area at the lowest setting needed using care not to significantly increase the depth or width of the field.
- Use the side of the electrode rather than the tip in order to maintain greater control of the depth.
- Following electrodessication, curette the tumor base again until a firm base is obtained. This will extend the wound margin by approximately 1 mm.
- For low risk basal and squamous cell carcinomas, repeat with 3 rounds of curettage followed by electrodessication.
- Place sterile petroleum jelly over the site and cover the site with an adhesive bandage.
- The site should be kept moist with petroleum jelly and covered until re-epithelialized.

of pressure for several minutes often controls bleeding. Identification of the bleeding vessel and compression while performing cautery is usually very effective. An assistant who can hold pressure and wick away blood that is obscuring the surgical field is critical in this process.

A second concern is postprocedure bleeding. As the vasoconstriction due to epinephrine wears off, bleeding may occur minutes or hours later. Even a small amount of blood may cause anxiety in a patient. The patient should be advised of this possibility and given clear instructions to apply firm constant pressure for a minimum of 15 minute. If the bleeding does not stop after this process, medical care should be sought either with the clinician who performed the procedure or at an urgent care facility. The development of a hematoma under a closed wound, if large and firm warrants evacuation, cautery, and resuturing of the wound. Antibiotics should be strongly considered in prevention of the infection.

Cardiac Devices

Part of patient screening should include questions regarding the presence of a pacemaker or implantable cardiac defibrillator. The use of monopolar electrodessication has a risk for triggering or damaging these devices. Electrocautery (heat cautery) or bipolar cautery should be used instead.

Infection

In general, cutaneous surgery performed in an outpatient setting carries a low risk of infection.[23,24] Infection is more

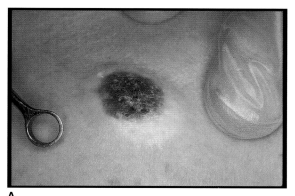

A

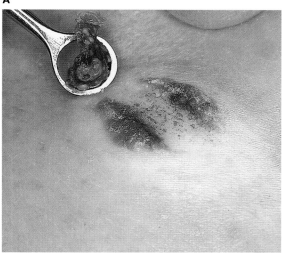

B

⏶ **Figure 7-6.** A, B. Curettage. A. Wheal produced by lidocaine with epinephrine throughout and adjacent to a seborrheic keratosis. B. A curette is stroked across the lesion with firm pressure.

likely in wounds that have been exposed to the environment, or in certain body areas such as distal extremities, areas near body orifices and the ear.

Depending on the wound location and the exposure risk, topical or oral antibiotics individually or in combination may be appropriate. When to use prophylaxis and what type of prophylaxis to use is often a topic of debate among experts and its specific application is beyond the scope of this text.

Importantly, some non prescription topical antibiotic ointments (e.g., bacitracin, neosporin) have a significant risk of allergic contact dermatitis. Whenever a wound becomes more inflamed with the use of a topical antibiotic, an allergic contact dermatitis must be considered. Mupirocin ointment is less likely to cause allergic contact dermatitis.

Wound Dehiscence

Separation of the wound can occur if excessive tension is placed on a recently sutured wound or the strength of the healing scar is not adequate at the time of suture removal. Excisions at sites with a poor vascular supply, such as the leg, will often require a prolonged period of healing. Infection can also lead to an increase in wound pressure and loss of wound integrity. Dehisced wounds can be resutured several days following a closure if the wound is cleaned and any risk for infection is addressed. The reclosed wound may require a drain if infection is present or anticipated. Resuturing should not be performed if an abscess is present. If the dehiscence occurs more than 24 hour after the excision, the re-epithelialized tissue from the center of the wound may need to be removed. A dehisced wound can also be re-excised and sutured or left to heal with secondary intention, but this may result in a significant scar.

REFERENCES

1. Alguire PC, Mathes BM. Skin biopsy techniques for the internist. *J Gen Intern Med.* 1998;13(1):46–54.
2. Elston DM, Stratman EJ, Miller SJ. Skin biopsy: Biopsy issues in specific diseases. *J Am Acad Dermatol.* 2016; (1):1–16. Erratum in: *J Am Acad Dermatol.* 2016 Oct;75(4):854.
3. Sleiman R, Kurban M, Abbas O. Maximizing diagnostic outcomes of skin biopsy specimens. *Int J Dermatol.* 2013; 52(1):72–78.
4. Sina B, Kao G F, Deng A C, Gaspari A. Skin biopsy for inflammatory and common neoplastic skin diseases: optimum time, best location and preferred techniques. A critical review. *J Cutan Pathol.* 2009;36(5):505–510.
5. Pickett H. Shave and punch biopsy for skin lesions. *Am Fam Physician* 2011;84(9):995–1002.
6. Nischal U, Nischal Kc U, Khopkar. Techniques of skin biopsy and practical considerations. *J Cutaneous Aesthet Surg.* 2008;1(2):107–111.
7. Bichakjian CK, Halpern AC, Johnson TM, et al. Guidelines of care for the management of primary cutaneous melanoma. *J Am Acad Dermatol.* 2011;65(5):1032–1047.
8. Frank M, Benedetto AV, Electrosurgery and Hemostasis. In Kantor J, *Dermatologic Surgery.* New York, NY: McGraw-Hill; 2018
9. Eisen D, Dermatologic Surgery. In Alikhan A, Hocker T, *Review of Dermatology.* New York, NY: Elsevier.
10. Smith C, Srivastava D, Nijhawan RI. Optimizing patient safety in dermatologic surgery. *Dermatol Clin.* 2019;37(3):319–328.
11. Zelickson BR, Goldberg LH, Rubenzik MK, Wu WJ. Finer needles reduce pain associated with injection of local anesthetic using a minimal insertion injection technique. *Dermatol Surg.* 2018;44(2):204–208.
12. Kazi R, Govas P, Slaugenhaupt RM, Carroll BT. Differential analgesia from vibratory stimulation during local injection of anesthetic: A randomized clinical trial. *Dermatol Surg.* 2020;46(10):1286–1293.
13. Fosko SW, Gibney MD, Harrison B. Repetitive pinching of the skin during lidocaine infiltration reduces patient discomfort. *J Am Acad Dermatol.* 1998; 39(1):74–78.
14. Zuber T J. Fusiform excision. *Am Fam Physician.* 2003;67(7):1539–1544, 1547.

15. Miller CJ, Antunes MB, Sobanko JF. Surgical technique for optimal outcomes: Part I. Cutting tissue: incising, excising, and undermining. *J Am Acad Dermatol.* 2015;72(3):377–387.

16. Miller CJ, Antunes MB, Sobanko JF. Surgical technique for optimal outcomes: Part II. Repairing tissue: suturing. *J Am Acad Dermatol.* 2015;72(3):389–402.

17. Andrews M D. Cryosurgery for common skin conditions. *Am Fam Physician.* 2004;69(10):2365–2372.

18. Thai K, Fergin P, Freeman M, et al. A prospective study of the use of cryosurgery for the treatment of actinic keratoses. *Int J Dermatol.* 2004;43(9):687–692.

19. Connolly M, Bazmi K, O M. Cryotherapy of viral warts: a sustained 10-s freeze is more effective than the traditional method. *Br J Dermatol.* 2001;145(4):554–557.

20. Work Group; Invited Reviewers, Kim JYS, Kozlow JH, Mittal B, Moyer J, Olencki T, Rodgers P. Guidelines of care for the management of basal cell carcinoma. *J Am Acad Dermatol.* 2018;78(3):540–559.

21. Work Group; Invited Reviewers, Kim JYS, Kozlow JH, Mittal B, Moyer J, Olenecki T, Rodgers P. Guidelines of care for the management of cutaneous squamous cell carcinoma. *J Am Acad Dermatol.* 2018;78(3):560–578.

22. Goldman G. The current status of curettage and electrodesiccation. *Dermatol Clin.* 2002;20(3):569–578.

23. Liu A, Lawrence N. Incidence of infection after Mohs micrographic and dermatologic surgery before and after implementation of new sterilization guidelines. *J Am Acad Dermatol.* 2014;70(6):1088–1091.

24. Futoryan T, Grande D. Postoperative wound infection rates in dermatologic surgery. *Dermatol Surg.* 1995 J;21(6):509–514.

Dermatitis

Allison Smith
Sheilagh Maguiness
Sara Hylwa

INTRODUCTION TO CHAPTER

Dermatitis (eczema) refers to a heterogeneous group of inflammatory skin disorders that share similarities in clinical appearance and histopathologic findings but may have very different etiologies. It is a common disorder, affecting 1 in 5 people at some point in life. Dermatitis may be acute, subacute, or chronic. In its acute stage, dermatitis is marked by erythema, edema, and vesicles, while chronic dermatitis is characterized by lichenification, fissures, and scaling. Dermatitis can further be delineated as either endogenous (internal factors) or exogenous (external factors). Pruritus is a common symptom of all types of dermatitis.

CONTACT DERMATITIS

Contact dermatitis is an exogenous form of dermatitis divided into two major categories: Irritant contact dermatitis and allergic contact dermatitis (Table 8-1). Irritant contact dermatitis is more common (80% of cases) than allergic contact dermatitis (20%); however, these reactions are not mutually exclusive and may occur simultaneously in a particular patient. For example, contact allergy to a glove chemical may complicate irritant hand dermatitis due to irritating soaps used for hand washing. Furthermore, one product may act as both an irritant and allergen; a patient may have an allergic reaction to a preservative in a liquid soap as well as having an irritant reaction to a detergent in the soap. Common irritants include water, soap, industrial cleansers, and frictional forces; additional irritants are listed in Table 8-2. Common allergens are listed in Table 8-3.

IRRITANT CONTACT DERMATITIS

Introduction

Key points for irritant contact dermatitis

- ✓ Irritant contact dermatitis is the more common form of contact dermatitis; it causes 80% of occupational contact dermatitis.
- ✓ It is a non-immunologic response to chemicals or physical agent that causes direct damage to keratinocytes and disrupts the normal epidermal barrier, most commonly on the hands and forearms.
- ✓ Exposure to water, soaps, acids, alkalis, and friction are common causes.
- ✓ Avoidance of the irritant and use of moisturizers are important.

Table 8-1. Comparison of irritant contact dermatitis and allergic contact dermatitis.

	Irritant contact dermatitis	Allergic contact dermatitis.
Onset	Strong irritants – Within minutes. Weak irritants – Days to weeks.	Within 24–96 hours in sensitized individuals.
Resolution	May improve within days after exposure, some cases may persist.	Improves after 3-6 weeks away from exposure.
Mechanism	Nonimmune, sensitization not required; epidermal barrier disruption, epidermal cellular damage, pro-inflammatory mediators released from keratinocytes.	Immune-mediated, sensitization required. Antigen activated primed T-cells; sensitization phase typically takes 10-14 days but can occur immediately or after years.
Agent	Concentration dependent.	Not concentration dependent.
Diagnosis	Clinical.	Patch testing.

Table 8-2. Examples of common skin irritants and their sources.

Irritant	Examples of common sources
Acids	Organic acids (e.g., chromic, formic, hydrochloric, hydrofluoric, nitric, oxalic, sulfuric).
Alcohols	Antiseptics, waterless hand cleansers.
Alkalis	Organic alkalis (e.g., calcium oxide and potassium and sodium hydroxide).
Body fluids	Urine, feces, saliva.
Concrete	Wet cement.
Detergents	Hand soap, shampoo, dish detergents.
Fiberglass	Insulation.
Food	Fruit acids, meat enzymes, proteins, vinegar.
Metal salts	Metal working, pulp, steel, and paper manufacturing.
Physical agents	Temperature extremes, friction, humidity.
Plastic resins	Unpolymerized monomers in plastics industries.
Solvents	Turpentine, gasoline, kerosene, benzene.

Irritant contact dermatitis is the more common form of contact dermatitis. It is estimated that irritant contact dermatitis represents approximately 80% of occupational contact dermatitis. It may present as either acute or chronic dermatitis, with chronic cases being the most common. It affects any area of the body although is seen most often on the hands (particularly finger webs) and face.[1] Occupations at high risk include those involving repeated exposure to water and/or soap such as healthcare workers, janitorial services, and food industry employees or those involving exposure to solvents such as machinists.[2] Females, infants, the elderly, and those with atopic tendencies are also at increased risk for irritant contact dermatitis.

Pathogenesis

Irritant contact dermatitis is a non-immunologic response to chemicals or a physical agents that causes direct damage to keratinocytes and disrupts the normal epidermal barrier faster than its ability to repair itself. The development of irritant contact dermatitis does not require prior sensitization. Severity increases with duration, intensity, amount, and concentration of the irritant.[3] Skin susceptibility also plays a factor, as damaged skin lacks the proper oils and moisture, thus allowing irritants to penetrate more deeply and cause further damage. Any condition that impairs skin barrier function, such as atopic dermatitis or asteatotic dermatitis/dry skin is a risk factor for developing irritant contact dermatitis.

Clinical Presentation

History

History taking should include information regarding patient's occupation, hobbies, and personal care products. Timing of onset is helpful to distinguish acute versus chronic irritant contact dermatitis. Acute irritant contact dermatitis may present with immediate pain, burning, and pruritus and typically occur minutes to hours after exposure. This is more typical with strong irritants, such as acids and alkalis or frictional exposure.[1] Chronic irritant contact dermatitis is more common and typically develops weeks after exposure to weak irritants, such as hand soap. It may affect any individual, given sufficient exposure to irritants, but those with a history of atopic dermatitis are at higher risk because of disruption of the normal epidermal barrier. Pruritus, pain, and burning are common symptoms in this and all types of contact dermatitis.

Physical Examination

Acute irritant contact dermatitis is often well demarcated with a glazed appearance, along with erythema, swelling, blistering, and scaling. Subacute reactions exhibit crusting, scale, and hyperpigmentation. Chronic irritant contact dermatitis is often lichenified with fissures and scaling. Irritant reactions are usually confined to the site of contact

Table 8-3. Common allergens.

Allergen	Sources of allergen
Urushiol	Anacardiaceae family of plants: Poison ivy, poison oak, poison sumac, cashew nut, mango rind, Indian marking nut, Chinese lacquer tree, Japanese wax tree.
Nickel	Metal. Commonly found in metal / jewelry (white gold, 14-carat gold, chrome, bronze, brass, silvery metals), coins, keys, tools, clothing fasteners (buttons/snaps/zippers), personal care products (clippers, eyelash curlers, razors), musical instruments, medical implants. Dimethylglyoxime test detects the presence of nickel in metal objects.
Methylisothiazolinone and Methylchloroisothiazolinone (MCI/MI)	Preservative. Used in personal care products (soaps, shampoos, cosmetics, wet wipes, personal hygiene products, bath and baby products, hair coloring agents, and hair care products), toiletries, household cleaning products (dish soap, stain removers, detergents, fabric softeners, cleansers), paint, and household / craft glue including school glue. Sodium bisulfite can inactivate MCI/MI in paint for occupational problems.
Fragrance	Fragrances are widely used to add flavor or scent to a product. They may come from natural (animals or plants) or synthetic sources. Essential oils and botanicals are frequent sources of fragrances in products. Most common product to cause ACD from cosmetics. *Unscented or fragrance-free* products are not necessarily safe as they may also contain fragrance materials.
Formaldehyde	Preservative. In many personal care, household, certain vaccines, industrial products, plywood glue, leather glues, plastics, coatings, fiber board, nail polish, and Brazilian-style keratin hair straighteners. Fixative used in embalming. May be an irritant. Can be used as a textile finisher; found in clothing marketed as "permanent press", "wash and wear", "wrinkle free". Formaldehyde containing foods: aspartame (metabolized to formic acid), coffee (especially instant), smoked ham, cod, caviar; also in cigarette smoke.
Neomycin	Topical antibiotic. Most frequent antibiotic causing contact sensitivity. Found in triple antibiotic ointments and Neosporin. Can be found also in eye drops, ear drops, impregnated into some bandages, and as a preservative in some vaccines. Co-reactivity with bacitracin. Cross-reacts with gentamicin.
Bacitracin	Topical antibiotic. Found in triple antibiotic ointments, Neosporin, and Polysporin. Common co-sensitization with neomycin.
Paraphenylendiamine	Dye. Found in almost all permanent and semi-permanent hair dyes, black henna (not natural henna), and black rubber products (black rubber hoses, tires, tool grips). Can cross-react with other para-amino compounds, such as benzocaine anesthetics, PABA sunscreen, sulfa, aminobenzene, IPPD, azo textile dyes, sulfa medications (thiazide diuretics, sulfonylurea antidiabetics, sulfa containing antibiotics).
Cobalt	Metal. Commonly found in metal alloys used to make tools, keys, magnets, jewelry (darker silver), orthopedic and dental implants, implanted cardiac devices. Also can be used as a dye (blue green paint, blue tattoos, hair dyes, ceramic dyes). Part of vitamin B12. Added to cement to bind to chromate and decrease its sensitivity. Can be used in plastics and leather manufacturing. Co-sensitization with nickel. Cobalt spot test with disodium-1-nitroso-2-naphthol-3,6-disulfonate is available (turns orange-red).
Rubber Accelerators (e.g., carbamates, thiurams, diphenylguanidine, dialkyl thioureas)	Different from latex allergy (a Type-1 hypersensitivity reaction). Rubber accelerators are used in the manufacturing of many rubber products to speed up the liquid-to-solid rubber transformation, and then they get impregnated in the final rubber product. All rubber products can be suspect (gloves (including nitrile and neoprene), elastic, neoprene, shoes.

ACD, allergic contact dermatitis; IPPD, isopropyl-phenyl-phenylenediamine; PABA, para-aminobenzoic acid.

with the irritant. The most common locations are hands, forearms, eyelids, and face (Figures 8-1, 8-2, 8-3).

▶ Laboratory Findings

Skin biopsies will show dermatitis but cannot specify if it is an irritant contact dermatitis: they are helpful primarily to rule out non-eczematous conditions such as psoriasis. Skin scrapings for fungal elements or a scabies preparation will also rule out those conditions.

Diagnosis

Irritant contact dermatitis is a diagnosis of exclusion. A detailed history is useful in making the correct diagnosis. The typical patient presents with pruritic or painful dermatitis beginning approximately three months after low-grade irritant exposure (e.g., hand dermatitis in a nursing student) or shortly after exposure to a strong irritant or frictional exposure.

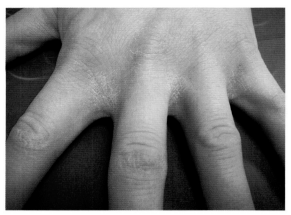

▲ **Figure 8-1.** Irritant contact dermatitis in finger webs from dish detergent. Subtle erythema and scale in the finger webs.

▷ Differential Diagnosis

✓ Allergic contact dermatitis: This may appear identical to irritant contact dermatitis. Allergic contact dermatitis is diagnosed by patch testing.

✓ Atopic dermatitis: Individuals with atopic dermatitis usually have a personal or family history of atopic dermatitis (childhood eczema), allergic rhinitis, or asthma.

✓ Photodermatitis: Occurs in sun-exposed areas. May coincide with or exacerbate irritant contact dermatitis.

✓ Plaque psoriasis and palmoplantar psoriasis

✓ Cutaneous fungal infections: Tinea infections present with annular plaques with a scaly border. Fungal hyphae causing tinea (corporis, manus, cruris, pedis) can be visualized on a potassium hydroxide (KOH) preparation from skin scrapings.

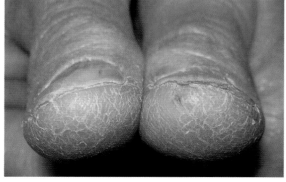

▲ **Figure 8-2.** Irritant contact dermatitis on fingertips from frequent hand washing with high detergent soap. Scale and fissures

✓ Other eczematous skin conditions: Nummular dermatitis, dyshidrotic eczema, lichen simplex chronicus.

✓ Uncommon conditions: Cutaneous T-cell lymphoma (mycosis fungoides).

Management

The management of irritant contact dermatitis is two-fold:

• Identification and removal of the irritant(s) (Table 8-2)

• Repair of the normal skin barrier

Once the causative irritant has been identified, patient education on avoidance is important. Vinyl gloves should be worn as a barrier to unavoidable irritant exposures such as dish soap and juice from citrus fruits. For repair of the skin barrier, emollients should be used 2–3 times a day or up to 20 times a day for the hands. Each water exposure should be immediately followed by application of an emollient to prevent dehydration of the skin. Cotton gloves over a heavy emollient such as petroleum jelly overnight may also be helpful.[4] Mild, unscented soaps, and moisturizers are recommended, as listed in Table 8-4. For cracks and

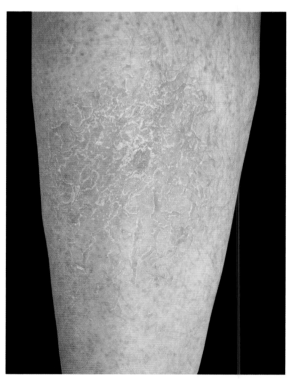

▲ **Figure 8-3.** Chronic irritant contact dermatitis on legs from long, hot showers. Eczema craquelê (cracked porcelain) pattern with erythema, scale and fine fissures on the lower leg.

Table 8-4. Selected gentle moisturizers and cleansers.

Moisturizers

- Petroleum jelly
- Aquaphor Healing Ointment
- Vanicream Skin Cream
- Eucerin Original Moisturizer Cream and Lotion
- Cetaphil Moisturizing Cream and Lotion
- CeraVe Cream and Lotion

Cleansers

- Cetaphil Gentle Skin Cleanser
- Dove Body Wash and Bar Soap (unscented / sensitive skin)
- CereVe Cleanser
- Vanicream Bar Soap
- Free and Clear Liquid Cleanser

fissures, application of superglue as a sealant may also be helpful. Mid-potency topical corticosteroid ointments or creams may be used twice a day as needed to treat symptoms as adjunctive therapy to frequent moisturization (Table 8-5). Oral antihistamines can also be used to control pruritus but will not affect the dermatitis. The sedating side effects of first generation antihistamines may be of benefit to aid in sleep.

Clinical Course and Prognosis

Clinical course in irritant contact dermatitis largely depends on the acuity and the ability to avoid the irritant in the future. Acute reactions typically peak minutes to hours following exposure and then begin to improve. Chronic reactions, as the name implies, may persist much longer.[3] Chronic dermatitis can greatly affect quality of life, particularly when involving the hands. It may lead to chronic pain and discomfort, avoidance of certain activities, and may require a change in occupation.

Indications for Consultation

Severe or persistent disease that does not respond to treatment.

Patient Information Sites

National Eczema Association www.nationaleczema.org/living-with-eczema/hand-eczema

▼ ALLERGIC CONTACT DERMATITIS

Introduction

Key points for allergic contact dermatitis

✓ Allergic contact dermatitis is a cell-mediated, delayed Type IV hypersensitivity reaction, resulting from contact with a specific allergen in a sensitized individual.

✓ It presents with pruritic vesicles or scaly lichenified plaques that correspond to the area of contact with the allergen.

✓ Mid- to high-potency topical corticosteroids (applied twice a day) are usually sufficient for treatment of the dermatitis.

✓ The allergen should be identified by history or patch testing and avoided indefinitely.

Allergic contact dermatitis is equally prevalent and incident across all age groups, although the causative allergen tends to differ from childhood to adulthood and is largely based on what allergens one is exposed to.[5] There is an increased prevalence in female over male patients, likely attributed to increased exposure to common allergens. The most common allergen causing allergic contact dermatitis in the United States is urushiol, the allergen in poison ivy, oak, and sumac. Of individuals patch tested by specialists in North America, the most common allergens are found in Table 8-3.

Table 8-5. Selected topical steroids for treatment of dermatitis.

1	Super potent	Clobetasol propionate	0.05% cream, gel ointment, solution.
2	High potency	Fluocinonide	0.05% cream, gel ointment, solution.
3,4,5	Mid potency	Triamcinolone acetonide	0.1% cream, ointment 0.025% ointment.
		Fluocinolone acetonide	0.025% cream, ointment. 0.01% solution.
6	Low potency	Fluocinolone acetonide	0.01 % oil.
		Desonide	0.05% cream, ointment.
7	Least potent	Hydrocortisone acetate	1% and 2.5% cream, ointment.

Pathogenesis

Allergic contact dermatitis is a cell-mediated, delayed Type IV hypersensitivity reaction, resulting from contact with a specific allergen to which a patient has developed a specific sensitivity. There are two main steps in developing allergic contact dermatitis: induction and elicitation. During the *induction* phase, also known as sensitization, an allergen penetrates the epidermis and is processed by antigen-presenting cells (Langerhans cells, dendritic cells, and macrophages). It is then presented on the cell surface as a human leukocyte antigen molecule to naïve T lymphocytes within regional lymph nodes. These T-lymphocytes differentiate into memory (effector) T-cells and undergo clonal expansion.[5] This initial phase is often asymptomatic and generally takes between 10 and 14 days. In the *elicitation* phase, re-exposure to the allergen causes activation of circulating effector T lymphocytes and aggregation within the skin containing the antigen. This results in a cytokine production cascade causing an inflammatory response.[7] Clinical manifestations usually occur within hours to days after allergen exposure. After removal of the allergen, allergic contact dermatitis typically persists for up to 3 weeks.

Clinical Presentation

Chief complaint is typically an intensely pruritic rash at the site of contact with the allergen. Pruritus should always be present for allergic contact dermatitis. As with irritant contact dermatitis, a detailed history regarding potential exposures is important. Questions regarding occupation, hobbies, and personal care products are helpful. Additionally, information regarding exacerbating or alleviating factors can help identify allergens (e.g., sun exposure, improvement when away from work, etc.).

▶ Physical Examination

The key physical exam features of allergic contact dermatitis are pruritic vesicles or scaly lichenified plaques that correspond to the area of contact with the allergen. The clinical presentation will vary depending on the acuity and severity of the reaction. The acute phase is typically confined to the area of direct exposure. This will classically present as papules or vesicles on an erythematous and edematous base (Figure 8-4 and 8-5). Recurrent contact with a causative allergen may lead to chronic disease and extend beyond the boundaries of direct contact.[5] Chronic allergic contact dermatitis manifests with xerosis, fissuring, and lichenified eczematous plaques.

Location of the reaction may provide clues to the causative allergen, for example, nickel allergy usually results in dermatitis at the earlobes, neck, and wrists if associated with jewelry, near the umbilicus if associated with belt buckles, or the thighs if associated with keys in one's pocket (Figure 8-6). Dermatitis in unexpected sites, especially the eyelids and face, may result from contact to allergens on the hands e.g. (fingernail polish) or scalp e.g. (hair products). Table 8-6 lists common allergens at selected body sites.

▶ Laboratory Findings

Skin biopsies are usually not diagnostic and are only helpful to rule out non-eczematous conditions such as psoriasis. Skin scrapings for fungal elements or a scabies preparation will rule out those conditions.

Diagnosis

History and physical examination are helpful in diagnosis of allergic contact dermatitis; however, the gold standard is patch testing. The allergen responsible for allergic contact dermatitis may be identified by patch testing with purified

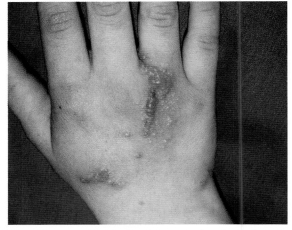

Figure 8-4. Acute allergic contact dermatitis from poison ivy on hand. Linear streaks of erythema and vesicles at sites of direct contact with urushiol.

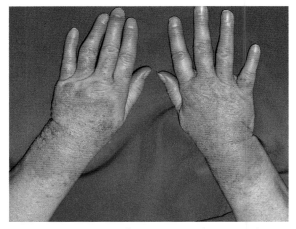

Figure 8-5. Acute allergic contact dermatitis due to latex in gloves. Erythematous, edematous, scaly, crusted plaques on the hands and wrists.

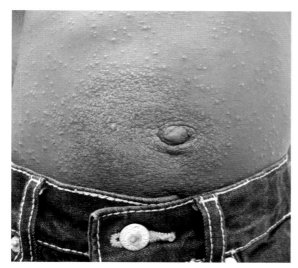

Figure 8-6. Allergic contact dermatitis due to nickel in metal button. Papules coalescing into a plaque around the umbilicus.

or specially prepared allergens. See Chapter 4 for details of patch testing. Patch testing typically occurs over 5–7 days. On the first day, allergens are applied to the upper back and taped in place. After 24–48 h, the patches are removed (Figure 8-7) and locations marked. The patch sites are read by the clinician at 2 days and 5–7 days. Allergic reactions manifest as palpable, pink-red, edematous, and/or vesicular-bullous plaques at the patch site.

After the identification of the allergen by patch testing, clinical relevance is determined by evaluating potential exposures to the allergen (identifying the ingredient in the patient's products used in the location of dermatitis). If the dermatitis clears after avoidance of the allergen, this is good evidence that the allergic reaction is clinically relevant. Improvement of allergic contact dermatitis typically requires at least 3 weeks and often up to 2 months of allergen avoidance.

Differential Diagnosis

✓ Irritant contact dermatitis: This may appear identical to allergic contact dermatitis.

✓ Atopic dermatitis: Individuals with atopic dermatitis usually have a personal or family history of atopic dermatitis (childhood eczema), allergic rhinitis, or asthma.

✓ Cutaneous fungal infections: Tinea infections usually present with annular plaques with a scaly border. Fungal hyphae can be visualized on a potassium hydroxide (KOH) preparation from skin scrapings.

✓ Other eczematous skin conditions: Nummular dermatitis, dyshidrotic eczema, lichen simplex chronicus.

✓ Uncommon conditions: Cutaneous T-cell lymphoma, dermatitis herpetiformis.

Table 8-6. Common skin allergens at selected body sites.

Body Site	Common Sources and Responsible Allergens
All Locations	Topical preparations (bacitracin, neomycin, corticosteroids, preservatives, emulsifiers). Personal care products (preservatives, emulsifiers).
Face	Cosmetics, personal care products (emulsifiers, preservatives). Hair products (shampoos / surfactants, fragrances, preservatives). Cell phones, eyeglasses, headsets (nickel). Consort/connubial contact from spouse/partner's products. Airborne allergens (fragrances, paints). Gold (from ring which then gets rubbed onto the skin of the face when touching the face).
Eyelids	Cosmetics (make-up, waxes, setting sprays). Nail products (nail polish, gel nails, acrylic nails). Eyelash curlers, tweezers (nickel). Eye drops (active ingredients, preservatives). Hair products (shampoos, conditioners, hair sprays). Airborne (fragrances).
Hands	Gloves (rubber most common). Hand soap/sanitizers. Tools/utensils (rubber, metals). Occupation-specific chemicals (e.g., hairdressers – hair dye).
Neck, shoulders	Jewelry (nickel, cobalt, gold). Hair products (surfactants, fragrances, preservatives).
Feet	Shoes (rubber accelerators, leather tanning agents, glue ingredients).
Under clothing only	Clothing dye (disperse blue dyes). Clothing finishes (formaldehyde resins).

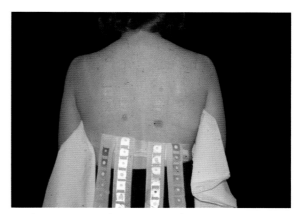

Figure 8-7. Patch testing. Patches are removed revealing 2 positive reactions to allergens.

Management

The management of allergic contact dermatitis is comprised of three steps:

- Identification of the allergen through patch testing
- Avoidance of the allergen
- Repair of the normal skin barrier

Patient education is important in promoting avoidance of the allergen. Even a small exposure of allergens up to every 3 weeks is enough to keep the dermatitis going. Thus, patient information sheets on specific allergens, customizable lists of allergen-free products (CAMP – Contact Allergen Management Plan), and individualized plans should be provided to patients to help them avoid their allergens. Helpful resources are available through the American Contact Dermatitis Society website (www.contactderm.org).

Mid-potency to high potency topical corticosteroids (Table 8-5) applied twice a day are usually sufficient for treatment of the dermatitis. Given the prolonged reaction in the skin with allergic contact dermatitis, a 2–3-week course is recommended. Restoration of the skin barrier with mild soaps and moisturizers is important, as listed in Table 8-4. An acute flare of widespread and extensive allergic contact dermatitis will respond to a 3-week tapering course of systemic corticosteroids. A standard adult dose consists of 40–60 mg of prednisone daily for 1 week, followed by a tapering dose over the next 2 weeks. Treatment with less than 3 weeks will usually result in rebound dermatitis, as this is a cell-mediated, delayed-type allergic reaction. Steroid sparing treatments, including topical calcineurin inhibitors or chronic immunosuppression should be considered for difficult cases and should be managed under the care of a dermatologist. Antihistamines may be helpful to abate pruritus but will not affect the dermatitis itself.

Clinical Course and Prognosis

Prognosis in allergic contact dermatitis is dependent upon identification and avoidance of causative allergen. Relapses tend to be very common, as allergens can be pervasive in everyday products. Risk factors for prolonged courses include long duration of dermatitis prior to diagnosis, atopy, and continuation in the same occupation. Allergic contact dermatitis can have a significant impact on quality of life, particularly in regards to emotional strain, symptom management, and occupation.[8] Pain, pruritus, embarrassment, workplace interference, and difficulty sleeping are commonly reported.[9] Poor prognosis is associated with the prolonged duration and extent of disease as well as those patients with primary hand involvement. Some studies suggest that increased education surrounding allergic contact dermatitis can improve a patient's quality of life.[10,11]

Indications for Consultation

Severe or persistent disease that does not respond to treatment.

Referral for patch testing should be considered when the diagnosis is unclear, has an unusual distribution, or when related to occupational exposures. Many general dermatologists perform limited patch testing of about 30 allergens. More extensive patch testing including 70 allergens is typically performed by specialized dermatologists for occupational and more difficult cases.

Patient Information Sites

American Contact Dermatitis Society
    www.contactderm.org

ATOPIC DERMATITIS

Introduction

Key points for atopic dermatitis

- ✓ Atopic dermatitis affects 20–25% of children in developed countries.
- ✓ It initially presents in children under age 2 and goes into remission in childhood or early adolescence in most patients, but it can persist into adulthood.
- ✓ The acute form presents with very pruritic, erythematous papules and/or vesicles with overlying excoriations and/or exudates. The chronic form presents with ill-defined, erythematous scaly, and lichenified plaques.
- ✓ Infants tend to have extensor involvement of the face, scalp, neck, and extensor extremities. Children and adults more often localize to the flexural surface.
- ✓ Most patients can be managed with moisturizers, topical steroids and topical calcineurin inhibitors.
- ✓ Patients and parents often have decreased quality of life issues.

Atopic dermatitis is a chronic, pruritic, inflammatory skin condition that affects 20–25% of children in developed countries. Most patients have onset of disease in early childhood. Up to 70% of children have a positive family history of atopic dermatitis, with relative risk increasing if both parents are affected. The diagnosis of atopic dermatitis is clinical. Diagnostic features have been proposed from consensus guidelines of care for atopic dermatitis.[12] The essential features for a diagnosis of atopic dermatitis are pruritus and the presence of eczematous dermatitis in typical areas. These include face and extensor areas in young children, and flexural dermatitis in any age group. [12] Associated comorbidities in patients with atopic dermatitis include other atopic diseases, namely, food allergies, asthma, and allergic rhinitis. These associations are not observed in every patient, and their relationship is complex. Other important comorbidities include sleep disturbance, occurring in greater than 60% of patients, depression and increased rates of attention- deficit/hyperactivity disorder (ADHD). The psychosocial impact of atopic dermatitis should not be minimized and include effects on physical health, emotional health, physical, and social functioning.[13,14]

Pathogenesis

The etiology of atopic dermatitis is multifactorial and complex. A combination of genetic, environmental, and immunologic factors lead to alterations in skin barrier function, immune response, and skin flora; these come together to produce the clinical manifestations of atopic dermatitis. The epidermal skin barrier prevents transepidermal water loss along with protecting the body from environmental irritants, allergens, and microbes. This barrier is made up of differentiated keratinocytes within a matrix of structural proteins, lipids, and enzymes. The structural protein filaggrin plays a key role in skin barrier function and is implicated in many disease processes, including atopic dermatitis.[15] Loss of function mutations in the filaggrin gene are a strong predisposing risk factor, with a nearly four-fold increase in atopic dermatitis.[16–18] Further studies have found that null mutations or homozygous filaggrin mutations are associated with increased disease severity and resistance to typical treatment.[19,20]

Not all cases of atopic dermatitis include a filaggrin mutation and multiple other genes have been proposed as possible contributors to disease pathogenesis. Gene mutations related to the differentiation of epithelial cell layers, cellular proteins including desmosomes and tight junctions, enzymes responsible for connective tissue remodeling and prevention of T-cell chemotaxis, as well as enzymes preventing transepidermal water loss have been identified.[21–24]

Immune dysregulation also plays a key role in the development of atopic dermatitis. The innate immune system includes physical barriers (particularly the epidermis), antimicrobial cytokines, and antigen presenting cells.[25] These antigen presenting cells contain toll-like receptors (TLR). Activation of these TLR leads to a cascade of inflammatory mediators and strengthening of the skin's barrier.[26,27] Reduced TLR function has been found in patients with atopic dermatitis, leading to altered inflammatory response and skin flora. The adaptive immune response also appears to play a role in atopic dermatitis pathophysiology. These patients have increased expression of Th2, Th22, and Th17 cytokines. These cytokines alter keratinocyte differentiation and promote epidermal hyperplasia, ultimately modulating the skin's epidermal barrier function.[28]

Another key player in the development of atopic dermatitis is altered skin flora and microbial colonization. Up to 90% of patients are colonized with *Staphylococcus aureus*, as compared to 5% in healthy individuals.[29] Other colonizers include *Streptococcus pyogenes*, herpes simplex virus, molluscum contagiosum, and *Malassezia* species. Colonization

with any of these potential pathogens is associated with increased severity and prolonged duration of disease.[30] *S. aureus* in particular confers poorer prognosis, mediated through the production of staphylococcal enterotoxins and toxic shock syndrome toxin-1. These toxins further modulate the immune response, induce T-cell proliferation, and decrease responsiveness to topical corticosteroids.[30]

The pathogenesis of atopic dermatitis is a complex interaction between genetics, immune regulation, skin barrier integrity, and skin flora. While many of the details remain unclear, this groundwork provides good data for which to guide therapies and future research.

Clinical Presentation

▶ History

The chief concern of the patient or parent of the patient is typically a recurrent pruritic skin eruption. Onset is important in diagnosis, as an earlier onset is supportive of atopic dermatitis. The location and distribution of the rash should also be discussed. Further history regarding chronicity or relapses is helpful. A personal or family history of atopy will also support the diagnosis.[12,30]

▶ Physical Examination

Important physical exam findings in atopic dermatitis include the morphology and location of eczematous lesions, which vary by stage and age, respectively.

Acute eczema consists of pruritic, erythematous papules, and/or vesicles with overlying excoriations and/or exudates (Figure 8-8). Acute eczematous plaques are more difficult to recognize in skin of color as erythema may not show that prominently (Figure 8-9). This is important to consider, so observing scale, crust and pigmentary changes in patients with skin of color is important in estimating the body surface area involved.

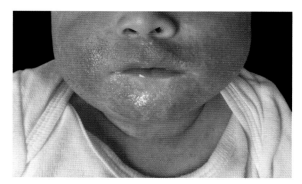

▲ **Figure 8-8.** Infantile atopic dermatitis. Classic appearance of infantile atopic dermatitis on the face of an infant with type I skin. Brightly erythematous, ill-defined plaque with scale, and yellowish crusting. Sparing of the nasal tip is common.

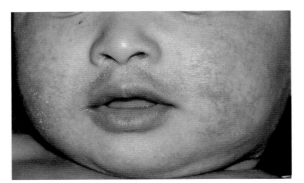

Figure 8-9. Infantile atopic dermatitis. Classic appearance of infantile atopic dermatitis in a 5 month of infant with type III-IV skin. Erythematous and hyperpigmented ill-defined plaques with scale and sparing of the nasal tip. Erythema may be more difficult to appreciate in skin of color.

Chronic eczematous plaques typically present as ill-defined, erythematous scaly, lichenified plaques with overlying hyper or hypopigmentation (Figures 8-10, 8-11) In patients with skin of color, chronic atopic dermatitis may manifest with a diffuse papular and lichenified variant with prominent postinflammatory pigmentary alterations (Figure 8-12).

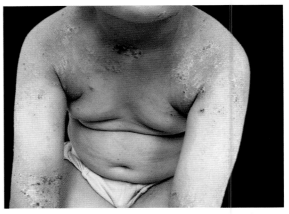

Figure 8-11. Chronic atopic dermatitis in children. Nine-year-old child with type III-IV skin and widespread, ill-defined erythematous, scaly, and crusted plaques. Upper chest and flexures tend to be affected.

Acute, subacute, and chronic plaques may occur in the same patient. Surrounding skin demonstrates xerosis/skin barrier dysfunction. Excoriations may be present. In children, periorbital skin folds maybe prominent (so-called Dennie Morgan folds). Other cutaneous features of atopic dermatitis including palmar hyperlinearity and keratosis pilaris (Figure 8-13).

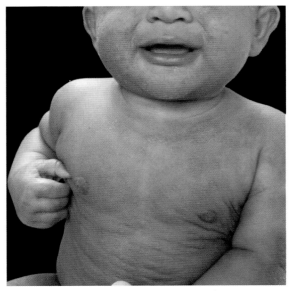

Figure 8-10. Chronic infantile atopic dermatitis. Nine-month-old child with chronic atopic dermatitis. Ill-defined erythematous lichenified plaques with hyper and hypopigmented plaques and patches from post-inflammatory change. Nipple involvement is typical. Chronic and significant pruritus.

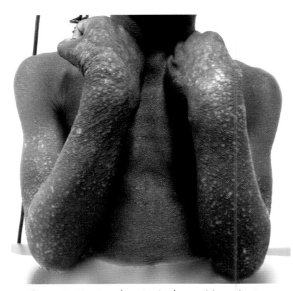

Figure 8-12. Papular atopic dermatitis variant, more common in skin of color. Ten–year-old male with type V skin. Widespread erythematous and hypopigmented papules coalescing into lichenified plaques. Papular variant of atopic dermatitis is more common in skin of color.

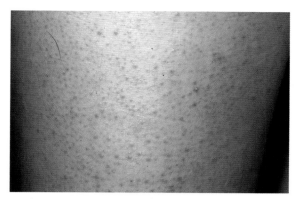

▲ **Figure 8-13.** Keratosis pilaris. 1–2 mm perifollicular papules on the extensor arms.

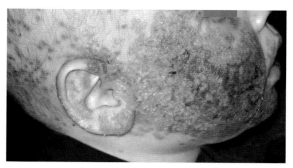

▲ **Figure 8-15.** Eczema herpeticum (HSV) in infant with atopic dermatitis. Erythematous, confluent papules and vesicles with "punched out" discrete erosions with hemorrhagic crusts.

The distribution of lesions is age dependent. Infants tend to have extensor involvement of the face, scalp, neck, and extensor extremities. Children and adults more often localize to the flexural surface. All age groups demonstrate relative sparing of the groin and axillary regions.[12]

As patients with atopic dermatitis have altered skin flora, physical examination may reveal a secondary infection of the primary lesions. *Staphylococcus aureus* is the most common cause of impetiginization and causes yellow or hemorrhagic crusting with erosions and drainage. Verruca vulgaris and molluscum contagiosum are also more common in atopic dermatitis. Not to miss findings include eczema herpeticum, caused by disseminated herpes simplex virus (HSV) in the setting of atopic dermatitis (Figure 8-14, 8-15). Lesions are widespread, "punched out" erosions and vesicles, often accompanied by fever, malaise, and/or lymphadenopathy. Eczema herpeticum requires emergent antiviral treatment and in many cases hospital admission. If eczema herpeticum is a consideration on the head and neck, herpes simplex virus polymerase chain reaction (PCR) and a viral culture should be obtained from

the base of a vesicle/erosion. If there is periorbital or nasal tip involvement, ophthalmology should be consulted to rule out herpetic keratitis, which may threaten vision.[30,31]

▶ Laboratory Findings

Lab work is not typically necessary or recommended in the evaluation of atopic dermatitis. If the diagnosis is unclear, potassium hydroxide (KOH) preparation, patch testing, or skin biopsy may be helpful. The histologic features of atopic dermatitis include epidermal edema (spongiosis) along with inflammatory cell infiltration within the dermis. Other lab work, such as serum IgE may be elevated, but is not recommended for diagnosis or disease monitoring.[12]

Diagnosis

Atopic dermatitis is a clinical diagnosis, based upon a patient's history, skin lesion morphology and distribution, and associated signs and symptoms. Essential features in the diagnosis include pruritus and eczema. The eczema with atopic dermatitis should have typical morphology and age-specific distribution. While it may be acute, subacute, or chronic, most history reveals a chronic, relapsing eczema. Other important features include an early age of onset, personal or family history of atopy, history of IgE reactivity, and xerosis. Helpful, but nonspecific findings include keratosis pilaris, hyperlinear palms, nipple dermatitis, and periorbital, perioral, or periauricular xerosis or lichenification.[12]

▶ Differential Diagnosis

In these differential diagnoses, it is important to consider that the following conditions may coexist, particularly in the patient with altered skin barrier protection:

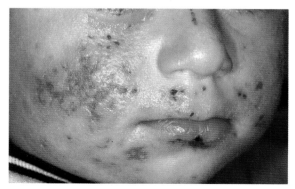

▲ **Figure 8-14.** Eczema herpeticum (HSV) in child with atopic dermatitis. Large erosion on erythematous base with multiple smaller crusted erosions on face of child

✓ Seborrheic dermatitis: This is a common differential diagnosis in infants. The most important comparison is that this has little to no pruritus associated. Lesions are yellow to pink with greasy scale, typically on the scalp, face, and neck.

✓ Contact dermatitis: Allergic or irritant contact dermatitis have similar appearing morphology to atopic dermatitis. Distinguishing features include localization of the dermatitis to an affected area or history of exposures. Patch testing may provide diagnostic clarity.

✓ Psoriasis: Well demarcated, persistent plaques with overlying scale. This most often affects the diaper area in infants.

✓ Tinea corporis: Well demarcated, scaly, annular plaques with a raised border and central clearing.

✓ Other differentials: Nummular dermatitis, lichen simplex chronicus, primary immunodeficiencies (Wiskott-Aldrich, hyperimmunoglobulin E syndrome), nutritional deficiencies, cutaneous T-cell lymphoma.

Management

The mainstay in atopic dermatitis treatment is repairing and maintaining the skin barrier, treating inflammation and superinfection. This is accomplished by addressing the clinical characteristics of eczema: dry skin, pruritus, inflammation, and infection. Depending on the severity of eczema, treatment may be aimed at prevention and decreasing overall inflammation or may be escalated to systemic therapies.

Bathing and moisturization, skin barrier maintenance: Restoring and maintaining the epidermal barrier is essential in treating atopic dermatitis. Diligent application of thick emollients helps restore moisture and prevent transepidermal water loss. This is an essential step in all stages and severity of atopic dermatitis, including inactive disease. Emollients have been shown to reduce disease severity and improve quality of life as well as decrease the need for topical steroids.[30,32] The choice of emollient is also important, as there are many options available. Lotion has a high water and alcohol content, which leads to evaporation, increased transepidermal water loss, and worsening xerosis. Creams and ointments (e.g., white petrolatum) are preferred for this reason. These should be applied at least twice a day, immediately after bathing, and after hand washing.

The frequency, duration, and methods for bathing in atopic dermatitis are widely discussed; however, there is insufficient evidence for conclusive recommendations at this time. Bathing has many benefits in atopic dermatitis, including hydrating the skin and clearing debris and allergens. In general, most pediatric dermatologists recommend a 5–10 min soaking bath in lukewarm water once daily. A soaking bath is preferred over showering. Non-soap, hypoallergenic, fragrance free cleansers are not essential, but may be used to wash the axilla, groin, hands, and feet, if desired. Soap should be avoided as it draws out proteins and lipids, worsening xerosis. Once out of the bath, pat the skin dry and apply emollients immediately to prevent further water evaporation. Dilute bleach baths either on a regular basis or used intermittently are effective in reducing *Staph aureus* infection or colonization in patients with atopic dermatitis and are quite useful in management (see below).

Topical corticosteroids: With the groundwork of maintaining skin barrier function, the next treatment steps aim to decrease cutaneous inflammation. Topical corticosteroids are considered first line treatment and are effective in treating and preventing inflammation. For an acute flare, a low to medium potency topical corticosteroid ointment twice a day for 2 weeks is recommended. Lower potency should be used on the face. As many patients with atopic dermatitis are children, it should be noted that children have a greater body surface area to weight ratio, thereby increasing absorption of topical corticosteroids. While rare, it is important to monitor for cutaneous side effects, such as striae, telangiectasias, and atrophy. Systemic side effects are very rare and no specific monitoring is necessary. Topical corticosteroids are safe, effective, and play an important part in atopic dermatitis management when used appropriately.[33]

Topical calcineurin inhibitors, such as tacrolimus or pimecrolimus, are another topical anti-inflammatory option. These act on activated T-cells to inhibit proinflammatory cytokine transcription. Low-potency formulations are approved for patients aged 2–15 years, and full potency formulations are available to patients over 15 years old. They may be used in conjunction with or as an alternative to topical steroids, although they are most often used as a second line, steroid sparing agent after treatment failure or intolerance of topical steroids.[12] For patients with active atopic dermatitis, these should be applied twice a day, although have also been shown to decrease relapses even when used 2–3 times weekly.[34] Despite initial concerns, these medications have demonstrated safety without increased risk of malignancy.[35]

Other topical treatments include crisaborole, which is a topical phosphodiesterase-4 inhibitor. This is an option to consider for adjunctive treatment, although further data is necessary regarding its efficacy and role to play in the management of atopic dermatitis.[36,37]

Managing infection/colonization: It is well known that patients with atopic dermatitis are often overtly infected or colonized with *Staphylococcus aureus*. If there is obvious yellowish crusting, fissuring of the skin or for extensive disease, a bacterial culture can be helpful in guiding the need for antimicrobial management. In these cases, treatment with systemic antibiotics (i.e., cephalosporins) may be helpful in calming an acute flare.

In cases of chronic colonization of the skin, dilute bleach (sodium hypochlorite) baths are very effective in reducing infection and subsequent disease severity. The mechanism of action for dilute bleach baths is unknown; however, there is some evidence that they may have an anti-inflammatory as well as an antimicrobial effect. Dilute bleach soaks are practical, safe, inexpensive, and do not lead to microbial resistance. They are an extremely useful adjunctive treatment.

General instructions are to add a half cup of bleach to a full tub of water or a one-fourth cup of bleach to a half tub of water and soak for 20 min. For smaller infant plastic tubs, 2 tablespoons of bleach is appropriate.

For overtly crusted or fissured skin, topical antibiotics such as mupirocin ointment twice a day can be helpful. In cases of methicillin-resistant *Staphylococcus aureus* (MRSA) infection, decolonization with intranasal mupirocin bid for 5 days monthly may also be utilized.

Wet wraps/dressings: For children and infants with severe, widespread disease, the initial use of wet wraps/wet dressings is a safe, inexpensive, and effective way to calm the skin. Several studies have demonstrated the utility of wet dressings, and though they are time consuming and cumbersome, they represent one of the fastest modalities to reduce the signs and symptoms of flaring atopic dermatitis. These can be done as an inpatient hospital treatment or at home.

After bathing, application of topical corticosteroids and a petrolatum-based emollient, wet dressings in the form of damp cotton pajamas can be applied to the skin. This can be followed with a dry pajama. If tolerated, children can remain in the wet dressing overnight, often with significant improvement in the skin and symptoms of pruritus by the next morning. Wet dressings can be done for days or up to 2 weeks at a time. Complications may include folliculitis or poor compliance, particularly in older children and adults.

Systemic treatment: When preventative and topical anti-inflammatory measures do not achieve disease remission, systemic therapies may be considered. Referral to dermatology is indicated at this point to help guide further treatment.

Dupilumab is a major development in the treatment of moderate to severe atopic dermatitis. It is a fully human monoclonal antibody that binds to the interleukin (IL)-4 receptor, inhibiting downstream signaling of IL-4 and IL-13, which are both cytokines produced by helper T lymphocytes.[38,39] This is an injected medication with an initial loading dose followed by a maintenance dose every other week. It has a favorable safety profile and may be used as long-term management of atopic dermatitis, particularly when compared to conventional immunosuppression. Dupilumab has been shown to lead to near or total disease remission with significant increase in quality of life and managing symptoms. Dupilumab is approved for use in adults and children as young as 6 years. It is an appropriate second line therapy when topical management has failed to yield long-term improvement.

Other systemic therapies include cyclosporine, azathioprine, methotrexate, mycophenolate mofetil, and interferon gamma. These medications are generally safe and well tolerated but require very close monitoring prior to initial doses and during therapy. Oral corticosteroids are not recommended for the management of atopic dermatitis. While they do improve symptoms, rebound flares with increased severity are commonly observed and thus should be avoided.[12] Given their known significant side effects, systemic corticosteroids are not a good short- or long-term option.

Phototherapy has good evidence supporting its use as maintenance therapy in atopic dermatitis.[12] There are many varieties of light therapy available and there is no definitive data supporting one particular form of light therapy over another. In general, narrow band ultraviolet light B (UVB) is preferred for its low-risk profile and efficacy, particularly when compared to natural sunlight. Phototherapy is, however, not an ideal choice for infants and children.

While not disease modifying, oral antihistamines are a systemic option available for symptomatic management of pruritus, particularly at night. First-generation sedating antihistamines such as diphenhydramine or hydroxyzine are more effective at managing symptoms than the second-generation antihistamines.

Clinical Course and Prognosis

A hallmark of atopic dermatitis is its chronic, relapsing course; however, with appropriate therapy, the majority of patients can be treated with topical therapies and some cases do spontaneously improve later in childhood or early adolescence. There is variable data on the persistence of atopic dermatitis into adulthood.[41–43] The majority outgrow it in childhood or early adolescence, but around 25% continue to have eczema in adulthood.[44] Risk factors for persistent disease include severity of disease, presence of genetic mutations, persistently elevated IgE and eosinophilia, associated rhinitis and/or asthma, early age of onset, and female gender.[45,46]

Atopic dermatitis has a significant impact on quality of life, more so than other chronic diseases of childhood such as asthma or type 1 diabetes.[40] As atopic dermatitis is primarily a disease of childhood, this burden falls on both patients and parents/caregivers. Pruritus and sleep disruption are major contributors to the decreased quality of life. Psychosocial issues, such as behavioral problems, mental health concerns, and social issues also contribute to morbidity. There are associations between patients with atopic dermatitis and increased risk of attention-deficit/hyperactivity disorder (ADHD), anxiety, and depression.[47,48] Time-consuming, complex, and occasionally expensive treatment regimens also cause significant stress and economic burden on patients and families. Fortunately, with appropriate therapy and education of patients and families, the burden of disease decreases and overall prognosis is favorable.[49,50]

Indications for Consultation

- Severe or persistent disease that does not respond to initial treatment with emollients and topical corticosteroids, particularly in children.

- Suspected atopic dermatitis in patients <2 months of age.

- Patients with suspected eczema herpeticum should be referred to dermatology and ophthalmology emergently and may require hospital admission if widespread or facial involvement.

Patient Information Sites

▼ NUMMULAR DERMATITIS

Introduction

Key points for nummular dermatitis

✓ Nummular dermatitis is a common skin disorder that presents with pruritic, round, scaly, or crusted plaques on the extremities in older adults.

✓ It can be managed with moisturizers and mid-potency to high-potency topical corticosteroids.

✓ It may become a chronic or relapsing disease.

Nummular is a Greek word meaning "coin." Nummular dermatitis is a common skin disorder that presents with "coin-shaped" plaques on the extremities. It is also commonly referred to as discoid eczema due to the shape of the plaques. It is more common in older individuals and is often associated with dry skin.

Pathogenesis

The pathophysiology of nummular dermatitis is unknown but thought to be linked to impaired skin barrier function. Decreased cutaneous lipid production, xerosis, bacterial colonization, contact allergy, increased tension, and immune mediation have all been proposed as possible causes.[51-56]

Clinical Presentation

▷ History

The patient typically complains of an itchy rash on the extremities.

▷ Physical Examination

The patient typically presents with round, light pink, scaly, thin, 1–3 cm plaques on the extremities (Figure 8-16). The plaques are typically uniform with no central clearing. The trunk may also be affected. The face and neck are not typically involved.

▷ Laboratory Findings

Skin biopsies are usually not diagnostic and are only helpful to rule out other disorders. Examination of a KOH preparation will be negative for fungal hyphae.

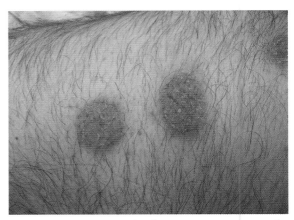

▲ **Figure 8-16.** Nummular dermatitis on arm. Round, scaly, crusted plaques.

Diagnosis

Nummular dermatitis is a clinical diagnosis. The key diagnostic features are pruritic, pink, scaly plaques, with no central clearing, commonly located on the arms and legs. The trunk may also be affected, although the face and neck should be spared.

▷ Differential Diagnosis

✓ Cutaneous fungal infections: Tinea corporis may present in circular plaques but these are typically annular (ring-shaped with central clearing). Fungal hyphae can be visualized on a KOH preparation from skin scrapings.

✓ Allergic and irritant contact dermatitis: Allergic and irritant contact dermatitis usually do not present in coin-shaped plaques. Allergic contact dermatitis is diagnosed by patch testing.

✓ Atopic dermatitis: Individuals with atopic dermatitis usually have a personal or family history of atopic dermatitis (childhood eczema), allergic rhinitis, or asthma. Atopic dermatitis does not usually present with the coin-shaped plaques.

✓ Other eczematous skin conditions including lichen simplex chronicus.

✓ Psoriasis: Typically, less pruritic and with increased scale when compared to nummular dermatitis.

✓ Uncommon conditions may include cutaneous T-cell lymphoma, subacute cutaneous lupus, granuloma annulare, psoriasis, or Bowen's disease.

Management

The management of nummular dermatitis includes the use of mid-potency to high-potency topical corticosteroids (Table 8-5) twice a day. For patients with isolated, persistent lesions, intralesional triamcinolone is an option. More severe or widespread disease may respond to phototherapy or systemic therapies under the guidance of a dermatologist.

Maintenance of skin barrier integrity with mild soap, emollients, and gentle skin care products is recommended as well.

Clinical Course and Prognosis

The clinical course in nummular dermatitis is favorable, with most patients achieving disease control and remission. In some patients, the course may be chronic and relapsing. Lesions may become dormant and recur in the same location or in adjacent areas.

Indications for Consultation

Severe or persistent disease that does not respond to treatment.

Patient Information

American Academy of Dermatology
    http://www.aad.org/skin-conditions/dermatology-a-to-z/nummular-dermatitis

DYSHIDROTIC DERMATITIS

Introduction

Key points for dyshidrotic dermatitis

✓ Dyshidrotic dermatitis is characterized by chronic, relapsing eruptions of small deep-seated vesicles along the sides of fingers, hand, and/or feet.

✓ Dyshidrotic dermatitis is managed with mid- to high-potency topical corticosteroids.

✓ It typically responds slowly to treatment and may become a chronic condition with intermittent flares.

Dyshidrotic dermatitis (sometimes called pompholyx) is a common pruritic, vesicular skin disorder of the palms and soles. Some experts consider dyshidrotic dermatitis and pompholyx to be distinct conditions although the terms are often used interchangeably.[18] In general, though, dyshidrotic dermatitis is characterized by chronic, relapsing eruptions of small deep-seated vesicles along the sides of fingers and hand. Pompholyx presents as explosive eruptions of large bullae on the hands. Dyshidrotic dermatitis is common, affecting approximately 1% of the general population,[57] whereas pompolyx is rare. Men and women are affected equally. It is most common among young adults, but can occur in any age group.

Pathogenesis

The term "dyshidrosis" (meaning "difficult sweating") is a misnomer, as the condition does not involve dysfunction of sweat glands. The cause is unknown and likely multifactorial. A few studies have found a link between flares of vesicular palmoplantar dermatitis and oral ingestion of nickel in nickel-allergic patients.[57] Similarly, exposure to contact irritants or allergens, particularly metals, has been associated with dyshidrotic dermatitis. Other case series describe an association with exposure to dermatophyte infection, intravenous immunoglobulin (IVIG), tobacco smoke, hyperhidrosis, or UV radiation.[58–63]

Clinical Presentation

▶ History

Typical presentation includes a history of pruritus followed by the sudden onset of pruritic vesicles on the palms and/or soles. History of patient's recent exposures is beneficial when considering other types of hand dermatitis.

▶ Physical Examination

Dyshidrotic dermatitis presents with grouped 2–5 mm vesicles, sometimes likened to "tapioca pudding" (Figure 8-17). The most common locations include lateral fingers, central palms, insteps, and lateral borders of the feet. Pompholyx presents as large, 1–5 cm bullae. Both present on a non-inflammatory base, with little surrounding erythema.

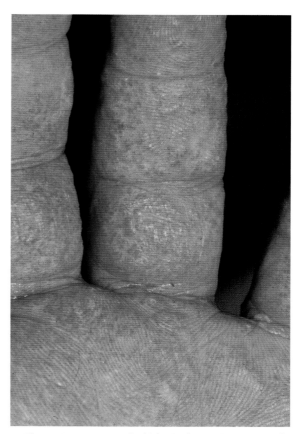

Figure 8-17. Acute dyshidrotic dermatitis. Grouped, tiny "tapioca –like" vesicles with minimal erythema.

▶ Laboratory Findings

Skin biopsies are usually not diagnostic and are only helpful to rule out other disorders. Examination of a KOH preparation will be negative for fungal hyphae.

Diagnosis

The key diagnostic features of dyshidrotic dermatitis are a history of pruritus and acute onset of small, grouped vesicles on the palms and/or soles.

▶ Differential Diagnosis

✓ Allergic and irritant contact dermatitis of the palms and soles: Allergic and irritant contact dermatitis usually are not limited to these locations and have surrounding erythema, scale, and eczematous plaques.

✓ Cutaneous fungal infections: Inflammatory tinea pedis caused by *Trichophyton mentagrophytes* may present with vesicles, but these typically have surrounding erythema. Fungal hyphae will be visualized on a KOH preparation from skin scrapings.

✓ Erythema multiforme: This can present with inflammatory, "bull's eye" lesions (3-zone targets) on the palms and soles. Skin biopsies will have specific findings.

✓ Scabies: This may present with vesicles and papules on the palms and soles, but usually there are burrows and more widespread lesions.

✓ Vesiculobullous diseases such as pemphigoid and pemphigus: Dyshidrotic eczema is typically non-inflammatory and only affects the palms and soles, whereas other vesiculobullous conditions have significant surrounding erythema and commonly affect multiple body sites.

Management

Dyshidrotic dermatitis is managed with mid- to high-potency topical corticosteroids (Table 8-5) twice a day. In individuals where sweat is a significant aggravating factor, iontophoresis or onabotulinumtoxin (Botox) injections may be helpful. In patients who have a strong positive reaction to nickel, a low-nickel diet can be considered.[64]

Clinical Course and Prognosis

Dyshidrotic eczema is typically a relapsing condition. With unclear pathogenesis, identifying eliciting factors in a patient can be difficult, increasing the chances of relapsing disease.

Indications for Consultation

Inflammatory bullae, severe or persistent disease that does not respond to treatment or extension to sites other than the palms and soles.

Patient Information

- American Contact Dermatitis Society—Low nickel diet: www.contactderm.org
- National Eczema Organization: https://nationaleczema.org/eczema/types-of-eczema/dyshidrotic-eczema/

LICHEN SIMPLEX CHRONICUS

Introduction

Key points for lichen simplex chronicus

✓ Lichen simplex chronicus is caused by chronic rubbing and scratching of the skin leading to thickening of the epidermis and fibrosis of the dermis

✓ It presents with chronic, intensely pruritic, lichenified plaques, mostly commonly found on the neck, or genitals or dorsum of the foot / ankle.

✓ Class 1 or 2 high to super-potent topical corticosteroid ointments or creams twice a day, but if often responds slowly to treatment and recurrence is common.

Lichen simplex chronicus is a term used to describe the clinical appearance of any long-standing and chronically pruritic skin condition. As a primary diagnosis, it exists without a known underlying condition or cause. As a secondary diagnosis, it results after years of scratching due to another condition, most commonly atopic dermatitis.

Pathogenesis

The exact pathophysiology is unknown. Chronic rubbing and scratching of the skin leads to thickening of the epidermis and fibrosis of the dermis. Chronic cutaneous nerve stimulation is hypothesized to result in nerve dysfunction; an "itch-scratch" cycle ensues perpetuating the need to rub and scratch affected areas. Lichen simplex chronicus is often seen in the setting of chronic atopic dermatitis.

Clinical Presentation

▶ History

The patient typically complains of localized areas of intensely pruritic skin. Sleep is often interrupted. In some cases, the chronic rubbing and scratching becomes a subconscious or compulsive habit.

▶ Physical Examination

Common locations for primary lichen simplex chronicus include the lateral neck, scrotum/vulva, and dorsal foot. The plaque is typically solitary, well-defined, pink to tan, thick, and lichenified (Figure 8-18). Secondary lichen simplex chronicus occurs at the sites of the underlying skin conditions such as in the antecubital and popliteal fossae in atopic dermatitis.

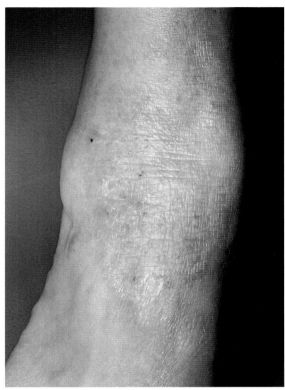

▲ **Figure 8-18.** Lichen simplex chronicus on leg. Thick ,erythematous well defined plaque with accentuation of skin markings.

▷ Laboratory Findings

Skin biopsies are usually not diagnostic and are helpful only to rule out other disorders.

Diagnosis

The key diagnostic features of lichen simplex chronicus are chronic, intensely pruritic, lichenified plaques, mostly commonly found on the neck, or genitals or dorsum of the foot/ankle.

▷ Differential Diagnosis

✓ Psoriasis: This usually presents with multiple symmetric lesions with elbows, knees, and scalp being commonly involved.

✓ Psychological disorders. Usually other signs of psychological disease are present.

✓ Squamous cell carcinoma: This can present as a hyperkeratotic plaque, but it is typically not pruritic and rarely becomes lichenified.

Management

Primary lichen simplex chronicus is typically managed with class 1 or 2 high to super potent topical corticosteroid ointments or creams twice a day (Table 8-5). Corticosteroid-impregnated tapes, such as flurandrenolide tape, which can be applied directly over the plaque, are often helpful. Oral antidepressants or antihistamines, especially doxepin, may benefit individuals with nighttime itching and sleep disturbance. It is important that patients become aware of the habit or compulsion to scratch or rub, replacing these activities with pushing on the skin, application of cool compresses and/or antipruritic creams such as those with menthol-camphor or pramoxine. In more severe cases, behavioral therapy may be of benefit.

The use of dupilumab for the treatment of chronic pruritic skin conditions such as prurigo nodularis or uncontrolled lichen simplex chronicus is reported. This is an emerging area of therapy and may be considered in recalcitrant cases.

Clinical Course and Prognosis

Lichen simplex chronic tends to have a chronic course with slow clearance in those patients motivated to treat the area aggressively and refrain from scratching.

Indications for Consultation

Severe or persistent disease that does not respond to treatment.

Patient Information Sites

National Eczema Association
    https://nationaleczema.org/eczema/types-of-eczema/neurodermatitis/

▽ PRURIGO NODULARIS

Introduction

Key points for prurigo nodularis

✓ Prurigo nodularis is an intensely pruritic, chronic dermatitis that is the result of result of the itch-scratch cycle.

✓ It is more common in patients with atopy, folliculitis, systemic diseases that cause pruritus and in neurologic or psychiatric disorders.

✓ It presents with firm hyperkeratotic papules, nodules, or plaques with clearly demarcated borders.

✓ Prurigo nodularis is difficult to manage even with high potency topical steroids it and typically becomes a chronic condition.

Prurigo nodularis is an intensely pruritic chronic dermatitis. It can be classified as a form of neurodermatitis. Its clinical manifestations are a result of the itch-scratch cycle; however, its underlying pathophysiology is poorly understood.[65] Many patients with prurigo nodularis have primary atopic tendencies, but prurigo is also seen in the context of other dermatologic disorders, systemic disease, infection, neurologic, or psychiatric disorders. There is limited epidemiologic data available. Prurigo nodularis is seen across all age groups, however, is most common in adults age 20–60 years old.[66]

Pathogenesis

The pathogenesis of prurigo nodularis is primarily attributed to cutaneous inflammation and neuronal dysplasia, although the mechanisms of these findings remain unclear. Skin biopsy reveals an increased number of nerve fibers and nerve endings within the dermis, also referred to as neural dermal hyperplasia; however, with a reduction in intraepithelial nerve fiber density. It is unclear what elicits the neural hyperplasia. The reduction in nerve fibers within the epithelium is likely secondary to persistent scratching as opposed to an endogenous neuropathy. This alteration of nerve fiber structure is likely of highest importance in the development of prurigo nodules. Pruritus is induced by the release of multiple inflammatory substances and neuropeptides, including interleukin-31 and substance P. Both of these substances have been shown to be increased in patients with prurigo nodularis.[65]

Clinical Presentation

History

Intense and persistent pruritus is the most common symptom in prurigo nodularis, although it may also be described as warm, cold, stinging, burning, or tingling. Further history should be obtained regarding a patient's occupation and potential exposures to rule out other differential diagnoses, such as allergic contact dermatitis. History regarding a patient's other health issues is important in diagnosing prurigo nodularis. A history of atopic tendencies, recent infection (particularly cutaneous infections such as scabies), chronic renal failure, diabetes mellitus, HIV, iron deficiency anemia, neurologic, or psychiatric disorders may be helpful in reaching the correct diagnosis and initiating a treatment plan.

Physical Examination

Prurigo lesions are typically firm hyperkeratotic papules, nodules, or plaques with clearly demarcated borders (Figure 8-19). The lesions may be erythematous, purpuric, hypopigmented, or hyperpigmented depending on how long they have been present. They often have secondary excoriation, ulceration, or scarring.[40] They are most commonly distributed across the extensor surfaces of the extremities and the trunk and spare unreachable areas that cannot be scratched. Lesions tend to be grouped together and are generally symmetric as opposed to unilateral. There may be only a few to >100 lesions present, depending on the severity.

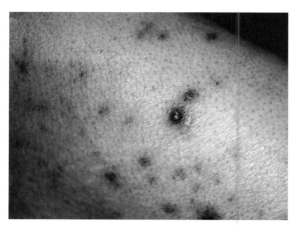

▲ **Figure 8-19.** Firm hyperpigmented papules on leg.

▶ Laboratory Findings

There are no typical lab findings in prurigo nodularis; biopsy may be helpful in determining a definitive diagnosis under the guidance of a dermatologist. There are an increased number of fibroblasts and capillaries along with T-cell, mast cell, and eosinophil infiltration within the dermis and hyperkeratosis within the epidermis, representative of fibrosis and inflammation.

Diagnosis

Diagnosis is typically made based on the clinical presentation, history, and physical examination. A biopsy may be useful in confirming diagnosis. Prurigo nodularis may be associated with other systemic diseases, further workup with a complete blood count with differential, metabolic panel, hemoglobin A1c, liver function tests, thyroid function tests, and human immunodeficiency virus (HIV) testing is often indicated.[66] A screening for depression, anxiety, or other psychological disease is helpful.[67]

▶ Differential Diagnosis

- ✓ Pemphigoid nodularis: Lesions similar to those of prurigo nodularis but with direct immunofluorescence (DIF) showing findings consistent with bullous pemphigoid.
- ✓ Dermatitis herpetiformis: symmetrical small very pruritic vesicular papules on the elbows, knees, buttocks, scalp in patients with celiac disease.
- ✓ Hypertrophic lichen planus. Thickened hyperkeratotic typically flat-topped plaques but can be nodular.
- ✓ Scabies: Pink-scaling patches or pink papules which can be diffuse or more localized to the finger webs, wrists, umbilicus, and genitals. Uncommon on face. Burrows can be clinically seen.
- ✓ Atopic dermatitis: Eczematous appearing skin typically in the flexures of the arms, leg, and neck. Can

be more widespread or affect localized areas like the eyelids, face, and hands.

✓ Contact dermatitis (irritant vs. allergic): Eczematous appearing papules/plaques in areas of contact with irritants/allergens.

Management

Treatment of prurigo nodularis is difficult and typically requires a prolonged treatment course. The mainstay in management is targeted at interrupting the itch-scratch cycle, which will ideally allow time for lesions to heal and improve quality of life. Emollients are a good initial therapy to help decrease pruritus and maintain the integrity of the skin barrier. Topical corticosteroids are used in treating pruritus and decreasing the hyperkeratotic nature of prurigo nodules. Higher potency steroids are necessary to adequately address thickened nodules and plaques. The use of occlusive dressings over topical steroid creams and ointments are helpful for further increasing efficacy and potency. Beyond topical steroids, first-line therapies included topical calcineurin inhibitors, topical calcipotriol, intralesional corticosteroids, and cryotherapy. Subsequent therapies which a dermatologist may use include cyclosporine, methotrexate, and narrowband ultraviolet B/psoralen ultraviolet B (UVB/PUVA) phototherapy. Next in line includes azathioprine and dupilumab.[68] Treating the neural component is also recommended. First line for this includes topical capsaicin or topical ketamine/amitriptyline/lidocaine compounded cream; next includes low-dose gabapentinoids, antidepressants such serotonin and norepinephrine reuptake inhibitors (SNRIs), selective serotonin reuptake inhibitors (SSRIs), tricyclic antidepressants (TCAs), and high-dose gabapentinoids.[68]

Initial oral therapy for pruritus is often oral antihistamines, although this is often not sufficient in abating symptoms. Next steps in the systemic management of pruritus include tricyclic antidepressants, such as amitriptyline or doxepin, anticonvulsants such as gabapentin or pregabalin, or opioid antagonists such as naltrexone. The use of dupilumab in the setting of prurigo nodularis is described with overall significant improvement. The use of dupilumab for chronic pruritic skin conditions poorly controlled with traditional therapies is an emerging therapeutic option.

Additional management in prurigo nodularis includes monitoring closely for secondary bacterial infection, which is common due to persistent scratching and subsequent skin breakdown.

Clinical Course and Prognosis

Prurigo nodularis is a chronic condition that often runs a long course. It has a significant impact on quality of life due to the severity of symptoms. It is also very difficult to treat effectively, which often causes further distress.

Indications for Consultation

Consultation to dermatology is recommended for further diagnostic clarity or for severe or persistent disease that is not improved with initial topical steroid treatment.

Patient Information Sites

Genetic and Rare Diseases Information Center https://rarediseases.info.nih.gov/diseases/7480/prurigo-nodularis

▼ **STASIS DERMATITIS**

Introduction

Key points for stasis dermatitis

✓ Stasis dermatitis is a common form of dermatitis in the elderly and is caused by chronic venous hypertension and venous insufficiency.

✓ It presents with chronically edematous lower extremities and bilateral erythematous, eczematous, and scaling hyperpigmented plaques usually on the lower leg especially on the ankles.

✓ Venous leg ulcers may develop in areas of chronic stasis dermatitis.

✓ Compression stockings and medium potency topical steroids are used for management.

Stasis dermatitis is a common form of dermatitis, caused by chronic venous hypertension and venous insufficiency.[69,70] It affects dependent areas and therefore often occurs on the lower extremities but can occur on the buttocks/sacrum in people who are bedbound.[71] It has many mimics and can be difficult at times to differentiate from cellulitis. Presentation ranges based on severity and duration of disease, with clinical findings including edema, hyperpigmentation, eczema, fibrosis, atrophy, and ulceration of the affected site(s). Risk factors include age, family history, female gender, obesity, and history of deep venous thrombosis.[72]

Pathogenesis

Chronic venous hypertension occurs as long-term sequelae from incompetent venous valves, valve destruction, or obstruction within the venous system.[69] This is a difficult cycle to break as rising venous pressures thereby produce more valvular destruction. Due to the small caliber of most superficial venous vessels, even a small increase in blood volume will cause an increase in pressure.[73] Venous hypertension produces histologic changes as well. Increased type I collagen, decreased type III collagen, decreased smooth muscle cells, and degeneration of the extracellular matrix all lead to weakening of the vessel wall.[74] Once the pathophysiology of the vessels is established, the clinical skin changes appreciated are mediated primarily by the chronic release of inflammatory markers. Expression of matrix metalloproteinases and other proteolytic enzymes leads to the breakdown of vessel walls, producing vascular permeability, edema, cutaneous ulcers, and poor wound healing.[75]

Clinical Presentation

▶ History

Patients typically experience chronic lower extremity edema with progressive overlying skin changes such as skin thickening sometimes progressing to elephantiasis, fibrosis sometimes progressing to bound-down skin of the extremity (i.e., lipodermatosclerosis). Patients usually have discoloration of the skin, typically hyperpigmentation due to postinflammatory pigment changes and/or hemosiderin deposition. Pruritus and/or pain are also frequently present. Inquire about any medical history including a history of congestive heart failure or deep venous thrombosis. Findings typically begin over the medial ankle and may extend to involve the entire lower extremity. The left lower extremity is more commonly involved than the right, but both may be involved.

▶ Physical Examination

Chronic stasis dermatitis typically reveals chronically edematous lower extremities with erythematous, eczematous, and scaling hyperpigmented patches or plaques (Figure 8-20).

Severe chronic stasis dermatitis may present with ulceration (Figure 8-21). Acute stasis dermatitis is often more brightly erythematous with inflammation, weeping, vesicles or bullae, and crusting. In both acute and chronic stasis dermatitis, the medial ankle is most frequently involved but may extend to involve the foot and upward toward the knee. It is often bilateral but may be unilateral as well (left more common than right). The upper extremity is very rarely involved, and typically only when associated with artificial arteriovenous fistulas for hemodialysis.[71]

▶ Laboratory Findings

There are no specific laboratory tests or work-up in stasis dermatitis. The absence of leukocytosis, normal C-reactive protein (CRP), and absence of other infectious markers will help differentiate stasis dermatitis from cellulitis or other skin/soft tissue infection, although these may co-exist. Venous doppler ultrasound is a useful adjunct in ruling in or out venous thromboembolism. Ankle-brachial index may also be indicated to rule out peripheral arterial insufficiency, which may also exist with venous insufficiency, and should be completed prior to the use of compressive therapy.

A skin biopsy is usually not indicated and should be considered carefully, as these patients typically have delayed and poor healing of the lower extremities. If pursued, biopsy reveals dilated blood vessels with extravasated

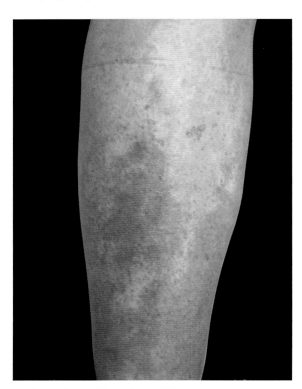

▲ **Figure 8-20.** Stasis dermatitis.

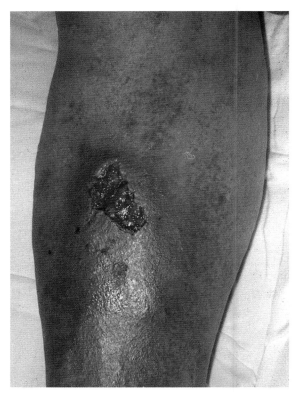

▲ **Figure 8-21** Stasis dermatitis with venous ulcer.

erythrocytes and hemosiderin deposition, parakeratosis, spongiosis, and fibrosis.

Diagnosis

Stasis dermatitis is a clinical diagnosis, although it poses quite a few diagnostic challenges. Routine lab work, particularly a complete blood count can help narrow the differential. Patients with venous insufficiency also have a higher prevalence of contact dermatitis; patch testing is helpful in confirming the accurate diagnosis.[76]

▶ Differential Diagnosis

✓ Cellulitis: Acute stasis dermatitis is most commonly misdiagnosed as cellulitis. Stasis dermatitis is typically bilateral and true bilateral cellulitis is rare. Cellulitis is typically warmer, more painful, and non-pruritic. It is accompanied by leukocytosis, tachycardia, and fever. It should be noted that stasis dermatitis can also be complicated by cellulitis; stasis dermatitis that has a sudden increase in drainage or weeping should have cellulitis considered as a diagnosis.

✓ Cutaneous fungal infections: Tinea corporis may present in circular plaques but these are typically annular (ring-shaped with central clearing). Fungal hyphae can be visualized on a KOH preparation from skin scrapings.

✓ Allergic and irritant contact dermatitis: Allergic and irritant contact dermatitis may be present in areas of stasis dermatitis. Allergic contact dermatitis is diagnosed by patch testing.

✓ Psoriasis: Typically, less pruritic and with increased scale when compared to nummular dermatitis.

✓ Lichen simplex chronicus: Well-defined pruritic lichenified plaques often with associated xerosis or scale. Due to chronic scratching/rubbing.

✓ Pretibial myxedema: Form of mucinosis in the skin almost always associated with Grave's disease characterized by thickened firm non-pitting plaques or nodules on the shins.

✓ Vasculitis: Palpable purpura of the lower extremities.

Management

Chronic stasis dermatitis is managed with diligent skin care and measures to improve venous hypertension. Leg elevation, exercise, and weight reduction along with compression therapy (if no history or findings of arterial disease in the extremity) are the mainstays in managing venous insufficiency. Gentle emollients and cleansers are recommended for symptomatic management.

Acute stasis dermatitis can be treated with topical mid- to high-potency corticosteroids. The course should be limited for 1–2 weeks. Wet dressings are useful to help decrease crusting in exudative dermatitis. Dressings should be saturated in saline or diluted anti-infective or drying solutions (such as aluminum acetate for weeping lesions) and applied 2–3 times daily.

Management should include evaluating for secondary bacterial infection and impetiginized lesions. Mupirocin is the preferred topical antibiotic ointment, if indicated. If signs or symptoms of more extensive skin or soft tissue infection, cultures should be collected in purulence is present. Empiric oral antibiotic coverage should focus on Gram-positive coverage, with an antibiotic such as trimethoprim-sulfamethoxazole or doxycycline.

If venous insufficiency progresses to venous ulcers the patient may require more extensive surgical management and have close follow up on wound care.

Clinical Course and Prognosis

Prognosis in chronic stasis dermatitis is typically prolonged. Diligent management of venous insufficiency improves prognosis significantly.

Indications for Consultation

Consultation is indicated for diagnostic clarity or severe, recalcitrant disease. Referrals to vascular surgery may also be beneficial.

Patient Information Sites

National Eczema Association
    https://nationaleczema.org/eczema/types-of-eczema/stasis-dermatitis/

▼ PHOTODERMATITIS

Introduction

Key points for photodermatitis

✓ *Phototoxicity* is a non-immune mediated response to direct tissue injury induced by a phototoxic agent and UV exposure; *photoallergy* is an immune-mediated reaction to a UVA-modified chemical.

✓ Photodermatitis presents with pruritic erythematous, scaly plaques on sun exposed areas of the face, upper chest, extensor arms and dorsal hands.

✓ Consistent photoprotection with sunscreens and UV protective clothing along with identification and avoidance of the phototoxic agent is important.

Photodermatitis, also referred to as photosensitivity, is an exaggerated response to sunlight, specifically to ultraviolet A (UVA) induced by a topical or systemic sensitizer. Exogenous types of photodermatitis can broadly divided into phototoxicity and photoallergy.[77] There are other varieties of idiopathic or innate photosensitivities, which are not discussed in depth in this section.[77] Phototoxicity is a non-immune mediated response to direct tissue injury induced by a phototoxic agent and UV exposure; photoallergy is an immune-mediated reaction to a UVA-modified chemical.[78] Both may occur in any Fitzpatrick skin type. Photodermatitis is often distinguished by its sun exposed distribution, although the differential includes many other types of dermatitis.

Pathogenesis

Phototoxicity occurs in a dose-dependent manner, depending both on the dose of the sensitizer and UV exposure. Most cases of phototoxicity are induced by systemic medications. Multiple processes may be occurring to predispose the skin to phototoxicity, including generation of reactive oxygen species, DNA cross-linking, activation of the inflammatory cascade, and induction of apoptosis.[78]

Photoallergy is a delayed type IV hypersensitivity in response to both a photoallergen and activation by UVA radiation. With the absorption of UV energy, the photoallergen is transformed to conjugate with a carrier protein and form a complete antigen. As with allergic contact dermatitis, this antigen is then taken up by epidermal Langerhans cells, transported to regional lymph nodes, and presented to T-lymphocytes. Photoallergy occurs when these T-lymphocytes are reactivated in the presence of antigen, circulate to the affected site, and initiate the inflammatory response.

Clinical Presentation

▶ History

Acute phototoxicity develops within hours after exposure to a phototoxic agent and UV radiation. Patients will typically report a burning or stinging sensation. Acute photoallergy presents with a pruritic, eczematous eruption 24–48 h following exposure to a photoallergen and UV radiation. Detailed history taking regarding medications and other possible sensitizers is important in making an accurate diagnosis and in management. The most common medications implicated in phototoxicity are tetracyclines, fluoroquinolones, and sulfonylureas. In photoallergy, hydrochlorothiazide, amiodarone, and chlorpromazine are common culprits. Certain drugs, such as doxycyclines, may cause both phototoxicity and photoallergy.[77]

▶ Physical Examination

Phototoxicity will affect sun-exposed areas and spare protected areas, such as the nasolabial folds, postauricular, submental areas, and areas covered by clothing (Figure 8-22).

Photoallergy may appear very similar to allergic contact dermatitis on physical examination; however, typically can be distinguished by distribution to sun exposed areas. If severe, photoallergy may extend beyond these boundaries,

although will be less severe than exposed regions.[77] Typical findings include erythema and edema and may include vesicles and bullae if severe.

▶ Laboratory Findings

There are no typical lab findings in the diagnostic workup of photodermatitis. If biopsy is indicated and pursued, it typically demonstrates necrotic keratinocytes, epidermal spongiosis, and dermal edema, with epidermal necrosis if severe.[5] Phototesting and photo patch testing are helpful to test for photosensitivity and photoallergic contact dermatitis, respectively.

Diagnosis

History of sun and photosensitizer exposure is important to obtain in making the correct diagnosis. Physical examination and distribution of the eruption also provides useful information regarding the type of photosensitizer involved. A topical photosensitizer will produce lesions only on the exposed areas, whereas a systemic photosensitizer will produce a more widespread eruption. The presence of pruritus may also be helpful to distinguish photoallergy versus phototoxicity.

Phototesting and photopatch testing provide more diagnostic certainty in photoallergy and may be performed under guidance of a dermatologist.[77]

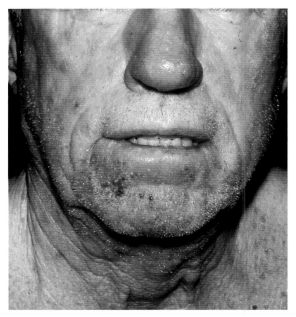

▲ **Figure 8-22.** Sulfamethoxazole-trimethoprim induced phototoxicity. Note sparing of area under nose and in nasolabial folds.

▶ Differential Diagnosis

✓ Allergic contact dermatitis: Similytar appearance but no association with but is not associated with UV light and not in a photodistributed distribution.

✓ Airborne allergic contact dermiatitis: Similar appearance and morphology but occurs only in areas that are exposed to air. Areas that are photoprotected (behind the ears, submental region) regions are affected in airborne contact allergy while these areas would be spared in photoallergic contact dermatitis.

✓ Irritant contact dermatitis: Similar eczematous appearance but no history of photoaggrevation and not in a photodistributed area.

✓ Polymorphous light eruption: Usually pruritic or otherwise uncomfortable rash usually on the forearms. The rash begins in spring and tend to wane over the course of the summer season.

✓ Chronic actinic dermatitis: Eczematous appearing rash typically on the face that is chronic in nature.

✓ Solar urticaria: Wheals which develop rather immediately with exposure to the sun.

Management

The management of photoallergy and phototoxicity is the same. The most important steps are careful and consistent photoprotection along with the identification and avoidance of the phototoxic agent. Guidance on photoprotection includes seeking shaded areas when outdoors, wearing photoprotective clothing (sleeves, pants, and hat), and sunscreen.[79] Broad-spectrum sunscreens with a high SPF (sun protective factor, 50+) are most effective and should be reapplied frequently. Mineral-based sunscreen and those tinted with iron oxides can protect from the most rays of light. If not easily identified, referral to dermatology for patch testing may be helpful. For those with photosensitivity, taking the oral supplement with *Polypodium leucotomos* can decrease one's sensitivity to the sun; it is *not*, however, a substitute for sunscreen but can act as an adjunct for certain patients.

Further management includes topical steroids, although systemic corticosteroids may be considered if severe.[77] There is discussion regarding the role of vitamin D supplementation in patients prone to photodermatitis, although data is limited.[77]

Clinical Course and Prognosis

Clinical course is typically limited in photodermatitis, although persistent hyperpigmentation may occur. Prognosis is otherwise favorable, particularly if the causative sensitizer is identified and careful sun protection is followed.

Indications for Consultation

Consultation to dermatology is indicated for diagnostic clarity or in severe, refractory cases.

Patient Information Sites

Mount Sinai Medical Center
https://www.mountsinai.org/health-library/condition/photodermatitis

▼ OCCUPATIONAL DERMATITIS

Occupational dermatitis is inflammation of the skin caused by the work environment. It accounts for 90% of all work-related skin diseases. Most cases (80%) are due to irritant contact dermatitis with the minority (20%) being due to allergic contact dermatitis. Acute, subacute, and chronic forms of dermatoses can all be a result of occupational exposures. Irritants in occupational contact dermatitis can come in many forms from substances contacting the skin directly or via the air (Table 8-7), or from mechanical forces, such as repetitive movements, friction, and vibration. Low humidity and cold temperatures can exacerbate these dermatoses. Hands are the primary site of involvement in occupational dermatitis. For the correct

Table 8-7. Common occupational skin irritants and allergens.

Common Occupational Skin Irritants
Water (especially wet work)
Soap, detergents, cleansers
Acids and alkalais
Solvents
Plants
Plastics and Resins
Metals
Particles (sand, fiberglass, sawdust)
Common Occupational Contact Allergens
Metals (especially nickel, cobalt, chromium)
Rubber accelerators (thiurams, carbamates, benzothiazoles, dialkyl thioureas)
Plastics and resins (bisphenol A, colophony)
Preservatives (formaldehyde and its releasers [quaternium-15, imidazolidinyl urea, diazolidinyl urea, bronopol, DMDM hydantoin], methylisothiazolinone/methylchloroisothiazolinone
Hair dyes (paraphenylenediamine)
Fragrances
Plants (compositae, sesquiterpene lactones, urushiol from poison ivy family of plants [*Toxicodendron*])

identification of occupational dermatoses, Mathias[80] has put forth criteria; if four of the criteria area present, occupational dermatitis is probable:

- Clinical appearance consistent with contact dermatitis.
- Workplace exposure to potential cutaneous irritants or allergens.
- Anatomical distribution consistent with cutaneous exposure related to the job.
- Temporal relationship between exposure and onset consistent with contact dermatitis.
- Nonoccupational exposures excluded as likely causes.
- Removal from exposure leads to improvement of dermatitis.
- Patch or provocation tests implicate a specific workplace exposure.

REFERENCES

1. Rashid RS, Shim TN. Contact dermatitis. *BMJ.* 2016;353:i3299.
2. Cashman MW, Reutemann PA, Ehrlich A. Contact dermatitis in the United States: epidemiology, economic impact, and workplace prevention. *Dermatol Clin.* 2012;30(1):87–98, viii.
3. Litchman G, Nair PA, Atwater AR, Bhutta BS. Contact Dermatitis. In: *StatPearls.* StatPearls Publishing; 2020.
4. Warshaw E, Lee G, Storrs FJ. Hand dermatitis: a review of clinical features, therapeutic options, and long-term outcomes. *Am J Contact Dermat.* 2003;14(3):119–137.
5. Kang S, Amagai M, Bruckner AL, et al. *Fitzpatrick's Dermatology in General Medicine.* 9th edition. McGraw-Hill. 2019.
6. Zug KA , Warshaw EM, et al. North American contact dermatitis group 2005-2006 patch test results . *Dermatitis.* 2009;20(3):149–160.
7. Kalish RS. Recent developments in the pathogenesis of allergic contact dermatitis. *Arch Dermatol.* 1991;127(10): 1558–1563.
8. Kadyk DL, McCarter K, Achen F, Belsito DV. Quality of life in patients with allergic contact dermatitis. *J Am Acad Dermatol.* 2003;49(6):1037–1048.
9. Holness DL, Nethercott JR. Is a worker's understanding of their diagnosis an important determinant of outcome in occupational contact dermatitis? *Contact Dermatitis.* 1991;25(5):296–301.
10. Veien NK, Hattel T, Laurberg G. Hand eczema: causes, course, and prognosis II. *Contact Dermatitis.* 2008;58(6):335–339.
11. Adisesh A, Meyer JD, Cherry NM. Prognosis and work absence due to occupational contact dermatitis. *Contact Dermatitis.* 2002;46(5):273–279.
12. Eichenfield LF, Tom WL, Chamlin SL, et al. Guidelines of care for the management of atopic dermatitis. *J Am Acad Dermatol.* 2014;70(2):338–351.
13. Kelsay K, Klinnert M, Bender B. Addressing psychosocial aspects of atopic dermatitis. *Immunol Allergy Clin North Am.* 2010;30(3):385–396.
14. Chamlin SL, Cella D, Frieden IJ, et al. Development of the Childhood Atopic Dermatitis Impact Scale: initial validation of a quality-of-life measure for young children with atopic dermatitis and their families. *J Invest Dermatol.* 2005;125(6):1106–1111.
15. Irvine AD, McLean WH, Leung DY. Filaggrin mutations associated with skin and allergic diseases. *N Engl J Med.* 2011;365(14):1315–1327.
16. O'Regan GM, Sandilands A, McLean WHI, Irvine AD. Filaggrin in atopic dermatitis. *J Allergy Clin Immunol.* 2009;124(3):R2–R6
17. Rodríguez E, Baurecht H, Herberich E, et al. Meta-analysis of filaggrin polymorphisms in eczema and asthma: Robust risk factors in atopic disease. *J Allergy Clin Immunol.* 2009;123(6):1361–1370.e7.
18. van den Oord RAHM, Sheikh A. Filaggrin gene defects and risk of developing allergic sensitisation and allergic disorders: systematic review and meta-analysis. *BMJ.* 2009;339:b2433–b2433.
19. Palmer CNA, Irvine AD, Terron-Kwiatkowski A, et al. Common loss-of-function variants of the epidermal barrier protein filaggrin are a major predisposing factor for atopic dermatitis. *Nat Genet.* 2006;38(4):441–446.
20. Chang J, Mitra N, Hoffstad O, Margolis DJ. Association of filaggrin loss of function and thymic stromal lymphopoietin variation with treatment use in pediatric atopic dermatitis. *J Am Acad Dermatol.* 2017;153(3):275.
21. Broccardo CJ, Mahaffey S, Schwarz J, et al. Comparative proteomic profiling of patients with atopic dermatitis based on history of eczema herpeticum infection and Staphylococcus aureus colonization. *J Allergy Clin Immunol.* 2011;127(1): 186–19411.
22. De Benedetto A, Rafaels NM, McGirt LY, et al. Tight junction defects in patients with atopic dermatitis. *J Allergy Clin Immunol.* 2011;127(3):773–786.e1-7.
23. Portelli MA, Hodge E, Sayers I. Genetic risk factors for the development of allergic disease identified by genome-wide association. *Clin Exp Allergy.* 2015;45(1):21–31.
24. Saunders SP, Goh CSM, Brown SJ, et al. Tmem79/Matt is the matted mouse gene and is a predisposing gene for atopic dermatitis in human subjects. *J Allergy Clin Immunol.* 2013;132(5):1121–1129.
25. Kuo I-H, Yoshida T, De Benedetto A, Beck LA. The cutaneous innate immune response in patients with atopic dermatitis. *J Allergy Clin Immunol.* 2013;131(2):266–278.
26. Kuo I-H, Carpenter-Mendini A, Yoshida T, et al. Activation of epidermal toll-like receptor 2 enhances tight junction function: implications for atopic dermatitis and skin barrier repair. *J Invest Dermatol.* 2013;133(4):988–998.
27. De Benedetto A, Agnihothri R, McGirt LY, Bankova LG, Beck LA. Atopic dermatitis: a disease caused by innate immune defects? *J Invest Dermatol.* 2009;129(1):14–30.
28. Leung DYM, Guttman-Yassky E. Deciphering the complexities of atopic dermatitis: shifting paradigms in treatment approaches. *J Allergy Clin Immunol.* 2014;134(4):769–779.
29. Roll A, Cozzio A, Fischer B, et al. Microbial colonization and atopic dermatitis. *Curr Opin Allergy Clin Immunol.* 2004;4(5):373–378.
30. Grey K, Maguiness S. Atopic Dermatitis: Update for Pediatricians. *Pediatr Ann.* 2016;45(8):e280–e286.
31. Nikkels AF, Pièrard GE. Treatment of mucocutaneous presentations of herpes simplex virus infections. *Am J Clin Dermatol.* 2002;3(7):475–487.
32. Grimalt R, Mengeaud V, Cambazard F. The steroid-sparing effect of an emollient therapy in infants with atopic dermatitis: a randomized controlled study. *Dermatology.* 2007;214(1):61–67.

33. Hong E, Smith S, Fischer G. Evaluation of the atrophogenic potential of topical corticosteroids in pediatric dermatology patients. *Pediatr Dermatol.* 2011;28(4):393–396.

34. Breneman D, Fleischer AB, Abramovits W, et al. Intermittent therapy for flare prevention and long-term disease control in stabilized atopic dermatitis: A randomized comparison of 3-times-weekly applications of tacrolimus ointment versus vehicle. *J Am Acad Dermatol.* 2008;58(6):990–999.

35. Siegfried E, Jaworski C, Hebert J. Topical calcineurin inhibitors and lymphoma risk: evidence update with implications for daily practice. *Am J Clin Dermatol.* 2013;14(3):163–178.

36. Paller AS, Tom WL, Lebwohl MG, et al. Efficacy and safety of crisaborole ointment, a novel, nonsteroidal phosphodiesterase 4 (PDE4) inhibitor for the topical treatment of atopic dermatitis (AD) in children and adults. *J Am Acad Dermatol.* 2016;75(3):494–503.e6.

37. Ahmed A, Solman L, Williams HC. Magnitude of benefit for topical crisaborole in the treatment of atopic dermatitis in children and adults does not look promising: a critical appraisal. *Br J Dermatol.* 2018;178(3):659–662.

38. Blauvelt A, de Bruin-Weller M, Gooderham M, et al. Long-term management of moderate-to-severe atopic dermatitis with dupilumab and concomitant topical corticosteroids (LIBERTY AD CHRONOS): a 1-year, randomised, double-blinded, placebo-controlled, phase 3 trial. *Lancet.* 2017;389(10086):2287–2303.

39. Deleuran M, Thaçi D, Beck LA, et al. Dupilumab shows long-term safety and efficacy in patients with moderate to severe atopic dermatitis enrolled in a phase 3 open-label extension study. *J Am Acad Dermatol.* 2020;82(2):377–388.

40. Beattie PE, Lewis-Jones MS. A comparative study of impairment of quality of life in children with skin disease and children with other chronic childhood diseases. *Br J Dermatol.* 2006;155(1):145–151.

41. Mortz CG, Andersen KE, Dellgren C, Barington T, Bindslev-Jensen C. Atopic dermatitis from adolescence to adulthood in the TOACS cohort: prevalence, persistence and comorbidities. *Allergy.* 2015;70(7):836–845.

42. Burr ML, Dunstan FDJ, Hand S, Ingram JR, Jones KP. The natural history of eczema from birth to adult life: a cohort study. *Br J Dermatol.* 2013;168(6):1339–1342.

43. Thorsteinsdottir S, Stokholm J, Thyssen JP, et al. Genetic, clinical, and environmental factors associated with persistent atopic dermatitis in childhood. *J Am Acad Dermatol.* 2019;155(1):50–57.

44. Thomsen SF. Epidemiology and nuatral history of atopic diseases. Eur Clinc Respir J. 2015;2:eCollection 2015.

45. Rystedt I. Prognostic factors in atopic dermatitis. *Acta Derm Venereol.* 1985;65(3):206–213.

46. Katoh N, Hirano S, Kishimoto S. Prognostic factor of adult patients with atopic dermatitis. *J Dermatol.* 2008;35(8):477–483.

47. Chen M-H, Su T-P, Chen Y-S, et al. Is atopy in early childhood a risk factor for ADHD and ASD? a longitudinal study. *J Psychosom Res.* 2014;77(4):316–321.

48. Patel KR, Immaneni S, Singam V, Rastogi S, Silverberg JI. Association between atopic dermatitis, depression, and suicidal ideation: A systematic review and meta-analysis. *J Am Acad Dermatol.* 2019;80(2):402–410.

49. Broberg A, Kalimo K, Lindblad B, Swanbeck G. Parental education in the treatment of childhood atopic eczema. *Acta Derm Venereol.* 1990;70(6):495–499.

50. Staab D, von Rueden U, Kehrt R, et al. Evaluation of a parental training program for the management of childhood atopic dermatitis. *Pediatr Allergy Immunol.* 2002;13(2):84–90.

51. Bonamonte D, Foti C, Vestita M, Ranieri LD, Angelini G. Nummular eczema and contact allergy: a retrospective study. *Dermatitis.* 2012;23(4):153–157.

52. Krupa Shankar DS, Shrestha S. Relevance of patch testing in patients with nummular dermatitis. *Indian J Dermatol Venereol Leprol.* 2005;71(6):406–408.

53. Khurana S, Jain VK, Aggarwal K, Gupta S. Patch testing in discoid eczema. *J Dermatol.* 2002;29(12):763–767.

54. Schena D, Papagrigoraki A, Girolomoni G. Sensitizing potential of triclosan and triclosan-based skin care products in patients with chronic eczema. *Dermatol Ther.* 2008;21 Suppl 2:S35–38.

55. Aoyama H, Tanaka M, Hara M, Tabata N, Tagami H. Nummular eczema: An addition of senile xerosis and unique cutaneous reactivities to environmental aeroallergens. *Dermatology.* 1999;199(2):135–139.

56. Truong A, Le S, Kiuru M, Maverakis E. Nummular dermatitis on guselkumab for palmoplantar psoriasis. *Dermatol Ther.* 2019;32(4):e12954.

57. Lofgren SM, Warshaw EM. Dyshidrosis: epidemiology, clinical characteristics, and therapy. *Dermatitis.* 2006;17(4):165–181.

58. de Boer EM, Bruynzeel DP, van Ketel WG. Dyshidrotic eczema as an occupational dermatitis in metal workers. *Contact Dermatitis.* 1988;19(3):184–188.

59. Jain VK, Aggarwal K, Passi S, Gupta S. Role of contact allergens in pompholyx. *J Dermatol.* 2004;31(3):188–193.

60. Lodi A, Betti R, Chiarelli G, Urbani CE, Crosti C. Epidemiological, clinical and allergological observations on pompholyx. *Contact Dermatitis.* 1992;26(1):17–21.

61. Chen J-J, Liang Y-H, Zhou F-S, et al. The gene for a rare autosomal dominant form of pompholyx maps to chromosome 18q22.1-18q22.3. *J Invest Dermatol.* 2006;126(2):300–304.

62. Pitché P, Boukari M, Tchangai-Walla K. Factors associated with palmoplantar or plantar pompholyx: a case-control study. *Ann Dermatol Venereol.* 2006;133:139.

63. Guillet MH, Wierzbicka E, Guillet S, Dagregorio G, Guillet G. A 3-year causative study of pompholyx in 120 patients. *Arch Dermatol.* 2007;143(12):1504–1508.

64. Veien NK. Restriction of nickel intake in the treatment of nickel-sensitive patients. *Curr Probl Dermatol.* 1991;20:203–214.

65. Zeidler C, Yosipovitch G, Ständer S. Prurigo nodularis and its management. *Dermatol Clin.* 2018;36(3):189–197.

66. Saco M, Cohen G. Prurigo nodularis: Picking the right treatment. *J Fam Pract.* 2015;64(4):221–226.

67. Dazzi C, Erma D, Piccinno R, Veraldi S, Caccialanza M. Psychological factors involved in prurigo nodularis: A pilot study. *J Dermatol Treat.* 2011;22(4):211–214.

68. Elmariah S Kim B, Berger T *et al.* Practical approaches for diagnosis and management of prurigo nodularis: United States expert panel consensus. *J Am Acad Dermatol* 2021;84:747–760.

69. Sundaresan S, Migden MR, Silapunt S. Stasis dermatitis: Pathophysiology, evaluation, and management. *Am J Clin Dermatol.* 2017;18(3):383–390.

70. Sippel K, Mayer D, Ballmer B, et al. Evidence that venous hypertension causes stasis dermatitis. *Phlebology.* 2011;26(8):361–365.

71. Deguchi E, Imafuku S, Nakayama J. Ulcerating stasis dermatitis of the forearm due to arteriovenous fistula: a case report and review of the published work. *J Dermatol*. 2010;37(6): 550–553.

72. Beebe-Dimmer JL, Pfeifer JR, Engle JS, Schottenfeld D. The epidemiology of chronic venous insufficiency and varicose veins. *Ann Epidemiol*. 2005;15(3):175–184.

73. Browse NL. The etiology of venous ulceration. *World J Surg*. 1986;10(6):938–943.

74. Sansilvestri-Morel P, Rupin A, Badier-Commander C, et al. Imbalance in the synthesis of collagen type I and collagen type III in smooth muscle cells derived from human varicose veins. *J Vasc Res*. 2001;38(6):560–568.

75. Herouy Y, May AE, Pornschlegel G, et al. Lipodermatosclerosis is characterized by elevated expression and activation of matrix metalloproteinases: implications for venous ulcer formation. *J Invest Dermatol*. 1998;111(5):822–827.

76. Erfurt-Berge C, Geier J, Mahler V. The current spectrum of contact sensitization in patients with chronic leg ulcers or stasis dermatitis - new data from the Information Network of Departments of Dermatology (IVDK). *Contact Dermatitis*. 2017;77(3):151–158.

77. Coffin SL, Turrentine JE, Cruz PD. Photodermatitis for the Allergist. *Curr Allergy Asthma Rep*. 2017;17(6):36.

78. Kerr A, Ferguson J. Photoallergic contact dermatitis. *Photodermatol Photoimmunol Photomed*. 2010;26(2):56–65.

79. Jansen R, Osterwalder U, Wang SQ, Burnett M, Lim HW. Photoprotection: part II. Sunscreen: development, efficacy, and controversies. *J Am Acad Dermatol*. 2013;69(6):867.e1-14; 881–882.

80. Mathias CGT. Contact dermatitis and workers' compensation: criteria for establishing occupational causation and aggravation. *J Am Acad Dermatol*. 1989;20:842–8.

Psoriasis and Other Papulosquamous Diseases

Jing Liu

INTRODUCTION TO CHAPTER

Psoriasis, seborrheic dermatitis, pityriasis rosea, and lichen planus are diseases that present with papulosquamous lesions (scaly papules and plaques). Although these diseases may have a similar morphology, their underlying etiologies vary. Secondary syphilis, cutaneous T cell lymphomas, and connective tissue disease may also present with papulosquamous lesions and should be included in the differential diagnosis.

PSORIASIS

Introduction

Key points for psoriasis

- ✓ Psoriasis is a common, chronic inflammatory disease that typically presents with scaly red to salmon pink plaques on the elbows, knees, scalp, lower back, and gluteal cleft.
- ✓ About 1/3 of patients with psoriasis will develop psoriatic arthritis during their lifetime.
- ✓ Cardiometabolic disease, gastrointestinal diseases, kidney disease, and mood disorders are common comorbidities in patients with psoriasis.
- ✓ Most patients with mild to moderate psoriasis can be managed with topical medications and/or phototherapy.

Psoriasis is a common, chronic, inflammatory, immune-mediated disease. Clinicians and patients have long been vexed by this ancient affliction. Although most medical literature prior to Willan (1757–1812) lumped psoriasis, leprosy, eczema, and other inflammatory dermatoses into a confusing menagerie, Celsus gave a convincing account of psoriasis vulgaris almost 2,000 years ago. His description included many of the morphologic features that physicians today utilize to diagnose psoriasis, including: the "ruddy" or salmon-colored plaques with silvery scales that often are associated with punctate hemorrhage or "erosions" when removed.[1]

More than 7.5 million adults (2.1% of the population) in the United States are affected and 30% of these individuals will develop psoriatic arthritis.[2] About 1.5 million patients are considered to have moderate to severe disease.

Psoriasis may have a significant negative impact on the patient's quality of life. Patients often are self-conscious, depressed, or frustrated over the appearance of their skin. Studies have found that between 5 and 10% of psoriasis patients suffer from depression, anxiety, and other mental health comorbidities.[3]

Psoriasis spans all socio-economic groups, and its prevalence varies by geographic location. Historically, the disease is more common in the northern latitudes. The rate of psoriatic disease is lower in African-Americans compared to European-Americans.[2]

Pathogenesis

The primary cause of psoriasis is dysregulation of the cell mediated, adaptive immune response, but a genetic predisposition along with environmental triggers are also postulated to play a role. A positive family history for psoriasis can be found in 35% of patients[4] and HLA-Cw6 is a well-researched gene implicated in psoriasis.

The dysregulation seen in psoriasis is likely triggered by hyperactivity of the innate immunological surveillance system to environmental antigens. In genetically predisposed individuals, the Th1 pathway response is over-stimulated and this overproduction of Th1 related cytokines along with interleukin -12, 17, and 23 causes hyper-proliferation of epidermal keratinocytes. These events lead to the formation of the psoriatic plaques.[5]

In the pediatric population, IL 22 was found to be more elevated in psoriatic plaques compared to adults.[6] Several environmental factors may interact with polygenic inheritance patterns and account for the variable expression of psoriatic disease. Some of these factors are postulated to be streptococcal pharyngitis (guttate psoriasis), stressful life events, low humidity, Human Immunodeficiency Virus (HIV), trauma, medications, cold climates, and obesity. Diets high in fish oils seem to be protective against the development of psoriasis.[2,4]

Clinical Presentation

▶ History

Most patients with mild to moderate psoriasis are asymptomatic, but pruritus is common in patients with severe or widespread disease. Psoriasis can initially present at any age, but onset typically occurs within a bimodal age distribution of ages 18–39 and ages 50–69 years.[4] Patients may give a history of joint pain and swelling, especially in the fingers and toes.

▶ Physical Examination

Psoriasis can vary in appearance and distribution. However, there are clues in the physical examination that allow the clinician to properly diagnose psoriasis and identify its subtypes.

- *Plaque-type psoriasis vulgaris* accounts for 90% of all cases. The primary lesion is a scaly, red to salmon pink-colored papule that expands centrifugally to form a similarly colored plaque (Figure 9-1). It is usually covered by a white or silvery scale that, when removed, may show pinpoint bleeding (Auspitz sign). The border may be red and with time central clearing may occur, with the plaques taking on an annular or arcuate configuration. Plaque-type psoriasis is usually on extensor surfaces such as the knees and elbows (Figure 9-2), and often involves the gluteal cleft, lumbosacral region and the umbilicus. Psoriasis may also affect the scalp (Figure 9-3). Psoriatic plaques may occur in an area after trauma, pressure, or injury. This is known as the Koebner phenomenon.

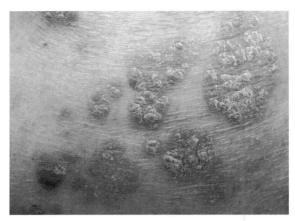

▲ **Figure 9-1.** Psoriasis. Pink plaques with silver white scale. Note small area of bleeding in plaque with scale removed.

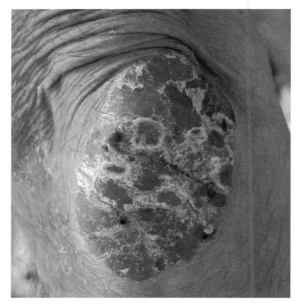

▲ **Figure 9-2.** Psoriasis. Red plaque on elbow with scale partially resolved after treatment with topical steroids.

- *Inverse psoriasis* presents with thin pink plaques with minimal scale in the axillae (Figure 9-4), inguinal and inframammary area and in body folds of the trunk. It may occur in conjunction with typical plaque psoriasis or it may be the only manifestation of psoriasis.
- *Guttate psoriasis* occurs in less than 2% of cases, but it is a common psoriatic subtype in young adults. It is characterized by small "droplet-like" thin pink to

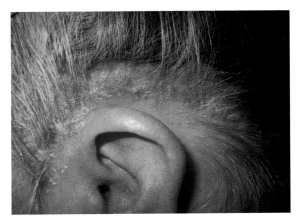

▲ **Figure 9-3.** Scalp psoriasis. Pink plaque with white scale along the hairline above the ear.

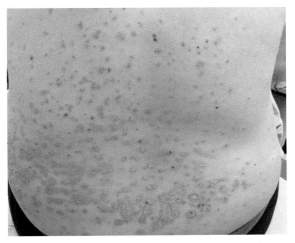

▲ **Figure 9-5.** Guttate psoriasis. Pink papules and plaques with fine white scale.

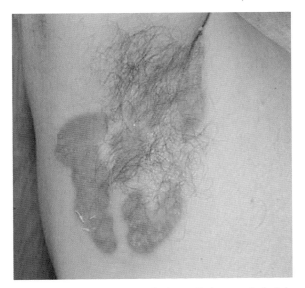

▲ **Figure 9-4.** Inverse psoriasis. Well demarcated pink plaques with no scale in axilla.

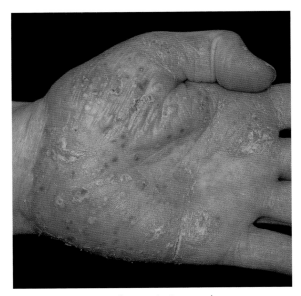

▲ **Figure 9-6.** Pustular psoriasis on palm. Erythematous plaque with pustules.

salmon-colored papules and plaques surmounted by a fine, white scale (Figure 9-5). The distribution is often similar to that of classic pityriasis rosea, favoring the trunk, abdomen, upper thighs, and fading toward the acral surfaces and sparing the palms and soles.

- *Pustular psoriasis* is an acute variant of the disease that presents with small, monomorphic sterile pustules surmounting painful, inflamed, and erythematous papules. Fever, systemic symptoms, and an elevated white blood cell count often accompany generalized pustular psoriasis. Acral pustules, usually without systemic symptoms, characterize palmoplantar pustulosis

(Figure 9-6) which is a milder, but more common presentation of pustular psoriasis.

- *Erythrodermic psoriasis* is a skin reaction pattern of total body redness and desquamation of the skin. There are many causes of erythroderma and it is not specific to psoriasis. The massive shedding of skin that occurs during an erythrodermic flare of psoriasis can result in infection, hypothermia, protein loss, hypoalbuminemia, dehydration, and electrolyte disturbances.[4]

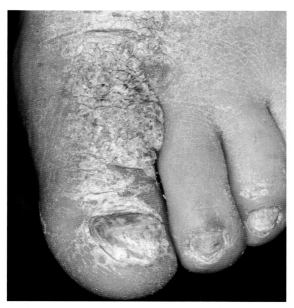

▲ **Figure 9-7.** Psoriasis with nail dystrophy. Thick scaly plaque on great toe with thick, discolored nail plate.

- *Psoriatic nails* can be seen in up to 50% of patients with psoriasis. It may be the only manifestation of psoriasis. It is recognized that nail disease is more closely linked with psoriatic joint disease. Up to 90% of patients with psoriasis have nail disease.[4] Nail dystrophies associated with psoriasis include pitting, onycholysis (nail plate separation), oil spots (yellow-orange subungual discoloration), thickening, and subungual debris (Figure 9-7). Splinter hemorrhages may also be present.

Laboratory Findings

Blood work is generally not necessary to make a diagnosis of psoriasis. Pustular flares of psoriasis during pregnancy may be associated with hypocalcemia. A biopsy is often helpful if the diagnosis is unclear. A punch biopsy of a plaque or pustule often supports the diagnosis. A biopsy is warranted in any patient not responding as expected to conventional therapy. The microscopic findings of common plaque-type psoriasis are epidermal hyperplasia, parakeratosis, thinning of the granular layer, epidermal infiltration of neutrophils and occasional "Munro's abscesses" (intraepithelial collections of neutrophils).

Diagnosis

The key diagnostic clinical features of plaque psoriasis are red to pink plaques with silver white scale present on the elbows, knees, scalp, and lower back and legs.

Table 9-1 Differential diagnosis of diseases presenting with papulosquamous lesions.

Diseases	Clinical Presentation
Psoriasis	Asymptomatic or mildly pruritic, pink-red plaques with white scale on scalp and extensor extremities. Bimodal age of onset at 22 and 55 years old.
Seborrheic dermatitis	Asymptomatic or mildly pruritic pink patches with fine greasy white scale on the scalp, eyebrows, ears, nasolabial folds and central chest. More common in infants or after age 40.
Pityriasis rosea	Asymptomatic 1–2 cm oval thin plaques with a fine central scale, larger 2–10 cm "herald patch" may precede rash. Lasts 6–8 weeks. More common in teens and young adults.
Nummular dermatitis	Pruritic well defined pink scaly plaques on extremities but not necessarily on elbows and knees.
Lichen planus	Pruritic violaceous flat-topped papules on volar wrists, forearms, ankles and lower back.
Subacute cutaneous lupus	Uncommon. Annular erythematous scaly plaques in sun exposed areas on trunk.
Tinea corporis	Asymptomatic or mildly pruritic pink scaly plaques with a scaly border and central clearing.
Secondary syphilis	Asymptomatic scaly papules or plaques on palms, soles and trunk. History of preceding genital ulcer.
Cutaneous T cell lymphoma (mycosis fungoides)	Uncommon. Asymptomatic or mildly pruritic scaly well-defined plaques with random distribution. Lesions may also be annular or arcuate and are chronic and persist in the same location. Typically presents after age 50.

Differential Diagnosis

√ The differential diagnosis of psoriasis includes other papulosquamous diseases (Table 9-1).

Management of Cutaneous Psoriasis in Adults

- *Topical steroids* are the first line treatment of mild to moderate psoriasis. They act as a foundation on which a therapeutic regimen is developed for more severe diseases. While topical regimens demonstrate efficacy in clinical trials, the response to these agents in everyday practice is often not impressive. Frequently, this is a result of poor compliance. Ointments are the most

Table 9-2 Examples of topical medications for psoriasis

Generic Name	Formulations	Uses
Clobetasol	cream, gel, ointment, solution, foam, shampoo 0.05%.	Super to high potency steroids for use on localized areas of thick plaques on extremities and trunk twice a day initially for 2-4 weeks and then alternate with calcipotriene or calcitrol. Use solutions and foams and/or shampoos for scalp.
Betamethasone dipropionate	cream, gel ointment, solution 0.05%.	
Fluocinonide	cream, ointment 0.05%.	
Triamcinolone	cream, ointment 0.1%.	Mid potency steroid for chronic use to widespread plaques on extremities and trunk twice a day.
Desonide	cream, ointment 0.05%.	Low potency steroids for use on psoriasis face, groin, axillae in adults or psoriasis in children twice a day.
Hydrocortisone	Cream, ointment 2.5%, 1%.	
Tacrolimus	Ointment 0.03% 0.1%.	Psoriasis on face, axillae, groin and genitals twice a day.
Pimecrolimus	Cream 1 %.	
Calcipotriol	Cream, solution 0.005%.	Typically used in combination therapy with topical steroids in adults. Weekly dose should not exceed 100 g.
calcitriol	Ointment.	
Calcipotriene + Betamethasone dipropionate	Ointment, suspension, spray.	For use in adults >18 years old for up to 4 weeks. Should not be used on face, axillae or groin. Weekly dose should not exceed 100 g.
Tazarotene	Cream, gel 0.05%, 0.1%.	For use on thick plaques in adults in combination with topical steroids. Pregnancy category X.
Salicylic acid	Gel 3%, 6%; Solution 3%, shampoo 3%. Ointment 10%.	For use in thick plaques in combination with topical steroids.

effective vehicles for psoriasis, but they can stain clothing and bedding. Creams are better patient-accepted vehicles for the face, neck, and hands. Solutions and foams are appropriate for the scalp. Table 9-2 contains commonly used topical medications for psoriasis.

It is often advisable to begin therapy with one simple agent. In plaque-type psoriasis which covers limited areas of the body, super-potent topical steroids, such as clobetasol or betamethasone are usually necessary to treat thick plaques.[7] Scalp disease often requires ultra-potent steroids in solution or foam vehicles. A simple regimen utilizing topical clobetasol 0.05% or betamethasone 0.05% twice a day for 2–4 weeks is an easy way to achieve control of disease. A less potent topical steroid and more cost-effective agent such as triamcinolone, when utilized regularly, may be more effective than intermittent use of high potency topical steroids. In areas of thin skin such as the face, neck, axillae, groin, genitals, and body folds, class lower potency steroids such as hydrocortisone 2.5%, desonide 0.05%, and hydrocortisone valerate 2.5% should be used.[7]

After finding the preferred vehicle and topical regimen for a patient, closely spaced follow-up visits improve adherence and will provide the clinician an opportunity to encourage continued compliance, and fine tune the regimen based on the patient's condition.

- *Topical vitamin D analogs,* such as calcipotriol, calcipotriene, or calcitriol can be used in patients who do not respond to the use of monotherapy with topical steroids.[8] These medications can be alternated by day (vitamin D analog Monday through Thursday and clobetasol Friday through Sunday) or by application (vitamin D analog in morning and clobetasol at bedtime). Topical vitamin D analogs may cause hypercalcemia; therefore the weekly dose should be under 100 mg.

- *Topical calcineurin-inhibiting agents* are also quite useful for treatment of psoriasis.[8] Tacrolimus ointment (0.1% for adults, 0.03% for children) may sting temporarily after application but seems to have slightly more efficacy than topical pimecrolimus. Because these medications are not corticosteroids, they do not cause skin atrophy, glaucoma, or many other steroid-related side effects. Thus, they are an effective and safe way to treat psoriasis on the face, in the skin folds, and around the eyes. In the United States, these medications are Food and Drug Administration (FDA) approved only for atopic dermatitis.

- *Tazarotene* (gel or cream, 0.05% or 0.1%) is a retinoid. It can be used as a steroid-sparing agent in a manner similar to the vitamin D analogs, but this agent tends to cause more inflammation than calcipotriene. Therefore, patients may find that tazarotene fits best into their regimen when applied in conjunction with topical steroids. Tazarotene is in pregnancy category X.

- *Keratolytic topical products* can be used in the setting of hyperkeratotic, scaly plaques to remove scale and facilitate penetration of a topical steroid and/or vitamin D analog. Salicylic acid, urea, and lactic acid are agents that can be added to a regimen for this purpose. Salicylic acid comes as a cream, gel, ointment, or shampoo in concentrations that range from 2% to 10%.

- *Topical coal tar products* have an anti-inflammatory effect in psoriasis and can be used in conjunction with topics steroids and keratolytic agents. Several brands of nonprescription coal tar shampoos are available.

- *Emollients* may aid treatment of psoriasis. They can improve efficacy and lower the economic burden of other topical agents by softening the stratum corneum through hydration and reduction of superficial scale. A daily bath in warm water, followed by application of petrolatum and supplemented by two or three further applications of a moisturizer during the day is a beneficial addition to any treatment regimen.

- Narrowband ultraviolet B (UVB) phototherapy for moderate and severe psoriasis, is a safe and effective treatment especially when paired with topical treatments[9]. Phototherapy utilizes the anti-inflammatory effects of ultraviolet radiation, however here the difference is that a specific wavelength of ultraviolet radiation is used that is considered safe with minimal risk of developing skin cancer.[9] These treatments are often done 2–3 times per week and are continued as needed. These are usually done in dermatology clinics.

- *Oral medications* may be prescribed by dermatologists for psoriasis that does not respond to topical therapy or UVB phototherapy. These include acitretin and immunomodulating therapies such as, methotrexate, apremilast, and cyclosporine[9]. Acitretin is an oral retinoid that helps to normalize keratinocyte turnover. Adverse effects include xerosis, elevated liver function tests, hyperlipidemia, and hair loss. Acitretin is contraindicated in women of childbearing age due to risk of teratogenicity.

- *Biologic agents* for psoriasis can be used in some patients with psoriatic arthritis and moderate to severe psoriasis who have not been controlled with topical therapy and/or phototherapy. These medications are usually prescribed and monitored by dermatologists and/or rheumatologists. They are typically self-administered by patients using various injection devices.

Biologic agents block specific parts of the inflammatory pathways in psoriasis resulting in significant clearing of psoriatic lesions within months of use. The most commonly used agents are tumor necrosis factor (TNF-α) inhibitors and agents that block interleukins (IL 12 and 23 or IL 17-A). Table 9-3 reviews certain features of some biologic agents.

The American Academy of Dermatology and the National Psoriasis Foundation published detailed guidelines in 2019 covering the use of biologics in psoriasis.[10] They recommend the following baseline testing before the use of biologic agents: complete blood count (CBC) with differential, complete metabolic profile, test for tuberculosis (TB) such as Quantiferon Gold with follow-up chest radiograph if TB test is positive, serologic tests for hepatitis B and C and HIV testing depending on patient's risk factors. Patients on biologic agents require regular follow-up visits and laboratory monitoring that varies with the agent used and the patient's history.

Several new biologic agents for psoriasis have been FDA approved and new agents are being developed. Also, other classes of medications such as Janus kinase (JAK) inhibitors and small molecule agents which modulate proinflammatory cytokines are some evolving options for treatment of psoriasis.

Management of Pediatric Psoriasis

There is a dearth of evidence regarding treatment of psoriatic disease in children. The lack of good, double-blinded, placebo-controlled trials is not specific to psoriasis treatment, but it does make predicting the future consequences of one's therapeutic decisions in this population quite murky. Most of the principles discussed above with regard to adults still hold for the pediatric population. In the pediatric population one must, of course, consider long-term side effects due to lengthy exposure to immuno-modulators. There's emerging evidence for safety and efficacy for use of biologics in treating psoriasis in pediatric population.[11]

Psoriatic Arthritis

Every patient with psoriasis should be specifically screened for joint disease and enthesitis[4] (inflammation of the tendon insertions). History of morning stiffness, joint tenderness, swelling, sausage digits, and involvement of the peripheral small joints is characteristic (Table 9.4). The hands are the most common site of involvement. Enthesitis usually occurs at the insertion sites of the Achilles tendon, the plantar fascia and ligament attachment points of ribs, spine, and pelvis. Psoriatic arthritis can present at any age, but most often begins between the ages of 30–50 years.

Comorbidities in Patient With Psoriasis

There is strong association between psoriasis, cardiometabolic disease, gastrointestinal diseases, kidney disease, malignancy, infection, and mood disorders.

Table 9-3. Examples of biologic agents for psoriasis.

Features	Etanercept	Adalimumab	Ustekinumab	Secukinumab	Ixekizumab
Mechanism of action	Human fusion protein, TNF type II receptor and Fc region of IgG1. Adheres to soluble TNF-α.	Recombinant, fully human monoclonal antibody to TNF-α (soluble and bound).	Human monoclonal antibody to p40 subunit of IL-12 and IL-23.	Human monoclonal antibody that binds to the protein interleukin (IL)-17A.	Humanized monoclonal antibody that binds to the protein interleukin (IL)-17A.
Indications FDA approved for	Plaque psoriasis. Psoriatic arthritis.	Plaque psoriasis. Psoriatic arthritis. Hidradenitis suppurativa.	Plaque psoriasis. Psoriatic arthritis.	Plaque psoriasis. Psoriatic arthritis.	Plaque psoriasis. Psoriatic arthritis.
Side effects	Injection site reactions. Infections: Most commonly viral URIs. Risk of invasive fungal infections, and TB. Rheumatologic: Development of lupus erythematosus (+ANA, +ds-DNA) (infliximab most commonly). Neurologic: Worsening of MS, optic neuritis, transverse myelitis, Guillain-Barre Cardiac: CHF Hematologic: rare hematologic toxicity. Increased risk of malignancy leukemia/lymphoma.		General: Injection site reactions (1%). arthralgias, fatigue. Infections: Upper respiratory infections and nasopharyngitis (most common for all agents). Neurologic: Headache (common) Reversible posterior leukoencephalopathy syndrome (rare).	Infection: Most common: Increased risk of mild infections: upper respiratory tract infections / nasopharyngitis. Increased risk of fungal infections (tinea/mucocutaneous candidiasis). Injection site reaction. Headache. Diarrhea. Rare side effects, exacerbation of Crohn's disease.	
Contraindications	Live vaccine in 4 places in this row. Active infection, history of demyelinating disease, CHF (NYHA class III or IV heart failure), TB or other granulomatous disease. history of fungal disease. Lives vaccines. Active infection, history of demyelinating disease, CHF (NYHA class III or IV heart failure), TB or other granulomatous disease, history of fungal disease.		Lives vaccines. Active infection Hypersensitivity reaction.	Lives vaccines. Crohn's Disease Active, chronic, or latent infections Immunosuppression. Depression / suicidal behavior.	Lives vaccines. Crohn's Disease. Active, chronic, or latent infections Immunosuppression.

ANA, antinuclear antibody; CHF, congestive har failure; IL, interleukin; MS, multiple sclerosis; NYHA, New York Heart Association; TB, tuberculosis; TNF, tumor necrosis factor;URI, upper respiratory infection.

Psoriasis is an independent risk factor for atherosclerosis, coronary artery disease, myocardial infarction, stroke, and cardiovascular mortality.[12,13] Patients with psoriasis are more likely to be obese and have diabetes, hypertension, dyslipidemia, fatty liver disease, and a history of tobacco use. This cardiovascular risk has also been demonstrated in the pediatric population. Children with psoriasis have been found to have 5 of 10 cardiovascular risk factors that are strongly associated with the development of metabolic syndrome later on in life.[12] Furthermore, patients with psoriasis who are also overweight tend to have more severe disease that is recalcitrant to treatment.

Psoriasis also has a major impact on mental and emotional well-being. Mood disorders including depression, anxiety, and suicidality are more prevalent in this group compared to the general population.[3,14]

Common pathways have been implicated in psoriasis and inflammatory bowel disease.[15] A large meta-analysis study of over 7 million study participants demonstrated patients with psoriasis had significant increased risk of Crohn's disease and ulcerative colitis compared to the general population.

The chronic inflammation of the skin has also been linked to malignancies in particular lymphomas. In a meta-analysis of 112 studies with over 2 million patients, there was a slightly increased risk of developing skin cancer and lymphomas.[16]

Recognition of the comorbid disease burden associated with psoriasis is essential for comprehensive medical care for patients with this chronic skin disorder.

Table 9.4 Classification of psoriatic arthritis

Type of Psoriatic Arthritis	Clinical Findings
Mono and symmetric oligoarthritis	• Most common presentation of psoriatic arthritis. • Asymmetric oligoarthritis of small joints of hands, feet. • DIP and PIP joints commonly involved. • Intense inflammation can lead to sausage digits.
Distal interphalangeal joints	• Involvement of DIP joints only. • Classic, but an uncommon presentation of psoriatic arthritis
Rheumatoid arthritis-like	• Symmetric polyarthritis that involves small and medium sized joints DIP, PIP, MCP, wrist, ankle, elbow. • May be different to distinguish from RA clinically.
Arthritis mutilans	• Least common presentation. • Rapid and progressive joint inflammation and destruction. • Osteolysis.
Spondylitis and sacroiliitis	• Inflammation of axial, knee, and sacroiliac joints • Patient may be HLA-B27 positive and have associated uveitis and IBD.

DIP, distal interphalangeal; HLA, human leukocyte antigen; IBD, Inflammatory bowel disease; MCP, metacarpophalangeal; PIP, proximal interphalangeal.

Potential Causes of Flares of Psoriasis

Group A beta-hemolytic streptococci infection can act as an environmental trigger for guttate psoriasis particularly in the pediatric population.[4] Many clinicians will obtain an anti-streptolysin-O, anti-hyaluronidase, anti-DNase-B, and streptozyme titer along with streptococcal cultures of the throat and peri-anal area as part of the initial work-up of pediatric psoriasis. Other commensal organisms on the skin may play a role in specific variants of psoriasis. Management of these microbes can be an adjunct to psoriatic treatment.

Common medications that may exacerbate psoriasis include beta-blockers, angiotensin converting enzyme (ACE) inhibitors, nonsteroidal anti-inflammatory drugs, lithium, interferon, and antimalarials.[4] Systemic corticosteroids, although providing short-term benefit in control of psoriasis, are not recommended. They can trigger pustular psoriasis and abrupt discontinuation of the systemic steroids commonly exacerbates psoriasis.

Psychiatric comorbidities such as anxiety and depression may exacerbate psoriasis. Stress is also a common trigger of psoriasis.[3] Thus, psoriatic patients may benefit from psychological intervention.

Clinical Course and Prognosis

Psoriasis is a chronic inflammatory condition with relapsing clinical course. The disease is unpredictable and often flaring with stress, illness, and other triggers such as medications. Although there is no cure, proper medication can significantly improve symptoms. Given the strong association with systemic and mental health conditions, it is important to properly counsel patients and family members on natural history and appropriate management of the condition.

Indications for Consultation

Dermatological consultation is indicated when topical medications have not been effective and ultraviolet light or systemic therapy is needed. These therapies include office- or home-based narrow band ultraviolet B or A light therapy, light therapy with psoralens (PUVA), acitretin, methotrexate, biologics (etanercept, adalimumab, alefacept, infliximab, ustekinumab, golimumab, etc.), and cyclosporine.[9]

Pregnant or lactating women with psoriasis should be co-managed by obstetrics and dermatology.[17]

All systemic comorbidities should be monitored and discussed with patients, with consultation to specialists when appropriate as discussed above. Rheumatologic consultation is indicated if signs or symptoms of psoriatic joint disease or enthesis are present.

Patient Information

- American Academy of Dermatology Psoriasis Resource Center
https://www.aad.org/public/diseases/psoriasis
- The National Psoriasis Foundation https://www.psoriasis.org
- Arthritis and Psoriasis www. rheumatology.org
- The Arthritis Foundation www. arthritis.org
- National Institute of Arthritis and Musculoskeletal and Skin Diseases Information Clearinghouse www niams. nih.gov

▼ SEBORRHEIC DERMATITIS

Introduction

Key point for seborrheic dermatitis

- ✓ Seborrheic dermatitis is a very common skin disorder that presents with simple dandruff or with erythematous plaques with a white, greasy scale on the scalp and sometimes on the central face and chest.
- ✓ *Malassezia* yeast species and sebum are associated with the development of seborrheic dermatitis.
- ✓ Most patients can be managed with topical steroids and medicated shampoos.

Seborrheic dermatitis is a common skin disorder that involves the scalp and other areas of high sebaceous gland activity such as the central face and chest. It can present at any age, but its peak incidence occurs in infants and in middle-aged adults. Seborrheic dermatitis is more prevalent and more severe in patients with acquired immunodeficiency syndrome (AIDS) and neurological disorders.

Pathogenesis

Etiology is dependent on three factors, sebum, *Malassezia* yeast and individual susceptibility. Recent work has revealed that *Malassezia* globosa and *Malassezia* restricta predominate and that oleic acid alone can initiate dandruff-like desquamation.[18]

Clinical Presentation

History

The patient typically complains of a dry, scaly, or flaky itchy scalp.

Physical Examination

Infants usually present with "cradle cap," pink to yellow macules and patches with white greasy scales on the scalp. The face, trunk, and diaper areas may also be affected. Adolescents and adults also present with scalp involvement most commonly with "dandruff," white flakes with no erythema (Figure 9-8). Moderate to severe seborrheic dermatitis is characterized by erythematous plaques with white greasy scales which may involve the forehead, eyebrows, eyelash line, nasolabial folds, and ears (Figure 9-9) and less commonly the upper chest and intertriginous areas.

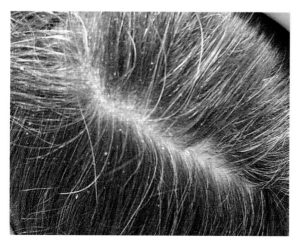

▲ **Figure 9-8.** Seborrheic dermatitis. Loose white flakes with no erythema on scalp

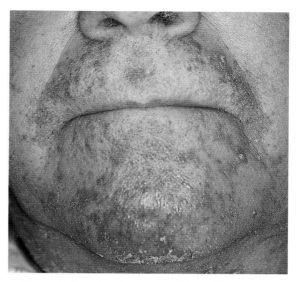

▲ **Figure 9-9.** Seborrheic dermatitis. Erythema and scale in the nasolabial folds and chin.

Laboratory Findings

Skin biopsies are usually not diagnostic and are only helpful to rule out other disorders.

Diagnosis

The key diagnostic clinical features of seborrheic dermatitis are pink plaques with fine greasy white scale on the scalp, eyebrows, nasolabial fold, and ears.

Differential Diagnosis

✓ The differential diagnosis includes other papulosquamous diseases (Table 9-1)

✓ Atopic dermatitis: Atopic children and to some degree adults may have scaly lesions in the scalp; however, they usually have other areas of involvement on the extremities, particularly in the flexural regions.

✓ Tinea Capitis: Trichophyton tonsurans fungal infections in children, especially in African-American children may be indistinguishable from seborrheic dermatitis. Fungal cultures or KOH examinations are needed to clarify the diagnosis.

✓ Other common diseases include rosacea and contact dermatitis.

✓ Uncommon diseases: Dermatomyositis, Langerhans cell histiocytosis (children).

Management

- Mild scalp seborrheic dermatitis can often be controlled with over the counter shampoos containing zinc pyrithione, selenium sulfide, coal tar, salicylic acid, or ketoconazole. Patients should be instructed to shampoo 3–5 times a week.
- Moderate to severe scalp disease can be treated with prescription shampoos that contain selenium sulfide 2.5% ketoconazole 2%, or clobetasol 0.05%. Topical steroid solutions such as fluocinonide 0.05% can be used sparingly twice a day.[19]
- Facial involvement can be managed with sparing use of hydrocortisone 1% cream daily and/or topical antifungal agents such as clortrimazole 1%, cream, miconazole 2% cream, and ketoconazole 2% cream. Tacrolimus ointment and pimecrolimus cream are commonly used for facial diseases. However, they only are FDA approved for use in atopic dermatitis.

Clinical Course and Prognosis

Seborrheic dermatitis usually responds well to treatment, but it is a chronic condition requiring long-term therapy. It can often flare with changes in season and stress. Although it has minimal systemic association and impact on physical health, severe cases and symptoms can cause great deal of distress in the affected individuals. Proper counseling is important for treatment adherence and patient compliance.

Indications for Consultation

Severe or persistent disease that does not respond to treatment, especially in children in whom the presence of persistent seborrheic dermatitis could indicate more serious underlying disease.

Patient Information

- American Academy of Dermatology https://www.aad.org/public/diseases/a-z/seborrheic-dermatitis-overview
- PubMed Health. www.ncbi.nlm.nih.gov/pubmed-health/PMH0001959/

PITYRIASIS ROSEA

Introduction

Key points for pityriasis rosea

✓ Pityriasis rosea is an acute, asymptomatic, self-limited rash that presents on the trunk with oval, pink plaques with a fine central scale.

✓ Human Herpes Virus (HHV)-6 and/or HHV-7 are proposed possible causes.

✓ Pityriasis rosea resolves spontaneously with 6 to 8 weeks in most patients.

Pityriasis rosea is an acute, self-limited papulosquamous exanthema which generally lasts between 6 and 8 weeks (average 45 days), resolving on its own. Cases are frequently noted in clusters, with no seasonal preference. Patients are typically young adults, average age at presentation is 10–35 years old, and females are slightly more affected (1.5:1).[20]

Pathogenesis

The etiology of pityriasis rosea remains an area of debate. Several factors suggest an infectious agent based on the clustering of cases, self-limited nature, and rare recurrences. The current proposed pathogen is Human Herpes Virus (HHV)-6 and/or HHV-7 with either a reactivation or primary infection.[20,21] Some support for this theory has come from the increased incidence in pregnancy, a relative immunosuppressed state, as well as studies identifying HHV-6 and HHV-7 using polymerase chain reaction (PCR) in the affected individual's skin. Pregnant women who develop pityriasis rosea within 15 weeks of gestation may have an active HHV-6 infection and may have a premature delivery with neonatal hypotonia or even fetal death.[22]

Clinical Presentation

▶ History

The most commonly reported symptom is mild pruritus. Occasionally a viral-like constitutional prodrome or symptoms of an upper respiratory infection may precede the onset of cutaneous lesions.

▶ Physical Examination

Pityriasis rosea typically presents initially with a single herald patch which is a pink, oval, 2–10 cm plaque with central fine collarette scale (Figure 9-10).

The subsequent lesions are smaller (1–2 cm) pink papules and plaques on the trunk and extremities. They also have fine central or a collarette of scale. They typically develop in the lines of cleavage (Langer's), symmetrically and result in a "Christmas tree" distribution. The face, scalp, hands, and feet are usually spared. Lymphadenopathy may be present. Pigmented skin alters the color of lesions with a violet-grey color spectrum as opposed to pink. It is more common to see involvement on the head in darker pigmented individuals as well.

Reported variants include papular, vesicular, urticarial, purpuric, inverse pityriasis rosea, and absent or numerous herald patches. In skin of color patients, a papular variant is more commonly seen.

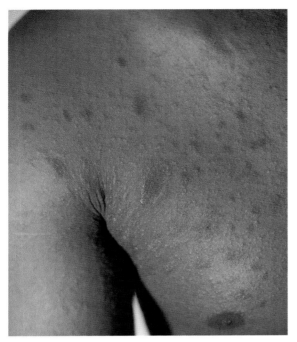

▲ **Figure 9-10.** Pityriasis rosea. Herald patch with collarette scale and multiple smaller lesions with similar morphology.

▶ Laboratory Findings

As pityriasis rosea is a clinical diagnosis made by history and physical, laboratory studies are usually unnecessary. However, if there is diagnostic uncertainty, a skin biopsy or a potassium hydroxide KOH scraping should be done. A rapid plasma reagin (RPR) should be done in any patient at risk for syphilis.

Diagnosis

The key diagnostic clinical features of pityriasis rosea are an initial herald patch, an oval plaque with a collarette scale followed by a symmetric, secondary eruption in a "Christmas tree" pattern.

▶ Differential Diagnosis

✓ The differential diagnosis includes other papulosquamous diseases (Table 9-1)

✓ Drug-related eruptions: Barbiturates, captopril, clonidine, metronidazole, penicillamine, isotretinoin, levamisole, non-steroidal anti-inflammatory drugs (NSAIDs), omeprazole, terbinafine.

✓ Vaccine-related eruptions: A handful of vaccinations have rare reported occurrences of pityriasis rosea-like eruptions, these are: diphtheria, pneumococcal, Hepatitis B, and tuberculosis.

✓ Other: Viral exanthems, pityriasis lichenoides chronica, lichen planus, erythema dyschromicans perstans.

Management

Pityriasis rosea is a self-healing, self-limited benign eruption, therefore treatment is not required. The most important "intervention" is patient education and reassurance. The diffuse, rapid eruption is often disconcerting to patients and parents. In fact, a study on the impact of pityriasis rosea on quality of life showed that concerns of etiology and infectivity had greater impact than rash severity.[23] Reassurance of the self-limited, not contagious nature of the eruption is important.

Additionally, no treatments can be recommended on the basis of evidence-based medicine. A recent Cochrane review showed insufficient evidence for nearly all tried interventions such as emollients, topical antihistamines, steroids, light therapy, and antimicrobials.[24] Based on the proposed correlation with HHV-6 and HHV-7 acyclovir has been studied at both high and low doses but is not commonly used.[21]

If treatment is needed, it is empiric and focuses on symptomatic relief, namely controlling pruritus.[13,14] Regular application of emollients can be helpful. Lotions with camphor, menthol, pramoxine, or oatmeal could provide added antipruritic benefit. Use of sedating (diphenhydramine, hydroxyzine) and non-sedating (cetirizine) antihistamines can also provide relief. Medium potency topical steroids such as triamcinolone or fluocinonide, may provide an additional antipruritic benefit as well as improve the inflamed appearance of lesions. In more severe or recalcitrant disease systemic steroids may be considered. Phototherapy (usually narrow-band UVB) may provide symptomatic relief, but requires a referral to a treatment center, and has not been shown to decrease the duration of disease.

Clinical Course and Prognosis

Pityriasis rosea is a self-limited disease with a benign clinical course. It may take up to a few months for the rash to resolve. Treatment is mostly geared toward symptomatic relief. In skin of color patients, postinflammatory hyperpigmentation will commonly occur secondary to the inflammation. This may linger for many months after pityriasis rosea has resolved and can take up to 6 months or longer for skin color to fully normalize. In pregnant women, during the first trimester, it is recommended for patients to follow up with their obstetrician to rule out any fetal abnormalities.

Indications for Consultation

Severe or nonresolving case with recalcitrant pruritus. Additionally, in light of the recent question of obstetric complications a referral for pregnant patients to Maternal Fetal medicine or alerting the patient's obstetrician may be prudent.[22]

Patient Information

American Academy of Dermatology
https://www.aad.org/public/diseases/a-z/pityriasis-rosea-treatment

▼ LICHEN PLANUS

Introduction

Key points for lichen planus

✓ Lichen planus is a relatively uncommon skin disorder that usually affects those between ages 30–60 years.

✓ It presents with itchy flat-topped firm papules on the flexor wrists, forearms, ankles, lower back and genitals. In the oral cavity net-like white streaks may be seen.

✓ Certain medications and hepatitis C may trigger lichen planus.

✓ Lichen planus usually resolves within 1–3 years, but medium potency topical steroids are usually needed to control symptoms.

Lichen planus is a relatively uncommon papulosquamous skin disorder. It affects all age groups but is most common between the ages of 30–60 years.[25] Children and infants can be affected but infrequently. There are no gender or racial predispositions.

Pathogenesis

Lichen planus is thought to occur as a result of an immune dysfunction with altered surface keratinocyte antigen presentation and subsequent cytotoxic T-cell reaction.[26] A genetic susceptibility has been proposed. The skin eruption has been associated with systemic drugs and Hepatitis C virus, but a definitive cause has not been identified. Common drugs linked to lichen planus are gold, antibiotics, diuretics, and antimalarials.[26]

Clinical Presentation

▶ History

Patients usually present with a complaint of itching and onset of red bumps. The pruritus can range from mild to

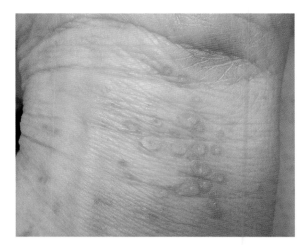

▲ **Figure 9-11.** Lichen planus. Violaceous flat-topped papules on flexural wrist.

severe with an occasional patient having no symptoms. If lichen planus affects the mouth, symptoms such as burning or stinging on exposure to hot or spicy foods is sometimes elicited.

▶ Physical Examination

The primary lesions of lichen planus are violaceous flat-topped firm papules (Figure 9-11). These may be scaly, round, or polygonal in shape. The lesions are distributed symmetrically, typically on the flexor wrists, forearms, ankles, lower back, and genitals (Figure 9-12). Mucous membrane lichen planus is often present and appears as net-like white streaks on the buccal mucosa (Wickman's striae) (Figure 33-33). Oral ulceration may be present. Scalp lesions with a scarring alopecia may be the only manifestation of the disease. A unique feature of lichen planus is its ability to Koebnerize (Figure 9-13). This phenomenon is triggered by trauma, with resultant lichen planus observed in the area of injury. Sometimes generalized and localized hypertrophic forms occur. Hypertrophic lichen planus most often involves the anterior shins and the papulo-nodules show marked hyperkeratosis.

▶ Laboratory Findings

The most useful diagnostic test is a skin biopsy. The biopsy shows a uniform band-like lymphocytic infiltrate at the base of the epidermis. In some instances, the histologic finding can suggest drug-induced lichen planus.[25]

Diagnosis

The key diagnostic clinical features of lichen planus are pruritic flat-topped papules on the flexor areas, lower back, and ankles.

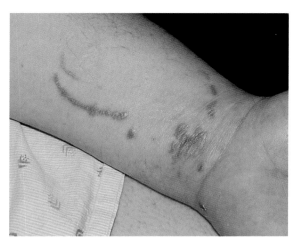

▲ **Figure 9-12.** Lichen planus. Linear streaks of papules demonstrating the Koebner response.

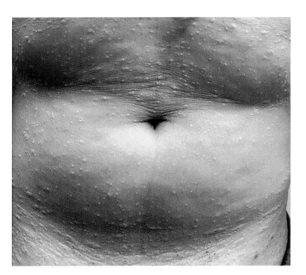

▲ **Figure 9-13.** Lichen planus/lichenoid drug rash. Discrete and confluent pink papules on abdomen.

▶ Differential Diagnosis

✓ The differential diagnosis includes other papulosquamous diseases (Table 9-1).

✓ Scabies: Presents with tiny, excoriated papules, and/ or vesicles in many of the same areas as lichen planus.

✓ Lichenoid drug rash: May be indistinguishable from lichen planus (Figure 9-13).

Clinical Course and Prognosis

Common cutaneous forms of lichen planus will often resolve within a few years. However, various subtypes including mucosal, hypertrophic, and nail disease can have a chronic course and often are challenging to treat. In individuals with oral and genital mucosal involvement, there is significant higher risk of developing squamous cell carcinoma. Therefore, the patient should seek treatment from dermatology and oral medicine for management. Long-term follow up is recommended to screen for development of cancer.

Management

Removal of the offending agent is the first step, if one is identified. Drug-induced lichen planus and hepatitis C are common conditions that may present with a lichenoid skin eruption.[26,27] Lichen planus can be treated with medium-potency corticosteroids applied to the affected area once to three times daily.[27] When the eruption is controlled, the frequency of drug use can be reduced or eliminated. If corticosteroids are used for prolonged periods, care must be taken to avoid drug-induced secondary changes such as atrophy.

Indications for Consultation

Unusual presentations or widespread distribution of a lichenoid eruption should be considered for consultation. Additionally, moderate to severe oral disease may require consultation with a specialist.

Patient Information

American Academy of Dermatology
    https://www.aad.org/public/diseases/a-z/lichen-planus-overview

▼ REFERENCES

1. Pusey WA. The history of dermatology. Springfield IL, Baltimore, Md C.C. Thomas;1933.
2. Scotti L, Franchi M, Marchesoni A, Corrao G. Prevalence and incidence of psoriatic arthritis: A systematic review and meta-analysis. *Semin Arthritis Rheum.* 2018 Aug;48(1):28–34.
3. Geale K, Henriksson M, Jokinen J, Schmitt-Egenolf, M. Association of skin psoriasis and somatic comorbidity with the development of psychiatric illness in a nationwide Swedish study. *JAMA Dermatol.* 2020; 156(7):795.
4. Armstrong AW, Read C. Pathophysiology, clinical presentation, and treatment of psoriasis. *JAMA.* 2020;323(19): 1945–1960.
5. Lynde CW, Poulin Y, Vender R, Bourcier M, Khalil S. Interleukin 17A: toward a new understanding of psoriasis pathogenesis. *J Am Acad Dermatol.* 2014 Jul;71(1):141–150.
6. Kwa L, Kwa MC, Silverberg JI. Cardiovascular comorbidities of pediatric psoriasis among hospitalized children in the United States. *J Am Acad Dermatol.* 2017;77(6): 1023–1029.

7. Elmets CA, et al. Joint AAD-NPF Guidelines of care for the management and treatment of psoriasis with topical therapy and alternative medicine modalities for psoriasis severity measures. *J Am Acad Dermatol.* 2021;84(2):432–470.

8. Lin AN. Innovative use of topical calcineurin inhibitors. *Dermatol Clin.* 2010;28(3):535–545.

9. Elmets CA, et al. A. Joint American Academy of Dermatology-National Psoriasis Foundation guidelines of care for the management and treatment of psoriasis with phototherapy. *J Am Acad Dermatol.* 2019; Sep;81(3):775–804.

10. Mentor A. Joint AAD-NPF guidelines of care for the management and treatment of psoriasis with biologics. *J Am Acad Dermatol.* 2019; 80:1029–1072.

11. Lansang P, Bergman JN, Fiorillo L, Joseph M, Lara-Corrales I, Marcoux D, McCuaig C, Pope E, Prajapati VH, Li SZJ, Landells I. Management of pediatric plaque psoriasis using biologics. *J Am Acad Dermatol.* 2020;82(1):213–221.

12. Lockshin B, Balagula Y, Merola JF. Interleukin 17, inflammation, and cardiovascular risk in patients with psoriasis. *J Am Acad Dermatol.* 2018;79(2):345–352.

13. Lockshin B, Balagula Y, Merola JF. Interleukin 17, inflammation, and cardiovascular risk in patients with psoriasis. *J Am Acad Dermatol.* 2018;79(2):345–352.

14. Read C, Armstrong AW. Association between the mental health of patients with psoriasis and their satisfaction with physicians. *JAMA Dermatol.* 2020; 156(7):754–762.

15. Fu Y., Lee C., Chi C. Association of psoriasis with inflammatory bowel disease. *JAMA Dermatol.* 2018;154(12), 1417–1423.

16. Vaengebjerg S, Skov L, Egeberg A, Loft ND. Prevalence, incidence, and risk of cancer in patients with psoriasis and psoriatic arthritis. *JAMA Dermatol.* 2020;156(4): 421-429.

17. Bae YC, Van Voorhees AS, Hsu S, et al. Review of treatment options for psoriasis in pregnant or lactating women: From the Medical Board of the National Psoriasis Foundation. *J Am Acad Dermatol.* 2012; 67(3):459–477.

18. Xu J, Saunders CW, Hu P et al. Dandruff-associated Malassezia genomes reveal convergent and divergent virulence traits shared with plant and human fungal pathogens. *Proc Natl Acad Sci USA,* 2007;104(47):387–396.

19. Naidi L, Rebora A. Clinical practice. Seborrheic dermatitis. *N Engl J Med.* 2009;360(4):387–396.

20. Gonzalez LM, Allen R, Janniger CK, and Schwartz RA. "Pityriasis rosea: an important papulosquamous disorder." *Int J Dermatol.* 2005; 44 (9):757–764.

21. Drago F, Broccolo F, Rebora A. Pityriasis rosea: an update with a critical appraisal of its possible herpes viral etiology. *J Am Acad Dermatol.* 2009; 61 (2): 303–318.

22. Drago F, Broccolo F, Zaccaria E, Malnati M, Cocuzza C, Lusso P, Rebora A. Pregnancy outcome in patients with pityriasis rosea. *J Am Acad Dermatol.* 2008;58(5Suppl 1):S78–S83.

23. Chuh AA, Chan HH. "Effect on quality of life in patients with pityriasis rosea: is it associated with rash severity?" *Int J Dermatol.* 2005;44(5):372–377.

24. Chuh AA et al. "Interventions for pityriasis rosea." *Cochrane Database Syst Rev.* 2007;18(2): CD005068.

25. Boyd AS, Neldner KHG. Lichen planus, *J Am Acad Dermatol.* 1991;25(4):593–619.

26. Tziotzios C, Lee JYW, Brier T, et al. Lichen planus and lichenoid dermatoses: Clinical overview and molecular basis. *J Am Acad Dermatol.* 2018;79(5):789–804.

27. Tziotzios C, et al. Lichen planus and lichenoid dermatoses: Conventional and emerging therapeutic strategies. *J Am Acad Dermatol.* 2018;79(5):807–818.

Acne, Rosacea, and Related Disorders

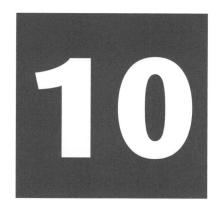

Yi Gao
Ronda Farah

INTRODUCTION TO CHAPTER

Acne and related pilosebaceous disorders rarely cause serious systemic symptoms, but these common skin diseases are often chronic, requiring long term therapy and can cause significant psychosocial distress. These disorders arise from abnormalities associated with the pilosebaceous unit, which is comprised of the hair shaft, hair follicle, and sebaceous gland.

ACNE

Introduction

Key points for acne

✓ Acne affects approximately 85% of people between 12 and 24 years of age and can persist into adulthood in up to 50% of affected individuals.

✓ Mild to moderate acne can be managed with topical medications (e.g., topical retinoids, topical benzoyl peroxide and topical clindamycin) and oral antibiotics if needed.

✓ Severe recalcitrant acne that is unresponsive to conventional therapy usually responds to oral isotretinoin.

✓ Patients with acne have higher rates of depression, anxiety, low self-esteem, and suicidal ideation.

Acne is one of the most prevalent skin disorders, affecting approximately 40–50 million individuals yearly in the United States.[1] Although all age groups may be affected by its variants, acne affects approximately 85% of people between 12 and 24 years of age, of which 20–40% have moderate to severe disease.[2] Preadolescent acne affecting children 7–11 years of age has become more common with the recent trend for earlier puberty.[3] While typically seen in adolescence, acne may persist into adulthood in up to 50% of affected individuals.[1]

Acne can have a profound effect on the quality of life,[4–6] and affected individuals have higher rates of depression, anxiety, low self-esteem, and suicidal ideation.[7] The risk of suicidal ideation and other mental health problems has been shown to be elevated in those with higher self-perceived acne severity.[8,9]

The precise role of genetics in the pathogenesis of acne remains an active area of investigation. The number, size, and activity of sebaceous glands are inherited, and studies have demonstrated an association between moderate to severe acne and a family history of acne.[10] Genome-wide associated studies (GWAS) have identified genes encoding components of transforming growth factor-β (TGF-β), inflammatory mediators, and regulators of androgen metabolism that may be implicated in those with a genetic predisposition to developing acne.[11]

The relationship between diet and acne is gradually being elucidated. Studies have identified skim milk,[12] whey protein,[13] and a high glycemic-load diet[14] as possible risk

113

factors for more severe acne. Vitamin B12 supplementation has been shown to be a possible trigger for acne through alteration of the transcriptome of the skin microflora.[15] A recent study demonstrated that consumption of milk, sugary beverages, and fatty and sugary foods are associated with acne in adults.[16]

Pathogenesis

Acne vulgaris is an inflammatory disorder of the pilosebaceous unit. The pathogenesis of acne is complex and involves the interplay of a variety of factors.[1,17]

- Hyperproliferation and adhesion of follicular keratinocytes in the lower portion of the infundibulum creates a keratin plug (microcomedo).
- Sebum production is stimulated by androgens including dihydrotestosterone (DHT) and testosterone produced by the gonads and dehydroepiandrosterone sulfate (DHEA-S) produced by the adrenal glands as well as locally within the sebaceous gland via 3β-hydroxysteroid dehydrogenase (HSD), 17β-HSD, and 5α-reductase in the hair follicle.
- *Cutibacterium acnes* (formerly *Propionibacterim acnes*)[18] is a Gram-positive, anaerobic rod found within the sebaceous follicle. *C. acnes* is a predominant organism that is usually considered commensal in the microbiome of facial skin and produces porphyrins (primarily coproporphyrin III) that exhibits coral red fluorescence under Wood's lamp illumination. Studies have documented increased levels of *C. acnes* on the facial skin of acne patients, but *C. acnes* density does not correlate with clinical severity.[19] *C. acnes* triggers the release of enzymes and inflammatory mediators through the Toll-like receptor 2 (TLR2) pathway including interleukin (IL)-1α, IL-8, IL-12, tumor necrosis factor α (TNF-α), and matrix metalloproteinases (MMPs) in patients with acne.[20]
- Inflammation leads to comedo rupture which releases keratin, sebum, *C. acnes*, and cellular debris into the surrounding dermis, which further intensifies inflammation forming a pustule (if neutrophils predominate) or inflamed papules, nodules, or cysts (due to lymphocytes and macrophages).

Clinical Presentation

▶ History

Acne usually initially presents at the onset of puberty on sites with high sebaceous gland activity including the face and upper trunk and has a chronic clinical course. Comedones on the central face can progress into inflammatory papules, pustules, and nodules that can be painful and may lead to permanent disfigurement and scarring.

▶ Physical Examination

Acne lesions can be categorized as non-inflammatory and inflammatory based on clinical appearance. Non-inflammatory acne is characterized by comedones. Inflammatory acne presents with papules, pustules, and nodules of variable severity (ranging from moderate to severe). Although the terms "cystic" and "nodulocystic" are used to describe severe acne, acne lesions are not true cysts as they do not have an epithelial lining. Acne is typically clinically classified based on the predominant lesion type seen on examination, although multiple morphologies may present simultaneously.[1]

- *Comedonal acne:* Closed comedones (whiteheads) are small (~1 mm), skin-colored papules with no follicular opening or associated erythema and may be subtle and better appreciated with palpation or tangential lighting (Figure 10-1). Open comedones (blackheads) have a dilated follicular opening filled with a central dark keratotic core (Figure 10-1). Melanin deposition and lipid oxidation may be responsible for the black color.
- *Papulopustular acne:* Erythematous inflamed 2–5 mm papules and/or pustules filled with white purulent material (Figure 10-2).
- *Nodular acne:* As the severity of lesions progress, nodules form and become inflamed, indurated, and painful, eventually resulting in deep fluctuant cyst-like lesions that can coalesce and form inflamed plaques and sinus tracts that may drain purulent fluid (Figure 10-3). These lesions often cause permanent scarring.

Erythema and postinflammatory hyperpigmentation often persist for weeks to months after the resolution of

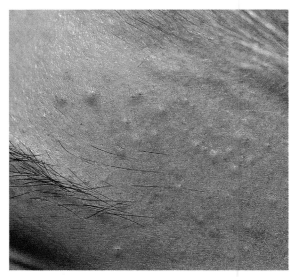

▲ **Figure 10-1.** Acne. Open and closed comendones on forehead.

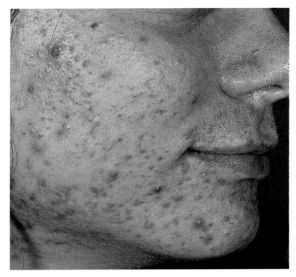

▲ **Figure 10-2.** Acne. Papules, pustules and open comendones.

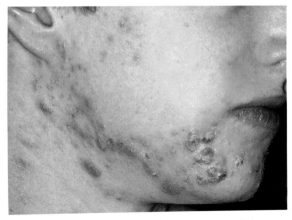

▲ **Figure 10-3.** Acne. Large inflammatory nodules with early sinus tract formation.

inflammatory acne lesions and can be cosmetically bothersome. Deeper inflammatory lesions may leave permanent scars which may be pitted (icepick scars), atrophic (boxcar and rolling scars), or hypertrophic.

> ## Acne Variants and Special Considerations

- *Neonatal acne (neonatal cephalic pustulosis)* occurs in >20% of healthy newborns at 2 weeks of age and generally resolves within the first 3 months of life. Small papules and pustules without comedones are seen on the cheeks, forehead, eyelids, and chin. *Malassezia* yeast has

been implicated as a potential etiology given favorable treatment responses to topical ketoconazole.

- *Infantile acne* presents at 2–12 months of age[21] and develops as a result of intrinsic androgen production. In contrast to neonatal acne, comedones and inflammatory nodules can occur (Figure 10-4). Androgen levels typically decrease by 12 months of age until adrenarche. Patients with infantile acne should be assessed for signs of hyperandrogenism, precocious puberty, or abnormal growth.

- *Solid facial edema* (Morbihan disease) is a disfiguring presentation seen in severe acne vulgaris that involves soft tissue swelling that leads to distortion of the midline face.

- *Acne fulminans* is the most severe form of acne and presents with rapid development of nodular and suppurative acne lesions in association with systemic symptoms including fever, arthralgias, myalgias, hepatosplenomegaly, and malaise (Figure 10-5). Osteolytic bone lesions (often on the clavicle and sternum) as well as laboratory abnormalities including elevated erythrocyte sedimentation rate (ESR), proteinuria, leukocytosis, and anemia may be present. Acne fulminans can be associated with late-onset congenital adrenal hyperplasia and anabolic steroid use, and can paradoxically be seen when initiating high dose isotretinoin for severe acne without concomitant oral corticosteroids.[22]

- *Acne conglobata* is a severe form of nodular acne with an eruptive onset without systemic manifestations and can be recalcitrant to treatment. It can be seen in association with related diseases of follicular occlusion including hidradenitis suppurativa, pilonidal sinus, and dissecting cellulitis of the scalp.

- *Acne associated with endocrinologic abnormalities* may warrant laboratory evaluation (total and free testosterone, dehydroepiandrosterone sulfate (DHEAS),

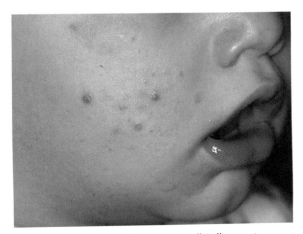

▲ **Figure 10-4.** Infantile acne. Small inflammatory papules and comedones on cheek.

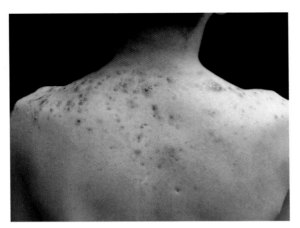

▲ **Figure 10-5.** Acne fulminans. Inflammatory papules, nodules and cysts with scaring on back and neck.

17-hydroxyprogesterone, and luteinizing hormone/follicle stimulating hormone (LH/FSH) ratio, particularly in female patients with other signs of hyperandrogenism (e.g., precocious puberty, hirsutism, androgenetic alopecia, infertility, irregular menses). Individuals at risk for the development of more severe acne that is recalcitrant to standard therapy include those with XYY syndrome (Jacobs syndrome), polycystic ovarian syndrome (PCOS), hyperadrenalism, hypercortisolism, and precocious puberty. Importantly, severe acne has been observed in transgender men (female-to-male) taking formulations of testosterone, particularly upon initiation of hormonal therapy. Although topical agents and oral antibiotics remain first-line for treatment, many transgender men will ultimately require isotretinoin, which creates psychological barriers as these patients are required to register by sex assigned at birth rather for iPledge, the U.S. FDA-mandated program to reduce fetal exposure.[23]

- *Acneiform eruptions* are characterized by lesions that resemble acne, but can affect unusual sites on the body, have a sudden onset, and are monomorphic.[24] They can occur from various medications[25] (systemic corticosteroids, cyclosporine, lithium, and chemotherapeutic medications such as epidermal growth factor inhibitors[26]), exposure to chemicals (chloracne), hair products (pomade acne), and physical occlusion (acne mechanica).

- *Gram-negative folliculitis* occurs in patients with acne treated with long-term oral antibiotics, mainly tetracyclines. Pustules or nodules spread outwards from the nares and lower cheeks, and culture reveals species including *Klebsiella, Enterobacter, Proteus,* or *Escherichia coli.* These patients benefit from oral isotretinoin or oral antibiotics such as amoxicillin or trimethoprim-sulfamethoxazole (TMP-SMX).[27]

Diagnosis

The diagnosis of acne is clinical and based on the examination findings of comedones and/or inflammatory papules, pustules, or nodules.

▶ Differential Diagnosis

✓ Milia: 1–2 mm white superficial cysts often on the eyelids and cheeks. Milia can resemble closed comedones.

✓ Keratosis pilaris: Common benign finding in children that may persist into adulthood. Presents with 1–2 mm hyperkeratotic follicular papules typically on the cheeks and upper arms and is caused by abnormal keratinization in the hair follicle.

✓ *Pityrosporum* folliculitis: Monomorphic itchy papules and pustules on the upper back, chest, forehead, and neck due to infection of the pilosebaceous unit by lipophilic *Malassezia* yeasts. Facial lesions can resemble closed comedones and inflammatory papules.

✓ Boils: Also known are furuncles if solitary and carbuncles if grouped. Painful red pus-filled nodules around follicles that usually form in pre-existing bacterial folliculitis.

✓ Rosacea: Erythema, telangiectasias, inflammatory papules, and/or pustules on central face. No comedones.

✓ See Table 10-1 for additional differential diagnoses.

Management

There are many factors to consider in the treatment of acne including the following:

- Age, gender, skin color, and risk of pregnancy during treatment.

- Type, severity, extent, and location of acne lesions.

- Presence of scarring and postinflammatory pigmentary changes.

- Effectiveness of current and previous treatments (prescription and over-the-counter).

- Current medications (corticosteroids, oral contraceptives, anabolic steroids, epidermal growth factor receptor (EGFR) inhibitors).

- Potential risks, adverse reactions, and contraindications of treatment.

- Factors that may affect adherence or compliance including motivation, occupation, and lifestyle, as well as use of cosmetics, sunscreens, cleansers, and moisturizers.

- Cost of medications and office visits (generic dermatologic medications are approximately 55% cheaper than brand-name medications).[28]

Table 10-1. Differential diagnosis for pilosebaceous disorders.

Disease	Clinical Findings	Notes
Acne	Comedones, inflammatory papules and/or pustules or nodules typically on the face. May also occur on neck and upper trunk.	Onset after puberty but may persist into adulthood.
Rosacea	Erythema, telangiectasias, inflammatory papules and/or pustules on central face. No comedones.	Onset usually after age 30. Chronic course.
Perioral Dermatitis	Perioral erythema with or without scale with papules and/or pustules.	Most common in females ages 20-45. May recur.
Folliculitis	Perifollicular inflammatory papules or pustules in hair bearing areas.	Onset after puberty. May recur intermittently or be chronic.
Boils (furuncles and carbuncles)	Painful red nodules around follicles that may contain pus and can progress to form abscesses.	Usually originates in pre-existing bacterial folliculitis. Often resolves after systemic antibiotics.
Hidradenitis Suppurativa	Inflammatory papules and abscesses in the inframammary region, axillae, and inguinal areas. Sinus tracts and scarring may be present.	Onset in early 20s. Chronic course.

- Perceived acne severity, associated level of distress, and individual risk-benefit ratio of treatment with potential side effects.

Several topical and oral medications are available for the treatment of acne. Table 10-2 lists formulations and brand names of several commonly used topical medications. Table 10-3 provides an overview of oral antibiotics that are commonly used to treat moderate to severe acne. Table 10-4 summarizes recent treatment guidelines for acne from the American Academy of Dermatology.[1,17,29] **Women who are pregnant, trying to conceive or are breastfeeding should discuss the use of any potential acne medication with their primary care/ obstetric care provider.**

Acne Medications

Topical retinoids are vitamin A derivatives that are the mainstay of acne treatment. They act by binding to various retinoic acid receptors to decrease cohesiveness of the keratinocytes in follicles, reduce and prevent comedones, and stimulate anti-inflammatory effects. They are effective as monotherapy for comedonal acne and in combination with other medications for all other forms of acne. Although most topical retinoids are available by prescription, adapalene 0.1% gel is available over the counter. Dryness, redness, and peeling are common side effects with initial use, but these often resolve or improve with continued use. Topical retinoids have been associated with photosensitivity and increased risk for sunburn. It is best to start with a low concentration and increase as tolerated. Published guidelines recommend the use of retinoids for maintenance therapy.[1,29]

Benzoyl peroxide is an antibacterial and comedolytic agent that may prevent antibiotic resistance in *C. acnes* when used in combination with oral or topical antibiotics.[1,29,30] Benzoyl peroxide is widely available in many types of vehicles in over-the-counter and prescription

formulations. Lower concentrations are usually better tolerated, less irritating, and as effective as high conentrations.[31] It may cause irritant or allergic contact dermatitis and can bleach fabrics. Tretinoin may be oxidized and inactivated by co-administration with benzoyl peroxide, so it is recommended that they are applied at different times.

Topical antibiotics such as clindamycin are effective medications for inflammatory acne lesions when combined with retinoids and benzoyl peroxide. They are typically not used as a monotherapy for acne due to the risk of developing antibiotic resistance.

Topical combination acne medications typically contain a retinoid, benzoyl peroxide, and or a topical antibiotic. In general, they are more expensive than each individual component, but may enhance patient compliance.[1]

Azelaic acid has antibacterial and comedolytic effects on acne. It also may decrease postinflammatory hyperpigmentation in patients with darker skin tones.[32]

Salicylic acid is a comedolytic agent that is available in various over-the-counter formulations. Both wash-off and leave-on preparations are well tolerated, but clinical trials demonstrating efficacy are limited.[33]

Dapsone gel can be used for inflammatory acne, particularly for women with adult-onset acne.

Topical sulfur products have been used for many years in the treatment of acne. It has been shown to have keratolytic, antibacterial, and anti-inflammatory properties and is often combined with sodium sulfacetamide.

Oral antibiotics are typically used for moderate to severe acne. Doxycycline and minocycline are the most commonly used oral antibiotics for acne because of their antibacterial and anti-inflammatory effects. Tetracyclines should not be used by women who are pregnant or breastfeeding or by children under 8 years old. Doxycycline and minocycline are generally considered first-line therapy for acne, if an oral antibiotic is indicated. Sarecycline is a newer

Table 10-2. Examples of topical acne medication for males and non-pregnant, non-breastfeeding females.

Generic Name	Formulation Examples	Notes
Topical Retinoids		
Tretinoin*	Cream: 0.025%, 0.05%, 0.1% Gel: 0.01%, 0.025%, 0.04%, 0.1%	Start treatment with lower concentrations applied at night. May be drying.†
Adapalene	Cream: 0.1% Gel: 0.1%, 0.3% Lotion: 0.1%	Differin 0.1% gel available OTC. May be better tolerated than tretinoin. Apply daily or nightly.†
Tazarotene*	Cream: 0.05%, 0.1% Gel: 0.05%, 0.1% Foam: 0.1% Lotion: 0.045%	More effective, but more irritating than other topical retinoids. Apply nightly.†[81,82]
Trifarotene	Cream: 0.005%	Novel topical retinoid FDA-approved for facial and truncal acne.[83,84]
Benzoyl Peroxide		
Benzoyl Peroxide*	Cream: 10% Gel: 2.5%, 4%, 5%, 8%, 10% Wash: 2.5%, 5%, 7%, 10%	Many OTC formulations. May reduce bacterial resistance to antibiotics. May cause irritant or allergic contact dermatitis.
Topical Antibiotics		
Clindamycin*	Gel, lotion, foam, pledget: 1%	Most effective of the topical antibiotics.
Minocycline	Foam: 4%	Recently approved for moderate to severe acne.[85] Apply once daily.
Dapsone	Gel: 5%, 7.5%	Apply twice daily. May turn skin orange if used with benzoyl peroxide.
Erythromycin*	Gel, ointment, solution, pad: 2%	Not recommended as monotherapy as antibiotic resistance may develop. Apply twice daily.
Miscellaneous		
Azelaic acid	Cream: 10%, 20% Gel, foam: 15%	10% cream available OTC. Has comedolytic effects and can be helpful in correcting dyspigmentation. Apply twice daily.
Salicylic Acid*	Cream, gel, wash, pads: 0.5-2%	Many OTC formulations. Apply thin layer 1–3 times daily. May cause dryness.
Sodium Sulfacetamide*	Lotion: 10% Cream: 10% Foam: 9.8% Gel: 10% Wash: 10%	May be drying.
Sodium Sulfacetamide and sulfur*	Cream: sodium sulfacetamide 10% and sulfur 2%, 5% Foam: sodium sulfacetamide 10% and sulfur 5% Wash: sodium sulfacetamide 10%, sulfur 1%,	Has antibacterial and keratolytic effects. Use twice daily. May have a sulfur odor.
Combination Medications		
Tretinoin + Clindamycin	Gel: tretinoin 0.025% and clindamycin 1.2%	Apply nightly.†
Adapalene + Benzoyl Peroxide	Gel: adapalene 0.1% and benzoyl peroxide 2.5%	Apply daily.†
Benzoyl Peroxide + Clindamycin*	Gel: benzoyl peroxide 2.5%, 3.75%, 5% + Clindamycin 1%, 1.2%.	Apply twice daily.

Table 10-2. Examples of topical acne medication for males and non-pregnant, non-breastfeeding females. (*Cont.*)

Generic Name	Formulation Examples	Notes
Benzoyl Peroxide + Erythromycin*	Gel: benzoyl peroxide 5% + erythromycin 3%	Apply twice daily.
Benzoyl Peroxide + Hydrocortisone	Lotion: benzoyl peroxide 5%, 7% + hydrocortisone 0.5%, 1%	Reduces irritation from benzoyl peroxide. Apply 1 to 3 times daily.

*indicates generic availability for some or all formulations.
†indicates theoretic risk of teratogenicity with systemic absorption.[79,80]
OTC, over the counter.

Table 10-3. Oral antibiotics used for acne and other pilosebaceous diseases in males and non-pregnant, non-breastfeeding females.

Medication	Formulations	Dosing	Notes
Tetracycline*	250, 500 mg	500 mg once daily to twice daily.	Take on an empty stomach. Avoid in pregnancy and children <8 years old.
Doxycycline*	50, 100 mg	50–100 mg once daily to twice daily.	May cause photosensitivity and dyspepsia. Avoid in pregnancy and children <8 years old.
Minocycline*	50, 100 mg	50–100 mg once daily to twice daily.	Can be taken with food. Potential side effects include skin discoloration, dizziness, tinnitus, hepatitis, and lupus-like syndromes. Avoid in pregnancy and children <8 years old.
Sarecycline	60, 100, 150 mg	60–150 mg once daily (weight-based)	Novel oral tetracycline antibiotic. May help reduce risk of antibiotic resistance due to targeted antimicrobial activity. Avoid in children <9 years old.[86]
Erythromycin*	125, 250, 333 mg	250–500 mg once to twice daily.	Off-label treatment of acne. May cause gastrointestinal upset and diarrhea. Risk of QT prolongation.
Azithromycin*	500 mg	Pulsed dosing: 500 mg once daily for 4 days per month for 3 months, 500 mg once daily for 3 days in first week followed by 500 mg once weekly for 10 weeks.	Off-label treatment of acne. Dosing regimens in clinical trials use pulse-dosing. Risk of QT prolongation.
Trimethoprim Sulfamethoxazole (TMP/SMX)*	TMX 80, 160 mg and SMX 400, 800 mg	1 to 2 single- or double-strength tablets once to twice daily.	Off-label treatment of acne. Potential side effects include photosensitivity, pancytopenia, liver damage, and mild to severe drug eruptions. Renal dosing adjustment required. Avoid in pregnant and breastfeeding women.
Amoxicillin*	250, 500 mg	250 mg twice daily up to 500 mg 3 times a day.	Renal dosing adjustment required.
Cephalexin*	500 mg	500 mg twice daily.	Renal dosing adjustment required.

*Indicates generic availability for some or all formulations.

FDA-approved oral tetracycline with a narrower spectrum of antibacterial activity that specifically targets *C. acnes*. Studies show that it may cause fewer adverse events and have a lower risk for inducing bacterial resistance.[34,35] All tetracyclines can cause photosensitivity. Minocycline can be associated with tinnitus, vertigo, and blue-gray pigment deposition in the skin and teeth.

Macrolides including erythromycin and azithromycin have also been used as off-label treatments for acne, but may lead to a higher risk of bacterial resistance and can cause cardiac conduction abnormalities (QT-prolongation).[29] Per the American Academy of Dermatology guidelines, the use of oral antibiotics other than those in tetracycline and macrolide classes are not routinely recommended for acne.[29]

Table 10-4. Treatment algorithm for management of acne vulgaris in adolescents and young adults who are not pregnant or breastfeeding.[29,*]

	Mild	Moderate	Severe
1st Line Treatment	Benzoyl Peroxide (BP) -or- Topical Retinoid -or- Topical Combination Therapy** BP+ Antibiotic or Retinoid +BP + Antibiotic	Topical combination therapy** BP+ Antibiotic or Retinoid + BP or Retinoid +BP + Antibiotic -or- Oral Antibiotic + Topical Retinoid + BP -or- Oral Antibiotic + Topical Retinoid + BP+ Topical Antibiotic	Oral antibiotic + Topical Combination Therapy** BP + Antibiotic or Retinoid + BP or Retinoid + BP + Antibiotic -or- Oral isotretinoin
Alternative Treatment	Add Topical Retinoid or BP (if not on already) -or- Consider Alternate Retinoid -or- Consider Topical Dapsone	Consider Alternate Combination Therapy -or- Consider Change in Oral Antibiotic -or- Add Combined Oral Contraceptive or Oral Spironolactone (Females). -or- Consider Oral Isotretinoin	Consider Change In Oral Antibiotic -or- Add Combined Oral Contraceptive Or Oral Spironolactone (Females) -or- Consider Oral Isotretinoin

*Reproduced with permission from Zaenglein AL, Pathy AL, Schlosser BJ, et al: Guidelines of care for the management of acne vulgaris, J Am Acad Dermatol. 2016 May;74(5):945-973.
**The double asterisks (**) indicate that the drug may be prescribed as a fixed combination product or as a separate component. BP,Benzoyl peroxide.

Trimethoprim/sulfamethoxazole (TMP-SMX) can be used as a second-line antibiotic for short-term treatment, but potential severe side effects include photosensitivity, pancytopenia, liver damage, and Stevens-Johnson syndrome/toxic epidermal necrolysis (SJS/TEN). This antibiotic should be limited to those who cannot use tetracycline or who are refractory to standard treatments.[29]

Although data supporting their use are limited, penicillins and cephalosporins can be used as alternative treatments. Gastrointestinal disturbance (nausea, diarrhea, abdominal pain), vaginal candidiasis, and mild drug eruptions can occur with chronic use of all oral antibiotics. Commonly recommended dosing regimens are detailed in Table 10-4.[36]

The development of *C. acnes* antibiotic resistance in the treatment of acne is noted in guidelines as an increasing concern.[1,17,29,30] *In general, guidelines recommend that treatment should be limited to 3 to 4 months and discontinued as soon as inflammatory lesions have resolved.* Monotherapy is strongly discouraged.[29]

Hormonal agents such as combination oral contraceptive pills (estrogen and progestin) can lead to improvement in acne through inhibition of ovarian androgen production by suppression of ovulation and estrogen-mediated down-regulation of sebogenesis,[29] but they have several potential risks including hypertension, venous thromboembolism, and pulmonary embolism.[37] Estrostep, Ortho-Tri-Cyclen,

Yasmin, and Yaz are FDA approved in the United States for women ≥15 years with moderate acne who also want to be on contraception. Spironolactone is an oral antiandrogen that may also improve acne, but also has potential risks including hypotension, abnormal menses, breast tenderness, and hyperkalemia.[29] Spironolactone can cause feminization of a male fetus and should not be taken during pregnancy. Women with acne on the lower face and jaw may benefit from hormonal intervention. Patients should be evaluated by their primary care provider or gynecologist prior to the use of oral contraceptives.

Oral isotretinoin is FDA-approved for patients with severe recalcitrant acne who are unresponsive to conventional therapy. It can also be used for poorly responsive acne not improving with combined oral and topical treatment, acne that causes scarring, and acne that induces psychological distress. It is the most effective treatment for acne and may lead to remission that can last for months to years. Isotretinoin is a teratogen with extremely high risk for severe birth defects if taken during pregnancy in any amount, even for a short period of time, which is the reason it can only be prescribed by clinicians who participate in a strictly regulated distribution program (iPLEDGE). Because of the complexity of the iPLEDGE program and the risks of treatment, referral to dermatology is usually warranted for patients who are potential candidates for isotretinoin. Sometimes patients will require a second course. There are many other potential adverse effects associated with isotretinoin which commonly include skin, eye, and mucosal dryness, arthralgias, hypertriglyceridemia, liver damage, and mood disturbance. Evidence-based guidelines still recommend the use of isotretinoin for appropriate patients.[1,17,29]

Basics of Acne Management

- Topical acne medications should be applied sparingly to all areas of active acne and to areas of chronic past involvement. Patients should wait a few minutes after washing before applying the medication.
- If irritation develops with the use of a topical acne medications, the frequency of application can be reduced and a noncomedogenic moisturizer can be added.
- Patients with acne should use noncomedogenic makeup and sunscreens and gentle cleansers. Scrubs and physical abrasives should be avoided.
- Benzoyl peroxide gel or wash should be used with topical or oral antibiotics to reduce the risk of bacterial resistance to antibiotics.
- Most topical medications will begin to improve acne after 6–8 weeks of use. It may take several more weeks before their maximum benefit is reached. Therefore, it is important not to discontinue or switch treatments until consistent use fails to produce improvement.
- When possible, oral antibiotics should be discontinued when inflammatory acne lesions resolve, usually within 3–4 months.
- Dietary modifications including limiting the intake of milk, whey protein, and foods high in fat and sugar content may be of benefit.[13,16,38]

Patient Adherence Issues

The term "adherence" has effectively replaced "compliance" as the former implies that there is a willingness to follow a management plan formulated and agreed upon by both the patient and the clinician. In the treatment of teenagers with acne, it is especially important to determine motivation for pursuing treatment. Adherence can be improved through counseling on the etiology of acne, educating patients on appropriate use of medications, addressing cost and access issues, and gauging self-perceived acne severity. It is also important to address psychosocial issues related to patient lifestyle and occupation with their primary care provider and mental health professionals as needed. In light of the COVID-19 pandemic, many dermatologists have transitioned to managing acne through teledermatology and virtual visits, which not only reduces potential viral exposures and transmission, but may also increase access to dermatologic care for patients who face barriers to making in-person clinic appointments.[39]

Surgical Treatment

Comedo extraction can improve the cosmetic appearance of acne and aids in maximizing effectiveness of comedolytic agents. Contents of open and closed comedones can be expressed with a comedo extractor. Penetrating the surface of closed comedones with a #11 blade or 18-gauge needle allows easier extraction. Intralesional corticosteroid injection (triamcinolone acetonide 2–5 mg/mL) can improve the appearance and associated tenderness of inflamed nodules. Photodynamic therapy using topical 5-aminolevulinic acid with various light sources (blue or red light) or methyl aminolevulinate with red light can be used to treat acne. Lasers such as pulsed dye laser (PDL), 1450 nm diode laser, or neodymium:YAG laser can be of benefit for inflammatory acne.[40] Low-concentration superficial chemical peels with α-hydroxy acids (glycolic acid), salicylic acid, and trichloroacetic acid can help reduce comedones, are generally well tolerated by individuals of all skin types, and can be performed in a clinic setting (see Chapter 34).[41]

Management of Acne Scars

Scarring from acne can be very distressing. Laser resurfacing (fractionated and ablative), dermabrasion, and deeper chemical peels may help reduce the heterogeneous texture of the skin surface and smooth out depressed scars. For discrete depressed scars, superficial injection of soft tissue filler such as hyaluronic acid, poly-L-lactic acid, and calcium hydroxyapatite can be temporarily beneficial (see Chapter 34). Surgical subcision, microneedling, punch grafting, and full-thickness surgical excision may also be utilized to improve the cosmetic appearance of acne scars.[42]

Clinical Course and Prognosis

Acne usually starts around adolescence and may persist into adulthood with a chronic course in many of the affected individuals. Mild to moderate acne typically responds to topical acne medications and oral antibiotics, but severe acne may require treatment with isotretinoin. Inadequately treated acne can cause permanent scarring and disfigurement as well as significant psychosocial distress.

Indications for Consultation

Patients with acne who do not respond to therapy or those who may be candidates for isotretinoin therapy should be referred to dermatology.

Patient Information

The American Academy of Dermatology
    https://www.aad.org/public/diseases/acne

▼ ROSACEA

Introduction

Key points for rosacea

✓ Rosacea is a common inflammatory disease which usually occurs in adults ages 30–50 years of age and typically persists with intermittent flares.

✓ It usually presents with a gradual onset of facial redness, flushing, or "pimples" on the central face and it can involve the eyes.

✓ Papular/pustular rosacea usually responds to topical therapy such as metronidazole. Oral doxycycline or minocycline can be added if topical therapy is not effective. Phymatous changes can be permanent and disfiguring.

Rosacea is a common inflammatory skin disease that often affects convex surfaces of the central face (cheeks, nose, chin, and forehead). Rosacea usually occurs in adults aged 30–50 years and typically persists with intermittent flares. It is more common in women, but men tend to have more severe disease.[43] It is seen most often in fair-skinned individuals of Northern European heritage, but can also occur in darker-skinned patients. The psychosocial impact of rosacea has been demonstrated through survey studies which have found that among patients with severe symptoms, a high percentage experience depression, anxiety, and overall decreased quality of life related to cosmetic disfigurement, painful burning sensations, and negative impacts on professional interactions.[44]

Pathogenesis

The exact pathogenesis of rosacea is unknown, but several potential factors have been identified.[43,45]

- *Immune factors:* Upregulation of proinflammatory cytokines through Toll-like receptor 2 (TLR2) in response to extrinsic stimuli that leads to cleavage of cathelicidin into LL-37 which activates nuclear factor kappa B (NF-kB) and promotes leukocyte chemotaxis and angiogenesis.[46]

- *Vascular hyperreactivity and neurogenic inflammation:* Various stressors including ultraviolet radiation, microbial antigens, trauma, emotional stress, and hormones stimulate the release of various neurotransmitters and neuropeptides that activate transient receptor potential (TRP) ion channels to release vasoactive neuropeptides such as substance P and calcitonin gene-related peptide (CGRP) which may contribute to vasodilation, flushing, increased skin sensitivity, and inflammation.[47]

- *Demodex folliculorum:* A mite found in the facial pilosebaceous unit of most adults is present in larger numbers in patients with rosacea.[48]

- *Genetics:* Individuals with a family history of rosacea are more likely to develop rosacea, with monozygotic twin studies suggesting a 40–50% genetic contribution.[49]

- *Triggers:* Sunlight exposure, exercise, hot or cold weather, emotional stress, topical steroids, spicy foods, alcohol, and caffeine have all been identified as potential triggers for rosacea flares.

Clinical Presentation

▶ History

Patients often report a gradual onset of facial redness, flushing, or "pimples" on the central face. A history of general sensitivity to skin care products is common, and the patient may have a history of topical steroid use. Burning, stinging, tearing, or foreign-body sensation are common complaints in ocular rosacea.[45]

▶ Physical Examination

In 2002, the National Rosacea Society (NRS) assembled an expert committee and developed a classification system based on the clinical morphology to provide a framework for understanding and managing rosacea. The four main subtypes of rosacea were previously designated as erythematotelangiectatic, papulopustular, phymatous, and ocular.[45] The subtypes were widely utilized and construed as distinct disorders, ignoring frequent simultaneous occurrences of one or more subtypes. Given the significant insights gleaned from research on the pathogenesis of rosacea over the years, the NRS convened another committee to update the standard classification to include new parameters for diagnosis and assessment on the basis of positive predictive value as supported by rosacea experts.[50] Rosacea's diverse features are also likely part of a continuum of inflammation that may not be clinically visible, which suggests that the common presentation of flushing and fixed centrofacial erythema may or may not progress to papules and pustules, and may only potentially lead (in a small proportion of cases) to subsequent phymas.[51] The new classification includes diagnostic phenotypes and major phenotypes based on observable characteristics that can result from intrinsic and environmental influences.

▶ Diagnostic Phenotypes

- *Fixed centrofacial erythema* in a characteristic pattern that may periodically intensify (Figure 10-6). Persistent redness of the facial skin is the most common sign of

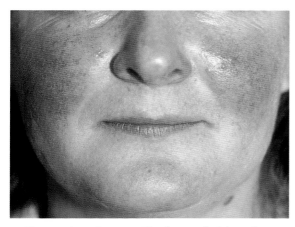

▲ **Figure 10-6.** Rosacea. Fixed centrofacial erythema affecting the nose, cheeks, and chin with telangiectasias on nose.

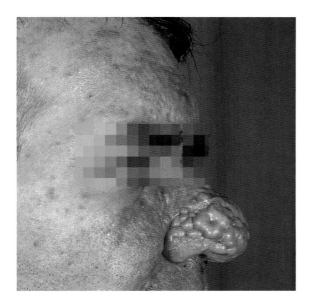

▲ **Figure 10-7.** Rosacea. Phymatous changes of the nose (rhinophyma) with multiple irregular nodules distorting normal structural architecture. Erythematous papules are also seen on the central face.

rosacea; however, erythema may be more difficult to detect in darker skin types.

- *Phymatous changes*: Patulous follicles, skin thickening and fibrosis, glandular hyperplasia, and bulbous appearance of the nose (Figure 10-7). It can also affect the forehead, chin, or ears.

▶ Major Phenotypes

- *Papules and pustules:* Dome-shaped red papules with or without pustules on the central face (Figure 10-8). Nodules may also occur, but comedones are typically absent.
- *Flushing:* Prolonged flushing within seconds to minutes in response to neurovascular triggers is common.
- *Telangiectasia:* Telangiectasias are commonly seen in rosacea. Detection can be improved with a dermatoscope.
- *Ocular manifestations:* Ocular rosacea can occur in the context of mild, moderate, or severe dermatologic disease, and can also appear independently without skin manifestations. Ocular findings include lid margin telangiectasias, interpalpebral conjunctival injection, spade-shaped infiltrates in the cornea, scleritis, and sclerokeratitis. Other nonspecific ocular signs include blepharitis and chalazion, conjunctivitis, "honey crust" and cylindrical collarette accumulation at the base of the lashes, irregularity of the lid margin architecture, and evaporative tear dysfunction (rapid tear breakup time). Symptoms include burning, stinging, photosensitivity, and gritty sensation.[45]

▶ Secondary Phenotypes

- *Burning or stinging* may occur on erythematous skin with or without scale
- *Edema:* Facial edema may accompany or follow prolonged erythema or flushing due to postcapillary extravasation during inflammation and may last for days. As in acne, solid facial edema can also occur with rosacea.

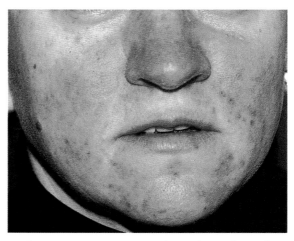

▲ **Figure 10-8.** Rosacea. Papules and pustules with erythema and telangiectasias on cheek.

- *Dry appearance*: Central facial skin may be dry, rough, and scaly. Rosacea may coexist with seborrheic dermatitis.

Laboratory Findings

Laboratory studies are generally not indicated, but occasionally skin biopsies can be utilized to confirm the diagnosis in atypical presentations or confirm a high burden of *Demodex folliculorum*.

Diagnosis

At least one diagnostic phenotype or two major phenotypes are required for the diagnosis of rosacea.

Differential Diagnosis

✓ Chronic sun damage: May very closely resemble or co-occur with rosacea, but papules and pustules are not present and areas such as the neck are also affected.

✓ Systemic lupus erythematosus (SLE): The malar "butterfly" rash of SLE may closely resemble centrofacial erythema and flushing in rosacea, but no papules or pustules are seen.

✓ *Demodex* folliculitis: *Demodex folliculorum* mites are normally found in hair follicles and sebaceous glands, but a very high number of mites can cause inflamed red papules on the face and neck. Many features overlap with rosacea, but it is considered clinically distinct in that it presents with a unilateral distribution, smaller and more superficial papules and pustules, follicular scale, pruritus, and generally lacks persistent erythema.[52]

✓ See Table 10-1 for additional differential diagnoses.

Management

Treatment was previously based on the subtype of rosacea. New treatment guidelines based on phenotype in which the choice of treatment is no longer limited to a particular clinical subtype but rather based on the patient's clinical symptoms.[53]

- *Transient erythema, persistent erythema, and telangiectasia*: These phenotypes are usually unresponsive to topical metronidazole and oral tetracyclines. Avoidance of triggers can help reduce concomitant flushing which may exacerbate the appearance of fixed centrofacial erythema. Topical α-adrenergic agonists including brimonidine 0.33% gel and oxymetazoline 1% cream are FDA-approved and improve erythema by promoting blood vessel constriction. However, these creams are often not covered by insurance and can be cost-prohibitive. There is also a risk of rebound erythema. Intense pulsed light (IPL), PDL, and Nd:YAG lasers can help reduce telangiectasias by selective

Table 10-5. Topical medications for the treatment of rosacea.

Medication	Formulations	Dosing
Brimonidine	Gel: 0.33%	Apply once daily. Risk of rebound erythema. May cause irritation.
Oxymetazoline	Cream: 1%	Apply once daily. Risk of rebound erythema. May cause irritation.
Metronidazole*	Lotion: 0.75% Gel: 0.75%, 1% Cream: 0.75%, 1%	Apply twice daily for 0.75% formulations and once daily for 1% formulations.
Azelaic acid	Gel: 15%	Apply twice daily.
Ivermectin	Cream: 1 %	Use once daily. Avoid in pregnancy and lactation.

*Indicates generic availability for some or all formulations.

photothermolysis of hemoglobin. Some guidelines recommend systemic oral β-adrenergic receptor blockers such as carvedilol which can constrict cutaneous vessels through β2-adrenergic receptors.[54]

- *Papules and pustules*: Topical metronidazole (first line therapy), azelaic acid, and ivermectin are recommended for this phenotype (Table 10-5). 1% ivermectin cream is effective in eradicating *Demodex* and is also anti-inflammatory. Other medications that may be of benefit include topical clindamycin, erythromycin, and tretinoin (Table 10-2). Doxycycline and minocycline are recommended in cases that are unresponsive to topical medications (Table 10-3). Once daily dosing may be sufficient, and most patients require only 2–3 weeks of oral tetracycline therapy on an intermittent basis.

- *Phymatous rosacea:* This phenotype can be improved with aggressive systemic treatment with oral tetracyclines or isotretinoin in early stages. Electrosurgery and ablative lasers are recommended for local treatment.

- *Ocular rosacea:* Artificial tears, lid hygiene, ocular cyclosporine (Restasis 0.05% ophthalmic emulsion), oral tetracyclines, and involvement of ophthalmology are indicated.

General Recommendations for Patients With Rosacea

- All topical steroids and any facial products causing irritation should be discontinued. Topical steroid withdrawal may cause an initial flare.

- Sun protection with broad brimmed hats and sunscreen is highly recommended.

- When possible, triggers for rosacea should be limited or avoided.

Clinical Course and Prognosis

Rosacea is often chronic with an unpredictable course of progression. Different phenotypes have variable responses to topical and oral medications. Phymatous skin changes can lead to permanent disfigurement.

Indications for Consultation

Patients with severe or persistent rosacea or with phymatous rosacea should be referred to dermatology. An ophthalmology referral is appropriate for patients with ocular rosacea.

Patient Information

- National Rosacea Society www.rosacea.org
- American Academy of Dermatology https://www.aad.org/public/diseases/rosacea

PERIORAL DERMATITIS

Introduction

Key points for perioral dermatitis

✓ Perioral dermatitis is a common acneiform eruption that usually affects women 20–45 years of age.

✓ It presents with discrete monomorphic papules and pustules on an erythematous base with or without scale distributed symmetrically around the mouth with a clear zone between the vermilion border and the affected skin.

✓ It is often triggered and or exacerbated by the use of topical corticosteroids

✓ Topical medications such as pimecrolimus, tacrolimus, metronidazole, and topical antibiotics are usually effective treatments.

Perioral dermatitis is a common acneiform eruption that usually affects women aged 20–45 years, but it can affect all adults and children.[55] It typically responds to treatment, but may recur. It is commonly misdiagnosed as contact dermatitis and treated with topical steroids which exacerbate the disease.

Pathogenesis

The pathogenesis of perioral dermatitis is unknown, but several associations have been identified including usage of topical and inhaled corticosteroids,[56] oral contraceptives, menstruation, pregnancy, certain skincare products, fluorinated toothpaste, and emotional stress.[55] *Candida* and *Demodex* mites have also been isolated from lesions, but it is unclear whether they cause disease.

Clinical Presentation

▶ History

Patients usually complain of a rash or pimples around the mouth with discomfort or burning. Usage of topical corticosteroids on the face commonly precedes the manifestation of perioral dermatitis.

▶ Physical Examination

Lesions consist of discrete monomorphic papules and pustules on an erythematous base with or without scale distributed symmetrically around the mouth with a clear zone between the vermilion border and the affected skin (Figure 10-9). The nasolabial folds and skin around the lateral canthi (periorbital dermatitis) may also be affected.

▶ Laboratory Findings

Laboratory studies and skin biopsies are generally not indicated.

Diagnosis

Perioral dermatitis is a clinical diagnosis based on skin examination findings and clinical history.

▶ Differential Diagnosis

✓ Allergic or irritant contact dermatitis: Presents with erythema and scale without papules or pustules. Usually due to lip products and involves the lips as well as other areas on the face.

✓ See Table 10-1 for additional differential diagnoses.

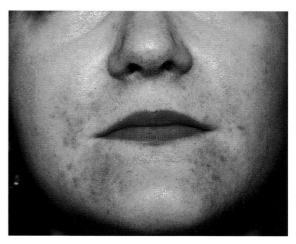

▲ **Figure 10-9.** Perioral dermatitis. Multiple erythematous papules around the mouth with an area of uninvolved skin along the border of the lips.

Management

All topical steroids and associated skincare products should be discontinued. Although abrupt withdrawal of topical steroids may cause a temporary flare in symptoms, they should not be resumed. Topical tacrolimus 0.1% ointment and pimecrolimus 1% cream can be used to control flares. Topical erythromycin, clindamycin, azelaic acid, and metronidazole have also been shown to be of benefit. In severe cases, oral tetracyclines can lead to clearance (Table 10-3).[57]

Clinical Course and Prognosis

Perioral dermatitis generally improves with topical treatment and discontinuation of topical corticosteroids, but some severe cases will require treatment with oral tetracyclines. Rarely, the disease can become persistent and chronic.

Indications for Consultation

Severe or persistent disease that does not respond to therapy warrants dermatology referral.

Patient Information

The American Academy of Dermatology
www.aad.org/public/diseases/a-z/perioral-dermatitis

▼ FOLLICULITIS

Introduction

Key points for folliculitis

✓ Folliculitis is very common disorder of the hair follicle that can affect individuals of all ages.

✓ Bacteria and certain fungal species are the most common causes, but many other infectious and noninfectious etiologies exist.

✓ Folliculitis typically presents with follicular-based pustules and/or inflammatory papules on any hair bearing area, but most commonly on the trunk, buttocks, thighs, axillae, face, and scalp.

Folliculitis is a very common disorder of the hair follicle that can affect individuals of all ages. It can be secondary to a wide range of infectious agents or caused by a variety of irritants or medications and is often is seen as an incidental finding on skin examination.

Pathogenesis

Folliculitis can be caused by infectious or noninfectious etiologies.[58]

- *Bacteria* are the most common cause of folliculitis. *Staphylococcus aureus* (Figure 10-10), *Streptococcus,*

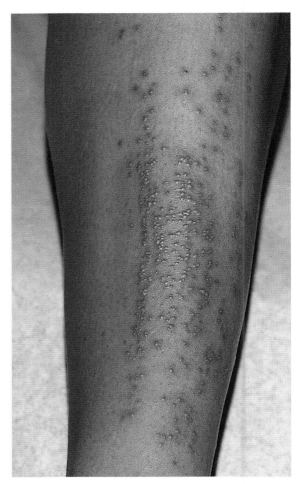

▲ **Figure 10-10.** Folliculitis. Multiple pustules in streaks which developed after shaving legs with a razor blade. A culture isolated coagulase positive *Staphylococcus aureus*

Pseudomonas aeruginosa (hot tub folliculitis) (Figure 10-11), and other Gram-negative organisms are frequent causes.

- *Fungal folliculitis* caused by *Malassezia/Pityrosporum orbiculare* species is common and can become chronic without appropriate treatment with antifungals (Figure 10-12). Candida and dermatophyte infections can also cause folliculitis on focal areas of the body.

- *Demodex folliculorum* mites are normally found in hair follicles and sebaceous glands, but when present in high numbers they may cause a follicular rash on the face and other body areas. Skin scrapings and biopsies reveal numerous *Demodex* mites.

- *Mechanical folliculitis* can be caused by hair being tightly pulled back (traction folliculitis), hair removal by

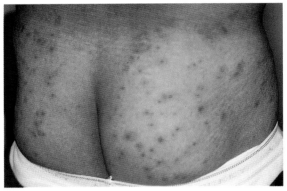

▲ **Figure 10-11.** Pseudomonas folliculitis. Multiple erythematous papules on buttocks after use of hot tub; usually caused by exposure to contaminated water with inadequate amounts of chlorine.

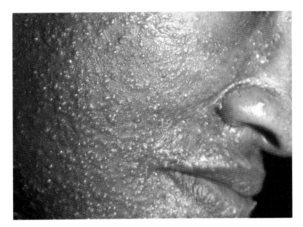

▲ **Figure 10-12.** *Malassezia/Pityrosporum* folliculitis. Monomorphic papules and pustules on face.

shaving, waxing, or plucking chronic friction from tight clothing, and ingrown hairs (pseudofolliculitis barbae) (Figure 10-13 secondary folliculitis may develop in patients who scratch areas of dermatoses.

- *Irritant folliculitis* can occur following application of topical medications and ointments which lead to follicular occlusion. It can be exacerbated by application in a direction opposite that of hair growth.
- *Herpes simplex folliculitis* can occur in men with a history of recurrent localized facial herpes simplex who shave with a razor blade. This presents with rapid development of grouped follicular pustules and vesicles in the beard area.
- *Drug-induced folliculitis* (See "Acneiform eruptions").
- *Eosinophilic folliculitis:* Immunosuppression (HIV)-associated eosinophilic pustular folliculitis is a pruritic

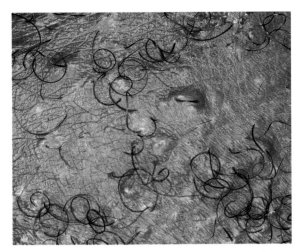

▲ **Figure 10-13.** Pseudofolliculitis barbae. Multiple perifollicular papules in beard of Black patient due to curved hair fibers reentering the skin.

papulopustular follicular eruption affecting the face, scalp, and upper trunk seen in the setting of HIV/AIDS as well as in other immunosuppressed patients. It typically occurs in HIV patients with CD4 counts <200 cells/mm³ and may also be a manifestation of immune reconstitution inflammatory syndrome (IRIS).

Diabetic and immunocompromised patients are more susceptible to folliculitis, often with presentations that are more widespread or usual.

Clinical Presentation

▷ History

Patients with folliculitis usually complain of pruritic or tender papules and pustules.

▷ Physical Examination

Folliculitis typically presents with follicular-based pustules and/or inflammatory papules on any hair bearing area, but most commonly on the trunk (Figure 10-14), buttocks, thighs, axillae, face, and scalp. It favors areas of occlusion with terminal hairs. Lesions of *Staphylococcal* folliculitis may occasionally coalesce into large, crusted plaques (sycosis barbae). Gram-negative folliculitis presents with pustules on the central face and may resemble acne. *Pseudomonas* folliculitis appears within a few hours of exposure and is most prominent in areas covered by a bathing suit (Figure 10-11). *Demodex* folliculitis resembles rosacea but may be unilateral and scaly without centrofacial erythema. *Malassezia/Pityrosporum* folliculitis typically occurs on the trunk of young adults and is worsened by

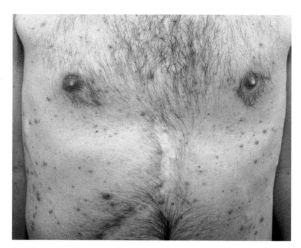

▲ **Figure 10-14.** Folliculitis. Multiple perifollicular papules and pustules on trunk.

sweating and occlusion (Figure 10-12). Pseudofolliculitis barbae (Figure 10-13) occurs in the beard area of men who shave, particularly in those with darker skin and curly hair.

▶ Laboratory Findings

Microbial cultures from intact pustules may or may not isolate the causative organism. Of the infectious etiologies, *Staphylococcus aureus* is the most common. A KOH preparation of follicular contents can help identify yeast and dermatophytes. A viral polymerase chain reaction (PCR) or culture from a follicular pustule or vesicle can aid in the diagnosis of herpes simplex folliculitis. In some cases, a skin biopsy can be helpful in identifying the specific cause.

Diagnosis

Diagnosis of folliculitis is made based on skin examination findings and clinical history.

▶ Differential Diagnosis

✓ Keratosis pilaris: Common benign finding in children that may persist into adulthood. Presents with 1–2 mm hyperkeratotic follicular papules typically on the cheeks and upper arms and is caused by abnormal keratinization in the hair follicle.

✓ See Table 10-1 for additional differential diagnoses.

Management

Appropriate treatment depends on the severity of disease and underlying cause. For culture-negative cases, topical acne medications including benzoyl peroxide, topical clindamycin,

and oral tetracyclines can be used. Mild cases of bacterial folliculitis may be managed with topical antibacterial washes and soaks (e.g., chlorhexidine, bleach). Dilute acetic acid soaks can be used to treat folliculitis due to *Pseudomonas*. Recalcitrant cases of gram-negative folliculitis can be treated with topical gentamicin, oral fluoroquinolones, or isotretinoin. *Malassesia/Pityrosporum* folliculitis usually responds to topical ketoconazole cream or shampoo, but severe cases can be treated with oral fluconazole or itraconazole. Oral terbinafine or griseofulvin can be used for dermatophyte folliculitis. Herpes simplex folliculitis is treated with oral acyclovir or valacyclovir for 5–10 days. Topical 1% ivermectin cream is effective for *Demodex* folliculitis.

Clinical Course and Prognosis

Disease course is highly dependent on the underlying cause. Folliculitis has a wide spectrum of severity, but usually will improve with targeted topical and oral medications.

Indications for Consultation

Patients with severe or persistent disease may benefit from consultation with dermatology or infectious disease.

Patient Information

The American Academy of Dermatology
www.aad.org/public/diseases/a-z/folliculitis

▼ HIDRADENTIS SUPPURATIVA

Introduction

Key points of hidradenitis suppurativa

✓ Hidradenitis suppurativa is a chronic inflammatory follicular disorder of apocrine gland-bearing skin, usually affecting the axillae, inframammary folds, and anogenital regions.

✓ The reported prevalence ranges from 1 to 4%, and it is more common in women.

✓ It presents initially after puberty with a gradual onset of painful, persistent, or recurrent boil-like lesions in the axillae and or inguinal area.

✓ Patients usually have multiple comorbidities and many quality of life issues.

✓ Management can be complex and typically requires a team-based approach.

Hidradenitis suppurativa (HS), also known as acne inversa, is a chronic inflammatory follicular disorder, typically involving intertriginous sites, including the axillae, inframammary folds, groin, and buttocks. The reported prevalence ranges from 1 to 4%, and it is more common in women.[59,60] Onset usually occurs shortly after puberty with a gradual decrease in activity after age 50. In its most severe form, hidradenitis suppurativa can be debilitating and result in considerable discomfort, embarrassment, and markedly impaired quality of life due to painful nodules, recurrent abscesses, draining tunnels, and hypertrophic scars.[61]

Pathogenesis

The pathogenesis of hidradenitis suppurativa is thought to stem from inflammation of the hair follicle. Follicular rupture releases keratin and bacteria, inciting a vigorous chemotactic response and abscess and sinus tract formation.[59] Apocrine involvement may occur secondary to dermal inflammation. Despite the temporal relationship to puberty, hyperandrogenism is usually not found.

Tumor necrosis factor (TNF)-α is an inflammatory mediator that is significantly increased with levels correlating with increasing disease severity. The role of TNF-α in hidradenitis suppurativa is multifactorial:

- TNF-α increases the ratio of T_{H}-17 to regulatory T cells which leads to release of IL-17, IL-22, interferon-γ (IFN-γ), and IL-2.
- TNF-α acts on adipocytes and muscle cells to induce defects in insulin signaling.
- Smoking increases nicotine-mediated eccrine gland secretion, expression of matrix metalloproteinases (MMPs), follicular plugging, and increased TNF-α.
- TNF-α induces upregulation of toll-like receptors (TLRs) and MMPs, further stimulating inflammation that leads to tissue injury.[63]

Other notable cytokines involved in the pathogenesis of hidradenitis suppurativa are IL-17, IL-1β, IL-12, IL-23, and IL-6.[64] 30–40% of patients with hidradenitis suppurativa have a positive family history. Mutations in genes involved in γ-secretase production (NCSTN, PSEN1, PSENEN), which are essential for immune function and hair follicle maturation result in an autosomal dominant familial form of HS with incomplete penetrance.[65]

Although the primary etiology of hidradenitis suppurativa is not infectious, significant alterations in the cutaneous microbiome have been found in patients with hidradenitis suppurativa. Lesional skin consists predominantly of *Corynebacterium*, *Porphyromonas*, and *Peptoniphilus* species, while non-lesional skin has *Acinetobacter* and *Moraxella* species.[66] Polymicrobial colonization, particularly with biofilm-forming bacteria, is common in hidradenitis suppurativa likely due to chronic inflammation and a functionally compromised skin barrier.[67]

Clinical Presentation

▶ History

Patients typically report a gradual onset of persistent or recurrent boil-like lesions in the axillae and or inguinal area.

The lesions may be very painful and may be misdiagnosed as infectious abscesses. Individual lesions may heal with scarring, but new lesions typically appear in the same area. With repeated flares, recurrent abscesses form draining tunnels and nodular scars. Some women with hidradenitis suppurativa experience perimenstrual flares or flares following pregnancy, suggesting a hormonal component to HS.

Patients with hidradenitis suppurativa have a *high comorbidity burden* and should be screened for the following conditions: hypertension, obesity, dyslipidemia, metabolic syndrome, polycystic ovarian syndrome (PCOS), inflammatory arthropathies, inflammatory bowel disease, and tobacco use have all been shown to be independently associated with hidradenitis suppurativa.[68] Patients with hidradenitis suppurativa are at increased risk for adverse cardiovascular events[69] and malignancies.[70] Long-standing lesions of hidradenitis suppurativa, typically in the buttock and groin, can transform into squamous cell carcinoma.[71] Hidradenitis suppurativa is part of the follicular occlusion tetrad (acne conglobata, dissecting cellulitis of the scalp, pilonidal cyst, and hidradenitis suppurativa) and patients with HS should also be screened for these associated conditions.[64]

Patients with hidradenitis suppurativa also have increased risk of anxiety, depression, and sexual dysfunction and should be screened for these related mental health conditions.[69] For those patients with chronic pain, psychological distress, and mental illness, recent guidelines suggest also screening for suicidal ideation and substance misuse.[69]

▶ Physical Examination

While disease presentation may vary, characteristic lesions are deep-seated nodules that expand to form abscesses that can progress to draining tunnels, bridged scars, and open "tombstone" comedones favoring the axillae and inguinal area (Figures 10-15, 10-16). The breasts, inframammary

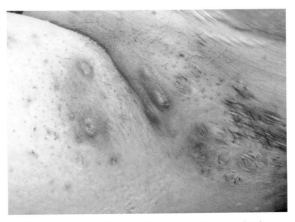

▲ **Figure 10-15.** Hidradenitis suppurativa. Multiple inflamed nodules and scars in axilla.

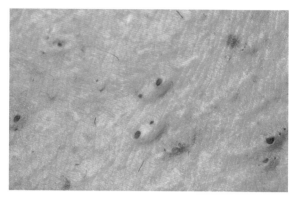

▲ **Figure 10-16.** Hidradenitis suppurativa. Single and double giant comedones.

folds, perineal area, buttocks, inner thighs, postauricular region, and posterior neck may also be involved. The Hurley staging system is most commonly used and consists of a 3-stage classification of disease designed to help guide treatment,[73] but limitations include lack of measures to assess disease activity or treatment response. Several additional scoring systems have been developed to quantify disease activity and response to treatment (modified Sartorius score, HS Severity Score Index, and HS Clinical Response).

- *Hurley stage I (mild):* Single or multiple isolated abscesses or nodules without tunnels or scarring (Figure 10-11).
- *Hurley stage II (moderate)*: Nonconfluent, recurrent abscesses or nodules with 1 or more tunnels and scarring separated by normal skin.
- *Hurley stage III (severe):* Diffuse boils with multiple interconnected tunnels and no intervening normal skin. Approximately 1% of patients progress to this stage.[60]

▶ Laboratory Findings

Bacterial cultures are usually negative, but secondary infections with *Staphylococcus aureus* and other organisms may occur.

Diagnosis

Hidradenitis suppurativa is diagnosed clinically based on characteristic lesions, predilection for flexural sites, and lesion recurrence.

▶ Differential Diagnosis

✓ Boils: Also known are furuncles if solitary and carbuncles if grouped. Painful red pus-filled nodules around follicles that usually form in pre-existing bacterial folliculitis and can progress to form abscesses.

✓ *Staphylococcal* abscesses: Usually presents with a more exophytic isolated red, inflamed, and tender nodule. Patients may have constitutional symptoms of fever and malaise.

✓ See Table 10-1 for additional differential diagnoses.

Management

Management is typically guided by disease severity and activity.[61,74,75]

- *Hurley stage I (mild)*

  Topical and oral antibiotics as listed in Table 10-3. Specifically, topical clindamycin has demonstrated efficacy in mild hidradenitis suppurativa most helpful for treatment of inflammatory papules and pustules. In terms of oral antibiotics, tetracyclines and clindamycin with rifampin have been the most extensively studied. While tetracyclines can be used for prolonged periods of time in some patients, clindamycin and rifampin combinations are typically only used for short periods of time for flares.

  Intralesional triamcinolone can be injected into early inflammatory lesions, but data supporting this is conflicting.

  Spironolactone, an antiandrogen medication, has demonstrated efficacy for some female patients, with potentially better responses in those patients with perimenstrual flares and those with a history of PCOS.

- *Hurley stage II (moderate)*

  In addition to therapeutic interventions for Hurley stage I, immunosuppressive agents targeting specific inflammatory mediators and cytokines can be utilized. Adalimumab, a tumor necrosis factor (TNF)-α is currently the only federal drug administration (FDA) approved medication for hidradenitis suppurativa. Other systemic medications used for recalcitrant hidradenitis suppurativa include, other TNF inhibitors (e.g., infliximab), dapsone, cyclosporine, and other biologics including 1L-17, IL12/23, and IL-1alpha inhibitors.[78] Oral retinoids have limited utility, due to their disappointing efficacy for HS compared to acne. Acitretin may be considered as a second or third line agent.

- Hurley Stage III (severe).

  This stage rarely improved with medical therapy alone. Surgical procedures such as local excisions and de-roofing with or without secondary intention healing may be indicated.[59] At this stage, patients are typically referred to plastic or dermatologic surgery for wide local excision and reconstruction of the affected area.

- General measures

  Weight loss for overweight or obese patients, smoking cessation, antiseptic cleansers and washes (chlorhexidine, benzoyl peroxide), and loose-fitting cotton clothing are recommended.

Clinical Course and Prognosis

Hidradenitis suppurativa usually has a chronic relapsing/remitting progressive course and can lead to severe morbidity due to intermittent flares and associated scarring. Mild cases may be responsive to topical and oral medications, but severe disease may be recalcitrant to even aggressive systemic treatments.

Indications for Consultation

Patients with moderate to severe disease should be managed through a multidisciplinary team-based approach with primary care, dermatology, and surgery. Coordination of care may be difficult as patients with more severe disease often go to urgent care clinics or emergency departments for management of acute flares.

Patient Information

- Hidradenitis Suppurativa Foundation
www.hs-foundation.org
- The American Academy of Dermatology
www.aad.org/public/diseases/a-z/hidradenitis-suppurativa-overview

REFERENCES

1. Thiboutot D, Gollnick H, Bettoli V, et al. New insights into the management of acne: an update from the Global Alliance to Improve Outcomes in Acne group. *J Am Acad Dermatol*. 2009;60(5 Suppl): S1-50.
2. Karimkhani C, Dellavalle RP, Coffeng LE, et al. Global skin disease morbidity and mortality: an update from the Global Burden of Disease Study 2013. *JAMA Dermatol*. 2017;153(5):406-412.
3. Tan JKL, Bhate K. A global perspective on the epidemiology of acne. *Br J Dermatol*. 2015;172 Suppl 1:3-12.
4. Chernyshov PV, Zouboulis CC, Tomas-Aragones L, et al. Quality of life measurement in acne. Position paper of the European Academy of Dermatology and Venereology task forces on quality of life and patient oriented outcomes and acne, rosacea and hidradenitis suppurativa. *J Eur Acad Dermatol Venereol*. 2018;32(2):194-208.
5. Rapp SR, Feldman SR, Graham G, Fleischer AB, Brenes G, Dailey M. The Acne Quality of Life Index (Acne-QOLI): development and validation of a brief instrument. *Am J Clin Dermatol*. 2006;7(3):185-192.
6. Hazarika N, Rajaprabha RK. Assessment of life quality index among patients with acne vulgaris in a suburban population. *Indian J Dermatol*. 2016;61(2):163-168.
7. Ramrakha S, Fergusson DM, Horwood LJ, et al. Cumulative mental health consequences of acne: 23-year follow-up in a general population birth cohort study. *Br J Dermatol*. 2016;175(5):1079-1081.
8. Halvorsen JA, Stern RS, Dalgard F, Thoresen M, Bjertness E, Lien L. Suicidal ideation, mental health problems, and social impairment are increased in adolescents with acne: a population-based study. *J Invest Dermatol*. 2011;131(2):363-370.
9. Loney T, Standage M, Lewis S. Not just "skin deep": psychosocial effects of dermatological-related social anxiety in a sample of acne patients. *J Health Psychol*. 2008;13(1):47-54.
10. Ghodsi SZ, Orawa H, Zouboulis CC. Prevalence, severity, and severity risk factors of acne in high school pupils: a community-based study. *J Invest Dermatol*. 2009;129(9):2136-2141.
11. Navarini AA, Simpson MA, Weale M, et al. Genome-wide association study identifies three novel susceptibility loci for severe acne vulgaris. *Nat Commun*. 2014; 5:4020.
12. LaRosa CL, Quach KA, Koons K, et al. Consumption of dairy in teenagers with and without acne. *J Am Acad Dermatol*. 2016;75(2):318-322.
13. Bowe WP, Joshi SS, Shalita AR. Diet and acne. *J Am Acad Dermatol*. 2010;63(1):124-141.
14. Kwon HH, Yoon JY, Hong JS, Jung JY, Park MS, Suh DH. Clinical and histological effect of a low glycaemic load diet in treatment of acne vulgaris in Korean patients: a randomized, controlled trial. *Acta Derm Venereol*. 2012;92(3):241-246.
15. Kang D, Shi B, Erfe MC, Craft N, Li H. Vitamin B12 modulates the transcriptome of the skin microbiota in acne pathogenesis. *Sci Transl Med*. 2015;7(293):293ra103.
16. Penso L, Touvier M, Deschasaux M, et al. Association between adult acne and dietary behaviors: findings from the NutriNet-Santé Prospective Cohort Study. *JAMA Dermatol*. 2020;156(8):854.
17. Nast A, Dréno B, Bettoli V, et al. European evidence-based (S3) guidelines for the treatment of acne. *J Eur Acad Dermatol Venereol*. 2012;26(s1):1-29.
18. Dréno B, Pécastaings S, Corvec S, Veraldi S, Khammari A, Roques C. Cutibacterium acnes (*Propionibacterium acnes*) and acne vulgaris: a brief look at the latest updates. *J Eur Acad Dermatol Venereol JEADV*. 2018;32 Suppl 2:5-14.
19. Leyden JJ, McGinley KJ, Mills OH, Kligman AM. Propionibacterium levels in patients with and without acne vulgaris. *J Invest Dermatol*. 1975;65(4):382-384.
20. Nagy I, Pivarcsi A, Koreck A, Széll M, Urbán E, Kemény L. Distinct strains of Propionibacterium acnes induce selective human beta-defensin-2 and interleukin-8 expression in human keratinocytes through toll-like receptors. *J Invest Dermatol*. 2005;124(5):931-938.
21. Eichenfield LF, Krakowski AC, Piggott C, et al. Evidence-based recommendations for the diagnosis and treatment of pediatric acne. *Pediatrics*. 2013;131 Suppl 3:S163-186.
22. Gualtieri B, Panduri S, Chiricozzi A, Romanelli M. Isotretinoin-triggered acne fulminans: a rare, disabling occurrence. *G Ital Dermatol E Venereol Organo Uff Soc Ital Dermatol E Sifilogr*. 2020;155(3):361-362.
23. Ginsberg BA. Dermatologic care of the transgender patient. *Int J Womens Dermatol*. 2016;3(1):65-67.
24. Dessinioti C, Antoniou C, Katsambas A. Acneiform eruptions. *Clin Dermatol*. 2014;32(1):24-34.
25. Momin SB, Peterson A, Del Rosso JQ. A status report on drug-associated acne and acneiform eruptions. *J Drugs Dermatol JDD*. 2010;9(6):627-636.
26. Li T, Perez-Soler R. Skin toxicities associated with epidermal growth factor receptor inhibitors. *Target Oncol*. 2009;4(2):107-119.
27. Böni R, Nehrhoff B. Treatment of gram-negative folliculitis in patients with acne. *Am J Clin Dermatol*. 2003;4(4):273-276.
28. Payette M, Grant-Kels JM. Generic drugs in dermatology: Part II. *J Am Acad Dermatol*. 2012;66(3):353.e1-353.e15.
29. Zaenglein AL, Pathy AL, Schlosser BJ, et al. Guidelines of care for the management of acne vulgaris. *J Am Acad Dermatol*. 2016;74(5):945-973.

30. Chon SY, Doan HQ, Mays RM, Singh SM, Gordon RA, Tyring SK. Antibiotic overuse and resistance in dermatology. *Dermatol Ther.* 2012;25(1):55-69.

31. Sagransky M, Yentzer BA, Feldman SR. Benzoyl peroxide: a review of its current use in the treatment of acne vulgaris. *Expert Opin Pharmacother.* 2009;10(15):2555-2562.

32. Kircik LH. Efficacy and safety of azelaic acid (AzA) gel 15% in the treatment of post-inflammatory hyperpigmentation and acne: a 16-week, baseline-controlled study. *J Drugs Dermatol JDD.* 2011;10(6):586-590.

33. Shalita AR. Comparison of a salicylic acid cleanser and a benzoyl peroxide wash in the treatment of acne vulgaris. *Clin Ther.* 1989;11(2):264-267.

34. Haidari W, Bruinsma R, Cardenas-de la Garza JA, Feldman SR. Sarecycline review. *Ann Pharmacother.* 2020;54(2):164-170.

35. Moore AY, Del Rosso J, Johnson JL, Grada A. Sarecycline: a review of preclinical and clinical evidence. *Clin Cosmet Investig Dermatol.* 2020;13:553-560.

36. Zaenglein AL, Graber EM, Thiboutot DM. Acne vulgaris and acneiform eruptions. In: Goldsmith LA, Katz SI, Gilchrest BA, Paller AS, Leffell DJ, Wolff K, eds. *Fitzpatrick's Dermatology in General Medicine.* 8th ed. The McGraw-Hill Companies; 2012. Accessed August 24, 2020. accessmedicine.mhmedical.com/content.aspx?aid=56046904

37. In brief: FDA warning about drospirenone in oral contraceptives. *Med Lett Drugs Ther.* 2012;54(1389):33.

38. Silverberg NB. Whey protein precipitating moderate to severe acne flares in 5 teenaged athletes. *Cutis.* 2012;90(2):70-72.

39. Villani A, Annunziata MC, Abategiovanni L, Fabbrocini G. Teledermatology for acne patients: How to reduce face-to-face visits during COVID-19 pandemic. *J Cosmet Dermatol.* 2020;19(8):1828.

40. Abyaneh M-AY, Griffith RD, Falto-Aizpurua L, Arora H, Nouri K. Lasers for acne. In: *Pediatric Dermatologic Surgery.* John Wiley & Sons, Ltd; 2019:207-221.

41. Kontochristopoulos G, Platsidaki E. Chemical peels in active acne and acne scars. *Clin Dermatol.* 2017;35(2):179-182.

42. Soliman YS, Horowitz R, Hashim PW, Nia JK, Farberg AS, Goldenberg G. Update on acne scar treatment. *Cutis.* 2018;102(1):21;25;47;48.

43. Baldwin HE. Diagnosis and treatment of rosacea: state of the art. *J Drugs Dermatol JDD.* 2012;11(6):725-730.

44. Kini SP, Nicholson K, DeLong LK, et al. A pilot study in discrepancies in quality of life among three cutaneous types of rosacea. *J Am Acad Dermatol.* 2010;62(6):1069-1071.

45. Gallo RL, Granstein RD, Kang S, et al. Standard classification and pathophysiology of rosacea: The 2017 update by the National Rosacea Society Expert Committee. *J Am Acad Dermatol.* 2018;78(1):148-155.

46. Yamasaki K, Gallo RL. The molecular pathology of rosacea. *J Dermatol Sci.* 2009;55(2):77-81.

47. Helfrich YR, Maier LE, Cui Y, et al. Clinical, histologic, and molecular analysis of differences between erythematotelangiectatic rosacea and telangiectatic photoaging. *JAMA Dermatol.* 2015;151(8):825-836.

48. Chang Y-S, Huang Y-C. Role of Demodex mite infestation in rosacea: a systematic review and meta-analysis. *J Am Acad Dermatol.* 2017;77(3):441-447.e6.

49. Aldrich N, Gerstenblith M, Fu P, et al. Genetic vs environmental factors that correlate With rosacea: a cohort-based survey of twins. *JAMA Dermatol.* 2015;151(11):1213-1219.

50. Tan J, Almeida LMC, Bewley A, et al. Updating the diagnosis, classification and assessment of rosacea: recommendations from the global ROSacea COnsensus (ROSCO) panel. *Br J Dermatol.* 2017;176(2):431-438.

51. Holmes AD, Steinhoff M. Integrative concepts of rosacea pathophysiology, clinical presentation and new therapeutics. *Exp Dermatol.* 2017;26(8):659-667.

52. Forton FMN, De Maertelaer V. Papulopustular rosacea and rosacea-like demodicosis: two phenotypes of the same disease? *J Eur Acad Dermatol Venereol.* 2018;32(6):1011-1016.

53. Juliandri J, Wang X, Liu Z, Zhang J, Xu Y, Yuan C. Global rosacea treatment guidelines and expert consensus points: The differences. *J Cosmet Dermatol.* 2019;18(4):960-965.

54. Hsu C-C, Lee JY-Y. Pronounced facial flushing and persistent erythema of rosacea effectively treated by carvedilol, a nonselective β-adrenergic blocker. *J Am Acad Dermatol.* 2012;67(3):491-493.

55. Lipozencic J, Ljubojevic S. Perioral dermatitis. *Clin Dermatol.* 2011;29(2):157-161.

56. Peralta L, Morais P. Perioral dermatitis -- the role of nasal steroids. *Cutan Ocul Toxicol.* 2012;31(2):160-163.

57. Tempark T, Shwayder TA. Perioral dermatitis: a review of the condition with special attention to treatment options. *Am J Clin Dermatol.* 2014;15(2):101-113.

58. Luelmo-Aguilar J, Santandreu MS. Folliculitis: recognition and management. *Am J Clin Dermatol.* 2004;5(5):301-310.

59. Danby FW, Margesson LJ. Hidradenitis suppurativa. *Dermatol Clin.* 2010;28(4):779-793.

60. Jemec GBE. Clinical practice. Hidradenitis suppurativa. *N Engl J Med.* 2012;366(2):158-164.

61. Alikhan A, Sayed C, Alavi A, et al. North American clinical management guidelines for hidradenitis suppurativa: A publication from the United States and Canadian Hidradenitis Suppurativa Foundations: Part I: Diagnosis, evaluation, and the use of complementary and procedural management. *J Am Acad Dermatol.* 2019;81(1):76-90.

62. Garg A, Papagermanos V, Midura M, Strunk A, Merson J. Opioid, alcohol, and cannabis misuse among patients with hidradenitis suppurativa: A population-based analysis in the United States. *J Am Acad Dermatol.* 2018;79(3):495-500.e1.

63. Frew JW, Hawkes JE, Krueger JG. A systematic review and critical evaluation of inflammatory cytokine associations in hidradenitis suppurativa. *F1000Research.* 2018;7:1930.

64. Goldburg SR, Strober BE, Payette MJ. Hidradenitis suppurativa: epidemiology, clinical presentation, and pathogenesis. *J Am Acad Dermatol.* 2020;82(5):1045-1058.

65. Ingram JR. The Genetics of Hidradenitis Suppurativa. *Dermatol Clin.* 2016;34(1):23-28.

66. Ring HC, Thorsen J, Saunte DM, et al. The follicular skin microbiome in patients with hidradenitis suppurativa and healthy controls. *JAMA Dermatol.* 2017;153(9):897-905.

67. Ring HC, Bay L, Nilsson M, et al. Bacterial biofilm in chronic lesions of hidradenitis suppurativa. *Br J Dermatol.* 2017;176(4):993-1000.

68. Shlyankevich J, Chen AJ, Kim GE, Kimball AB. Hidradenitis suppurativa is a systemic disease with substantial comorbidity burden: a chart-verified case-control analysis. *J Am Acad Dermatol.* 2014;71(6):1144-1150.

69. Garg A, Malviya N, Strunk A. Comorbidity Screening in hidradenitis suppurativa: Evidence-based recommendations from the US and Canadian Hidradenitis Suppurativa Foundations. *J Am Acad Dermatol.* 2021;84:

70. Jung JM, Lee KH, Kim Y-J, et al. Assessment of overall and specific cancer risks in patients with hidradenitis suppurativa. *JAMA Dermatol.* 2020;156(8):844-853.

71. Chapman S, Delgadillo D, Barber C, Khachemoune A. Cutaneous squamous cell carcinoma complicating hidradenitis suppurativa: a review of the prevalence, pathogenesis, and treatment of this dreaded complication. *Acta Dermatovenerol Alp Pannonica Adriat.* 2018;27(1):25-28.

72. Kridin K, Shani M, Schonmann Y, et al. Psoriasis and hidradenitis suppurativa: a large-scale population-based study. *J Am Acad Dermatol.* Published online November 28, 2018.

73. Hurley H. Axillary hyperhidrosis, apocrine bromhidrosis, hidradenitis suppurativa and familial benign pemphigus. Surgical approach. In: *Roenigk & Roenigk's Dermatologic Surgery: Principles and Practice.* 2nd ed. CRC Press; 1996.

74. Rambhatla PV, Lim HW, Hamzavi I. A systematic review of treatments for hidradenitis suppurativa. *Arch Dermatol.* 2012;148(4):439-446.

75. Alikhan A, Sayed C, Alavi A, et al. North American clinical management guidelines for hidradenitis suppurativa: A publication from the United States and Canadian Hidradenitis Suppurativa Foundations: Part II: Topical, intralesional and systemic medical managment . *J Am Acad Dermatol.* 2019;81:91-101.

76. Golbari NM, Porter ML, Kimball AB. Antiandrogen therapy with spironolactone for the treatment of hidradenitis suppurativa. *J Am Acad Dermatol.* 2019;80(1):114-119.

77. Matusiak L, Bieniek A, Szepietowski JC. Acitretin treatment for hidradenitis suppurativa: a prospective series of 17 patients. *Br J Dermatol.* 2014;171(1):170-174.

78. Savage KT, Flood KS, Porter ML, Kimball AB. TNF- inhibitors in the treatment of hidradenitis suppurativa. *Ther Adv Chronic Dis.* 2019;10:2040622319851640.

79. Kong YL, Tey HL. Treatment of acne vulgaris during pregnancy and lactation. *Drugs.* 2013;73(8):779-787.

80. Leachman SA, Reed BR. The use of dermatologic drugs in pregnancy and lactation. *Dermatol Clin.* 2006;24(2):167-197, vi.

81. Chien A. Retinoids in acne management: review of current understanding, future considerations, and focus on topical treatments. *J Drugs Dermatol JDD.* 2018;17(12):s51-55.

82. Butler DC, Heller MM, Murase JE. Safety of dermatologic medications in pregnancy and lactation: Part II. Lactation. *J Am Acad Dermatol.* 2014;70(3):417.e1-10; quiz 427.

83. Tan J, Miklas M. A novel topical retinoid for acne: trifarotene 50 μg/g Cream. *Skin Ther Lett.* 2020;25(2):1-2.

84. Tan J, Thiboutot D, Popp G, et al. Randomized phase 3 evaluation of trifarotene 50 μg/g cream treatment of moderate facial and truncal acne. *J Am Acad Dermatol.* 2019;80(6):1691-1699.

85. Paik J. Topical minocycline foam 4%: a review in acne vulgaris. *Am J Clin Dermatol.* 2020;21(3):449-456.

86. Leyden JJ, Sniukiene V, Berk DR, Kaoukhov A. Efficacy and safety of sarecycline, a novel, once-daily, narrow spectrum antibiotic for the treatment of moderate to severe facial acne vulgaris: results of a phase 2, dose-ranging study. *J Drugs Dermatol JDD.* 2018;17(3):333-338.

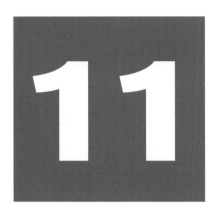

Bacterial Infections

Christina L. Boull

INTRODUCTION TO CHAPTER

Within hours after birth, the skin's surface becomes a host for a vast assortment of microorganisms.[1] Species of staphylococcus, corynebacterium, *Propionibacterium acnes*, and a multitude of other bacteria, yeast, and fungi begin to colonize the skin, each organism with a predilection for specific body sites.[2] The skin's microbiome changes over time modified by environmental exposures and hormonal shifts. A growing volume of studies highlight the essential function of the skin's microorganisms in protecting us from pathogens and regulating the immune system.[3] A pathogenic shift in the skin flora, or dysbiosis, has been described in acne, atopic dermatitis, and chronic wounds, but is likely to contribute to many other disease processes.[2]

The host immune system is an essential factor in influencing the microbiome, but the interactions are complex and differ by disease process. For example, individuals with atopic dermatitis tend to have decreased microbiome diversity with a lower prevalence of bacterial species that are anti-inflammatory.[4] In contrast, diabetic ulcers that are deeper or chronic demonstrate more microbial diversity than those that are more shallow or present for a shorter duration.[5] Ongoing research in this field will help to highlight the interface between the human microbiome and disease pathogenesis. In most cases, our microbiome is protective, serving as an important component of the skin's barrier function. Disruption of this barrier caused by mechanical trauma or intrinsic cutaneous disease alters the skin's biodiversity and inflammatory pathways allowing for skin infections to propagate.[2]

Most bacterial skin infections are caused by coagulase positive *Staphylococcus aureus* or group A beta hemolytic streptococci. These common skin infections previously resulted in serious illness and death until the 1950s when penicillin became widely available. By the early 1960s scattered cases of methicillin-resistant staphylococcus (MRSA) were already emerging. From the late 1960s to the mid-1990s, MRSA infections became a major problem especially in large urban hospitals. In the past decade, improved infection control measures have decreased hospital acquired MRSA infections, but community acquired cases have continued to increase.

Syphilis has been called "the great masquerader" and "the great imitator" based on the many varied presentations of the cutaneous and systemic findings. Patients with secondary syphilis usually present with rashes that mimic common papulosquamous skin diseases but can manifest skin findings that mimic almost any cutaneous disorder.

IMPETIGO

Introduction

Key points for impetigo

✓ *Staphylococcus aureus* is the most common cause, but group A beta hemolytic streptococci including the nephritogenic strains may also cause impetigo.

✓ Impetigo presents with a red macule or papule that quickly becomes a vesicle which ruptures resulting in erosions with honey-colored crusts.

✓ Removal of the crusts and topical antibiotics are sufficient therapies for most patients.

Impetigo is a common, highly contagious, and superficial skin infection. Nonbullous impetigo accounts for the majority of cases. It occurs in children of all ages, as well as adults, whereas the bullous form is most common in newborns. Impetigo is limited to the epidermis.

Pathogenesis

Staphylococcus aureus is the most common cause of both bullous and nonbullous impetigo. Group A beta hemolytic streptococci including the nephritogenic strains may also cause impetigo.[6] Nasal colonization by staphylococcus or cutaneous colonization by streptococci typically precede cutaneous inoculation.[6]

Clinical Presentation

▶ History and Physical Examination

- Nonbullous impetigo begins as a single red macule or papule that quickly becomes a vesicle. The vesicle ruptures, forming erosion and the contents dry to produce the characteristic honey-colored crust (Figure 11-1). Nonbullous impetigo typically occurs on the face or extremities.

- Bullous impetigo begins as a superficial vesicle that rapidly progresses to a flaccid bulla, with sharp margins and no surrounding erythema (Figure 11-2). When the bulla ruptures, a moist yellow crust forms. Impetigo is often spread to surrounding areas by autoinoculation. Bullous impetigo usually arises on grossly normal skin and favors moist intertriginous areas, such as the diaper area, axillae, and neck folds.

- Ecthyma is an uncommon variant of impetigo that begins as a typical impetigo infection, often on the lower legs. The infection then spreads deeper into the dermis forming ulcers that are covered by a thick crust (Figure 11-3). It is more common in young children, immunosuppressed patients and in patients with poor hygiene.

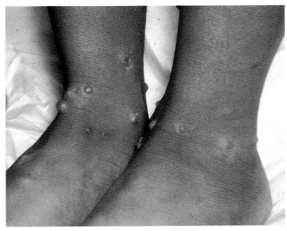

▲ **Figure 11-2.** Bullous impetigo. Multiple superficial bullae on ankles and feet.

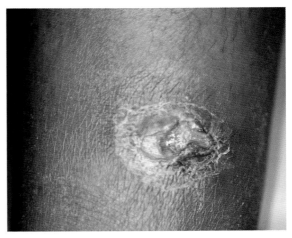

▲ **Figure 11-3.** Ecthyma. Ulcer partially covered with thick crust.

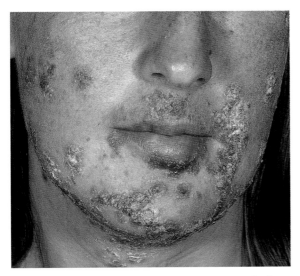

▲ **Figure 11-1.** Extensive impetigo on face. Multiple yellow white crusts.

▶ Laboratory Findings

Bacterial cultures from the infected areas are usually positive for *S. aureus* or streptococci.

Diagnosis

The key diagnostic clinical features of impetigo are honey-colored crusts or bullae.

▶ Differential Diagnosis

✓ Herpes simplex: Presents with grouped vesicles on the lips, perioral, and genital region. It can exist concomitantly with impetigo.

✓ Atopic dermatitis: Presents with pruritic, scaly, or crusted papules and plaques in patients with a history of atopy. Impetigo may occur concomitant with atopic dermatitis.

✓ Varicella (chicken pox): Presents with fever and widespread vesicles with surrounding erythema.

✓ Other: Perioral dermatitis, insect bites, tinea infections, abrasions, lacerations, thermal burns, erythema multiforme, dermatitis herpetiformis, burns, bullous fixed drug eruptions, staphylococcal scalded skin syndrome, bullous tinea pedis, and bullous insect bites. In adults, bullous pemphigoid and pemphigus are in the differential.

Management

The superficial crusts should be removed with gentle cleansing. An antimicrobial wash may be used. Wet dressings can help to remove thicker crusts (see Chapter 6). Topical antibiotics are favored for treatment of localized infections as they are equally effective as oral antibiotics.[6,7] Mupirocin cream or ointment should be applied 3 times a day for 7–14 days. Retapamulin ointment may be used in adults and children 9 months and older twice daily for 5 days.

Severe or widespread impetigo may require oral antibiotics, such as cephalexin, dicloxacillin, clindamycin, amoxicillin/clavulanate, minocycline, or doxycycline. Treatment should be tailored to microbial sensitivity patterns.

Clinical Course and Prognosis

Impetigo usually responds well to the treatment but may be recurrent. Impetigo may resolve with postinflammatory hyper or hypopigmentation. Ecthyma ulcers may heal with scarring.

Indications for Consultation

Severe or persistent disease that does not respond to therapy

Patient Information

American Academy of Dermatology: https://www.aad.org/public/diseases/a-z/impetigo-overview

▼ BOILS

Introduction

Key point for boils

✓ Methicillin sensitive *Staphylococcus aureus* is the most common cause of boils in the general population.

✓ Boils caused by MRSA are more common in hospitals and nursing homes and in patients who have diabetes or atopic dermatitis.

✓ Large boils should be lanced and drained.

A boil (furuncle) is a deep-seated inflammatory nodule that develops around a hair follicle, often from a preceding superficial folliculitis. A carbuncle is two or more confluent boils.

Pathogenesis

Coagulase positive *Staphylococcus aureus* is the most common cause of boils and carbuncles. The organism may be methicillin sensitive (MSSA) or methicillin resistant (MRSA).

MRSA infections may be acquired in healthcare facilities such as hospitals and nursing homes or more commonly in the community. In one study of 12 United States emergency departments, MRSA infections were responsible for 38% to 84% of purulent skin and soft tissue infections.[8]

Clinical Presentation

▶ History

Patients report a rapidly enlarging tender "pimple" or boil. The patient may give a history of risk factors such as crowded living conditions, infected family members, diabetes, obesity, atopic dermatitis, or inherited or acquired immune deficiency.

▶ Physical Examination

A boil starts as a hard, tender, red nodule with an overlying folliculocentric pustule. The nodule enlarges and becomes painful and fluctuant after several days (Figures 11-4, 11-5). Rupture may occur, with extrusion of pus.

▶ Laboratory Findings

Cultures from pus within the lesion or from drainage are usually positive for MSSA or MRSA.

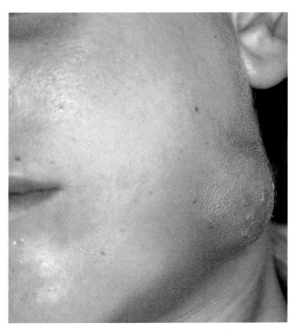

▲ Figure 11-4. Staphylococcal boil on jawline.

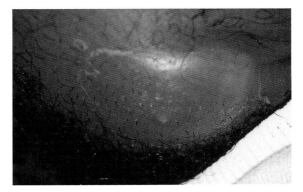

▲ Figure 11-5. Furuncle. Staphylococcal boil evolving into an abscess in suprapubic area.

Diagnosis

The key diagnostic clinical feature of a boil is a tender, fluctuant cyst, or nodule.

▷ Differential Diagnosis

✓ Ruptured epidermal inclusion cyst: This may very closely resemble a staphylococcal boil, but when lanced, the cyst contains thick white keratinous material.

✓ Acne cyst: This may also closely resemble a staphylococcal boil, but other signs of acne such as comedones should be present.

✓ Hidradenitis suppurativa: Presents with cysts limited to intertriginous areas of the body.

✓ Other: Deep fungal infections, dental abscess, kerion.

Management

Small boils may be managed with a trial of warm moist compresses to promote drainage. For larger lesions, the most important management is incision with a scalpel blade (#11 is recommended) and drainage with evacuation of the contents and probing of the cavity to break up loculations. Bacterial cultures of the fluid should be collected. The wound can be packed with iodoform gauze to encourage further drainage. The surgical site should be covered with a dry dressing.[9]

Patients with central facial disease, multiple lesions, immunosuppression, lesions greater than 5 cm, or with surrounding cellulitis or fever may require systemic antibiotics. Patients who are very young or very old may also require systemic antibiotics. Recommended oral antibiotics for MSSA infections include dicloxacillin, cephalexin, clindamycin, doxycycline, minocycline, and trimethoprim sulfamethoxazole. Medications recommended for MRSA include clindamycin, doxycycline, minocycline, and trimethoprim sulfamethoxazole.[9] Antibiotic selection should be adjusted based on microbial sensitivities.

Clinical Course and Prognosis

Boils typically heal over the course of 1–2 weeks after drainage. Patients with recurrent boils who are carriers of MSSA or MRSA should be treated with intranasal mupirocin (Bactroban) ointment twice a day for 5 days each month. This approach has been reported to decrease recurrence rates by approximately 50%.[9]

Indications for Consultation

Severe or persistent or recurrent disease that does not respond to therapy.

Patient Information

Centers of Disease Control and Prevention www.cdc.gov/mrsa/
    Derm Net NZ: https://dermnetnz.org/topics/boil/

▼ CELLULITIS

Introduction

Key points for cellulitis

✓ Most cases of cellulitis are caused by *Staphylococcus aureus* and group A streptococcus.

✓ Cellulitis presents with the acute onset of localized tenderness and erythema with ill-defined borders.

✓ Treatment for most common forms of cellulitis includes empiric treatment with penicillinase-resistant penicillin, first generation cephalosporin, amoxicillin-clavulanate (Augmentin), a macrolide, or a fluoroquinolone antibiotic.

Cellulitis is an acute infection of the dermis and subcutaneous tissue. It is a common cause of outpatient medical visits and inpatient hospital admissions, accounting for 10% of infectious disease related United States hospitalizations from 1998 to 2006.[10] Unfortunately, many of these diagnoses are inaccurate resulting in a huge financial burden on the healthcare system. It is estimated that approximately 30% of hospital admissions for a diagnosis of cellulitis are actually for cellulitis mimics that do not require hospitalization. This translates into an estimated $195–$515 million dollars in avoidable healthcare spending annually in the United States alone.[11] Careful consideration of potential alternative diagnoses and early consultation with the dermatology service can ensure appropriate patient care.[12]

Pathogenesis

Most cases of cellulitis are caused by *Staphylococcus aureus* and group A streptococcus. However, in certain situations other organisms may be involved, such as Gram-negative organisms in cellulitis originating from a toe web fissure or *Haemophilus influenza* in young infants.[13]

Risk factors for cellulitis include skin trauma or a leg ulcer or fissured toe webs which can serve as a portal of entry for pathogenic bacteria. Other risk factors include chronic venous or arterial insufficiency, edema, surgery, IV drug use, body piercing, human and animal bites, diabetes, hepatic cirrhosis, immunosuppression, and neutropenia.[13]

Clinical Presentation

History

Classic features include rubor (erythema), dolor (pain), calor (warmth), and tumor (edema). Other symptoms include fever, chills, and malaise.

Physical Examination

Cellulitis typically begins with the acute onset of localized tenderness and erythema with ill-defined borders. Cutaneous edema may cause a dimpled (peau d'orange) texture of the skin surface. Overlying vesicles, bullae, hemorrhage, and crust may form (Figure 11-6). Less common findings include ascending lymphangitis and regional lymphadenopathy. Bilateral cellulitis is uncommon and should prompt consideration of alternative diagnoses. While most cases are mild, severe cellulitis may cause serious systemic findings including confusion, tachycardia, fever, and hypotension.

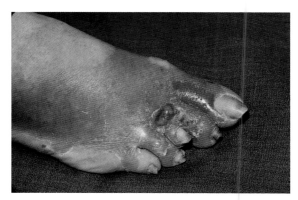

▲ **Figure 11-6.** Cellulitis. Erythematous tender area with crusts and bullae on foot.

Some other clinical presentations of less common types of cellulitis are listed in Table 11-1.

▶ Laboratory Findings

The diagnosis of cellulitis is generally made in the clinical setting. If indicated, cultures from exudate or blistered areas can be done with a culturette swab or cultures can be obtained by aspirating the affected skin. A skin punch biopsy of affected skin may also be cultured. However, these techniques often do not isolate the pathogenic organism. If cultures are positive, they usually show Gram-positive microorganisms, primarily *Staphylococcus aureus*, group A or group B streptococci, *Streptococcus viridans*, *Streptococcus pneumoniae*, *Enterococcus faecalis*, and less commonly, Gram-negative organisms such as *Hemophilus influenzae and Pseudomonas aeruginosa*.[13]

Other lab findings may include leukocytosis and elevated inflammatory markers.

Diagnosis

The key diagnostic clinical feature of cellulitis is a painful, warm, red, edematous, and ill-defined plaque. A recently described prospectively validated predictive tool, the asymmetry, leukocytosis, tachycardia, age $\geq$ 70 years score (ALT-70) has been shown to increase the accuracy of cellulitis diagnoses made in the emergency room and inpatient settings.[14] Points are assigned as follows:

- Unilateral (as opposed to bilateral) presentation (3 points)
- Leukocytosis with white blood cell count >/= 10,000/μL (1 point)
- Tachycardia with heart rate >/= 90 bpm (1 point)
- Age >/= 70 years (2 points)

A score of 5–7 points is associated with a true cellulitis more than 80% of the time, whereas a score of less than

Table 11-1. Less Common Types of Cellulitis

Types of cellulitis	Presentation	Organism(s)
Erysipelas	Sharply defined red, edematous plaque, usually on face or legs (Figure 11-7).	Group A, or less commonly B,C or G streptococci or rarely *S. aureus*
Periorbital (preseptal) cellulitis	Painful erythema and edema on the eyelid and periorbital area, more common in children Figure 11-8).	*S aureus, Streptococcus pyogenes, Haemophilus influenzae*
Ecthyma gangrenosum	Painful blue-grey thick eschar over an ulcer in an immunocompromised patient.	*Pseudomonas aeruginosa*
Perianal cellulitis (dermatitis)	Sharply marginated bright red, painful erythema surrounding the anus (Figure 11-9). More common in young children.	*Streptococcus pyogenes*
Blistering distal dactylitis	Tense non-tender bullae filled with seropurulent fluid on the palmar distal fingertips, more common in children.	Group A streptococcus, occasionally *S. aureus* or Group B streptococcus
Streptococcal intertrigo	Similar presentation to perianal strep cellulitis, but it occurs in body fold areas such as the axillae and inguinal area.	*Streptococcus pyogenes*
Crepitant cellulitis (gas gangrene)	Rapid development of edema, crepitus and bullae.	Clostridia species usually *C. perfringens*
Gangrenous cellulitis (necrotizing fasciitis)	Indurated painful erythema with bullae (Figure 11-10) quickly progressing into a large black eschar and necrosis of the skin, fascia or muscle.	Polymicrobial including Group A Streptococcus and anaerobes

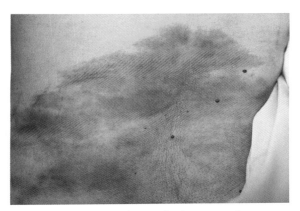

▲ **Figure 11-7.** Erysipelas. Red edematous plaque on back.

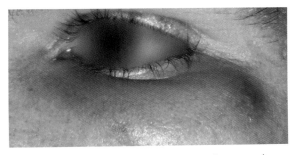

▲ **Figure 11-8.** Periorbital cellulitis. Erythema and edema below the eye.

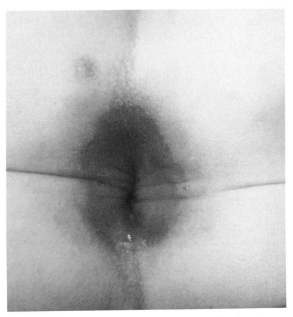

▲ **Figure 11-9.** Perianal cellulitis in a child. Sharply marginated bright red painful erythema surrounding the anus.

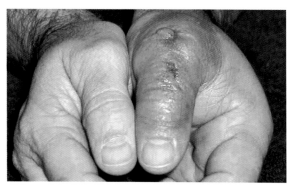

▲ **Figure 11-10.** Necrotizing fasciitis. Sudden onset of painful area with erythema, edema and bullae.

3 points would suggest an alternative diagnosis for more than 80% of patients. A dermatology consult should be considered for those with an intermediate score of 3–4.

▶ Differential Diagnosis

✓ Acute allergic contact dermatitis: Usually presents with pruritic, but not painful red plaques, with more than one area involved. Often well-marginated.

✓ Stasis dermatitis: Presents with bilateral chronic dermatitis on the lower legs, with red/brown pigment. Cellulitis may be concomitant.

✓ Thrombophlebitis/deep vein thrombosis (DVT): Presents with calf pain, erythema, usually no fever or chills, abnormal ultrasound of the leg vessels/

✓ Other: Gout, herpes zoster, insect bite, erythema migrans, erythema nodosum, panniculitis, eosinophilic cellulitis, fixed drug eruption, lipodermatosclerosis, polyarteritis nodosa, and Sweet's syndrome.

MANAGEMENT

Treatment for most common forms of cellulitis includes empiric treatment with a penicillinase-resistant penicillin, first generation cephalosporin, amoxicillin-clavulanate (Augmentin), a macrolide, or a fluoroquinolone antibiotic.[13] See the above section on boils for recommendations on systemic treatment for MRSA.

Localized disease can be treated in the outpatient setting, whereas extensive disease may require intravenous administration in an inpatient setting. Ancillary measures include elevation of the involved limb to reduce swelling. One should also identify and treat the underlying portal of entry of the cellulitis (e.g., tinea pedis, leg ulcer). Imaging studies and emergent surgical consultation are needed if crepitant or necrotic cellulitis is suspected.

Clinical Course and Prognosis

Episodes of cellulitis may result in permanent damage to lymphatic channels and subsequent worsened chronic edema. Preventative strategies include use of compression garments, emollients to improve skin barrier function, and diuretics when appropriate.

Indications for Consultation

Given the frequency of misdiagnosis of cellulitis early dermatology consultation should be obtained for patients with bilateral disease, those without systemic signs of infection, or those not responding to standard treatments. Patients with non-reassuring vital signs, altered mental status, high fevers, crepitant or necrotic cellulitis should be hospitalized.

Patient Information

Up To Date:
   https://www.uptodate.com/contents/skin-and-soft-tissue-infection-cellulitis-beyond-the-basics

▼ LYMPHANGITIS

Introduction

Lymphangitis is caused by inflammation of the lymphatic channels in the deep dermis. A variety of infectious and noninfectious causes have been described. Noninfectious causes include lymphangitic spread of malignancies (lymphangitis carcinomatosa), and granulomatous intestinal lymphangitis associated with Crohn disease.[15] Bacterial lymphangitis is the most common infectious variant but fungal, filarial, or mycobacterial lymphangitis should be considered in the appropriate clinical setting.

Pathogenesis

Acute bacterial lymphangitis usually occurs at sites proximal to a cutaneous injury or soft tissue infection. Pathogens are directly inoculated into the lymphatic channels and spread proximally toward regional lymph nodes. Individuals with lymphedema, congenital lymphatic malformations, or damaged lymphatic systems from surgery or injury have a higher risk of developing lymphangitis. *Streptococcus pyogenes* and *Staphylococcus aureus* are the most common pathogens. *Nocardia brasiliensis* may enter the skin via a cat scratch or puncture from plant material. Zoonotic pathogens include *Pasteurella multocida* from animal bites, *Erysipelothrix rhusiopathiae* from contact with animal butchering or aquariums, *Francisella tularensis* from tick bites or contact with infected animals, and *Bacillus anthracis* from contact with animal hides or wool.[15]

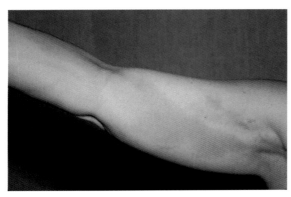

▲ **Figure 11-11.** Lymphangitis. Erythematous streak on the flexor surface of the arm.

Clinical Presentation

▶ History and Physical Examination

Acute bacterial lymphadenitis typically presents as rapidly advancing erythematous streaking moving from a distal area of skin injury or infection toward regional lymph nodes (Figure 11-11). The overlying skin is tender and there is often associated lymphadenopathy. Fever may be present. Nodular lymphangitis consists of a slow progression of subcutaneous nodules along lymphatic tracts (sporotrichoid spread). The nodules may ulcerate. This presentation is more typical of nocardia, tularemia, fungal, and atypical mycobacterial infections.

▶ Laboratory Findings

Leukocytosis or elevated inflammatory markers may be seen in some patients. In cases of nodular lymphangitis, a skin biopsy should be obtained for histopathologic analysis and for tissue culture. Bacterial, mycobacteria, and fungal cultures should be obtained.

Diagnosis

The diagnosis of acute bacterial lymphangitis is made clinically in the setting of erythematous streaking of the skin overlying lymphatic channels. Nodular lymphangitis or lymphangitis not responsive to systemic antibiotics should prompt skin biopsy.

▶ Differential Diagnosis

✓ Erysipelas: Indurated well-circumscribed erythematous plaques which do not typically follow the lymphatic channels. Erysipelas may be the nidus for lymphangitis.

✓ Lymphangitis carcinomatosa: Indolent progressive lymphangitic streaking in a patient with a systemic malignancy.

✓ Thrombophlebitis: Tender subcutaneous nodule or cord at the site of an intravenous (IV) site or IV drug use, or in those with a hypercoagulable state.

✓ IV infiltration/ extravasation: Leakage of intravenous fluid into the surrounding tissues can produce a tender subcutaneous nodule at the site. Extravasation of acidic, basic, or hyperosmotic solutions.

✓ Phlebitis: Linear streaking erythema at an IV insertion site resulting from inflammation of the vessel.

Management

Systemic antimicrobials with coverage of staphylococcus and streptococcus are the first-line treatment for acute bacterial lymphangitis.[15] Please see information from the preceding cellulitis section for further details. A detailed exposure history should be obtained in patients with nodular lymphangitis. Treatment should be guided by biopsy and tissue culture results.

Clinical Course and Prognosis

Acute bacterial lymphangitis responds quickly to antibiotic therapy. Those with an underlying predisposition to lymphangitis should monitor their skin closely to ensure that there are no skin breaks that could serve as bacterial entry sites. Nodular bacterial lymphangitis responds to the treatment once the correct microorganism is identified, but surgical debridement may be needed in recalcitrant cases.

Indications for Consultation

Consultations to dermatology and infectious disease should be considered for nodular lymphangitis as a tissue culture should guide antimicrobial therapy.

Patient Information

https://emedicine.medscape.com/article/966003-overview

| ▼ ERYTHRASMA |

Introduction

Key points for erythrasma

✓ *Corynebacterium minutissimum*, a Gram-positive bacillus is the cause of erythrasma.

✓ It presents with well-marginated pink brown patches in skin folds or web spaces.

✓ Topical clindamycin solution, erythromycin gel, or benzoyl peroxide wash are first-line therapies.

Erythrasma is a common bacterial infection that favors the interdigital spaces, umbilicus, axillae, crural, inframammary, and intergluteal folds. Generalized forms have been reported in individuals with diabetes mellitus.[13]

Pathogenesis

Corynebacterium minutissimum, a Gram-positive bacillus, is the causative bacteria. It thrives in warm, moist areas of the body. Erythrasma is more prevalent in warm climates and in individuals with advanced age, poor hygiene, increased sweating, obesity, and diabetes mellitus.[13] It can be found in isolation or in conjunction with other infections or dermatoses that favor the same anatomical sites, such as dermatophyte or candida infections, contact dermatitis, and inverse psoriasis.[16]

Clinical Presentation

History and Physical Examination

Patients present with well-marginated pink to brown patches in skin folds or web spaces. Central clearing may be noted. There is often overlying scaling and fissuring and the surrounding skin may be macerated. Usually the lesions are not symptomatic, but they can be mildly pruritic. The web spaces of the 3rd, 4th, and 5th toes and the inguinal folds are the most common sites of erythrasma. Illumination with a Wood's lamp will reveal coral red fluorescence (Figure 11-12).

Laboratory Findings

Bacterial cultures or gram stains may be obtained but are rarely needed.

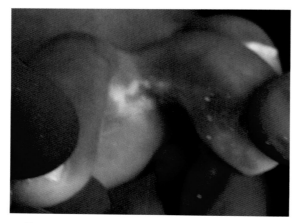

▲ **Figure 11-12.** Erythrasma. Wood's lamp reveals coral red fluorescence in toe web.

Diagnosis

Examination with Wood's lamp in conjunction with a characteristic distribution is usually adequate to diagnose erythrasma.

▶ Differential Diagnosis

✓ Tinea: Annular scaling pruritic patches and plaques. Some variants may fluoresce green or blue-green. Skin scraping will show fungal elements.

✓ Candidal intertrigo: Erythematous macerated patches favoring the interdigital spaces, crural and submammary folds, and under the abdomen. Erythema is ill-defined and satellite papules may be present.

✓ Inverse psoriasis: Well-marginated pink plaques in the axillae, inguinal creases, genital area, and gluteal cleft. Look for other signs of psoriasis including nail dystrophy, and plaques on the extensor surfaces, scalp, post-auricular sulci, or in the umbilicus.

✓ Inverse lichen planus: Asymptomatic or mildly pruritic violaceous plaques in the skin folds which may have overlying reticulate white striations.

✓ Contact dermatitis: Pink ill-defined pruritic scaling plaques which may be located in the axillary vault or pillars.

✓ Seborrheic dermatitis: Ill-defined scaling salmon pink plaques in the skin folds. Look in more common sites including the scalp, conchal bowls, eyebrows, and glabella for similar lesions.

Management

Erythrasma typically resolves with the use of topical antibiotics. Topical clindamycin solution, erythromycin gel, or benzoyl peroxide wash are first-line therapies. Systemic treatment with oral clindamycin, a macrolide, or tetracycline antibiotic can be considered for rapid clearance or for severe or widespread infections.[13]

Clinical Course and Prognosis

Erythrasma clears quickly with most treatments. Those with predisposing factors may experience recurrences so antimicrobial soaps can be used preventatively.

Indications for Consultation

Multiple dermatoses mimic erythrasma and may present concurrently. Consultation should be obtained when erythrasma fails to resolve with standard treatments.

Patient Information

SYPHILIS

Introduction

Key points for syphilis

✓ Syphilis is a sexually transmitted disease caused by *Treponema pallidum*, a spirochetal bacterium.

✓ The primary lesion is a non-tender, indurated, firm ulcer (chancre), with a raised border on the genitals.

✓ Secondary syphilis presents with pink, violaceous or red-brown macules and papules on the face, trunk and extremities including the palms and soles, mimicking many common papulosquamous skin diseases.

✓ Up to 30% of patients with untreated syphilis go on to develop tertiary syphilis which primary affects the central nervous system and the cardiovascular system.

✓ A single intramuscular dose of Benzathine penicillin G 2.4 million units is recommended for primary, secondary, and early latent syphilis.

Syphilis is a sexually transmitted disease with a worldwide distribution. Incidence dropped dramatically after the introduction of penicillin as treatment and reached a nadir in 2001, but the Centers for Disease Control and Prevention (CDC) has reported resurgence in recent years. Rates escalated initially among men who have sex with men. More recently incidence has also spiked in women and in men who have sex with women.[17] Cases of congenital syphilis have increased as a result.[17] Syphilitic skin eruptions may manifest various morphologies, often mimicking other skin conditions, such as pityriasis rosea, psoriasis, lichen planus, exanthems, etc., giving cutaneous secondary syphilis the name "the great masquerader."

Pathogenesis

Syphilis is an infection caused by *Treponema pallidum*, a spirochetal bacterium. Approximately one-third of people who come in contact with a primary syphilis lesion (chancre) become infected.[18] After inoculation through skin or mucous membranes, the bacterium spreads throughout the body via the lymphatic system and blood.

Clinical Presentation

▶ History and Physical Examination

Syphilis progresses through active and latent stages and in some cases progresses to a tertiary stage.[18]

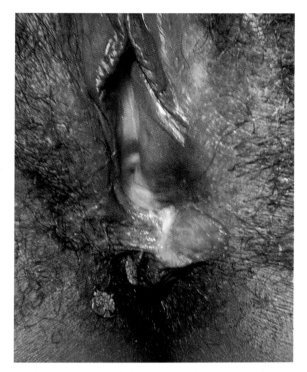

Figure 11-13. Syphilis. Primary chancre on vulva presenting as a superficial ulcer.

- Primary stage

  At the site of entry, 10–90 days (average 3 weeks) after infection, a dusky red macule appears and evolves into a papule. Surface necrosis occurs with progression to a non-tender, indurated, firm ulcer (chancre), with a raised border (Figure11-13). Multiple chancres may form. Nontender regional lymphadenopathy may occur. Chancres spontaneously heal in 2–10 weeks.

- Secondary stage and latent stages

  Untreated patients may progress to secondary syphilis. Systemic symptoms, such as fever, malaise, sore throat, generalized lymphadenopathy, myalgia, and headache develop 4–10 weeks after onset of infection. Within a few days, a pink, violaceous or red-brown macular, papular, or more typically a papulosquamous eruption appears on the face, trunk (Figure 11-14), and extremities; often including the palms and soles (Figure 11-15). The eruption may become follicular, pustular, annular, nodular, or plaque-like and may be pruritic. A patchy, "moth-eaten" and/or diffuse alopecia may develop.

  Superficial erosions (mucous patches) are seen in the mouth, throat, and genitalia. Wart-like moist papules (condylomata lata) may appear in the anogenital area. Chancres of primary syphilis may be concurrent with secondary syphilis. Patients are highly infectious.

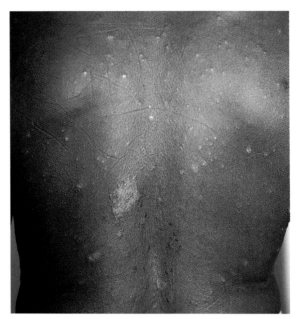

▲ **Figure 11-14.** Secondary syphilis on back. Multiple scaly papules.

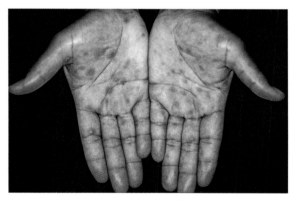

▲ **Figure 11-15.** Secondary syphilis on palms: pink and tan macules and papules.

Without treatment, the symptoms and eruptions clear within 3–12 weeks, but may relapse at a later time. Most relapses occur within 1 year (early latent stage). After 1 year (late latent stage) relapse is unlikely. During latent stages syphilis can still be spread from a pregnant woman to her fetus.[18]

• Tertiary syphilis

Up to 30% of patients with untreated syphilis go on to develop tertiary syphilis which primarily affects the central nervous system and the cardiovascular system and is not contagious. Symptoms may not develop for 20–40 years postinfection.

▶ Laboratory Findings

Nontreponemal blood tests, such as the rapid plasma reagin (RPR) or venereal disease research laboratory test (VDRL), are useful for screening, but may be negative in early primary syphilis, or show false-positive results. Biologic false positive results can occur, usually with a low titer (<1: 8). Positive reactions need to be confirmed with a treponemal test such as fluorescent treponemal antibody absorbed [FTA-ABS] test, *T. pallidum* passive particle agglutination [TP-PA] assay, or enzyme immunoassays [EIAs]. Some laboratories use a reverse screening algorithm, initially testing by treponemal tests, with reflex nontreponemal testing. This approach can identify previously treated or inadequately treated individuals.[19]

Serous material obtained from a chancre and examined with a dark-field microscope can detect the spirochete. A skin biopsy of primary or secondary lesions may detect *T. pallidum*, using special stains.

Diagnosis of Primary Syphilis

The diagnostic feature is a painless indurated ulcer in the genitals, rectum, or mouth.

▶ Differential Diagnosis of Primary Syphilis

• Chancroid: Presents with very painful ulcers or erosions that are not indurated.
• Herpes simplex: Presents with grouped vesicles or erosions. Cultures and Tzanck smear are diagnostic.
• Other: Lymphogranuloma venereum, trauma, fixed drug eruption, and ulcerated genital carcinoma.

Diagnosis of Secondary Syphilis

The diagnostic features are pink to rust colored macules and/or papules on the trunk, palms, and soles.

▶ Differential Diagnosis of Secondary Syphilis

• Pityriasis rosea: Presents with oval, scaly papules, or plaques with a collarette scale located on the trunk in a parallel sloping arrangement similar to evergreen branches. A larger herald lesion is usually present, and palms and soles are not involved.
• Guttate psoriasis: Present with pink papules or plaques with subtle to silvery scale, primarily on the trunk. Palms and soles are usually not involved with this form of psoriasis.
• Other: Tinea corporis, tinea versicolor, lichen planus, pityriasis lichenoides, drug eruptions, primary human

immunodeficiency virus (HIV) infection, erythema multiforme, viral exanthems, nummular dermatitis, folliculitis, and alopecia areata. Mucous membrane lesions may mimic lichen planus, aphthae, hand-foot-mouth disease, herpangina, and angular cheilitis.

Management

A single intramuscular dose of Benzathine penicillin G 2.4 million units is recommended for primary, secondary, and early latent syphilis. Longer treatment courses are needed for those with late latent and neurosyphilis. See CDC publication for treatment of penicillin Allergic Individuals or For Special Cases.[19]

Clinical Course and Prognosis

Follow-up laboratory testing is recommended at 3 and 6 months after treatment, and then every 6 months for 2 years. Patients with syphilis often have other sexually transmitted diseases including HIV and should be tested and treated for these diseases and counseled on safe sex practices. Cases of syphilis should be reported to the local health department for follow-up and identification of sexual contacts.

Indications for Consultation

Significant doubt about the diagnosis, immunosuppressed patient or patient with advanced disease.

Patient Information

Centers for Disease Control and Prevention http://www.cdc.gov/std/syphilis/default.htm

REFERENCES

1. Mueller NT, Bakacs E, Combellick J, et al. The infant microbiome development: mom matters. *Trends Mol Med.* 2015;21(2):109-17.
2. Byrd AL, Belkaid Y, Segre JA. The human skin microbiome. *Nat Rev Microbiol.* 2018;16(3):143.
3. Belkaid Y, Segre JA. Dialogue between skin microbiota and immunity. *Science.* 2014;346(6212):954-9.
4. Fyhrquist N, Ruokolainen L, Suomalainen A, et al. Acinetobacter species in the skin microbiota protect against allergic sensitization and inflammation. *J Allergy Clin Immunol.* 2014;134(6):1301-9.
5. Gardner SE, Hillis SL, Heilmann K, et al. The neuropathic diabetic foot ulcer microbiome is associated with clinical factors. *Diabetes.* 2013;62(3):923-30.
6. Hartman-Adams H, Banvard C, Juckett G. Impetigo: diagnosis and treatment. *Am Fam Phys.* 2014;90(4):229-35.
7. Stevens DL, Bisno AL, Chambers HF, et al. Practice guidelines for the diagnosis and management of skin and soft tissue infections: 2014 update by the infectious diseases society of America. *Clin Infect Dis.* 2014; 59(2):147-59. PMID: 24973422
8. Talan D A, Krishnadasan A, Gorwitz R J, et al. Comparison of *Staphylococcus aureus* from skin and soft-tissue infections in US emergency department patients, 2004 and 2008. *Clin Infect Dis.* 2011;53(2):144-149.
9. Atanaskova N, Tomecki K J. Innovative management of recurrent furunculosis. *Dermatol Clin.* 2010;28(3):479-487.
10. Bailey E, Kroshinsky D. Cellulitis: Diagnosis and management. *Dermatol Ther.* 2011;24(2):229-239.
11. Weng QY, Raff AB, Cohen JM, et al. Costs and consequences associated with misdiagnosed lower extremity cellulitis. *JAMA Dermatol.* 2017;153(2):141-6.
12. Li DG, Di Xia F, Khosravi H, et al. Outcomes of early dermatology consultation for inpatients diagnosed with cellulitis. *JAMA Dermatol.* 2018;154(5):537-43.
13. Pearson ER, Margolis DJ in Kang S. 2018 Fitzpatrick's Dermatology, 2-Volume Set (EBOOK). McGraw Hill Professional.
14. Raff AB, Weng QY, Cohen JM, et al. A predictive model for diagnosis of lower extremity cellulitis: A cross-sectional study. *J Am Acad Dermatol.* 2017;76(4):618-25.
15. Spelman D. Lymphangitis. In: UpToDate, Sexton DJ (Ed), UpToDate, Waltham, MA. (Accessed on September 4th, 2020).
16. Janeczek M, Kozel Z, Bhasin R, et al. High Prevalence of Erythrasma in Patients with Inverse Psoriasis: A Cross-sectional Study. *J Clinv Aesthet Dermatol.* 2020;13(3):12.
17. CDC website https://www.cdc.gov/std/stats18/syphilis.htm
18. James WD, Berger T, Elston D, 2015. Andrews' diseases of the skin: clinical dermatology. Philadelphia.
19. CDC website https://www.cdc.gov/std/tg2015/syphilis.htm

12

Fungal Infections

Andrea Bershow

▼ INTRODUCTION TO CHAPTER

Most superficial fungal infections of the skin are caused by dermatophytes or yeasts. They rarely cause serious illness, but fungal infections are often recurrent or chronic in otherwise healthy people. The availability of effective over the counter antifungal medications has been helpful to consumers with true fungal infections, but many of these medications are used by people who may actually have other skin diseases such as dermatitis. One of the main diagnostic problems with fungal infections is that they closely resemble dermatitis and other inflammatory disorders. Clinicians and patients both over and under diagnose fungal infections. A few simple clinical points can help avoid misdiagnoses.

- Many inflammatory skin diseases such as nummular dermatitis present with an annular (ringworm) pattern and are often misdiagnosed as tinea corporis.
- Dermatitis and dermatophyte infections on the feet have a very similar appearance. However, the presence of toe web scale or maceration and nail plate thickening is more characteristic of a fungal infection.

- Half of all nail disorders are caused by fungal infections. The other causes of nail disease such as psoriasis and lichen planus may appear very similar to fungal infections.
- Fungal infections are rare on the hands, but when they do occur, they may be almost indistinguishable from irritant contact dermatitis or dry skin.
- Fungal infections on the scalp are uncommon after puberty.
- The diagnosis of a suspected fungal skin infection should be confirmed with a potassium hydroxide (KOH) examination, Periodic Acid Schiff (PAS) stain on skin or nail plate biopsies, or fungal culture.

▼ INTRODUCTION TO DERMATOPHYTE INFECTIONS

Dermatophytes can penetrate and digest keratin present in the stratum corneum of the epidermis, hair, and nails. Superficial dermatophyte infections are a common cause of skin disease worldwide, especially in tropical areas. The names of the various dermatophyte infections begin with "tinea," which is a Latin term for "worm." The second word in the name is the Latin term for the affected body site.

- Tinea capitis-scalp
- Tinea barbae-beard
- Tinea faciei-face
- Tinea corporis-trunk and extremities
- Tinea manuum-hands
- Tinea cruris-groin
- Tinea pedis-feet
- Tinea unguium (onychomycosis)-nails

Three dermatophyte genera and nine species are responsible for most infections in North America and Europe.

- *Trichophyton: rubrum, tonsurans, interdigitale, verrucosum, schoenleinii*
- *Microsporum: canis, audouinii, gypseum*
- *Epidermophyton: floccosum*

The species within these genera may be further classified according to their host preferences.

- Anthropophilic- human
- Zoophilic- animal
- Geophilic- soil

Infections can occur by direct contact with infected hosts or fomites.

Dermatophyte infections can mimic many common skin rashes. Therefore, it is important to confirm the diagnosis of a suspected fungal infection with a microscopic examination using KOH or with cultures.

Proper specimen collection is very important as outlined in Table 12-1. False negative results can occur when specimens are taken from the wrong site, or when insufficient volume is collected, or when the patient has been using antifungal medications.

Most dermatophyte infections can be confirmed by performing a KOH examination (Table 12-1). However, fungal cultures may be needed, especially in scalp infections. Nail infections should be diagnosed either by scraping the subungual debris under the nail plate for a KOH exam, or by clipping the nail and sending it for staining with periodic acid-Schiff (PAS). Culture of the subungual debris can be performed but is not a sensitive or reliable method for diagnosis of onychomycosis. Nail plate clippings should not be sent for culture; send only the subungual debris.

Table 12-1. Specimen Collection for Potassium Hydroxide (KOH) Examination for Superficial Fungal Infections.

Equipment needed

- # 15 scalpel blade (for skin and nails), small (1 to 2 mm) metal excavator curette (for nails), tweezers or needle holder, swab or gauze (for scalp and hair).
- Microscope, glass slides, cover slip, 20% potassium hydroxide solution (plain or with dimethyl sulfoxide (DMSO) or dyes such as Chlorazol Black E or Chicago Sky Blue).
- If specimens are submitted for culture, a sterile urine container or petri dish is needed for transport of the specimens to the laboratory. Modified Sabouraud's agar, such as Dermatophyte Test Medium (DTM) or Mycosel ™ or Mycobiotic™ should be available if specimens will be directly placed onto fungal media.

Techniques for specimen collection

- **Skin:** Select an area of scale from the edge of the lesion. Clean the area with an alcohol pad. Gently scrape off the scale using a #15 scalpel blade onto a glass slide or sterile urine container. If the lesions are vesicular (i.e., vesicular tinea pedis), trim off the roof of a vesicle with iris scissors and submit that as a specimen.
- **Nails:** Scrape the subungual debris under the nail plate using a small metal skin or ear curette or a #15 scalpel blade.
- **Scalp**: Pluck involved hairs with a needle holder or tweezers, cut the hair saving the proximal 1 to 2 cm of the hair fiber and bulb. Scalp scales can be collected for culture using a bacterial transport swab that has been pre-moistened by the transport media or sterile gauze or a sterile toothbrush. The involved areas of the scalp should be vigorously rubbed with these devices.

Examination of specimens

- Place the skin scales or proximal hair fibers on a glass slide and cover the specimen
- Cover with 2-4 drops of 20% KOH solution (plain or with dimethly sulfoxide (DMSO) or Chlorazol Black E or Chicago Sky Blue) to partially dissolve keratin. Apply a cover slip.
- Let the slide sit for 20 minutes.
- Lower the condenser on the microscope and decrease the intensity of the light.
- Scan the entire preparation at low power (10 X) magnification looking for branching septate hyphae (Figure 12-7) or pseudohyphae and spores (Figures 12-18 and 12-24). These may be slightly refractile and are easier to view if using Chlorazol Black E or Chicago Sky Blue. Switch to higher power (20 X magnification) to confirm findings.
- Be aware of the many causes of false positive examinations, such as clothing fibers, hair fibers, and the cell walls of keratinocytes, which can look like hyphae. Also, air bubbles and oil droplets can look like spores.

Cultures for dermatophytes are usually done on modified Sabouraud's agar, such as dermatophyte test media (DTM) or Mycosel or Mycobiotic. DTM contains an indicator dye that turns red within 7–14 days in the presence of dermatophytes. Identification of the specific species may be helpful in certain cases of tinea capitis and in the identification of zoophilic infections which require treatment of the host animal. Specimens for culture can be placed in a sterile petri dish or in a sterile urine cup and transported to the lab for placement on agar. If agar plates are available at the site of care, the specimens can be placed directly into the agar.

TINEA CAPITIS

Introduction

Key points for tinea capitis

- ✓ Tinea capitis is uncommon after puberty.
- ✓ It presents with areas of hair loss with broken hair fibers, or grey scales or pustules or as generalized dandruff like scale with no alopecia.
- ✓ Oral griseofulvin or terbinafine are recommend therapies.

Tinea capitis (ringworm of the scalp) is a superficial dermatophyte infection of the hair shaft and scalp. It is most common in children 3–7 years of age and is uncommon after puberty. It is more common in boys than girls, and more common in African American children compared to children of other ethnicities.[1] One study of 200 urban children showed a 4% overall incidence of asymptomatic colonization and a 12.7% incidence in African American girls; however, incidence is reportedly decreasing in recent years.[1,2] Tinea capitis is endemic in many developing countries, and can be associated with crowded living conditions.

Pathogenesis

Trichophyton tonsurans causes 90% of the cases of tinea capitis in North America and in the United Kingdom.

Trichophyton tonsurans fungal spores are confined within the hair shaft (endothrix) (Figure 12-1) and their presence can lead to hair breakage, creating 'black dots" on the scalp. The spores are spread by person-to-person contact and by fomites such as combs, brushes, and pillows.

Microsporum canis is a more common pathogen in Europe, especially in the Mediterranean region.[3] Its fungal spores are present primarily on the surface of the hair shaft (ectothrix). The spores are spread by contact with an infected person, or animal, such as a dog or cat or by contact with a contaminated object, such as a hat or comb.

Clinical Presentation

▶ History

The clinical presentation depends on the pattern of tinea capitis. It may vary from mild pruritus, with flaking and no hair loss, to multiple scaly areas of alopecia, with erythema, pustules, or posterior cervical lymphadenopathy.

▶ Physical Examination

There are six patterns of tinea capitis:

- Dandruff-like adherent scale, with no alopecia.
- Areas of alopecia dotted with broken hair fibers which appear like black dots (Figure 12-2).
- Circular patches of alopecia with gray scales. This is most commonly seen in *Microsporum* infections.

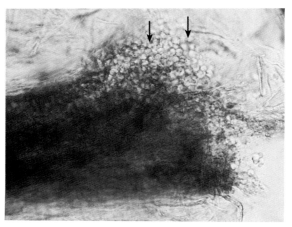

▲ **Figure 12-1.** Fungal spores within hair fiber (ectothrix) in KOH preparation of *T tonsurans* infection. Pseudohyphae and spores in tinea versicolor infection.

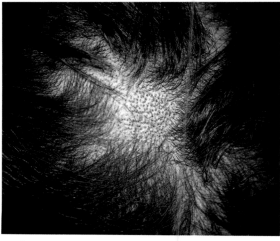

▲ **Figure 12-2.** Tinea capitis. Area of alopecia with multiple broken hair fibers forming "black dot" pattern.

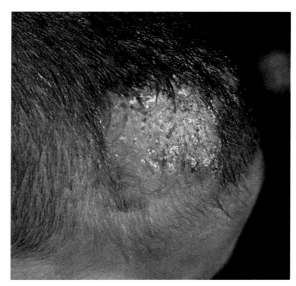

▲ **Figure 12-3.** Kerion on child's scalp. Thick boggy plaque with pustules.

- "Moth-eaten" patches of alopecia with generalized scale.
- Alopecia with scattered pustules.
- Kerion, a boggy, thick, tender plaque with pustules (Figure 12-3) which is caused by a marked inflammatory response to the fungus. This is often misdiagnosed as a tumor or boils.

Occipital lymphadenopathy is often present in patients with tinea capitis. Green blue fluorescence with Wood's light examination is seen in *Microsporum* infections, due to the ectothrix nature of the dermatophyte. Wood's light examination of tinea capitis caused by *Trichophyton tonsurans* is negative, because the fungal spores are within the intact hair shaft.

▶ Laboratory Findings

KOH examination or cultures of the proximal hair fiber and scalp scales should be performed to confirm the diagnosis. Table 12-1 lists some child friendly techniques for specimen collection of scalp scales and techniques for collection of the proximal hair shaft.

KOH examination of the proximal hair fiber of *Trichophyton tonsurans* infections shows large spores within the hair shaft (endothrix) (Figure 12-1). *Microsporum* infections have smaller spores, primarily on the surface of the hair shaft (ectothrix). KOH evaluation of hair fiber specimens can be difficult, and inter-evaluator variability is common.

Use of DTM cultures is a non-specific way of confirming dermatophyte infection. A color change in the media (from yellow to red) is usually noted within 2 weeks if a dermatophyte is present. However, this gives no information on the specific organism. Other agar-based cultures can take up to 4–6 weeks. Species identification can also be done if needed, especially if a pet animal is thought to be the source, or in cases that have been resistant to treatment.

Diagnosis

The key diagnostic clinical features of tinea capitis are patches of alopecia (with scale or black dots) or diffuse scaling with no alopecia. It occurs primarily in children and occipital lymphadenopathy is often present.

▶ Differential Diagnosis

✓ Alopecia areata: Presents with alopecia, but there is no significant scale.

✓ Seborrheic dermatitis: Presents with mild pruritus and localized or diffuse erythematous scale on the scalp, typically there is no significant hair loss.

✓ Psoriasis: Presents with red, localized or diffuse silvery scaly plaques on the scalp. Similar plaques on the elbows and knees or elsewhere on the body are usually seen.

✓ Bacterial infections and tumors: These may closely resemble a kerion. However, tumors are rare in children and when they do occur, they should be biopsied to confirm the diagnosis.

✓ Other: Head lice, traction alopecia, trichotillomania, and Langerhans cell histiocytosis.

Management

Unlike other superficial fungal infections of the skin, tinea capitis does not respond to topical therapy alone. Systemic therapy is needed to penetrate the hair shaft and eradicate the infectious spores. Oral griseofulvin has been the gold standard of therapy for over 50 years based on cost and efficacy, and griseofulvin is the preferred antifungal medication for a kerion infection.[4] It should be taken with a fatty meal, or with whole milk or ice cream to improve absorption. Common side effects of griseofulvin include rash, headache, diarrhea, nausea, and vomiting. Elevated liver function tests are rare.

Meta-analysis suggests that oral terbinafine is more effective in *Trichophyton* infections, but griseofulvin is more effective in *Microsporum* infections.[4,5] Baseline liver enzyme tests are not necessary in pediatric patients.[6,7]

In addition, 2% ketoconazole shampoo and 1% or 2.5% selenium sulfide shampoo should be massaged into the scalp 2–3 times a week for 5–10 minutes during therapy to reduce surface fungal colony counts. This may be continued until clinical clearance or used on an ongoing basis to reduce the risk of recurrence.

It is important to clean combs, brushes, and hats to prevent reinfection. Reinfection can also occur if household contacts or pets remain infected.

The use of oral steroids for a kerion infection remains controversial. However, if significant hair loss is noted, they should be considered, as the inflammation which occurs with a kerion can result in scarring alopecia.

Clinical Course and Prognosis

Most patients can expect to be cured after a single course of treatment. Patients who experience hair loss can expect normal regrowth to begin after treatment; however, a small subset of patients with severe involvement could have permanent hair loss.

Indications for Consultation

Patients with severe or persistent disease that does not respond to treatment should be referred to dermatology.

Patient Information

Centers for Disease Prevention and Control.
https://www.cdc.gov/fungal/diseases/ringworm/symptoms.html

▼ TINEA CORPORIS

Introduction

Key Points for tinea corporis

- ✓ Tinea corporis presents as an annular lesion usually with central clearing.
- ✓ Widespread infections are more common in immunocompromised patients and those with diabetes.
- ✓ Most patients respond to topical antifungal medications.

Tinea corporis (ringworm) is a dermatophyte infection primarily of the skin of the trunk and limbs. It can occur at any age. Outbreaks are more frequent in daycare facilities and schools. Epidemics can occur in wrestlers. It is more common in hot and humid areas, farming communities and in crowded living conditions.

Pathogenesis

Tinea corporis is caused most frequently by the anthromorphilic fungi, *Trichophyton rubrum* or *Trichopyton interdigitale,* or the zoophilic fungus, M*icrosporum canis* which is spread by contact with cats and dogs and other mammals. These fungi can more easily infect inflamed or traumatized skin.

Clinical Presentation

▷ History

The patient usually complains of a mildly itchy, scaly papule that slowly expands to form a ring. Often there is a history of another family member with a tinea infection.

▷ Physical Examination

Tinea corporis presents initially as a red scaly papule that spreads outward, eventually developing into an annular plaque with a scaly, slightly raised, and well-demarcated border. The center of the lesion may partially clear, resulting in a "ring" or "bulls-eye" appearance (Figure 12-4).

Less common presentations include.[8]

- Tinea faciei: This is the term used for tinea infections that occur on the face, most often in children (Figure 12-5).

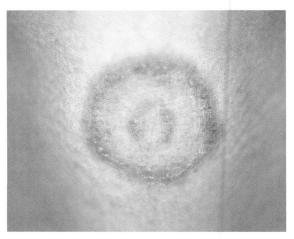

▲ **Figure 12-4.** Tinea corporis on arm. Annular plaque with sharply defined scaly border with a "bulls-eye" center.

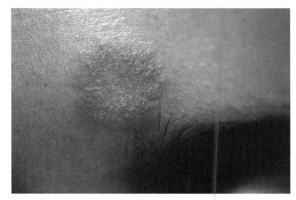

▲ **Figure 12-5.** Tinea faciei on a child's cheek. Annular plaque with scaly papules on border and central clearing.

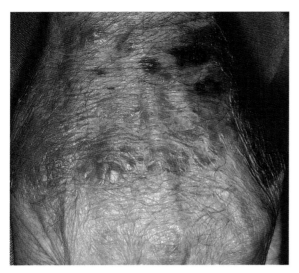

▲ **Figure 12-6.** Tinea incognito on hand. Tinea corporis infection treated with potent topical steroid resulting in purpura and multiple red dermal papules and plaques.

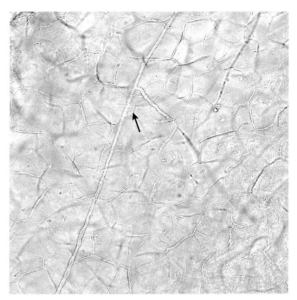

▲ **Figure 12-7.** Fungal dermatophyte hyphae with branches in a potassium hydroxide (KOH) preparation.

- Majocchi's granuloma: In rare instances, tinea corporis does not remain confined to the stratum corneum. Dermal invasion by hyphae following the hair follicle root can produce Majocchi's granuloma, which presents as perifollicular granulomatous papules or pustules typically on the shins or arms.
- Tinea incognito: This is an atypical presentation of tinea corporis that can occur when a dermatophyte infection has been treated with potent topical steroids or systemic steroids. It is characterized by dermal papules or kerion-like lesions with no inflammation, scaling or pruritus (Figure 12-6).

Laboratory Findings

KOH examination (Table 12-1) or cultures of scale from the edge of lesion(s) should be performed to confirm the diagnosis, because there are many other skin diseases, such as nummular dermatitis that present with red and scaly annular lesions.

KOH examination of infected scale shows branched septate hyphae (Figure 12-7). DTM cultures are usually positive within 2 weeks. If appropriate, a skin biopsy can be done to confirm the diagnosis. A periodic acid- Schiff stain (PAS) stain will show hyphae in the stratum corneum.

Diagnosis

The key diagnostic clinical features of tinea corporis are annular, ring-like lesions with central clearing and a red scaling border typically on the trunk or limbs.

Differential Diagnosis

✓ Nummular dermatitis: Presents with pruritic circular, coin-shaped, scaly plaques that have no central clearing.

✓ Atopic dermatitis: Presents with pruritic erythematous scaly plaques in patients with atopy.

✓ Tinea versicolor: Presents with multiple hyper- or hypopigmented asymptomatic macular lesions with very fine powdery scales on the upper trunk with no central clearing. A KOH examination reveals both spores and hyphae.

✓ Granuloma annulare: Presents as skin-colored, smooth, dermal papules in a circular distribution that may coalesce into annular plaques. These plaques can vary from one to several centimeters and they typically occur on the dorsum of the hands, feet, and lower extremities. They usually spontaneously resolve over 1–2 years. The lack of scale is an important differentiating feature.

✓ Other: Candidiasis, psoriasis, pityriasis rosea, erythema multiforme, fixed drug eruption, subacute cutaneous lupus, secondary syphilis, and erythema migrans (Lyme disease).

Management

Topical antifungal medications (Table 12-2) are effective for isolated lesions of tinea corporis.

Table 12-2. Topical medications for superficial fungal infections.

Medication	Formulations	Dosing	Nonprescription
Allylamines			
Naftifine	Cream, gel 2%.	Once a day.	No
Terbinafine	Cream, spray 1%.	Twice a day.	Yes
Imidazoles			
Clotrimazole	Cream, lotion, solution 1%.	Twice a day.	Yes
Econazole	Cream 1%.	Once a day.	No
Ketoconazole	Cream, gel, foam 2%.	Twice a day.	No
Miconazole	Cream, ointment, lotion, spray solution, powder 2%.	Twice a day.	Yes
Oxiconazole	Cream, lotion 2%.	Twice a day.	No
Sulconazole	Cream, solution 1%.	Once a day to twice a day.	No
Miscellaneous			
Butenafine	Cream 1%.	Once a day.	Yes
Ciclopirox	Cream, 0.77%, gel 3%, lotion 0.77%.	Twice a day.	No
Tolnaftate	Cream, lotion, solution, spray, powder 1%.	Twice a day.	Yes

They should be applied at least 1–2 cm beyond the visible advancing edge of the lesions. Treatment should be continued for 1–2 weeks after the lesions resolve. If the infection is extensive, or if it does not respond to topical therapy, oral griseofulvin or oral terbinafine can be prescribed.[9]

Bedding, towels, and clothing should be laundered and should not be shared with other individuals. Children with active infections should not participate in contact sports until the infection is treated and resolved. For those infected with zoophilic fungi, especially in cases of tinea faciei, it is important to identify the infected animal and have the animal treated appropriately by a veterinarian. Tinea corporis usually responds well to the treatment but can recur with repeated contact with the source of the organism.

Clinical Course and Prognosis

Most patients can expect to be cured after completing a course of topical treatment, but re-infection may occur. Some patients may require oral antifungal treatments if they have extensive disease or fail to clear with topical treatments.

Indications for Consultation

Patients with severe or persistent disease that does not respond to treatment should be referred to dermatology.

Patient Information

American Academy of Dermatology
    https://www.aad.org/public/diseases/a-z/ringworm-overview

▼ TINEA MANUUM

Introduction

Key Points for tinea manuum

✓ Tinea manuum presents with diffuse, subtle scales on the palms and is often misdiagnosed as dry skin.
✓ One or both hands may be involved; the fingernails may also be affected.
✓ Tinea pedis is often also present.

Tinea manuum is a dermatophyte infection that affects the palmar and dorsal aspects of the hands. It is more common in men and is rare in children. In most cases, there is preexisting tinea pedis.

Pathogenesis

Predisposing factors include manual labor, preexisting inflammatory conditions of the hands, hyperhidrosis, heat, and humidity. These can lead to a breakdown in the protective stratum corneum barrier of the epidermis allowing the dermatophytes to penetrate.

Tinea manuum may be acquired by direct contact with an affected person or animal, or from autoinoculation from fungal infections on the feet or groin. *Trichophyton rubrum*, *Trichophyton interdigitale*, and *Epidermophyton floccosum* are the species that commonly cause tinea manuum.

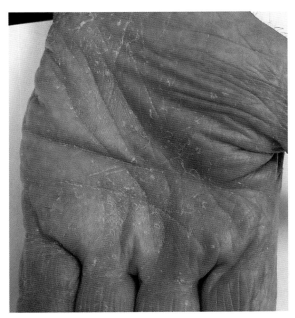

▲ **Figure 12-8.** Tinea manuum on the palm. Subtle diffuse fine scale.

Clinical Presentation

▷ History

Patients typically complain of chronic dryness on the palms or redness and scaling on the dorsa of the hands.

▷ Physical Examination

Tinea manuum can present with two patterns.

- Tinea on the palms presents with diffuse, fine scale (Figure 12-8). It frequently is associated with the *T. rubrum* moccasin type of tinea pedis. Tinea manuum is unilateral in about 50% of the cases. In some cases, there is a concomitant fungal infection of the fingernails.
- On the dorsal surface, tinea manuum usually presents in a ringworm pattern with an annular plaque with a red scaly border. Vesicles and red papules may be present.

▷ Laboratory Findings

KOH examination (Table 12-1) or cultures of scale should be performed to confirm the diagnosis of tinea manuum may be clinically indistinguishable from dermatitis. KOH examination of infected scale shows branched septate hyphae. DTM cultures are usually positive within 2 weeks.

Diagnosis

The key diagnostic clinical features of tinea manuum is an asymptomatic, fine, subtle, diffuse scale on one or both palms.

▷ Differential Diagnosis

- ✓ Irritant or allergic contact dermatitis: Usually bilateral and presents with erythematous, nonexpanding pruritic plaques on the dorsum of the hands. Fissures, erosions, and scales may also be present on the palms.
- ✓ Psoriasis: Presents with thick silvery plaques on the dorsum of the hands, usually associated with plaques elsewhere, such as the elbows and knees.

Management

Tinea infections of the dorsum of the hands usually respond to the use of topical antifungal medications (Table 12-2). Tinea infections of the palms that don't resolve with topical antifungal medications may require oral terbinafine or griseofulvin.[9]

It is also important to treat any accompanying tinea infection of the feet and nails.

Clinical Course and Prognosis

Most patients can expect to be cured after completing a course of topical treatment, but re-infection may occur. Some patients may require oral antifungal treatments if they have concomitant onychomycosis or fail to clear with topical treatments. If the patient has concomitant onychomycosis that can't be successfully treated, re-infection is common.

Indications for Consultation

Patients with severe or persistent disease that does not respond to treatment should be referred to dermatology.

Patient Information

American Academy of Dermatology
    https://www.aad.org/public/diseases/a-z/ringworm-overview

TINEA CRURIS

Introduction

Key point for tinea cruris

- ✓ Tinea cruris is most common in adult males
- ✓ It presents as a semi-circular plaque in the inguinal folds and medial upper thighs.

✓ Most patients respond to topical antifungal medications, but recurrence is common.

Tinea cruris (jock itch) is a dermatophyte infection of the inguinal, buttock, and perianal areas. It is three times more prevalent in men than in women. It rarely occurs in children. It is more common in hot and humid environments. Obesity and activities that cause increased sweating are risk factors.

Pathogenesis

Tinea cruris is predominantly caused by *Trichophyton rubrum, Trichophyton interdigitale,* and *Epidermophyton floccosum.* Sweating, tight or damp clothing produce maceration of the skin allowing the dermatophytes to easily penetrate into the epidermis. Autoinoculation commonly occurs from tinea pedis or onychomycosis. The organisms may also be transmitted from fomites present on items such as towels and sheets.

Clinical Presentation

▶ History

Patients usually complain of itching or redness in the groin area.

▶ Physical Examination

Patients present with pruritic, semi-circular, plaques with sharply defined scaly borders in the inguinal folds and the upper inner thighs (Figure 12-9). In more acute infections,

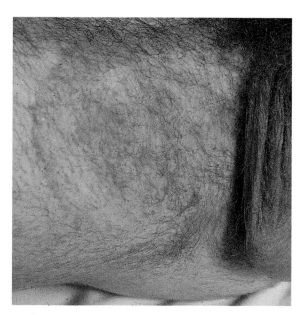

▲ **Figure 12-9.** Tinea cruris. Arc of erythema with scale on border, scrotum is not involved.

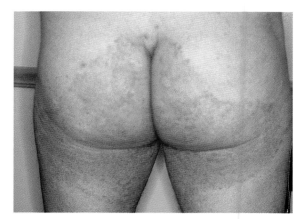

▲ **Figure 12-10.** Tinea cruris. Annular plaque of extension of tinea to posterior thighs and buttocks.

the lesions may be moist or have an eczematous appearance. Chronic infections with *Trichophyton rubrum* usually present with a dry, annular plaque with small follicular papules.

The penis and scrotum are **not** involved in contrast to candidiasis which can involve the penis and scrotum. The infection can spread to the lower abdomen, suprapubic area, perianal area, and buttocks (Figure 12-10). In those areas it has the appearance of a symmetrical, typical tinea corporis infection.

▶ Laboratory Findings

Collection of scale for laboratory testing may be difficult in the groin area because of moisture on the skin surface in that region. It is helpful, but not essential to confirm the diagnosis of tinea cruris with a KOH examination or fungal cultures.

KOH examination of infected scale shows branched septate hyphae. DTM cultures usually are positive within 2 weeks.

Diagnosis

The key diagnostic clinical features of tinea cruris are circular or semi-circular, pink, annular plaques with a distinct scaly border, most commonly found in the inguinal folds and the upper inner thighs.

▶ Differential Diagnosis

✓ Candidiasis: Presents as a deep red, moist plaque with satellite pustules. There is no central clearing. The scrotum is commonly affected and occasionally the penis is affected.

✓ Erythrasma: This is caused by *Corynebacterium minutissimum.* It appears as uniform, red to brown, macular lesions with no scale or central clearing. Borders are sharply demarcated, but not elevated. The lesions exhibit a bright coral red fluorescence on examination with a Wood's light.

✓ Seborrheic dermatitis: Presents with symmetrical, confluent, salmon pink, slightly scaly plaques on the inner thighs. Usually the scalp and central face are involved.

✓ Other: Psoriasis and lichen simplex chronicus.

Management

Most cases of tinea cruris can be successfully treated with topical antifungal medications preferably a cream or lotion (Table 12-2). Nystatin is not effective for dermatophyte infections. Absorbent powders such as miconazole powder are very helpful treatment adjuncts and can help prevent recurrences. Oral griseofulvin and oral terbinafine are reserved for refractory, widespread, or more inflammatory lesions.[9]

Coexisting tinea pedis and onychomycosis should be treated to prevent reinfection. Men should be instructed to wear loose fitting pants and boxer shorts.

Clinical Course and Prognosis

Tinea cruris usually responds well to treatment, but recurrences are common.

Indications for Consultation

Patients with severe or persistent disease that does not respond to treatment should be referred to dermatology

Patient information

American Academy of Dermatology
https://www.aad.org/public/diseases/a-z/ringworm-overview

TINEA PEDIS

Introduction

Key points for tinea pedis

✓ Tinea pedis is more commonly seen in adult males.

✓ Scales and fissures in the toe webs and or diffuse scaling on the plantar surface are the most common presentations.

✓ Most patients respond to topical antifungal medications, but recurrence is common.

Tinea pedis (athlete's foot) is one of the most common superficial fungal infections of the skin in developed countries. At least 10% of the world population is affected at any given time. It is more common in males and is uncommon in females and children. Risk factors include the use of communal pools and showers and occlusive shoes.

Pathogenesis

The skin of the soles has a thick keratinized layer and numerous eccrine sweat glands. The combination of abundant keratin sweat and occlusion with shoes creates a perfect environment for dermatophyte infections. Chronic non-inflammatory tinea pedis is usually caused by a *Trichophyton rubrum* infection. There may be a genetic predisposition for this type of tinea pedis. Vesiculobullous tinea pedis is usually caused by *Trichophyton* interdigitale.

Clinical Presentation

▷ History

Patients usually complain of itching and persistent scaling or less commonly blisters usually on the plantar surface or in the toe webs.

▷ Physical Examination

Patients may present with three patterns of tinea pedis:

• Interdigital pattern with scales, fissures, or maceration or malodor usually in the fourth and fifth web spaces (Figure 12-11). Secondary infection with Gram-negative or Gram-positive organisms may be present. The tinea infection may spread to the dorsum of the foot, creating scaly and annular plaques.

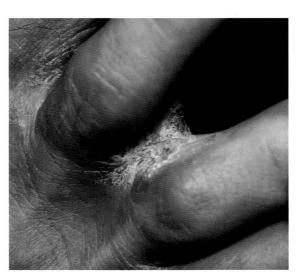

▲ **Figure 12-11.** Interdigital tinea pedis. Scale and small fissures.

- Moccasin pattern with diffuse, dry, silvery white scale on the soles extending up the sides of the foot (Figure 12-12). In its mildest form, tiny scattered arcs of scale are seen. Concomitant onychomycosis and tinea manuum may be present.
- Vesiculobullous pattern with vesicles and/or bullae on the plantar surface, especially instep areas, accompanied by inflammation and tenderness (Figure 12-13). Secondary bacterial infection in the blisters may progress into cellulitis or lymphangitis. A vesicular or dermatitic "id" reaction may occur on the palms or other body sites. This presentation is often misdiagnosed as dermatitis because of the presence of vesicles.

Accompanying fungal infections of the toenails are common in chronic tinea pedis. Concomitant tinea manuum may also be present.

Laboratory Findings

KOH examination (Table 12-1) or cultures of scale or the roof of a vesicle should be performed to confirm the

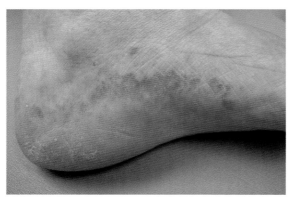

▲ **Figure 12-12.** Moccasin pattern tinea pedis. Plaque with scalloped scaley border.

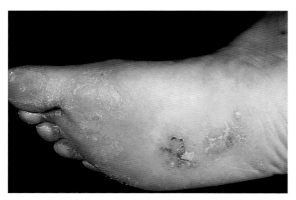

▲ **Figure 12-13.** Vesiculobullous pattern tinea pedis. Intact and collapsed vesicles on the instep of the foot.

diagnosis, as tinea pedis may be clinically indistinguishable from dermatitis. One exception is toe web scale or fissures, which are usually caused by fungus and may be diagnosed on the basis of clinical findings. KOH examination of infected skin shows branched septate hyphae. DTM cultures are usually positive within 2 weeks.

Diagnosis

The key diagnostic clinical features of tinea pedis are scaly plaques and/or blisters on the feet, and interdigital maceration or fissures.

▶ Differential Diagnosis

✓ Contact dermatitis: Presents with symmetrical erythematous plaques on the dorsa of the feet, usually caused by an allergy to one or several components in rubber, leather, or metal in shoes.

✓ Dyshidrotic eczema (pompholyx): Presents with numerous pruritic, symmetrical vesicles that resemble "tapioca pudding" on the sides of the soles and/or palms. It is more common in patients with hyperhidrosis.

✓ Psoriasis: Presents with two patterns on the feet; erythematous scaly plaques or painful symmetrical pustules. Nail dystrophy may be present in both patterns.

✓ Other: Interdigital soft corns, erythrasma, juvenile plantar dermatosis, and atopic dermatitis.

Management

Treatment options for tinea pedis include:

- Interdigital toe web infections will usually respond to various topical antifungal medications (Table 12-2). Lamb's wool padding (e.g., Dr Scholl's) in the web spaces and shoes with wider toe-boxes may also be needed to keep the web spaces dry.
- The dry, moccasin form of tinea pedis may respond to topical antifungal medications, but may require an oral antifungal medication to clear the infection. Recurrences are common.
- Acute vesiculobullous tinea pedis may be treated with Burrow's wet dressings (see Chapter 6) and topical or oral antifungal medications. Secondary bacterial infections should be treated with topical or oral antibiotics.
- Oral terbinafine or griseofulvin can be used if tinea pedis does not respond to topical antifungal medications.[9]

Patients with hyperhidrosis should use products such as aluminum chloride hexahydrate solution, tolnaftate powder, or miconazole powder. These powders should be sprinkled on the feet, in the shoes or in the socks daily. Patients should be advised to thoroughly dry their feet, especially in the toe webs with a towel or hair dryer after bathing. Sandals should be worn in communal showers and swimming pools.

It is important to treat recurrences and prevent reinfection in diabetic and immunocompromised patients. Fissures and erosions caused by tinea pedis can be a portal for the entry of bacteria that may cause cellulitis.

Clinical Course and Prognosis

Tinea pedis usually responds well to treatment, but recurrence is common, especially if onychomycosis is present, as it may act as a reservoir of infection.

Indications for Consultation

Patients with severe or persistent disease that does not respond to treatment should be referred to dermatology.

Patient Information

American Academy of Dermatology
    https://www.aad.org/public/diseases/a-z/ringworm-overview

ONYCHOMYCOSIS (TINEA UNGUIUM)

Introduction

Key points for onychomycosis

✓ Onychomycosis is most common in adult males.

✓ It presents with a thickened discolored nail plate that may be partially detached from the nail bed.

✓ Many other disorders may mimic a dermatophyte infection of the nail. The diagnosis should be confirmed by cultures, KOH examinations or histopathologic examination of a nail clipping.

✓ Oral terbinafine is the treatment of choice.

Onychomycosis is a very common nail disorder and accounts for about 50% of nail disease. The prevalence of onychomycosis in North Americans and Europeans is reportedly between 2 to 13% with the prevalence increasing with age.[9,10] Onychomycosis is rare in prepubertal children. In contrast, 60% of patients older than 70 years of age are affected.[11,12] Nondermatophyte molds are responsible for 1.5–6% of cases of onychomycosis.[12]

Onychomycosis is more common in patients who are male, immunosuppressed, diabetic, infected with human immunodeficiency virus (HIV) or who have poor circulation. Trauma or nail dystrophy also predisposes patients to fungal infection.[12]

Pathogenesis

The most common organisms that cause fungal infection of the nail include.[12]

- Dermatophytes: *Trichophyton rubrum*, *Trichophyton interdigitale*, *Epidermophyton floccosum*
- Nondermatophyte molds: *Acremonium*, *Aspergillus* species, *Cladosporium carrionii*, *Fusarium* species, *Onychocola canadensis*, *Scopulariopsis brevicaulis*, *Scytalidium dimidiatum*, *Scytalidium hyalinum*
- Yeasts: *Candida albicans*

Clinical Presentation

▶ History

Patients usually complain of thickening or discoloration of the nail plate. Pain or tenderness may be present. Patients often have a history of other fungal skin infections, especially tinea pedis and tinea manuum.

▶ Physical Examination

The initial findings are white/yellow or orange/brown streaks or macules under the nail plate. As the infection progresses, subungual hyperkeratosis, onycholysis (separation of the nail plate from the nail bed), and a thickened nail plate may develop.

There are four major patterns of infection:

- Distal subungual: Nails are dystrophic and thickened (Figure 12-14). Color changes are present (white, yellow, orange, or brown).
- Proximal subungual: Proximal portion of nail appears white, but not crumbly or chalky.
- White superficial: Nail plate appears white and chalky (Figure 12-15).
- Candida: Mild cases may produce nothing more than diffuse leukonychia (white spot(s) under the nail plate).

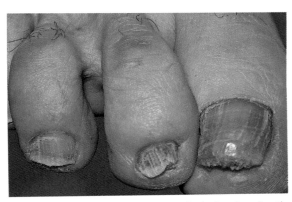

▲ **Figure 12-14.** Onychomycosis. Thick discolored nail plate and subungual hyperkeratosis.

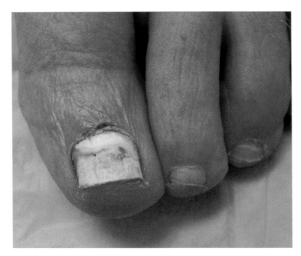

▲ **Figure 12-15.** White superficial onychomycosis. White chalky nail plate.

Severe cases may present with a yellow-brown discoloration, with a thick nail bed and lateral and proximal nail fold swelling. Onycholysis is common and subungual hyperkeratosis can occur.[12,13]

▶ Laboratory Findings

It is important to confirm the diagnosis of fungus prior to initiating treatment. Fungal cultures are not always necessary but can sometimes be helpful in distinguishing between dermatophytes, mold, and yeasts. A fungal culture is the least sensitive, but most specific, method for confirming a fungal infection. The most sensitive method to detect fungus is to clip the distal portion of the nail plate, place it in formalin, and send it for histopathologic examination; fungal elements stain positive with periodic acid Schiff stain (PAS) (Figure 12-16). A KOH preparation can be done in clinic (Table 12-1 and should demonstrate septate hyphae or arthroconidia. However, false negatives are common. These

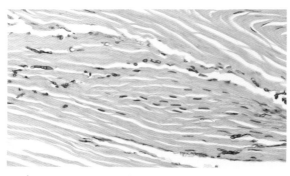

▲ **Figure 12-16.** Fungal hyphae in nail plate clipping. Histopathology with PAS stain.

tests are not sensitive, and they may need to be repeated serially, if negative and clinical suspicion remains high.[12]

Diagnosis

Nail disorders can be difficult to differentiate from one another based only on their clinical findings. It takes practice, and some investigation, to determine the correct diagnosis. To add to the confusion, many nail disorders can also be complicated by secondary infection, either fungal or bacterial.

▶ Differential Diagnosis

✓ Trauma. Should be suspected if only the first and or fifth toenails are involved. This is typically caused by pressure from shoes, or from traumatic sports such as running, tennis, or soccer.

✓ Psoriatic nail changes. Suspect psoriasis if there is nail pitting, and if there is a band of erythema on the nail bed adjacent to the onycholytic nail (if onycholysis is present).

✓ Suspect mold as the cause of onychomycosis when periungual inflammation is present and/or tinea pedis is absent.[13]

Management

Oral antifungals are the gold standard of treatment for onychomycosis,[14,15] but for many patients nontreatment is a viable option. Although oral antifungals are generally well-tolerated, patients may prefer not to risk the potential side effects of oral antifungal medications. Oral terbinafine has the highest cure rate of any onychomycosis therapy, with no significant difference in rate of adverse effects when compared to azoles, and a lower rate of adverse effects compared to griseofulvin.[14] It is recommended that liver function tests be obtained prior to the initiation of terbinafine, and every 6 weeks during treatment. Recently, the utility of ongoing laboratory monitoring beyond baseline during treatment with terbinafine has been questioned.[7] Topical nail lacquers (efinaconazole, tavaborole, ciclopirox) for treatment for onychomycosis are available, although the cure rates are significantly lower, the costs significantly higher, and the duration of treatment significantly longer.

It takes 4–6 months for a fingernail, and 12–18 months for the great toenail to grow out completely. As a result, patients will not see a completely normal nail plate until that length of time has passed. The first sign that treatment is working will be a transition to normal nail plate growth from the proximal nail fold, which, for the fingernails, can usually be seen within a few months of starting oral treatment.

Recurrence is common. One study showed that there was a lower recurrence rate in patients initially treated with oral terbinafine (12%) than those treated with itraconazole (36%).[16] The same study showed no benefit from long-term use of amorolfine nail lacquer (not available in the United States) on rate of relapse; however, most experts recommend continuing use of topical antifungal products to prevent reinfection. Patients should continue to use antifungal creams on their feet, or powders inside their shoes, at least 3 times a week after treatment with oral medications is completed.

Proximal subungual onychomycosis should prompt investigation for immunosuppression, specifically HIV infection. Candida onychomycosis is usually considered a sign of immunosuppression.[13]

Clinical Course and Prognosis

Treatment failure is common in onychomycosis with complete cure rates of approximately 50% for oral terbinafine, which is the most effective treatment for onychomycosis due to dermatophytes. Onychomycosis is recurrent in 10–53% of previously "cured" patients.[14,16,17] If patients develop recurrent disease, another course of treatment is indicated.

Indications for Consultation

- Patient not responding to the treatment.
- Patient preference for physical removal of the diseased nail plates.
- Underlying nail disease such as psoriasis that requires treatment.

Patient Information

American Academy of Dermatology
   https://www.aad.org/public/diseases/a-z/ringworm-overview

INTRODUCTION TO SUPERFICIAL YEAST INFECTIONS

Tinea versicolor and candida infections are caused by yeasts, which are ubiquitous organisms on the skin and in the environment. Cutaneous candida infections generally do not cause significant medical problems, but they can be the source for disseminated candidiasis in immunocompromised patients.

TINEA VERSICOLOR

Introduction

Key points for tinea versicolor

✓ Tinea versicolor is a common fungal infection caused by *Malassezia,* a lipophilic, dimorphic yeast.

✓ It presents with tan macules with a fine powder like scale on the upper trunk often leaving areas of hypopigmentation.

✓ Most patients respond to topical antifungal medications or selenium sulfide, but recurrence is common.

Tinea versicolor (pityriasis versicolor) is a common fungal infection caused by *Malassezia,* a lipophilic, dimorphic yeast. It is more prevalent in young adults but can occur at any age. It is more common in the summer months and in tropical areas.

Pathogenesis

Tinea versicolor is caused by *Malassezia furfur* and *Malassezia globosa,* which are saprophytes that normally colonize the skin.[18] After converting to their mycelial form, they spread into the superficial epidermis, resulting in the appearance of the rash. In humans, the seborrheic areas (scalp, face, back, and trunk) are always colonized by one or several species of the *Malassezia* genus.

Clinical Presentation

History

Patients usually present during the summer months with a history of asymptomatic, hypo- or hyperpigmented, scaly areas on the trunk. The patient's chief complaint is usually cosmetic, because these lesions do not tan with sun exposure.

Physical Examination

Macules with a fine powdery scale are seen on the upper arms, upper chest (Figure 10-17), back, and occasionally on the face. The initial lesions are 3–5 mm, oval, or

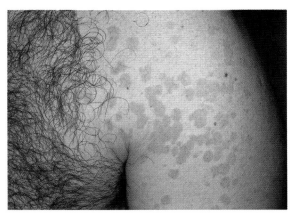

▲ **Figure 12-17.** Tinea versicolor on shoulder. Light brown macules with subtle scale.

round macules. Over the course of time, they may coalesce and cover more extensive areas of the body creating large irregularly shaped patches. The color of lesions varies from white to reddish-brown light tan. Other areas that can be affected include the neck, abdomen, pubis, and intertriginous areas. Facial lesions may be present primarily in children. Hypopigmentation is very conspicuous in dark-skinned individuals and the hypopigmentation may last for weeks or months until the area has repigmented through sunlight exposure.

Laboratory Findings

Wood's light examination shows a characteristic yellow/orange fluorescence. KOH examination of infected scale shows numerous strands of fungal hyphae (mycelia) and numerous spores commonly referred to as "spaghetti and meatballs" (Figure 12-18). Cultures are rarely done as it is difficult to grow malassezia on standard fungal culture media.

Diagnosis

The key diagnostic clinical features of tinea versicolor are white, reddish brown or tan macules, and patches with fine powdery scale on the upper trunk and upper arms.

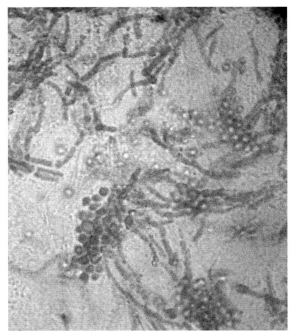

▲ **Figure 12-18.** Tinea versicolor demonstrating non-septated fungal hyphae(mycelia) and spores, referred to as "spaghetti and meatballs" in a Chicago Sky Blue and potassium hydroxide (KOH) preparation.

▶ Differential Diagnosis

✓ Seborrheic dermatitis: Presents with scaly, pink patches on the central trunk, usually the scalp and central face are involved. KOH examination is negative.

✓ Pityriasis rosea: Presents initially with a pink herald patch with a very fine peripheral scale (collarette scale). Approximately 1 week later, multiple similar but smaller lesions develop on the chest and back, usually in a "Christmas tree" pattern. KOH examination is negative.

✓ Vitiligo: Presents with macular areas of complete pigment loss, with no scale or other surface changes.

✓ Other: Secondary syphilis and lupus erythematosus.

Management

- 2.5% selenium sulfide lotion and 2% ketoconazole shampoo are a cost-effective first-line treatment. Ketoconazole shampoo lather should be applied to damp skin of all involved areas and left on for 5 minutes, then showered off daily for 3 consecutive days. Selenium sulfide lotion should be applied to involved areas and left on for 10 minutes, then showered off and reapplied in the same manner for 7 days. In warmer humid weather, the application of these medications may need to be repeated biweekly or monthly to prevent recurrence.

- Clotrimazole, miconazole, and ketoconazole creams are inexpensive treatment options.[19,20] The creams are applied nightly for 2–3 weeks and then repeated on a once a month basis to prevent recurrences. Oral antifungals such as itraconazole and fluconazole can be used for extensive cases in adults that do not respond to topical treatments. These have a higher incidence of adverse effects and are more expensive. [19,20]

Oral griseofulvin is not an effective therapy for tinea versicolor. Oral ketoconazole is no longer recommended due to the risk of hepatotoxicity[21] and QT prolongation resulting in ventricular dysrhythmias.

Clinical Course and Prognosis

Clinical improvement is not evident until 3–4 weeks after treatment. Patients should be advised that pigmentation changes will resolve slowly over several weeks with the aid of exposure to sunlight. Recurrence is common.

Indications for Consultation

The patient should be referred to dermatology for severe or persistent disease that does not respond to treatment.

Patient Information

American Academy of Dermatology
    http://www.aad.org/skin-conditions/dermatology-
a-to-z/tinea-versicolor

▼ CANDIDIASIS

Introduction

Key points for superficial candida infections

✓ Candida species can cause infections in the intertriginous areas and on mucosal surfaces.

✓ Candida infections are more common in elderly or immunosuppressed individuals.

✓ Most patients respond to topical anticandidal medications, but recurrence is common.

✓ Oral anticandidal medications may be needed for widespread or locally severe disease.

Candida albicans is often present as part of the normal flora in the mouth, gastrointestinal tract, and vagina. However, it can become a pathogen, especially in the vaginal tract and intertriginous areas. Risk factors for superficial candidiasis include infancy, pregnancy, aging, occlusion of epithelial surfaces (e.g., dentures, occlusive dressings), maceration, immunodeficiency, diabetes, obesity, and use of medications such as oral glucocorticoids and antibiotics.

Pathogenesis

Candida is a dimorphic yeast that has the ability to transform from a budding yeast phase to an invasive mycelia growth phase, which is necessary for tissue infection.

The most common cause of superficial candidiasis is *Candida albicans*. Occasionally, other species such as *Candida* glabrata, *tropicalis, krusei,* and *parapsilosis* can be pathogenic.[22]

Clinical Presentations of Intertriginous Candidiasis

▶ History

Patients usually complain of redness and itching in body fold areas or in moist areas.

▶ Physical Examination

Primary lesions appear as moist, erythematous, plaques with maceration with a predilection for moist, warm, or macerated areas of the body. Common sites include inframammary, axillary (Figure 12-19), and abdominal folds of the body, interdigital and groin/diaper region (Figure 12-20), and the head of the penis of uncircumcised men.

The periphery of the rash can show scaling and satellite pustules. Candidiasis is often pruritic.

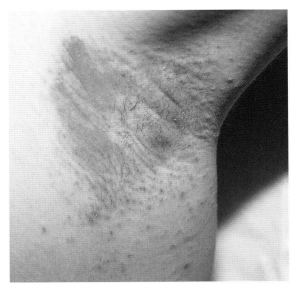

▲ **Figure 12-19.** Candida skin infection in axilla. Pink plaque surrounded by satellite pustules.

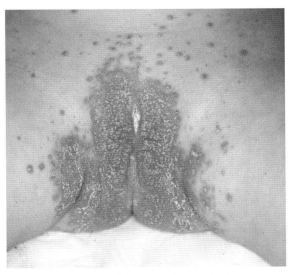

▲ **Figure 12-20.** Candida skin infection in diaper area of child. Erythematous plaque over the labia and inner thighs surrounded by satellite papules and pustules.

Clinical Presentation of Candida Paronychial Infections

▶ History

Patients complain of swelling and pain of the cuticle or nail folds. Chronic immersion of the hands in water is a risk factor.

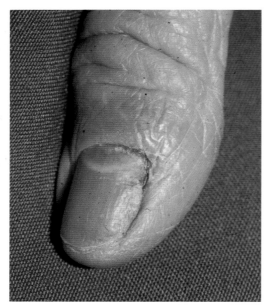

▲ **Figure 12-21.** Candia paronychial infection. Erythema and swelling of cuticle.

▶ **Physical Examination**

Cutaneous findings include erythema, swelling, and pain of the nail fold along with retraction of the cuticle (Figure 12-21). Acute paronychial infections are often bacterial, but chronic infection often involves a combination of bacterial and *Candida* species.

Clinical Presentation of Angular Cheilitis

▶ **History**

The patient typically complains of redness and sometimes pain in the corners of the mouth. It is more common in circumstances that result in increased moisture at the oral commissures, for example in lip lickers, elderly patients or those with poorly fitting dentures.

▶ **Physical Examination**

Angular cheilitis presents with painful, erythematous, scaly fissures in the oral commissures usually bilaterally (Figure 12-22). Angular cheilitis often is due to a combination of fungal and bacterial infection, for example, *Candida albicans* and *Staphylococcus aureus*.[20]

Clinical Presentation of Oral Candidiasis

▶ **History**

Oral candidiasis, commonly known as thrush, typically presents in infants, the elderly, or immunosuppressed

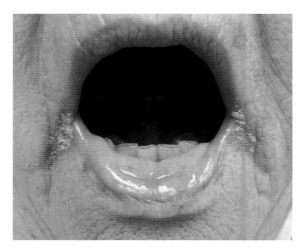

▲ **Figure 12-22.** Angular cheilitis. Erythema, scale and fissures in corners of the mouth.

individuals. Risk factors include use of dentures, inhaled corticosteroids, antibiotics, chemotherapy or radiation.[21] Most patients are asymptomatic or have the sensation of a dry mouth. Some patients experience pain.

▶ **Physical Examination**

Thrush presents with white plaques on the buccal mucosae, tongue and or palate, and may extend into the oropharynx (Figure 12-23). These plaques can be removed easily with a tongue depressor. The material can be placed on a glass slide for diagnosis using a KOH preparation.

Angular cheilitis presents with painful fissures of the oral commissures.

▶ **Laboratory Findings in Candida infections**

Candida albicans grows on bacterial media, but Sabouraud's agar is usually recommended. KOH examination shows numerous spores and pseudohyphae (Figure 12-24).

Diagnosis

The key diagnostic clinical features of candida skin infections are moist, erythematous plaques with satellite pustules usually in a body fold area.

▶ **Differential Diagnosis**

Differential diagnosis of cutaneous candidiasis

  ✓ Dermatophyte infection: In men, dermatophyte infections do not involve the penis and scrotum, while in candidiasis these areas may be affected.

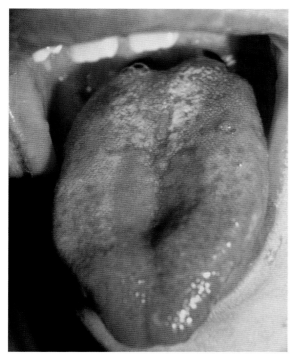

▲ **Figure 12-23.** Thrush. Candia infection on tongue. White plaques that can be easily removed.

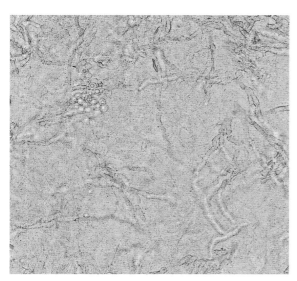

▲ **Figure 12-24.** Candida in KOH preparation. A cluster of spores and pseudohyphae.

✓ Erythrasma: Presents with erythema, with no satellite pustules and coral red fluorescence with Wood's light examination.

✓ Other: Contact dermatitis, inverse psoriasis.

Differential diagnosis for candidal paronychia includes bacterial or herpes viral paronychia.

Management

It is important to keep the affected areas dry and free of moisture. Powders such as 2% miconazole may be helpful in body fold areas. Mild cases of cutaneous candidiasis and paronychia can be treated with topical imidazole medications (Table 12-2) or nystatin cream.[23]

Treatment for oral candidiasis in non-immunosuppressed adults include clotrimazole troches, and nystatin oral suspension. Oral fluconazole can be used if there is no response to these treatments.

Management of Angular Cheilitis

Ensure an optimal environment; dentures should be properly fitted and cleaned, and oral hygiene maintained including treatment of dry mouth if needed. Treat with clotrimazole cream twice a day for 2–3 weeks along with petrolatum or zinc oxide for barrier protection. Topical mupirocin ointment twice daily is often used to treat any concomitant staphylococcal infection. Treatment may be repeated as needed. If no response to topical treatment, or difficulty adhering to a regimen, oral fluconazole may be used.

Clinical Course and Prognosis

Candida infections respond well to treatment, but recurrence is common.

Indications for Consultation

Patients with severe or persistent disease that does not respond to treatment should be referred to dermatology.

Patient Information

Centers for Disease Control and Prevention
    https://www.cdc.gov/fungal/diseases/candidiasis/index.html

DEEP FUNGAL INFECTIONS OF THE SKIN

Deep fungal infections can be seen in the skin as a result of dissemination from other organs or from primary inoculation.[24] These infections are relatively uncommon, but immunosuppressed patients are more susceptible. Deep fungal infections are often misdiagnosed as bacterial infections, warts, papulosquamous diseases, or tumors. Table 12-3 lists selected deep fungal infections.

Table 12-3. Deep Fungal Infections.

Deep Fungal Infection	Pathogenesis	History & Clinical Findings
Blastomycosis 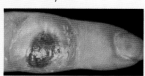	Caused by *Blastomyces Dermatitidis* in soil via pulmonary inhalation. Endemic in central USA especially in the Mississippi valley and Great Lakes areas.	Most commonly presents in skin after dissemination. Primary cutaneous infection is very rare and occurs after traumatic inoculation. Disseminated disease presents on the face or extremities with multiple papules, nodules or verrucous plaques which may ulcerate. Pustules and sinus tracts may be present. The primary cutaneous form presents as an indurated, erythematous, ulcerated papule or plaque at the site of inoculation with associated lymphadenopathy.
Coccidioidomycosis 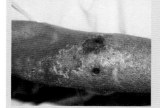	Caused by *Coccidioides immitis* and *C. posadasii* via inhaled dust, in California, southwest USA, Mexico and Central and South America	Infection is usually via inhalation. Direct cutaneous infection rarely occurs. Pulmonary infection presents with flu like symptoms, (Valley Fever), multiple papules, plaques or pustules and abscesses may be present. Pulmonary symptoms may be minimal.
Cryptococcosis 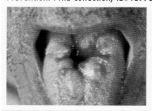	Mainly caused by *Cryptococcus neoformans* in soil and pigeon droppings. Present throughout the world and more common in immunosuppressed patients.	Most commonly lung, CNS and blood infections (90% of patients have only lung involvement) but can be primary skin infection or spread via hematogenous dissemination. Presents with various types of skin lesions including papules, vesicles, pustules, nodules, ulcers. More common in HIV and solid organ transplant patients. Can be seen as part of immune reconstitution syndrome.
Histoplasmosis (Reproduced with permission from Centers for Disease Control and Prevention. PHIL Collection, ID#18970) 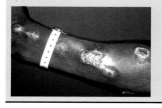	Caused by *Histoplasma capsulatum*, in soil of the central US and Canada, as well as areas of South America, Asia, Australia and Africa. Transmitted by inhalation or direct contact.	Systemic involvement of the lung, liver, lymph nodes, spleen and bone marrow. Skin involvement presents with various types of lesions including papules, plaques, nodules, and ulcers. Cutaneous involvement rare in immunocompetent individuals.
Sporotrichosis	Caused by dimorphic fungus of the Sporothrix genus, most commonly *Sporothrix schenckii,* found in soil and sphagnum moss. Infection occurs through traumatic implantation of the fungus, which classically is introduced via rose thorn, hay, or other plant material.	Initially begins with single nodule or eroded papule at the site of inoculation, usually on an extremity. Eventually multiple lesions may appear in a linear pattern consistent with lymphocutaneous spread. A fixed cutaneous form can also be seen, more commonly on the face in children. Less commonly, the infection may be systemic or disseminated. The systemic involvement most frequently seen is in the lungs, joints or CNS.

CNS, Central nervous system; HIV, Human immunodeficiency virus

REFERENCES

1. Mirmirani P, Tucker LY. Epidemiologic trends in pediatric tinea capitis: a population-based study from Kaiser Permanente Northern California. *J Am Acad Dermatol.* 2013;69(6):916-921.

2. Sharma V, Hall JC, Knapp JF, Sarai S, Galloway D, Babel DE. Scalp colonization by Trichophyton tonsurans in an urban pediatric clinic. *Arch Dermatol.* 1988; 124(10):1511-1513.

3. Ginter-Hanselmayer G, Weger W, Ilkit M, Smolle J. Epidemiology of tinea capitis in Europe: current state and changing patterns. *Mycoses.* 2007;50 Suppl 2:6-13.

4. Gupta AK, et al. Tinea capitis in children: a systematic review of management. *JEADV.* 2018; 32 (12): 2264-2274.

5. Chen X, Jiang X, Yang M, et al. Systemic antifungal therapy for tinea capitis in children. Cochrane Skin Group, ed. *Cochrane Database Syst Rev.* Published online May 12, 2016.

6. Gupta AK, Bamimore MA, Renaud HJ, Shear NH, Piguet V. A network meta-analysis on the efficacy and safety of mono-therapies for tinea capitis, and an assessment of evidence quality. *Pediatr Dermatol.* Published online September 8, 2020.

7. Stolmeier DA, Stratman HB, McIntee TJ, Stratman EJ. Utility of laboratory test result monitoring in patients taking oral terbinafine or griseofulvin for dermatophyte infections. *JAMA Dermatol.* 2018;154(12):1409-1416.

8. Degreef H. Clinical forms of dermatophytosis (ringworm infection). *Mycopatholgia.* 2008;166(5-6):257-65.

9. Ely JW, Rosenfeld S, Seabury Stone M. Diagnosis and man-agement of tinea infections. *Am Fam Physician.* 2014;90(10):702-710.

10. Scher RK, Tavakkol A. Sigurgeirsson B. et al. Onychomycosis: Diagnosis and definition of cure. *J Am Acad Dermat.* 2007;56(6):939-944.

11. Welsh O, Vera-Cabrera L, Welsh E. Onychomycosis. *Clin Dermatol.* 2010; 28(2):151-159.

12. Daniel III CR, Jellinek NJ. Commentary: the illusory tinea unguium cure. *J Am Acad Dermat.* 2010;62(3):415-417.

13. Scher RK, Daneil III CR. *Nails: Diagnosis Therapy Surgery.* 3rd ed. China: Elsevier Saunders; 2005:123-125,130-131.

14. Tosti A, et al. Treatment of nondermatophyte mold and can-dida onychomycosis. *Dermatol Clin.* 2003; 21(3):491-497.

15. Kreijkamp-Kaspers S, Hawke K, Guo L, et al. Oral antifungal medication for toenail onychomycosis. *Cochrane Database Syst Rev.* 2017;7(7):CD010031.

16. Iorizzo M, Piraccini BM, Tosti A. Today's treatment options for onychomycosis. *J Dtsch Dermatol Ges.* 2010;8(11): 875-879.

17. Piraccini BM, Sisti A, Tosti A. Long-term follow-up of toenail onychomycosis caused by dermatophytes after successful treatment with systemic antifungal agents. *J Am Acad Dermatol.* 2010: 62(3); 411-414.

18. Gupta A, Foley K. Antifungal Treatment for Pityriasis Versicolor. *JoF.* 2015;1(1):13-29.

19. Hu SW, Bigby M. Pityriasis versicolor: a systematic review of interventions. *Arch Dermatol.* 2010;146(10):1132-1140.

20. Bamford JT, Flores-Genuino RNS, Ray S, et al. Interventions for the treatment of pityriasis versicolor. Cochrane Skin Group, ed. *Cochrane Database Syst Rev.* Published online June 25, 2018.

21. Haegler P, Joerin L, Krähenbühl S, Bouitbir J. Hepatocellular Toxicity of Imidazole and Triazole Antimycotic Agents. *Toxicol Sci.* 2017;157(1):183-195.

22. Vila T, Sultan AS, Montelongo-Jauregui D, Jabra-Rizk MA. Oral Candidiasis: A Disease of Opportunity. *JoF.* 2020;6(1):15.

23. Taudorf EH, Jemec GBE, Hay RJ, Saunte DML. Cutaneous candidiasis – an evidence-based review of topical and sys-temic treatments to inform clinical practice. *J Eur Acad Dermatol Venereol.* 2019;33(10):1863-1873.

24. Hay RJ. Deep Fungal Infections. In: Kang S, Amagai M, Bruckner AL, Enk AH, Margolis DJ, McMichael AJ, Orringer JS. eds. *Fitzpatrick's Dermatology, 9e.* McGraw-Hill; Accessed October 15, 2020.

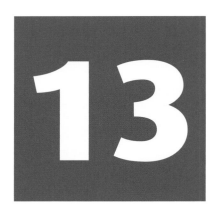

Viral Infections of the Skin

Erin Luxenberg

INTRODUCTION TO CHAPTER

Despite all the advances in antiviral therapy and the body's efficient immune system, the viruses that cause common skin infections continue to evade complete destruction. The herpes simplex and herpes zoster virus can persist in a dormant state in the dorsal root ganglia. The viruses that cause verrucae vulgaris (common warts) and molluscum contagiosum can persist for months to several years in the epidermis.

Herpes simplex and herpes zoster infections can cause significant illness and death especially in immunocompromised patients if the infection spreads to other organs. Common nongenital warts and molluscum contagiosum rarely cause significant problems in immunocompetent patients, but for various reasons most patients want treatment for these conditions. Genital warts are often asymptomatic and may be clinically undetectable; however, patients with oncogenic wart virus infections are at increased risk for anogenital and oropharyngeal cancers.[1]

HERPES SIMPLEX

Introduction

Table Key Points for Herpes Simplex

✓ Herpes simplex viruses (HSV-1 and HSV-2) are double - stranded DNA viruses that cause primary, latent and recurrent infections.

✓ HSV presents with painful grouped vesicles that often erode and develop crusts.

✓ Topical and oral HSV antiviral medications are most effective if given within 72 hours of the onset of symptoms.

Herpes simplex viruses (HSV) cause primary, latent, and recurrent infections and they are common infections worldwide. Human herpes virus-1 (HSV-1) typically infects the oral cavity, lips, and perioral skin and is usually acquired in childhood via nonsexual contact. Human herpes virus-2 (HSV-2) primarily infects the genital area and is almost always acquired via sexual contact. Nevertheless, HSV-1 is becoming a more common cause of genital herpes infections[1]. HSV has worldwide distribution but may be more common in less developed countries. Antibodies to HSV-1 are present in up to 85% of adults and antibodies to HSV-2 are present in 20–25% of adults.[2] However, many patients who have antibodies to HSV do not recall having had an infection.

Pathogenesis

HSV-1 and HSV-2 are human herpesviruses (HHV) which have double - stranded DNA and replicate within the nuclei of infected cells. HSV infects mucocutaneous tissue after direct contact or by way of secretions, mainly saliva in the case of HSV-1. The virus is transmitted via sensory nerves to the ganglia, where it may reside in a latent stage.

Recurrent infections are caused by reactivation of the virus, which travels back to the skin or mucous membranes resulting in an active infection. Immune mechanisms suppress the virus with clearing of the lesions in 1–2 weeks, but latency in the ganglia persists. Recurrent mucocutaneous infection may occur every few weeks to months to years via viral reactivation. Viral shedding may continue after the infection has clinically resolved.

Clinical Presentation

▶ History

Patients with orolabial HSV may complain of "fever after blisters or "cold sores" on the lips or perioral area or sores within the oral cavity. Patients with genital herpes may complain of pain or tingling in the genital area in the prodromal and active phase of the infection. Primary infection occurs 3–7 days following exposure. Localized pain, tenderness, and burning may be accompanied by fever, malaise, and tender lymphadenopathy. Vesicles develop, progressing to pustules and/or erosions. The eruption resolves in 1–2 weeks. Recurrent infection tends to be milder, with fewer vesicles and absent, or minimal systemic symptoms. Fever, sun exposure, and possibly stress may trigger recurrence of infection. Many individuals harboring HSV are asymptomatic.

▶ Physical Examination

HSV infections present with vesicles that tend to be grouped in clusters with underlying and surrounding erythema. Primary infections typically last about 12 days while recurrent infections will often last about a week.[3]

There are several presentations of HSV infections:

- HSV-1 most frequently affects the lip area (Figure 13-1), but may involve the buccal mucosa, gingiva, and oropharyngeal membranes. Primary infection may present as a gingivostomatitis in children, with fever, sore throat, and painful vesicles and ulcerative erosions on

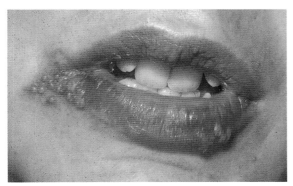

13-1. Herpes simplex on lips and oral commissure. Grouped vesicles.

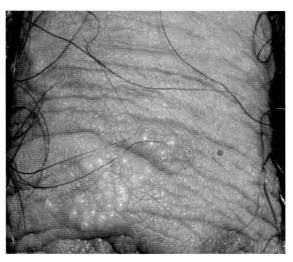

13-2. Herpes simplex on shaft of penis. Grouped vesicles.

the tongue, palate, gingiva, buccal mucosa, and lips. Patients may develop lymphadenopathy and an inability to eat. Recurrent eruptions are less severe, mostly affecting the vermilion border of the lip, and, less frequently, the perioral skin, nose, and cheeks. Patients may develop concomitant impetigo.

- HSV-2 usually affects the genital area and is the most common cause of genital ulcerations. The primary infection may be extremely painful with erosive vulvitis or vaginitis. The cervix, perineum, and buttocks may be involved with accompanying inguinal lymphadenopathy and dysuria. Affected men may develop an erosive balanitis. Recurrent genital infections can be subclinical or mild with few vesicles (Figure 13-2), clearing in 1–2 weeks. Most individuals found to be seropositive for HSV-2 have no reported history of genital herpes symptoms yet shed the virus and can transmit the virus to a partner.

- Fingers (herpetic whitlow) may be affected in children who suck their fingers or in healthcare workers from exposure to secretions (Figure 13-3).

- Herpes simplex keratitis is the second most common cause of corneal blindness in the United States. It presents with pain, redness, blurred vision, and photophobia.

- Primary neonatal infection usually develops after exposure to HSV in a mother's vaginal secretions during delivery, less commonly the virus is transmitted in utero. This is much more likely to occur when the mother has a primary infection. Infected healthcare workers can also transmit the virus to the neonate. Vesicles, if present, appear 4–7 days after birth and may be localized or widespread. The central nervous system

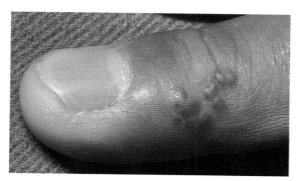

▲ **13-3.** Herpetic whitlow. Grouped vesicles on finger.

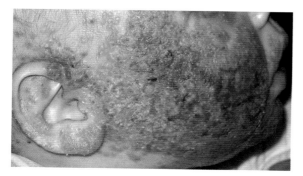

▲ **13-4.** Eczema herpeticum. Herpes simplex infection in child with atopic dermatitis. Confluent vesicles and papules with discrete erosions with hemorrhagic crusts.

and visceral organs can be affected, sometimes in the absence of skin lesions. Infected neonates may have significant morbidity and mortality.

- Patients with atopic dermatitis are at risk of developing eczema herpeticum, which is disseminated cutaneous HSV infection (Figure 13-4). This may begin as a herpes simplex infection on the lip, which rapidly spreads, or may develop after exposure to an individual with HSV infection.

▶ **Laboratory Findings**

Tzanck smears can be done by scraping the base of a lesion with a number 15 scalpel blade and spreading the contents on a glass slide. Microscopic examination after staining with a Wright or Giemsa stain reveals multinucleated epithelial giant cells. (Figure 13-5). A skin biopsy will show changes in the nuclei of keratinocytes characteristic of a viral infection. Viral cultures and Polymerase Chain Reaction (PCR) are sensitive and specific tests and can differentiate HSV-1 from HSV-2. The Western blot is a 99% sensitive and specific test for serologic status. In practice, the diagnosis of HSV infection is confirmed via DNA detection via PCR. A sterile swab is used to unroof a vesicle and the base is swabbed to isolate the epidermal cells containing the HSV.[4]

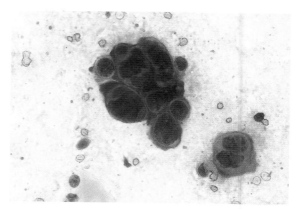

▲ **13-5.** Positive Tzanck smear in herpes simplex infection. Several giant multinucleated keratinocytes.

Diagnosis

The key diagnostic clinical features of herpes simplex are painful, grouped vesicles, or erosions on the face or genital area.

▶ **Differential Diagnosis**

For orolabial herpes

✓ Impetigo: Presents with flaccid vesicles with a honey colored crust, usually not recurrent in the same area.

✓ Aphthous stomatitis: Presents with painful 4–8 mm oral ulcers with white centers and sharp red borders.

✓ Other: Behcet's disease, diphtheria, herpangina (coxsackie virus infection), allergic contact dermatitis, Epstein Barr Virus (EBV) infection, oral candidiasis, and drug-induced mucositis.

For genital herpes

✓ Syphilitic chancre: Presents most commonly with a single nontender indurated ulcer.

✓ Other: Trauma, aphthae, chancroid, lymphogranuloma venereum, and granuloma inguinale.

Management

Mild and limited orolabial HSV in immunocompetent patients does not require therapy; however, moderate to severe disease can be treated with topical or oral medications as listed in Tables 13-1 and 13-2. Treatment should be initiated quickly after onset of symptoms, as these medications may not be helpful if started 72 hours after onset of symptoms.

The Centers for Disease Control and Prevention (CDC) has updated information for clinicians on the treatment of immunocompromised patients and for chronic suppressive treatment for genital herpes.[2] Immunocompromised

Table 13-1. Topical medications for oralabial herpes simplex

Generic Names	Dosage	Duration
5% **Acyclovir** ointment	Apply every 3 hours, 6 times a day	7 days
10% **Docosanol** cream otc	Apply 5 times a day	Up to 10 days
1% **Pencyclovir** cream	Apply every 2 hours while awake	4 days

individuals require higher doses of oral antiviral medications or may require intravenous therapy. Recurrent episodes of HSV-1 are less common after age 35. Recurrent episodes of genital herpes can have a major psychosocial impact on an affected individual. The American Social Health Association, www.ashastd.org and the CDC have patient-oriented information on these issues.[5]

Clinical Course and Prognosis

The clinical course of HSV is chronic and often relapsing. Relapses are often brought on by stress, infections, medication, or sun exposure. While no cure is currently available for HSV, patients who have more than four relapses of cutaneous lesions per year may benefit from suppressive therapy.

Indications for Consultation

Patients with ocular or systemic involvement and immunocompromised patients with widespread disease should be referred to the appropriate specialist.

Patient Information

- Centers for Disease Control and Prevention: www.cdc.gov/std/herpes/default.htm
- American Academy of Dermatology: aad.org/public/diseases/a-z/herpes-simplex-overview

▼ HERPES ZOSTER

Introduction

Table Key Points for Herpes Zoster

✓ Herpes zoster (shingles) is caused by the reactivation of a latent varicella (chicken pox) infection.

✓ Herpes zoster typically presents with painful grouped vesicles within a single unilateral dermatome. Pain may precede the lesions.

✓ Oral antiviral medications for herpes zoster are most effective if given within 72 hours of the onset of symptoms.

✓ Post-herpetic neuralgia can occur in 5% to 20% of patients and is more commonly seen in older (> 60 years old) or immunocompromised individuals.

✓ An adjuvanted recombinant zoster vaccine (RZV), Shingrex has an efficacy of 97% in reducing the risk of developing herpes zoster.

Herpes zoster (shingles) represents reactivation of latent varicella (chicken pox) infection. Persons with a history of primary varicella have a 20–30% lifetime risk of developing herpes zoster. Herpes zoster seldom affects children or adolescents. Incidence and severity increase after age 60 and in immunocompromised individuals.[6]

Pathogenesis

The varicella-zoster virus is a double- stranded DNA virus. Following a varicella infection, varicella-zoster virus may be retained in dorsal root ganglia in a latent form. Reactivation of the virus, leading to the cutaneous eruption in the distribution of the affected sensory nerve(s), may be induced by trauma, stress, fever, radiation therapy, or immunosuppression. Direct contact with vesicular fluid can result in varicella in a susceptible person.

Table 13-2. Oral medications for initial genital herpes and recurrent orolabial and genital herpes infections in immunocompetent adults.

Medication	Selected dosing options for herpes simplex infections.	Duration
Acyclovir	Initial genital: 200 mg every 4 hours, 5 times a day.	10 days
	Recurrent genital: 200 mg every 4 hours, 5 times a day.	5 days
Famciclovir	Initial orolabial: 250 mg every 8 hours.	7–10 days
	Recurrent orolabial: 1500 mg one dose.	1 day
	Recurrent genital: 1000 mg twice a day.	1 day
Valacyclovir	Initial genital: 1 gram twice a day.	10 days
	Recurrent genital: 500 mg twice a day.	3 days
	Recurrent orolabial: 2 g every 12 hours.	1 day

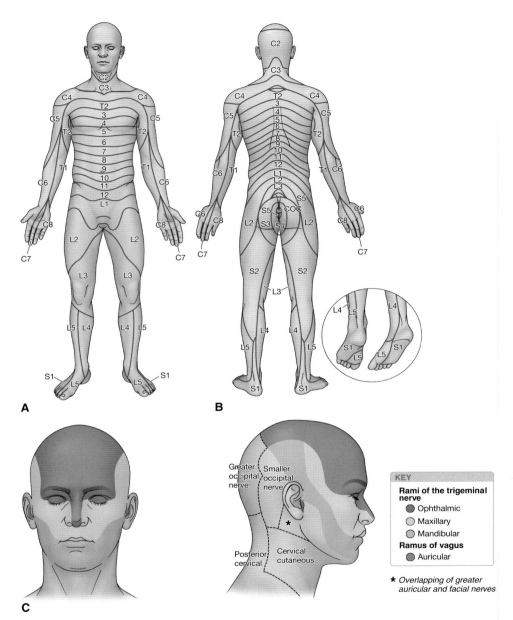

A

B

C

▲ **13-6.** Dermatomes. The cutaneous fields of peripheral sensory nerves. (Reproduced with permission from Wolff K, Johnson R, Saavedra AP, et al: Fitzpatrick's Color Atlas and Synopsis of Clinical Dermatology, 8th ed. New York, NY: McGraw Hill; 2017).

Clinical Presentation

▷ History

Herpes zoster often begins with intense pain, which may precede the eruption by one or a few days. Pruritus, tingling, tenderness, or hyperesthesia may also develop.

▷ Physical Examination

The eruption presents as grouped vesicles within the dermatome of the affected nerves, usually within a single unilateral dermatome (Figure 13-6). Any area of the body may be affected, but it is seen most frequently on the trunk (Figure 13-7).

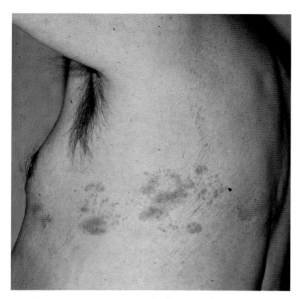

▲ **13-7.** Herpes zoster in 6th thoracic dermatome. Small vesicles on erythematous plaques.

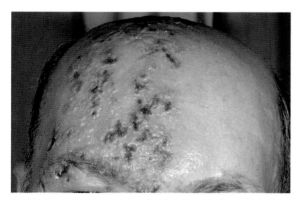

▲ **13-8.** Herpes zoster in distribution of the ophthalmic branch of the trigeminal nerve. Hemorrhagic crusts and erosions at sites of resolving vesicles.

Involvement of the trigeminal nerve, particularly the 1st (ophthalmic) division (Figure 13-8), occurs in 10–15% of patients. When vesicles develop on the tip or side of the nose indicating involvement of the nasociliary branch (Hutchinson's sign), the eye is more likely to be affected, sometimes resulting in blindness. Herpes zoster affecting the 2nd and 3rd division of the trigeminal nerve may produce symptoms, vesicles, and erosions in the mouth, ears, pharynx, or larynx. Facial palsy may develop with accompanying involvement of the ear and/or tympanic membrane with or without tinnitus, vertigo, and deafness (Ramsay Hunt Syndrome). Herpes zoster may involve adjacent dermatomes or become disseminated in immunocompromised patients (Figure 13-9).

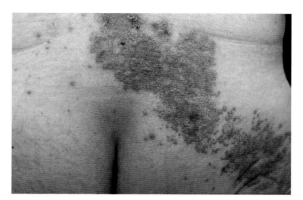

▲ **13-9.** Disseminated herpes zoster. Multiple confluent crusted erosions along L4, L5 and S1 dermatomes with scattered lesions extending beyond the midline of the trunk.

▶ Laboratory Findings

A Tzanck smear or skin biopsy may reveal characteristic multinucleated giant cells (Figure 13-5), which cannot be differentiated from those seen in herpes simplex infection. Viral cultures and PCR testing are more specific and sensitive tests for herpes zoster, with PCR being the preferred method of testing.

Diagnosis

The key diagnostic clinical features of herpes zoster are grouped painful vesicles on an erythematous base within a single dermatome.

▶ Differential Diagnosis

√ Herpes simplex: Presents with vesicles that are similar, but the lesions are not as painful, and they do not extend over an entire dermatome or may cross the midline.

√ The prodromal pain of herpes zoster can mimic headaches, myocardial infarction, pleuritic chest pain, or an acute abdomen.

√ Urticaria: Wheals last less than 24 hours and are more often itchy, may move and cross dermatomal boundaries.

√ Allergic contact dermatitis: Vesicles are not grouped, and eruption is extremely pruritic.

Management

Oral antiviral medications, if given early, may reduce the duration of the eruption and may reduce the risk and severity of acute pain and perhaps postherpetic neuralgia.

The treatments should be started within 72 hours of onset of symptoms. Recommended immunocompetent adult treatment oral doses (dose adjustment needed for renal insufficiency):

- Valacyclovir 1000 mg three times a day for 7 days.
- Acyclovir 800 mg five times a day for 7 to 10 days.
- Famciclovir 500 mg every 8 hours for 7 days.

Appropriate treatment for acute pain (acute neuritis) may be needed. Antiviral therapy may reduce the pain associated with acute neuritis, but the pain syndromes may still be severe. Nonsteroidal anti-inflammatory drugs (NSAIDs) and acetaminophen can be used alone or in combination for mild to moderate discomfort. For moderate to severe pain, opioid analgesics might be necessary.[7]

Persistent postherpetic neuralgia can have a negative impact on a patient's health and quality of life. It is associated with insomnia, anorexia, and depression, especially in the elderly.[8] Treatments may include topical lidocaine or capsaicin, antidepressants such as amitriptyline, desipramine and nortriptyline, and anticonvulsants such as carbamazepine, pregabalin, and gabapentin. Acupuncture and biofeedback may also be helpful.[9]

Two vaccines are available to prevent the development of herpes zoster. An adjuvanted recombinant zoster vaccine (RZV), Shingrix was approved in 2017. It has been found to be more effective than the older live vaccine (ZVL) Zostavax. While ZVL has been shown to reduce the risk of developing herpes zoster by 51% and the risk of postherpetic neuralgia by 67%, RZV has an efficacy of 97%.[10,11]

Clinical Course and Prognosis

The rash associated with herpes zoster usually resolves in 3–5 weeks, but symptoms may persist for a longer time, sometimes for many months or years (postherpetic neuralgia). This may occur in 5–20 % of patients but is rarely seen in those less than 40 years of age. Incidence increases with age. Symptoms resolve in 3 months in 50% of patients and in 1 year in 75% of patients.

Indications for Consultation

Patients with severe disease or systemic involvement and patients with postherpetic neuralgia who are not responding to treatment should be referred to the appropriate specialist. Patients with disseminated zoster, spanning more than one dermatome, likely need hospital admission for intravenous (IV) acyclovir treatment. Patients with eye involvement should be referred to ophthalmology.

Patient Information

- Centers for Disease Control and Prevention: www.cdc.gov/shingles/index.html

- American Academy of Dermatology: www.aad.org/public/diseases/a-z/shingles-overview

MOLLUSCUM CONTAGIOSUM

Introduction

Table Key Points for Molluscum

✓ Molluscum infections are caused by a member of the pox virus group, which contains double- stranded DNA.

✓ Lesions present as pearly, 2 to 10 mm dome shaped papules.

✓ Spontaneous resolution usually occurs in 6 to 9 months but lesions may persist for over a year.

Molluscum contagiosum is a benign viral infection of the skin and mucous membranes. The infection has a worldwide distribution and occurs in all ethnicities. Children are most frequently affected. In adults, it is mostly seen in the genital area and represents a sexually transmitted disease. It is more common and severe in patients with human immunodeficiency virus (HIV) infection, especially in patients with low CH4 counts.

Pathogenesis

Molluscum contagiosum is caused by a member of the pox virus group, which contain double- stranded DNA and replicate within the cytoplasm of epithelial cells. The virus is spread by direct skin-to-skin contact.

Clinical Presentation

▶ History

Small papules develop on the skin and sometimes on the genital mucous membranes usually 2–7 weeks after contact

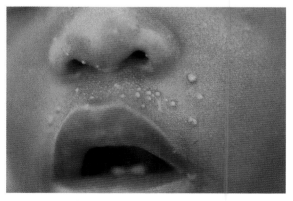

▲ 13-10. Molluscum contagiosum on face. 1 to 2 mm dome shaped papules.

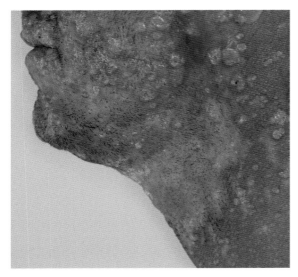

▲ 13-11. Molluscum contagiosum in immunosuppressed patient. Multiple umbilicated papules on face and neck.

with an infected individual. The lesions are typically initially asymptomatic, but pruritus and inflammation can develop.

▶ Physical Examination

The typical lesions present as pearly, 2–10 mm dome-shaped papules with a waxy surface (Figure 13-10) which often have a central umbilication and erythema around the rim. Papules may be larger and more extensively distributed in immunocompromised patients (Figure 13-11). The face, upper chest, and upper extremities are most frequently affected in children, whereas the anogenital, suprapubic, and thigh areas are the usual sites of infection in adults. [12]

▶ Laboratory Findings

The diagnosis can be confirmed by incising a lesion with a needle and squeezing out the core with gloved fingers or with a small curette. The core should be squashed between two glass slides to flatten the specimen. The specimen can be stained with Giemsa stain and examined for the presence of large, purple, oval bodies which are the viral inclusion bodies within the cytoplasm of keratinocytes. These inclusion bodies can also be seen in skin biopsy specimens.

Diagnosis

The key diagnostic clinical features of molluscum are small skin-colored papules with central umbilication.

▶ Differential Diagnosis

✓ Acne: Presents with papules, pustules, and cysts that could appear similar to molluscum. However, comedones should be present and there is no central umbilication of acne lesions.
✓ Folliculitis: Presents with small papules and/or pustules without umbilication.
✓ Milia: Can be found on the face of children but are much smaller pinpoint white papules.
✓ Other: Syringomas, flat warts, milia, cryptococcosis.

Management

A recent Cochrane review reported that no single treatment has been shown to be convincingly effective. [13] However, several options for therapy are commonly used.

Molluscum papules can be removed surgically using a small skin curette. They can also be incised with a needle and the contents expressed with gloved fingers or with a comedone extractor. Physical removal via curettage or extraction tends to be not only the most effective but also the most time-consuming treatment. It is not often tolerated in children. Liquid nitrogen cryotherapy can be used in a single pulse. 17% salicylic acid over the counter (OTC) products, which are normally used for common warts, can also be used. Additional options include cantharidin as well as imiquimod and keratolytics. [14] Spontaneous resolution typically occurs in 6–9 months but may take one to several years.

Public Health Issues

Because molluscum contagiosum is easily spread among children, parents and schools should be notified of the importance of trying to avoid direct skin-to-skin contact with affected children. There is also frequent spread in certain sports activities, particularly in wrestling. Therefore, coaches and participants should be educated about the infection. Individuals with involvement of the genital region should practice safe sex.

Clinical Course and Prognosis

Untreated lesions of molluscum can last up to 18 months but will generally resolve on their own. Once exposed to molluscum, most patients will rarely have subsequent infections.

Indications for Consultation

Patients with symptomatic lesions that have not responded to treatment.

Patient Information

American Academy of Dermatology: www.aad.org/public/diseases/a-z/molluscum-contagiosum-overview

▼ WARTS

Introduction

Table Key Points for Warts (verrucae vulgaris)

✓ Warts are caused by the human papillomavirus (HPV), a double-stranded DNA virus which has many distinct genotypes.

✓ HPV genotypes, such as 16, 18, 31 and 33 may be oncogenic, inducing malignant transformation to squamous cell carcinoma in the anogenital and oropharyngeal areas.

✓ There are multiple treatments for warts; with the exception of topical salicylic acid products none show consistent efficacy in controlled studies

✓ Choice of treatment depends on the location, size, number, and type of wart, as well as the age and cooperation of the patient.

Warts (verrucae vulgaris) represent one of the most frequently seen viral mucocutaneous infections. All age groups can be affected, but the incidence is higher in children and young adults. In immunocompromised individuals, warts are more common and widespread, more resistant to treatment, and more frequently progress to intraepithelial neoplasms. Wart infections can be seen worldwide and affect all ethnicities.

Pathogenesis

Warts are caused by the human papillomavirus (HPV), a double-stranded DNA virus with over 200 distinct subtypes. The virus infects keratinocytes in skin and mucous membranes by direct skin-to-skin contact or less commonly via fomites such as floors. Autoinoculation frequently occurs. Warts can spontaneously resolve after months to years in patients with intact cell mediated immunity. In two-thirds of infected individuals, warts regress within 2 years.

Some HPV genotypes that are found on normal skin and mucous membranes may induce wart development when patients become immunocompromised. Plantar and acral warts are typically caused by HPV types 1, 2, and 4. Nongenital warts occur in 10% of children and are present on 3.5% of adults at any given time.[15] Benign genital warts are most often caused by HPV types 6 and 11. Visible lesions may be found in up to 1% of sexually active adults, and subclinical infection may be present in up to 15% of individuals.[16]

Other HPV genotypes, such as 16, 18, 31, and 33 may be oncogenic, inducing malignant transformation to squamous cell carcinoma in the anogenital and oropharyngeal areas.[9]

Cervical cancer is the fourth most common cancer among women worldwide and nearly all cases can be attributed to HPV infection, most commonly types 16 and 18. HPV type 16 may also be the most common subtype found in HPV-associated oropharyngeal cancer as well as anal cancer.[17,18]

The link between HPV and specific types of cancer has been established based on several factors including the presence of viral oncogenes present in HPV and the identification of HPV within tumor specimens. The potential role of HPV in cutaneous squamous cell carcinoma is yet to be established, though there may be a link.[19-21]

Clinical Presentation

▶ History

Warts may develop on any skin or mucosal surface, most frequently affecting the hands, feet, and genitalia. Trauma to the skin may encourage inoculation of the virus. Widespread infection can be seen in immunocompromised individuals, specifically people with impaired cell-mediated immunity.

▶ Physical Examination

There are several clinical presentations for warts, depending on location and genotype.

• Verrucae vulgaris (common warts)

Skin colored, hyperkeratotic, exophytic, dome-shaped papules ranging in size from 1 to 10 mm. Mild erythema may be seen around the borders (Figure 13-12). The papules can be in a linear configuration, due to autoinoculation of the virus in an excoriation (Figure 13-13). Warts are most frequently seen on the hands but may involve other skin areas.

• Verrucae plantaris (plantar warts)

Verrucous or endophytic papules, 1–10 mm, affecting the plantar surface of the foot. Black or brown dots created

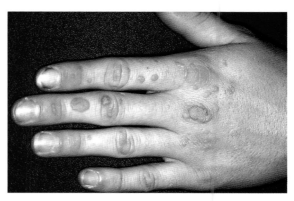

▲ **13-12.** Verrucae vulgaris on hands. Multiple hyperkeratotic papules and plaques

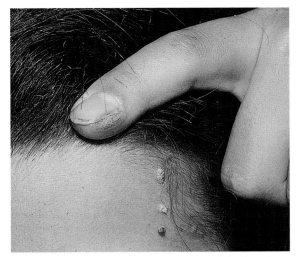

▲ **13-13.** Verrucae vulgaris on finger and forehead. Example of auto-inoculation of wart virus in an excoriation.

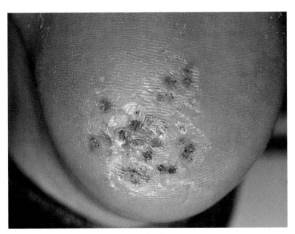

▲ **13-14.** Plantar warts. Multiple warts in mosaic pattern with brown dots caused by thrombosed capillaries.

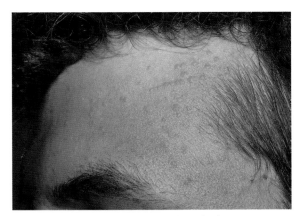

▲ **13-15.** Flat warts on forehead. Multiple 1-2 mm papules.

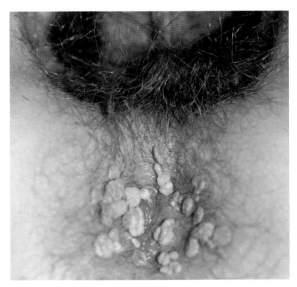

▲ **13-16.** Condyloma accuminata (genital warts). Multiple grouped pedunculated papules on the perineal body.

by thrombosed capillaries may be seen on the surface or after paring the warts (Figure 13-14).

- Mosaic warts

Localized confluent collection of small warts, usually seen on the palms and soles (Figure 13-14).

- Verrucae planae (flat warts)

Small, 1–3 mm, slightly elevated, flat-topped papules with minimal scale, frequently seen on the face and dorsal hands (Figure 13-15).

- Filiform/digitate warts

Pedunculated papules with finger-like projections arising from the skin's surface, frequently seen on the face and neck.

- Condyloma accuminata (genital or venereal warts)

Sessile, smooth-surfaced exophytic papillomas, which may be skin-colored, brown, or whitish (Figure 13-16). The papillomas may be pedunculated or broad-based, sometimes coalescing to form confluent plaques. There may be extension into the vagina, urethra, or anal canal.

▶ **Laboratory Findings**

Diagnosis is typically clinical. Warts on acral surfaces often obscure normal skin lines. Paring overlying hyperkeratotic skin will often reveal the classic black dots representing thrombosed capillaries. A skin biopsy may be done, especially if a carcinoma is suspected, or if the diagnosis is unclear. Histopathologic examination of a skin biopsy of an active wart infection is usually diagnostic.

Diagnosis

The key diagnostic clinical features of warts are 2–10 mm verrucous or smooth papules, usually present on the hands, feet, or genitals.

Differential Diagnosis

- Squamous cell carcinoma: Typically presents as an isolated papule or plaque that may ulcerate or appear inflamed. It usually occurs on sun exposed skin.
- Seborrheic keratosis: Presents with verrucous tan to dark brown papules or plaques that appear "stuck on" to the skin and are commonly seen in older adults. Skin-colored lesions on the dorsum of the hand may closely resemble warts.
- Corns and calluses: These lesions have no red or brown dots (thrombosed capillary loops) when pared. Corns often have translucent/white cores (Figure 13-17).
- Pearly penile papules: These are often confused with warts on the penis. They present with numerous 1–3 mm smooth papules in a linear arrangement on the corona and are seen in up to 10% of males.
- Acrochordon: Fleshy, skin-colored papules, often in the axilla and groin, with a less verrucous appearance than warts.

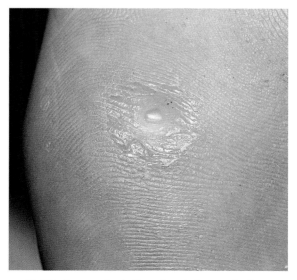

▲ **13-17.** Corn on foot. Hyperkeratotic papule that can mimic a wart, but after it is pared down it has a translucent base without the characteristic brown pinpoint dots or white opaque center typical of a wart.

Management of Nongenital Warts

Active treatment of cutaneous warts might not be necessary as warts will often resolve on their own with time. However, there are multiple treatments for warts, none showing consistent efficacy in controlled studies, with the exception of topical salicylic acid products.[22,23] Existing modalities mostly aim at destruction or removal of visible lesions or induction of an immune response to the virus. Antiproliferative treatments can be used as well. Choice of treatment depends on the location, size, number, and type of wart, as well as the age and cooperation of the patient. Induction of pain and the risk of scarring need to be considered. The patient and the treating clinician need to be persistent and patient with therapy as it may take up to 4–6 months for warts to resolve with the treatment. Patients should be made aware of the necessity for often prolonged treatment and the possibility of treatment failure or lesion recurrence.[22,23]

- Salicylic acid: Salicylic acid preparations are available as nonprescription solutions, gels, plaster, or patches. Compound W wart remover, Dr. Scholl's Clear Away, Duofilm, Mediplast, Occlusal, Trans-Ver-Sal, Wart Stick, and Wart-Off are examples of some available products with salicylic acid. The patients should follow the package instructions. Most preparations are applied at bedtime, after the wart(s) has been soaked in warm water and then pared down with an emery board. The induced irritation can cause an inflammatory immune response, which speeds resolution of the wart. Treatment may take up to 4–12 weeks to be effective.
- Topical immunotherapy: The idea behind topical immunotherapy is to induce an allergic response via a contact sensitizer thereby theoretically awakening the body's immune system to the wart virus. Dinitrochlorobenzene (DNCB), squaric acid, diphenylcyclopropenone (DPCP) can be used with and be beneficial in the treatment of refractory warts.
- Fluorouracil: FU may work by inhibiting wart proliferation. It can be used topically or intralesionally.
- Cantharidin: Cantharidin comes from the green blister beetle. When applied, it causes blistering of skin in an attempt to separate the wart from normal skin. However, this product is not currently FDA approved for use in the United States.
- Cryotherapy: Liquid nitrogen is applied to the wart by a healthcare provider using a Q-tip or a spray canister for 10–20 seconds or until a 2-mm-rim of white frost appears beyond the border of the wart. The treatment can be repeated 2–3 times during a visit (see Chapter 7). Repeat treatments can be done every 2–3 weeks if improvement is noted. Over-the-counter cryotherapy kits are available. Although the agent is not as cold as liquid nitrogen, these home kits can sometimes be successful in destroying warts. Patients must carefully

follow the package insert directions for use, to avoid injury.

- Procedures: Surgical excision, electrosurgery, and laser surgery may be used to successfully remove or destroy warts, but they may result in significant scarring and recurrence of the wart within or adjacent to the scar.
- Cimetidine: Cimetidine, besides being an H2 blocker, is known to stimulate T-lymphocyte cells which may help fight viral infections. Doses of 400 mg 2–3×/day may lead to clinical improvement and resolution of warts.[24]

Management of Genital Warts

In addition to the aforementioned treatments, the following options have been used with success in treating genital warts.[25]

- Imiquimod 5% cream (Aldara cream) is an immune response modifier, used primarily for genital warts. A thin layer of the cream is applied sparingly by the patient 3 times a week (e.g., Monday, Wednesday, Friday) to warts at bedtime and washed off in 6–10 hours for a maximum of 16 weeks. The cream may induce an inflammatory response prior to clearing of the warts.
- 25% podophyllin in tincture of benzoin is an antimitotic agent applied every 1–3 weeks to external genital warts by a healthcare provider. It should be washed off in 20 minutes to 2 hours. It should not be used in pregnant or lactating women.
- 0.5% podophyllotoxin (Condylox gel or solution) is a prescription medication that can be used at home by the patient. It is applied to external genital warts twice a day for 3 consecutive days per week, and then discontinued for 4 consecutive days for up to 4 weeks. It should not be prescribed to pregnant or lactating women.
- 15% sinecatechins (Veregen) ointment, a green tea extract and keratolytic, is applied 3 times a day to external genital warts until the warts are clear. It should not be used for more than 16 weeks. It should not be used in pregnant or lactating women or in children.

Prevention

Patients with anogenital warts need to use safe-sex practices. Sexual partners should be examined and treated as indicated.

While several HPV different vaccines have been developed, only the 9-valent (Gardasil 9) has been available in the United States since 2016. This vaccine targets HPV types 6 and 11, which cause about 90% of anogenital warts. In addition, it targets the "high risk" HPV subtypes 16 and 18, which cause about 70% of cervical cancers, as well as types 31, 33, 45, 52, and 58, which together are thought to cause an additional 20% of cervical cancer.

The vaccine is designed to prevent initial HPV infection thereby preventing HPV associated cervical, vulvar, vaginal, anal, oropharyngeal, and other head and neck cancers as well as genital warts. The American Cancer Society (ACS) recommends routine HPV vaccination between ages 9–12 years, with "catch-up" vaccination up to age 26 years. The combined use of HPV vaccination of all children between 9 and 12 years of age along with routine cervical cancer screening of all individuals with a cervix has the potential to eliminate cervical cancer in the population.[26,27]

Clinical Course and Prognosis

While nongenital warts can self-resolve without treatment, adherence to a treatment regimen will give patients the greatest chance of resolution. Genital warts are often recurrent, even after apparent resolution.

Indications for Consultation

Widespread warts that have not responded to therapy should be referred to dermatology. Females should be referred to gynecologist for cervical cancer screening. Persistent anal warts should be referred to colorectal surgery for further treatment and cancer screening.

Patient Information

▶ For nongenital warts

American Academy of Dermatology: www.aad.org/skin-conditions/dermatology-a-to-z/warts

▶ For genital warts

Centers for Disease Control and Prevention: www.cdc.gov/std/hpv

▼ REFERENCES

1. Fatahzadeh M, Schwartz RA. Human herpes simplex virus infections: epidemiology, pathogenesis, symptomatology, diagnosis, and management. *J Am Acad Dermatol.* 2007;57(5): 737-762.
2. Xu F, et al. Trends in herpes simplex virus type 1 and 2 seroprevalence in the United States. *JAMA.* 2006; 296(8);964.
3. Amir J, et al. The natural history of primary herpes simplex type 1 gingivostomatitis in children. *Pediatr Dermatol.* 1999;16(4)259.
4. Magaret AS et al. Optimizing PCR positivity criterion for detection of herpes simplex virus DNA on skin and mucosa. *J Clin Microbiol.* 2007;45(5):1618.
5. Workowski KA, Berman S. Sexually transmitted diseases treatment guidelines. *MMWR Recomm Rep.* 2010; 59(60):22-25.
6. Weinberg JM. Herpes zoster: epidemiology, natural history, and common complications. *J Am Acad Dermat.* 2007; 57(6 Suppl) :S130-5.
7. Dworkin RH, et al. Recommendations for the management of herpes zoster. *Clin Infect Dis.* 2007;44 Suppl 1:S1.

8. Sampathkumar P, Drage LA, Martin DP. Herpes zoster (shingles) and postherpetic neuralgia. *Mayo Clin Proc.* 2009; 84(3):274-80.

9. Christo PJ, Hobelmann G, Maine DN. Post-herpetic neuralgia in older adults: evidence-based approaches to clinical management. *Drugs Aging.* 2007; 24(1):1-19.

10. Oxman MN, Levin MJ, Johnson GR et al. A vaccine to prevent herpes zoster and postherpetic neuralgia in older adults. *N Engl J Med.* 2005; 352(22):2271-84.

11. Lal H et al. Efficacy of an adjuvanted herpes zoster subunit vaccine in older adults. *N Eng J Med.* 2015;372(22):2087.

12. Leftheriou LI, Ker SC, Stratman EJ. Diagnosis of atypical molluscum contagiosum:the utility of a squash preparation. *Clin Med Res.*2011;9(1):50-51.

13. van der Wouden JC, van der Sande R, van Suijlekom-Smit LW, Berger MY, Butler CC. Interventions for cutaneous mollscum contagiousum. *Cochrane Database Syst Rev.* 2009;CD004767.

14. Hanna D, et al. A prospective randomized trial comparing the efficacy and adverse effects of four recognized treatments of molluscum contagiosum in children. *Pediatr Dermatol.* 2006;23(6):574.

15. Beutner KR. Nongenital human papillomavirus infections. *Clin Lab Med.* 2000;20(2):423.

16. Gillison ML et al. Prevalence of oral HPV infection in the United States, 2009-2010. *JAMA.* 2012;307(7): 693.

17. Dunne EF, Friedman A, Datta SD, Markowitz LE, Workowski KA. Updates on human papillomavirus and genital warts and counseling messages from the 2010 Sexually Transmitted Diseases Treatment Guidelines. *Clin Infect Dis.* 2011;53 (Suppl. 3):S143-S152.

18. Frisch M, et al. Sexually transmitted infection as a cause of anal cancer. *N Engl J Med.* 1997;337(19):1350.

19. Koutsky L. Epidemiology of genital human papillomavirus infection. *Am J Med.* 1997;102(5A):3.

20. Zur Hausen H. Papillomaviruses causing cancer: evasion from host-cell control in early events in carcinogenesis. *J Natl Cancer Inst.* 2000;92(9):690.

21. Wang J et al. Role of human papillomavirus in cutaneous squamous cell carcinoma: A meta-analysis. *J Am Acad Dermatol.* 2014;70(4):621.

22. Kwok CS, Holland R, Gibbs S. Efficacy of topical treatments for cutaneous warts: a meta-analyis and pooled analysis of randomized controlled trials. *Brit J Dermatol.* 2011;165(2): 233-46.

23. Kwok CS, Gibbs S, Bennett C, Holland R, Abbott R. Topical treatments for cutaneous warts. *Cochrane Database Syst Rev.* 2012; Issue 9. Art. No.: CD001781. DOI: 10.1002/14651858. CD001781.pub3.

24. Glass AT, Solomon BA. Cimetidine therapy for recalcitrant warts. *Arch Dermatol.* 1996;132(6):680.

25. **Workowski KA, Bolan GA, Centers for Disease Control and Prevention. Sexually transmitted diseases treatment guidelines, 2015. *MMWR Recomm Rep.* 2015; 64:1.**

26. Marks DH, Katz KA. Vaccination Against Human Papillomavirus. *JAMA Dermatol.* Published online August 19, 2020.

27. Saslow D, et al. Human papillomavirus vaccination 2020 guideline Update: American Cancer Society Guideline Adaptation. *Ca Cancer J Clin.* 2020 70(4):274-280.

Infestations and Bites

Cindy Firkins Smith

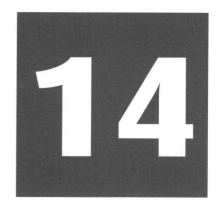

INTRODUCTION TO CHAPTER

Arthropods have always feasted on humans and humans have tried countless strategies to keep them from doing so. Although seldom causing any life-threatening physical illness, the societal burden of biting and sucking bugs is significant, costing millions of dollars, tremendous discomfort, and immeasurable emotional distress. They bite, we itch, we scratch, and these facts seem destined to endure.

SCABIES

Introduction

Table Key Points for Scabies

✓ Scabies is transmitted from person to person by direct skin contact.

✓ Scabies typically presents with intensely pruritic, excoriated papules on the hands, wrists, arms, trunk and genitals. The head, neck and feet may be affected in children.

✓ A burrow, a short, wavy line, is pathognomic of scabies.

✓ Permethrin 5% cream is considered the first line treatment for scabies.

✓ Patients should be advised that it may take up to 4 to 6 weeks for symptoms to resolve despite effective treatment.

Scabies is a common parasitic infection caused by the mite *Sarcoptes scabiei* var *hominis*. Transmission of the mite is primarily person-to-person by direct skin contact. Situations that result in more skin-to-skin contact, such as parents with small children, sexual activity, overcrowding, and institutional settings increase the prevalence of infestation. Although the scabies mite has not been shown to transmit any significant pathogens, the intense itching associated with the infestation, the risk of superinfection of excoriated skin and the fact that up to 300 million people may be affected worldwide annually makes scabies a significant public health problem.[1]

Pathogenesis

Sarcoptes scabiei is an obligate human parasite that completes its entire 30-day life cycle within the epidermis. The fertilized female weaves through the epidermis and leaves a trail of 60–90 eggs and feces (scybala), in her burrow (Figure 14-1). The eggs hatch into larvae which then mature into nymphs and adults. The rash and pruritus of scabies is a result of a hypersensitivity reaction to the mite and its detritus.

179

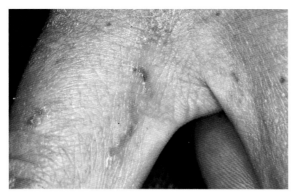

▲ **Figure 14 -1.** Burrow in a finger web: Thin curved ridge in the superficial epidermis created by a female mite.

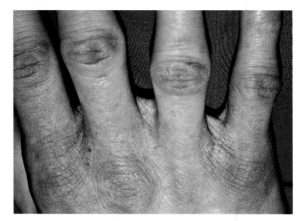

▲ **Figure 14 -2.** Scabies in finger webs: Excoriated papules with lichenification of skin due to chronic scratching.

The incubation period from infestation to pruritus can range from days to months. The first time an individual is infested it typically takes 2–6 weeks to become sensitized and develop symptoms, but in subsequent infestations, the previously hypersensitized individual can begin itching in as little as 1–3 days. Some infested individuals never develop hypersensitivity to the mite and never experience symptoms but can still transmit the infection; these are asymptomatic "carriers."

Clinical Presentation

▶ History

Intense pruritus is the main presenting complaint, although very young children who can't verbalize itching are often irritable and eat and sleep poorly. Adults often complain that the pruritus is worse at night. Family members and close contacts frequently report similar symptoms.

▶ Physical Examination

The patient presenting with scabies usually has a nondescript, excoriated, and papular dermatitis. The most common physical findings are papules, vesicles, pustules, or nodules. These typically occur on the trunk, arms, hands (Figures 14-2, 14-3) and genitals in adults and may also involve the head, neck, and feet in infants and young children (Figures 14-4, 14- 5). The burrow, a short, wavy line, is pathognomonic of scabies and is typically seen on the wrists, finger webs, and penis (Figures 14-1, 14-3).

Less common presentations include nodular, bullous, and crusted scabies.[2]

- Nodular scabies: This typically presents with a few salmon-colored pruritic nodules usually seen in the axillae, groin, and male genitalia. Nodular scabies is a hypersensitivity reaction that typically occurs after a successfully treated scabies infestation and does not necessarily indicate active infection.

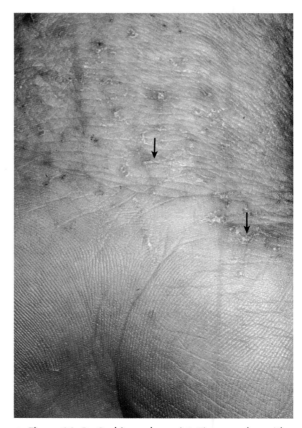

▲ **Figure14 -3.** Scabies volar wrist: Tiny papules with many curved and wavy burrows.

- Bullous scabies: While blisters commonly occur on the palms and soles of infants infested with scabies, bullous scabies is a more extensive bullous eruption most

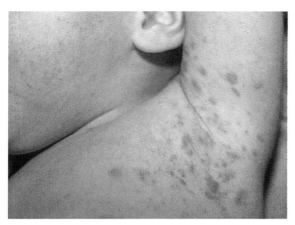

▲ **Figure 14-4.** Scabies in axillae of child: Papules and nodules.

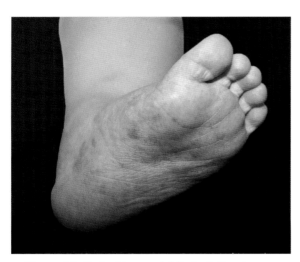

▲ **Figure 14-5.** Scabies on child's foot: Papules on plantar surface of foot.

commonly seen in elderly in adults. It is often confused with bullous pemphigoid.

- Crusted (Norwegian) scabies: This presents with thick, crusted, or scaly plaques and is often confused with psoriasis or extensive eczema. Crusted scabies typically affects the immunocompromised, elderly, disabled, or debilitated. These patients often do not exhibit typical pruritus and scratching and are often infested with thousands of mites. They are highly contagious.

▶ **Laboratory Findings**

Table 14-1 has instructions for collection and examination of a scabies preparation. The presence of a mite, eggs, or scybala in a scabies preparation confirms the diagnosis

Table 14-1. Scabies skin scraping

Equipment needed
• #15 scalpel blade, alcohol pad, mineral oil.
• Microscope, glass slide, cover slip.

Technique for specimen collection
• Select a burrow (Figure 14-1) or papule(s) (Figures 14-2 to 14-5) that have not been excoriated and swab the lesion(s) with an alcohol pad.
• Apply a small amount of mineral oil on the scalpel blade or on the lesion(s).
• Using firm pressure scrape the burrow or papules with a #15 scalpel blade and smear the contents on a glass slide.

Examination of specimen
• Cover the contents with 2-4 drops of mineral oil and apply a cover slip. Do not use KOH as this may dissolve the mite's fecal material.
• Scan the entire specimen at low power (10 X) for the presence of mites, eggs and or fecal material.

(Figures 14-6, 14-7). Scraping the skin for a scabies specimen is not always easy to do without injuring the patient, particularly if that patient is a squirming child; therefore, other identification techniques have been suggested.

Dermoscopy has shown to be a sensitive tool for mite identification.[3] Examination of suspicious areas with a dermatoscope allows for greater sensitivity in identifying curvilinear or serpiginous burrows.[4] The mite itself may be seen just beyond the leading edge of a burrow as a dark triangular structure, which corresponds to the head and anterior legs of the scabies mite. This is often referred to as the "delta wing sign" or the "jet with contrail" (Figure 14-8). Burrows can often be localized by rubbing a washable or dry erase marker over suspicious areas, letting it sit for a few minutes and removing the surface excess. Ink seeps

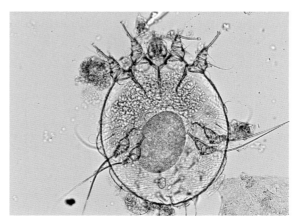

▲ **Figure 14-6.** Female *Sarcoptes scabiei* mite with ovum (egg).

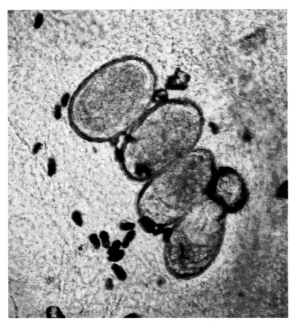

▲ **Figure 14-7.** Four eggs and scybala (feces) of female scabies mite. Microscopic view of skin scraping of burrow contents.

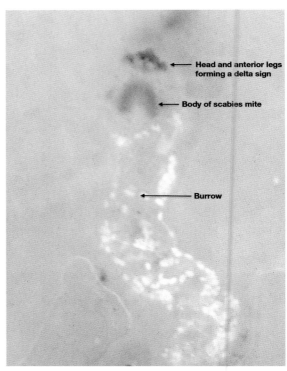

▲ **Figure 14-8.** Dermoscopy view of a scabies mite at the end of a burrow. The head and anterior legs of the mite form the "delta wing sign." Reproduced with permission from Juan Jaimes, MD.

into the burrows and makes them easy to identify. This is called the "burrow ink test" (Figure 14-9). When enhanced with dermatoscope examination, occasionally burrow contents such as eggs can be visualized (Figure 14-10). Another safe, inexpensive, and relatively sensitive way to identify burrow contents is to firmly apply adhesive tape to a burrow, pull it off rapidly, and then transfer the tape to a slide for microscopic identification.[3]

Diagnosis

The key diagnostic features of scabies are intensely pruritic papules, vesicles or burrows in the finger webs, wrists, breast, axillae, abdomen, or genitals. In children, the lesions can be in any location including the head, neck, or feet.

In 2018, the International Alliance for Control of Scabies (IACS) Delphi Panel established consensus criteria for the diagnosis of scabies as either, (1) confirmed, (2) clinical, or (3) suspected based on clinical criteria and mite identification. A confirmed diagnosis requires the direct visualization of mite or mite products by microscopy, dermoscopy, or videoscopy. IACS Criteria are summarized in Table 14-2.[5]

▶ Differential Diagnosis

Scabies should be considered in the differential diagnosis of any patient who presents with an intensely pruritic, eczematous rash of recent onset, especially if family members and other close contacts have similar complaints. Scabies is often misdiagnosed as the following diseases:

✓ Atopic dermatitis: Presents with scaly, often crusted, pruritic papules and plaques on the face, and flexural areas in patients with a personal or family history of atopy. Scabies may be difficult to diagnose in patients who have moderate to severe atopic dermatitis.

✓ Body and pubic lice: Present with pruritus and lice on the body or clothing.

✓ Other arthropod bites: There are no burrows present.

✓ Dermatitis herpetiformis: Presents with lesions very similar to scabies on the elbows, knees, and lower back. The genitals are not affected.

✓ Other: Fiberglass dermatitis, tinea corporis, drug rash, lichen planus, contact dermatitis, papular urticaria, dyshidrotic dermatitis, prurigo, delusions of parasitosis, and acropustulosis of infancy.

The differential diagnosis of crusted scabies would also include disorders of hyperkeratosis, such as psoriasis, seborrheic dermatitis, ichthyosis, and palmoplantar keratoderma.

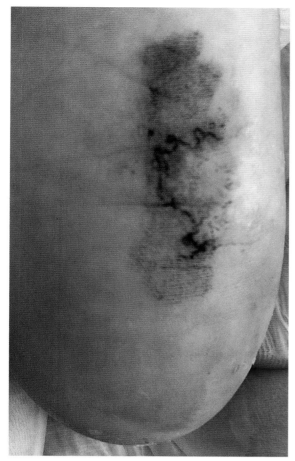

Figure 14-9. Ink burrow test for scabies demonstrating a serpiginous burrow on a child's foot. Reproduced with permission from Dr. Paolo Bartalini.

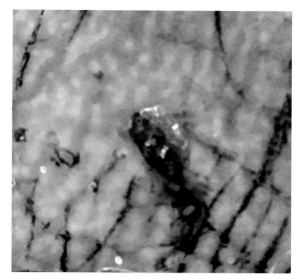

Figure 14-10. Ink burrow Test with dermatoscope view demonstrating scabies eggs in a burrow. Reproduced with permission from Dr. Paolo Bartalini.

Management

A patient can be treated based on a suspicious history and clinical presentation. Scabicides can be divided into topical and oral treatment. While scabies treatment-resistance and patient (or parent) desire to use "natural" treatment alternatives have both led to the study of new scabies treatments, no over the counter (nonprescription) or plant-based products have been tested and approved to treat scabies.

Table 14-3 outlines Centers for Disease Control (CDC) listed prescription scabies treatment options.[6] Permethrin 5% cream is considered the first line treatment for scabies. It is Federal Drug Administration (FDA) approved for children over 2 months and is Pregnancy Category B. Since less than 2% of applied permethrin cream is absorbed and is rapidly metabolized in adults via urinary excretion, it is considered safe and has few reported side-effects. Though

Table 14-2. Summary of 2018 IACS criteria for the diagnosis of scabies[5]

A	Confirmed Scabies	At least one of:
	A1	Mites, eggs, or feces of light microscopy of skin samples.
	A2	Mites, eggs, or feces visualized on individual using high-powered imaging device.
	A3	Mite visualized on individual using dermoscopy.
B	Clinical Scabies	At least one of:
	B1	Scabies burrows.
	B2	Typical lesions affecting male genitalia.
	B3	Typical lesions in a typical distribution and two history features.
C	Suspected Scabies	One of:
	C1	Typical lesions in a typical distribution and one history feature.
	C2	Atypical lesions or atypical distribution and two history features.
History Features:	H1	Itch.
	H2	Close contact with an individual who has itch or typical lesions in a typical distribution.

Table 14-3. Topical medications for scabies

Drug	Administration	Restrictions	Risks	Comments
TOPICAL				
Permethrin 5% cream (Elimite, Acticin)[6]	Apply from neck (include head and neck in infants and young children). Include skin folds (but not mucous membranes) and under nails. Wash off in 8 to 14 hours	FDA approved ≥ 2 months. Pregnancy Category B.	Mild, transient stinging or Burning.	**Considered treatment of choice for scabies.** CDC says 2 treatments one week apart may be needed.
Lindane 1% lotion (Kwell)[6]	As above	FDA approved for scabies. Infants, children, elderly or those ≤110 pounds are at greater risk for toxicity. Pregnancy Category C.	**Black box warning for seizure and death.** Contraindicated in patients with sores or inflamed skin in application areas.	Considered a 2nd or 3rd line therapy.[2]
Sulfur (5 to 10%) ointment[6,9]	Typically applied from neck down (head and neck in infants/young children) daily for 3 days. (Anecdotally, some recommend not showering/ bathing until treatment is complete.)	Considered safe.	Mild burning sensation. Occasional pruritus.	Smells like rotten eggs. Messy. Can stain. No proprietary prescription products in US. Can be pharmacist compounded. Multiple OTC products available on-line. Low cost; first line in developing countries.[4]
Benzyl Benzoate 25% emulsion[7]	Apply to clean, dry skin from neck down (head and neck in infants/children). Leave on 24 hours. Wash off with soap and warm water.[7]	Use only one application in children. Can be repeated in severe cases in adults one time only within 5 days.[7]	Stings. Don't use on open wounds, disrupted skin.[7]	Infants: Mix with 3 parts water. Children: Mix with equal parts water Low cost; first line in developing countries.[4]
Crotamiton 10% cream/lotion (Eurax)[6]	Apply for 24 hours, rinse and apply for 24 hours	FDA approved adults. Pregnancy Category C.	No safety issues.	Frequent treatment failures.

not FDA approved for use in neonates, multiple studies have found it to be effective and well-tolerated in infants younger than 2 months.[7] Other topical medications considered at higher risk, with less supporting data or more commonly used in other parts of the world include: lindane 1% lotion, benzyl benzoate 10% or 25% lotion, malathion 0.5% aqueous lotion, sulfur 6% to 33% cream, ointment or lotion, and synergized pyrethrin foams.[8–10]

Scabicide creams should be applied at bedtime and spread thoroughly from neck to soles, including under the fingernails and toenails. In children under age 2, permethrin cream should also be applied to the head and neck and mittens or socks should be placed on the hands to avoid rubbing the cream into the eyes. Patients should remove the cream after 8–14 hours by showering or bathing.

There is lack of consensus on how many treatments are required to eradicate scabies. Theoretically, when a scabicide kills both mites and eggs (is "ovicidal") one treatment should suffice. In practice, most sources recommend two treatments separated by 1–2 weeks. Ongoing repeated treatments with the same scabicide should be avoided and contribute to resistance.

Oral ivermectin, although not FDA approved for the treatment of scabies is easier to use in patients that have failed other treatments and may result in improved treatment compliance. The most recent Cochrane review comparing the equivalence of permethrin and ivermectin demonstrated that differences between efficacy and adverse effects were irrelevant.[11,12]

Crusted scabies requires a more aggressive approach, with a combination of 5% permethrin every 2–3 days for up to 2 weeks and oral ivermectin in 3–7 doses over approximately 1–4 weeks, depending on the severity of infection.[13] Topical keratolytics are often required in order to decrease the thickness of the scale and enable adequate topical scabicide penetration.[13]

Resistance to scabicides has been increasing throughout the years. Newer therapies being developed for the treatment of scabies include new drugs, insect growth regulators, vaccines, and "natural" products.[14] A variety of plant-based extracts and essential oils have been of particular interest, with tea tree oil *(melaleuca alternifolia)*, clove oil *(syzygium aromaticum)*, lippia oil (*Lippia multiflora*), neem oil (*Azadirachta indica*), and components or extracts, all showing some variable efficacy in in vitro scabicide studies.[14] While these products may ultimately offer some advantages in safety, acceptability, compliance, cost-effectiveness, reduced resistance and environmental persistence, they pose equally as many challenges as viable treatment alternatives, including variations in biological activity, challenges in skin permeability, contact dermatitis potential, commercial viability and the lack of well-conducted, controlled human studies.[15]

Nonspecific measures may be useful at reducing scabies itch. These include the following:

- Restoring the skin barrier through good skin care and emollient use.
- Using topical corticosteroids to reduce irritation, inflammation, and pruritus caused by the infestation, scratching, and occasionally the topical scabicides themselves.
- Prescribing a sedating antihistamine, such as diphenhydramine or hydroxyzine, to help patients sleep.[10]

While human scabies mites can remain viable and capable of infestation off the human body for up to 24–36 in normal room conditions, indirect, or fomite transmission (from clothing, bedding, and other environmental sources) is believed to play an insignificant role in all but the most serious forms of crusted scabies infestations.[16] Treating clothing and bed linen by washing at 60°C/140°F, freezing, or keeping them in a sealed bag for at least 48–72 hours, remains controversial. Some sources recommend treatment of clothing be restricted to severe cases and not be prescribed routinely, while other sources, including the CDC maintain this recommendation.[16,17] The use of insecticides and fumigants is not recommended.[17] Persons who had close contact with an infested individual should be evaluated and treated appropriately.

Clinical Course and Prognosis

The pruritus from scabies is a result of patient hypersensitivity and neither the immune response nor the itching resolves immediately after treatment. Patients should be advised at the time of initial evaluation that it takes up to 4–6 weeks for symptoms to resolve despite effective treatment. If pruritus persists beyond this interval, the patient should be reexamined and if evidence of active infestation is present, the possibilities of poor treatment compliance, reinfestation or mite scabicide resistance should be considered and addressed.

While scabies generally resolves completely and without sequelae, it is not uncommon for pruritus and sensations or belief of infestation to persist after successful treatment of disease. Usually this resolves with time and reassurance.

A fixed, unmistakable belief, despite lack of evidence, that one is infested is defined as delusions of parasitosis. Morgellons disease is a controversial entity that revolves around a fixed patient believe that there are "fibers," "hairs," or "worms" under the skin. There are two polarized points of view surrounding Morgellons. The first, supported by a 2012 CDC Study supports that Morgellons is a form of delusional mental illness, similar to delusional infestation.[18] The second is that Morgellons is a tickborne-infection *(primarily Borrelia burgdorferi)* induced dermopathy, characterized by multicolored filaments composed of keratin and collagen, that lie under, are embedded in, or project from skin.[19] Optimal treatment has not been determined.

Indications for Consultation

If symptoms persist despite two courses of appropriate therapy, consider dermatologic consultation. Several eczematous and vesiculobullous conditions can mimic the presenting signs and symptoms of scabies and occasionally scabies treatment can cause secondary dermatologic sequelae that require intervention. Delusions of parasitosis may occasionally require mental health professional intervention.

Patient Information

- Scabies. Centers for Disease Control. http://www.cdc.gov/parasites/scabies/biology.html.
- Scabies. MedlinePlus: Trusted Health Information for You. National Institutes of Health. https://medlineplus.gov/scabies.html
- Scabies. American Academy of Dermatology. http://www.aad.org/skin-conditions/dermatology-a-to-z/scabies

▼ LICE (PEDICULOSIS)

Introduction

Table Key Points for Lice

✓ Head, crab and body lice are obligate human parasites that feed exclusively on human blood and do not survive for long off their human host.

✓ Clinical findings are non-specific with erythema, papules, wheals, excoriations, hemorrhagic crusts and occasionally scale.

✓ The occipital scalp, posterior ears and neck are the most common sites involved with head lice; lower abdomen, pubic area, and thighs with crab lice; and back, neck, shoulders, and waist with body lice.

✓ Head lice have become resistant to many topical pediculicides.

Human lice are bloodsucking, wingless insects that have been feeding on mankind for thousands of years.[2] Head, crab, and body lice remain a bane in modern times, with hundreds of millions of cases of pediculosis worldwide annually.

Head lice are the most common of the three pediculosis and are a ubiquitous nuisance. They are found in people of all age, sex, race, and socioeconomic class. School children ages 3-11 years, especially girls with long hair and a propensity to share hair care tools and accessories are at greatest risk. African-American children are less commonly affected, perhaps because their hair shape or texture creates a less amenable environment for lice survival and reproduction.[20]

Crab (pubic) lice are transmitted primarily by sexual contact and the highest incidence is seen in men who have sex with men, ages 15-40 years.

Body lice give all lice a bad name. Not only are they associated with poor hygiene, they serve as disease vectors for epidemic typhus, relapsing fever, trench fever, and bacillary angiomatosis or endocarditis.[2,21]

Pathogenesis

All three lice species are obligate human parasites that feed exclusively on human blood and do not survive for long off their human host. They vary in size, shape, and preference for body area location.

• The head louse, *Pediculosis capitis,* as the name suggests, favors scalp hair. It is light, tan to medium brown, and is about the size of a sesame seed (Figure 14-11). Although it is unable to jump or fly, it moves extremely quickly and thus can be difficult to see. The female louse lives about 30 days and lays 5–10 eggs a day. Oval egg capsules or nits are cemented to hair shafts close to the scalp for warmth (Figure 14-12). Transmission is via direct contact or by fomites such as combs, brushes, hats, helmets, headphones; although static electricity and blow dryers have been shown to launch lice into the air, creating another possible mode of transmission.[22]

• Crab lice, *Phthirus pubis* are smaller and wider than head lice and resemble tiny crabs (Figure 14-13). Often referred to as pubic lice, this is a misnomer; as crab lice are adapted to ambulate over the entire body surface. The infestation can involve not only pubic hair but the scalp, eyebrows, eyelashes, moustache, beard, axillae, and perianal area.

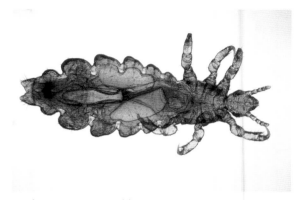

▲ **Figure14-11.** Head louse. Dorsal view of female head louse. Reproduced with permission from Centers for Disease Control and Prevention. PHIL Collection ID# 377, Dr. Dennis D. Juranek.

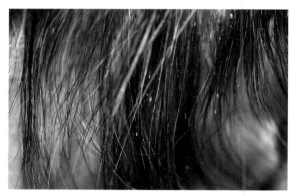

▲ **Figure14-12.** Nits attached to hair in head lice infestation.

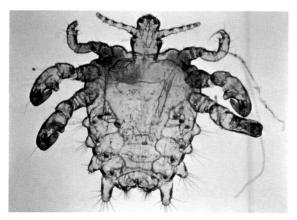

▲ **Figure14-13.** Crab louse. Reproduced with permission from Centers for Disease Control and Prevention. PHIL Collection ID# 4077, contributed by World Health Organization, WHO.

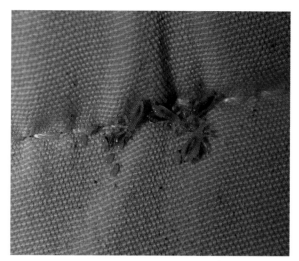

▲ **Figure 14-14.** Eggs of body lice in clothing seams. Figure 148.2. Reproduced with permission from Usatine RP, Smith MA, Mayeaux EJ, et al: The Color Atlas of Family Medicine, 3rd ed. New York, NY: McGraw Hill; 2019. Photo contributor: Richard P. Usatine, MD.

- The body louse, *Pediculosis corporis*, at 2–4-mm-long, is slightly larger than the head louse, but otherwise looks similar. It differs from head and crab lice in that while it feeds on humans it does not live on them; it lives in clothing and lays its eggs along the seams (Figure 14-14).

Clinical Presentation

▶ History

A patient with lice will usually present with intense itching in the area of infestation and a history compatible with exposure.

▶ Physical Examination

Clinical findings are nonspecific with erythema, papules, wheals, excoriations, hemorrhagic crusts, and occasionally scale. The occipital scalp, posterior ears, and neck are the most common sites involved with head lice; lower abdomen, pubic area, and thighs with crab lice; and back, neck, shoulders, and waist with body lice. Pyoderma and regional lymphadenopathy may be present. Maculae ceruleae, small bluish dots may be seen at the site of lice and flea bites.

Examining proximal hair shafts, or in the case of body lice, clothing seams can yield nits. Identifying a live louse is the only way to make a definitive diagnosis of active infection, but lice shy away from light and move very quickly, so this is not easy to do. Systematically wet-combing

detangled and lubricated hair with a specially designed nit comb has been shown to be a sensitive method to harvest and identify live lice. [23]

▶ Laboratory Findings

A skin biopsy demonstrates nonspecific inflammation.

Diagnosis

The key diagnostic features of pediculosis are the presence of lice or nits on hair or skin.

▶ Differential Diagnosis

For body and crab lice

✓ Scabies, flea bites, other arthropod bites. The individual lesions are similar to those of lice infestations, but the locations of the bites differ.

✓ Atopic dermatitis, folliculitis. No lice are seen on the body or clothing.

For head lice

✓ Seborrheic dermatitis: The flakes of skin are loose and not attached to the hair fibers.

✓ Residual hair styling products, hair casts. There is no pruritus.

Management for Body Lice

Body lice are usually successfully treated by bathing the patient and bagging and discarding infested clothing and bed linen. If clothing cannot be discarded it can be washed in hot water (at least 65°C/149°F) for 30 minutes, dry cleaned or hot ironed (especially in seams). If nits are found on body hair, the best treatment option is a single 8–10-hour application of 5% permethrin cream to the entire body, similar to scabies treatment.[24]

Management for Crab Lice

Crab lice are best treated topically with 5% permethrin cream applied overnight to all hairy areas, washed off in the morning and repeated 1 week later. Topical pediculicides cannot be applied to the eyelashes and treating this area is challenging. If possible, nits and lice can be physically removed with fingernails or a nit comb or ophthalmic-grade petrolatum ointment (only available by prescription) can be applied to the eyelid margins 2–4 times a day for 10 days. Regular petrolatum jelly (Vaseline) should not be used in this location because it can irritate the eyes.[24] Oral ivermectin is not FDA-approved for crab lice but has been suggested for patients with perianal or eyelid involvement or when topical treatment fails. The recommended dose is 200 mcg/kg, repeated 1 week later.[25] Individuals with crab lice should be evaluated for sexually transmitted diseases which often occur concomitantly.

Management for Head Lice

Head lice management can be challenging. Pediculicides remain the mainstay of treatment, but increased resistance to therapy, both by parents who are concerned about safety and by lice that have evolved to withstand insecticides, often confounds the healthcare provider. Pediculicides currently

employed for the treatment of head lice are reviewed in Table 14-4.[22,24–30] Most head lice treatments should be applied to dry hair (wetting the hair may cause lice to close their respiratory spiracles and make them less susceptible to treatment), are left on for 10 minutes and removed. Malathion, the exception, is left on for 8–12 hours. Most studied treatments kill live lice and not nits and need to be repeated 7–10 days after the first to treat newly hatched lice. While most treatments need to be repeated, there are two main exceptions. Malathion kills live lice and nits and it should be repeated only if live lice are noted. Lindane, which in **not** a first line treatment for head lice should be

Table 14-4. Topical medications for head lice

Drug	Administration	Restrictions	Risks	Comments
TOPICAL				
Pyrethrin/4% piperonyl butoxide lotion (e.g., RID)[24]	Apply to clean, dry hair. Leave on 10 minutes. Rinse. Repeat in 7 to 10 days.	FDA approved ≥ 2 months.	Do not use if allergic to ragweed/Chrysanthemum.	Resistance is common.[2,22] Kills lice, not nits.
Permethrin 1% lotion (Nix)[24]	Same as above.	FDA approved ≥ 2 months. Pregnancy Category B.	Same as above.	Kills lice, not nits. May kill newly hatched lice for several days.
Malathion lotion .5% (Ovide)[24]	Saturate clean, dry hair. Leave on 8-12 hours. Repeat 7-9 days only if LIVE LICE are present.	FDA approved ≥ 6 years. Pregnancy Category B.	Alcohol vehicle. Irritating to skin and eyes. **Highly flammable! Avoid heat source (e.g. hair dryers, curling irons).**	Strong odor. Less resistance than with permethrin or pyrethrins.[2,22] Kills lice, some nits.[24]
Benzyl alcohol 5% lotion[26]	Saturate clean, dry hair. Leave on 10 min, rinse. Repeat in 7 days.	FDA approved ≥ 6 months & < 60 years.[26] Pregnancy Category B.	Irritating to skin and eyes. Transient skin numbness.	Kills lice, not nits. Kills by lice asphyxiation, not neurotoxicity.[26]
Spinosad .09% suspension (Natroba)[27]	Apply to dry hair for 10 minutes, rinse; repeat in 7 days only if LIVE LICE are present.[27]	FDA approved ≥ 6 months. Pregnancy Category B.	Irritating to skin and eyes. (Contains benzyl alcohol.)[27]	Contains benzyl alcohol. More effective than permethrin.[28] Less resistance. Kills lice and nits.[24]
Ivermectin .05% lotion (SKLICE)[30]	Apply to dry hair. Rinse after 10 minutes. Retreat only if recommended by health care professional.	FDA approved ≥ 6 months. Pregnancy Category C.	Irritating to skin and eyes. Safety data would suggest that a second treatment is low risk.[29,20]	Kills lice, nymphs, not nits.[24] Up to 76% patients had no live head lice 14 days after one-time application.[29,30]
Lindane 1% shampoo (Kwell)[24]	Apply to clean, dry hair. Add small amount of water to create lather. Massage into hair for 4 minutes. Rinse thoroughly and comb with fine toothed comb to remove nits. Do NOT re-treat.	FDA approved for head lice. **American Academy of Pediatrics no longer recommends as a pediculocide.** Pregnancy Category C.	NOT recommended for 1st line treatment. Overuse, misuse, ingestion are neurotoxic. Do not use in premature infants, HIV, seizure disorders, pregnant or breast- feeding women, those with irritated skin, infants, children, elderly or anyone <110 pounds. Seizures reported after multiple uses. Rare with one use.	Resistance common. Banned in California. Use only as 2nd line for those who fail or cannot tolerate other therapies.

Table 14-5. Calculator for RID lotion[31]

Length of Hair	Quantity Needed
Short hair (ear length or shorter)	1 to 2 oz/treatment x 2 (30 to 60 g)
Medium hair (shoulder length)	2 to 3 oz/treatment x 2 (60 to 90 g)
Long hair (past shoulder length)	3 to 4 oz/treatment x 2 (90 to 120 g)

used for one treatment only because of its toxicity. Topical ivermectin may be effective after one treatment; persistent symptoms should prompt re-evaluation before a second treatment.

Parents, caregivers, or patients should be instructed to carefully read and follow the patient medication guidelines in the package inserts of pediculicides. The amount of product required depends on the hair length and required treatments, for example Table 14-5 has this information for Pyrethrin/4% piperonyl butoxide lotion (e.g., RID). Many other treatments have been suggested. Trimethoprim-Sulfamethoxazole has been studied in small trials and is recommended in combination with 1% permethrin for use in cases of multiple treatment failures or suspected lice resistance.[21]

A desire to avoid pediculicides as well as increasing resistance to existing medications have prompted interest in alternative therapies for head lice. In repeated studies outside the United States, dimethicone has shown activity against head lice, though it's mechanism of action has not been established and there is no data to support the effectiveness or safety of formulations available in the United States.[32,33] Home remedies, such as petroleum jelly, olive oil, and mayonnaise have generally been found to be ineffective, though these therapies may transiently suppress louse metabolic activity and give the false impression a cure.[29] Many plant-derived or essential oils have been studied in vitro for efficacy in the treatment of head lice. These include melaleuca or tea tree, cassia, eucalyptus, spearmint, anise, sesame, thyme, wild bergamot, clove, lavender, yunnan verbena, coconut, sunflower, ylang ylang, nerolidol, and others. Further study will be needed to demonstrate in vivo efficacy and safety, especially given the potential for contact sensitization and other potential severe adverse effects, including reports of seizures and systemic hypersensitivity.[34–37] Recently an industry dedicated to physically "nit-picking" or "bug-busting" lice infestations has been borne. Removal by fingers, nit combs, "bug-buster" heat-producing combs, and commercially available "egg-removal" products, when studied have been suboptimal in obtaining cure.[23]

Heavily infested children may serve as "super-spreaders" in school environments or close quarters and physical removal of live lice and nits may serve to reduce spread.[38]

Shaving the hair has been suggested as a chemical-free treatment option, but it can be emotionally traumatic for the child.[22] Clothing and linen used in the 2 days before treatment should be washed and dried at the hottest temperatures the fabrics can withstand, dry cleaned, or sealed in plastic bags for 2 weeks. Hair grooming utensils should be soaked in hot water (54.5°C/130°F) for 5–10 minutes and floor and furniture vacuumed.[24] Although the presence of nits often creates anxiety, current consensus is that affected children may return to school after their first treatment. The presence of nits should **not** exclude school attendance.[21,22]

Clinical Course and Prognosis

Pediculosis generally resolves completely and without any sequelae. As previously discussed in the section on scabies, if itching persists more than 4–6 weeks after treatment in the absence of signs of infestation, then delusions of parasitosis might be considered.

Indications for Consultation

Consultation should be considered when live lice persist after two appropriate treatments or when symptoms persist beyond 4–6 weeks. Patients should be advised that it may take several weeks for symptoms to abate even when the lice have been successfully treated and that the persistence of nits does not imply persistent active infection.

Patient Information

- Head Lice Fact Sheet: https://www.health.state.mn.us/diseases/headlice/headlice.html
- Lice. Mayo Clinic: https://www.mayoclinic.org/diseases-conditions/lice/symptoms-causes/syc-20374399
- Lice. Centers for Disease Control: http://www.cdc.gov/parasites/lice/

LYME DISEASE

Introduction

Table Key Points for Lyme Disease

✓ The Ixodes tick, *Ixodes scapularis,* also called the deer, or black-legged tick, is the primary vector of *Borrelia burgdorferi,* the organism which causes Lyme disease.

✓ Ixodes nymphs, which are most active in the spring, cause most of cases of Lyme disease. The nymphs are the size of a pinhead (2 mm or less), so they may go undetected while attached to human skin.

✓ In North America 90% of cases occur on the east coast between the states of Maine and Maryland, and in Minnesota and Wisconsin.

✓ Erythema migrans usually appears 7 to 10 days after inoculation and typically presents as a pink patch of up to 15 cm in diameter, often with central clearing.

✓ Doxycycline is the treatment of choice for most patients.

Newly discovered tickborne organisms, novel tick species and tick geographic expansion are all contributing to the increase of tickborne disease in the United States. While Lyme disease, most frequently caused by the spirochete *Borrelia burgdorferi*, remains the most commonly reported tickborne illness in the United States, over the past two decades seven new illness-inducing tickborne organisms have been identified: *Borrelia mayonii* (a rare cause of Lyme disease in the upper Midwest), *Borrelia miyamotoi, Ehrlichia ewingii, Ehrlichia muris eauclairensis,* Heartland virus, *Rickettsia parkeri,* and *Rickettsia* species 364D.[39,40,41] While the exact reasons for the geographic expansion of ticks and tickborne diseases are unclear, multiple factors may contribute: changing land use patterns, reforestation, suburban sprawl and climate change. As the number of counties in the United States considered at high risk for Lyme disease has expanded, the number of reported cases has tripled since the late 1990s.[39]

In North America, 90% of cases occur on the east coast between the states of Maine and Maryland, and in Minnesota and Wisconsin.[42] *Borrelia* species also cause disease in central and eastern Europe and eastern Asia, specifically *B. burgdorferi, afzelii, and garinii*.[41] The incidence of Lyme disease peaks in patients between the ages of 5–19 years and 55–69 years. The onset of Lyme disease in the United States usually occurs from May to November with a peak in June, July, and August. Erythema migrans is the characteristic annular plaque of Lyme disease.

Pathogenesis

The Ixodes tick, *Ixodes scapularis,* also called the deer, or black-legged tick, is the primary vector of *Borrelia burgdorferi* in the Eastern United States, as well as the causative agents of anaplasmosis and babesiosis (Figure 14-15). The number of counties in which *I. scapularis* is considered established has more than doubled in the past two decades, with most of the expansion in the North-Central and Northeastern states and emergence in the Ohio River Valley. The western black-legged tick *Ixodes pacificus* is the main vector of Lyme and anaplasmosis in the Western United States and is established primarily in coastal states along the Pacific Ocean (Washington, Oregon, California), and locally in cool or moist settings in more arid inland states (Arizona, Nevada Utah).[43]

The ixodes tick has a 2-year life cycle with larval, nymphal, and adult stages. The ticks feed once during

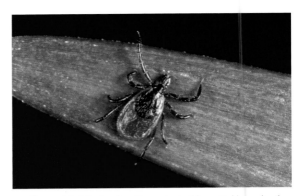

▲ **Figure14-15.** Ixodes Scapularis (deer tick) on leaf. Reproduced with permission from Centers for Disease Control and Prevention. PHIL Collection ID# 1669, Michael L. Levin, PhD.

each stage on various hosts and may acquire *B. burgdorferi* while feeding on an infected host. The white-tailed deer and white-footed mouse are common hosts, but other species of birds, mice, rats, raccoons, and rabbits may also be hosts. In humans, the affected tick usually needs to be attached and feeding for 48–72 hours to transmit the *Borrelia* organism.[44] Ixodes nymphs, which are most active in the spring, cause most cases of Lyme disease. The nymphs are the size of a pinhead (2 mm or less), so they may go undetected while attached to human skin.[44] Ixodes ticks are resourceful and if there is little to no snow cover and temperatures rise above freezing, it is possible to find an active adult tick searching for a host on a warm winter day.[45]

Clinical Presentation

▶ History

Lyme disease has protean manifestations, including dermatologic, rheumatologic, neurologic, and cardiac abnormalities, often making it a diagnostic challenge. The most common early clinical marker for the disease is erythema migrans (EM), the initial skin lesion that occurs in 60%–80% of patients. Typically, patients with suspicious skin findings will have a history of being in a wooded or grassy area in an endemic region within the prior month. The CDC keeps running surveillance data on endemic areas with Maine, New Hampshire, and Rhode Island leading the United States in 2018 with 83, 65.3, and 62.5 confirmed cases per 100,000 people in each state.[46] However, many patients will not recall having a tick bite.

▶ Physical Examination

Erythema migrans usually appears 7–10 days after inoculation. Typically, it presents as a pink macule or patch, but

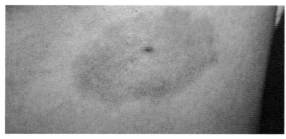

▲ **Figure14-16.** Erythema migrans on trunk: annular plaque with central clearing and central puncta from the bite.

it can be quite variable in appearance. It almost invariably expands, up to a diameter of about 15 cm, although the range can be from 3 to 68 cm (Figure 14-16). Often there is central clearing, but the lesion may be uniform throughout. Rashes that are warm and itchy and resolve within 48 hours are usually an allergic or hypersensitivity reaction to the tick bite and NOT borreliosis.[47,48]

Also occurring within 3–30 days after tick bite and considered "early" signs and symptoms of Lyme disease are: fatigue, fever, chills, headache, mildly stiff neck, arthralgia, or myalgia, and swollen lymph nodes. These symptoms are typically intermittent and may occur in the absence of erythema migrans.[47,48]

The initial lesion is at the site of the bite and is usually located on the legs, trunk, groin, or axillae. In children common sites include the head and neck. Erythema migrans resolves without treatment within 4–6 weeks.[44] The presence of erythema migrans, though common, is not universal in Lyme disease and both early and later symptoms can develop without recognizable skin findings.

Later signs and symptoms occur days to months after the tick bite. These can include the following:[49]

- Severe headaches and neck stiffness.
- Additional erythema migrans lesions on other areas of the body.
- Facial palsy (loss of muscle tone or droop on one or both sides of the face).
- Arthritis with severe joint pain and swelling, particularly the knees and other large joints.
- Intermittent pain in tendons, muscles, joints, and bones.
- Heart palpitations or an irregular heartbeat (Lyme carditis).
- Episodes of dizziness or shortness of breath.
- Inflammation of the brain and spinal cord, and/or
- Nerve pain, shooting pains, numbness, or tingling in the hands or feet.

Of these, neurological involvement is the second most common clinical manifestation of Lyme disease after erythema multiforme. Approximately 5% of people with untreated Lyme disease will develop neuroborreliosis, usually 4–6 weeks after tick exposure.[50]

▶ Laboratory Findings

The CDC currently recommends a two-step testing process for Lyme disease. Both steps are required and can be done using the same blood sample. If this first step is negative, no further testing is recommended. If the first step is positive or indeterminate (sometimes called "equivocal"), the second step should be performed. The overall result is positive only when the first test is positive (or equivocal) and the second test is positive (or for some tests equivocal).[51]

Traditionally, the two-step process included using a sensitive enzyme immunoassay (EIA) or immunofluorescence assay, followed by a western immunoblot assay if the first test yielded positive or equivocal results. On July 29, 2019, the FDA cleared several Lyme disease serologic assays with new indications for use, allowing for an EIA rather than western immunoblot assay as the second test in a Lyme disease testing algorithm.[51]

There are several key points to remember when testing patients suspected of having Lyme disease.[52]

- Antibodies can take several weeks to develop, and a test can return a false-negative result if performed too early in the course of disease. If symptoms persist and concerns exist that the patient was tested too early, the test may need to be repeated.
- Other infections or disorders can return a false-positive result. Table 14-6 lists possible causes of false-positive

Table 14-6. Causes of false-positive borrelia burgdorferi enzyme immunoassay results[48,51,52]

Other spirochetes	*Borrelia* relapsing fever agents *Treponema pallidum* (Syphilis) *Leptospira interrogans* Oral treponemes in subjects with gingivitis or periodontal diseases
Other tick-borne disease agents	*Anaplasma phagocytophilum* *Ehrlichia chaffeensis*
Other infections	*Helicobacter pylori* Epstein-Barr virus Parvovirus B19 HIV Infective endocarditis
Autoimmune Disorders	Systemic lupus erythematosus Rheumatoid arthritis
Other	Intravenous immunoglobulin administration

test results.[48,53] The two-step testing ensures a greater likelihood that a positive test result represents a true case of Lyme disease.

- Antibodies can persist for months to years after successful treatment, so a persistent positive test result cannot be used to determine cure.
- Some tests give results for two types of antibody, IgM and IgG. Positive IgM results should be disregarded if the patient has been ill for more than 30 days.

While the histopathologic features of erythema migrans are not specific, a skin biopsy obtained from the periphery of the lesion may be helpful in differentiating it from other similar appearing skin lesions, and a Warthin-Starry stain can sometimes demonstrate Borrelia spirochetes in the skin.[54]

Diagnosis

The CDC has established a set of uniform criteria that it uses to define Lyme disease for public health surveillance (Table 14-7). While these outline very specific criteria for diagnosis, they are not intended as strict criteria to be used by healthcare providers to make a clinical diagnosis or determine a patient's treatment needs. [47] In that case, the physician or healthcare provider should pursue his or her best judgment in the diagnosis and treatment.

> ### Differential Diagnosis of Erythema Migrans

✓ Bites from ticks, mosquitoes, bees, and wasps: Typically, the erythema associated with these bites does not exceed 5 cm in diameter. Mosquito bites frequently itch, and bee or wasp stings typically hurt. Erythema migrans is often asymptomatic.

✓ Erysipelas or cellulitis: The white blood cell count may be elevated and often the area is tender and there is no central clearing.

✓ Herald patch of pityriasis rosea: The diameter does not usually exceed 5 cm and there is a ring of scale within the lesion.

✓ Other: Fixed drug rash, tinea corporis, dermatitis, granuloma annulare, erythema multiforme.

Management

Treatment depends on the stage of the disease, the age of the patient, and relative contraindications associated with the recommended medications. In areas that are highly endemic for Lyme disease a single dose of doxycycline (200 mg for adults or 4.4 mg/kg for children of any age weighing less than 45 kg) may reduce the risk of acquiring Lyme disease after the bite of a high-risk tick.[55] There is no evidence that this will prevent disease, so when prescribing prophylactic treatment in high risk situations, patients must be warned to watch for symptoms that suggest Lyme disease, but benefits of prophylaxis may outweigh risks when the following are present:[55]

- Doxycycline is not contraindicated.
- The tick is identified as adult or nymph *Ixodes scapularis.*
- The time of attachment can be estimated as ≥36 hours (based on time of exposure or tick engorgement).
- Prophylactic antibiotic can be started within 72 hours of tick removal.
- Tick bite occurred in endemic county or state.

People who are appropriately treated in the early stages of Lyme disease usually recover rapidly and completely.[56] Erythema migrans should be treated empirically without waiting for serological confirmation. Antibodies to *B. burgdorferi* may take 4–8 weeks to be detected.[48] Table 14-8 summarizes the most recent CDC guidelines for the treatment of **localized (early)** Lyme disease.[56] These regimens are guidelines only and may need to be adjusted depending on a person's age, medical history, underlying health conditions, pregnancy status, or allergies.

Antibiotics commonly used for oral treatment include doxycycline, amoxicillin, or cefuroxime axetil. Macrolides azithromycin, clarithromycin, or erythromycin may be used, although they have a lower efficacy. People treated with macrolides should be closely monitored to ensure that symptoms resolve.[56]

The warning against the use of doxycycline in children less than 8 years old dates to the recognition in the 1970s that tetracyclines can cause permanent staining and hypoplasia of developing teeth.[57] This recognition and resultant fear lead to inadequate treatment, increased morbidity and even mortality in children with diseases for which doxycycline is the optimal treatment, notably Rocky Mountain Spotted Fever.[58] Doxycycline binds less readily to calcium than does tetracycline and in one retrospective cohort study of children younger than 8 years treated with doxycycline for Rocky Mountain Spotted Fever, there was no evidence of tetracycline-like tooth staining or enamel hypoplasia compared to control.[59,60]

Early Lyme disease, unlike Rocky Mountain spotted fever, is seldom fatal, and can be treated in children with antibiotics other than doxycycline, but given the CDC's statement about the safety of short-term use in children it would seem reasonable to use doxycycline for prophylaxis in all age groups.[58,59] People with certain neurological or cardiac forms of illness may require intravenous treatment with antibiotics such as ceftriaxone or penicillin. Refer to the references (Hu 2016; Sanchez 2016) for treatment of patients with disseminated (late) Lyme disease.[59,61,62]

Table 14-7. Summary of lyme disease 2017 case definition. Council of state and territorial epidemiologists position statement[47]*

Criteria for New Case of Lyme Disease

Early Manifestation

- Erythema Migrans (EM) is the most common marker that occurs in 60-80% of patients.
- Diagnosis must be made by a physician.
- EM begins as a red macule or papule and expands over a period of days to weeks to form a large round lesion, often with partial central clearing.
- EM must reach a diameter of greater than or equal to 5 cm across its largest diameter. Secondary lesions may occur.
- Annular erythematous lesions occurring within several hours of a tick bite represent hypersensitivity reactions; do NOT qualify as EM.
- Usually accompanied by other acute, usually intermittent symptoms, including fatigue, fever, headache, mildly stiff neck, arthralgia, or myalgia.
- Laboratory confirmation recommended for persons with no known exposure.

Late Manifestation (any of the following when alternative explanation is not found)

Musculoskeletal system: Recurrent, brief attacks (weeks/months) of objective joint swelling in one or a few joints, sometimes followed by chronic arthritis. NOT criteria for diagnosis includes chronic progressive arthritis not preceded by brief attacks, chronic symmetrical polyarthritis or solo diagnoses of arthralgia, myalgia, or fibromyalgia syndromes.
Nervous system: Any of the following (alone or in combination) not explained by other etiology: lymphocytic meningitis, cranial neuritis, particularly facial palsy (may be bilateral), radiculoneuropathy, encephalomyelitis (rarely). NOT criteria for diagnosis includes headache, fatigue, paresthesia, or mildly stiff neck alone.
Cardiovascular system: Acute onset of high-grade (2nd-degree or 3rd-degree) atrioventricular conduction defects that resolve in days to weeks (sometimes associated with myocarditis). NOT criteria for diagnosis include palpitations, bradycardia, bundle branch block, or myocarditis alone.

Laboratory Criteria for Diagnosis of Lyme Disease

A positive culture for *B. burgdorferi*, **OR**
A positive two-tier test. (This is defined as a positive or equivocal enzyme immunoassay (EIA) or immunofluorescent assay (IFA) followed by a positive Immunoglobulin M (IgM) or Immunoglobulin G (IgG) western immunoblot (WB) for Lyme disease) **OR**
A positive single-tier IgG WB test for Lyme disease. (While a single IgG WB is adequate for surveillance purposes, a two-tier test is still recommended for patient diagnosis.)

Criteria to Distinguish a New Case from an Existing Case (case not previously reported)

Exposure: ≤ 30 days before onset of EM, present in wooded, brushy, or grassy areas (i.e., potential tick habitats) of Lyme disease vectors in high risk geography/state. Travel history required. (https://www.cdc.gov/lyme/stats/tables.html)
High-incidence state= ≥10 confirmed cases/ 100,000 for prior 3 reporting years.
Low-incidence state= <10 confirmed cases/100,000.
History of tick bite is **not** required.

Case Classification

Suspected:
Erythema Migrans (EM) and NO known exposure and NO lab evidence of infection, **OR**
A case with evidence of infection but no clinical information available (e.g., a laboratory report).
Probable: Any other case of physician-diagnosed Lyme disease that has lab evidence of infection.
Confirmed:
EM with exposure in a high-incidence state), **OR**
EM with lab evidence of infection and a known exposure in a low incidence state, **OR**
Any case with at least one late manifestation that has lab evidence of infection.

*Modified with permission from CDC National Notifiable Disease Surveillance System (NNDSS).

Table 14-8. Treatment of early lyme disease[58]

Age Category	Drug	Dosage	Maximum	Duration (days)
Adults	Doxycycline	100 mg twice daily orally.	N/A	10-14
	Cefuroxime axetil	500 mg twice daily orally.	N/A	14
	Amoxicillin	500 mg three times daily orally.	N/A	14
Children	Amoxicillin	50 mg/kg/day orally, divided into two doses.	500 mg/dose	14
	Doxycycline	4.4 mg/kg/day orally, divided into 2 doses.	100 mg/dose	10-14
	Cefuroxime axetil	30 mg/kg/day orally, divided into 2 doses.	500 mg/dose	14

Prevention

The best way to treat Lyme disease is to avoid acquiring it. Instructions for prevention of Lyme disease include the following[39]:

- Avoid areas with high grass and leaf litter.
- Stay on trails.
- Use insect repellents containing DEET, picaridin, IR3535, oil of lemon eucalyptus, para-menthane-diol, or 2-undecanone.
- Use products that contain permethrin to treat clothing and gear, such as boots, pants, socks, and tents or look for clothing pre-treated with permethrin.
- Tuck pants into socks.
- Treat dogs for ticks.
- Bathe or shower as soon as possible after coming indoors.
- Conduct a full-body tick check using a hand-held or full-length mirror.
- Put dry clothes in a dryer on high heat for 10 minutes to kill ticks.

Tick Removal

If an attached tick is identified, it should be removed as soon as possible. The most recommended and successful tick-removal method is manual extraction.[63] Use a fine tipped, preferably slanted forceps or tweezer to grasp the tick as close to the skin surface as possible and pull upwards, away from the skin with slow and steady pressure. Usually, the tick will release. Avoid crushing, puncturing, or squeezing the tick's body, which may stimulate the tick to regurgitate contents into the attachment site. Don't twist or jerk, as this may result in separating of the tick's body from head/mouth parts with the latter remaining embedded in the skin. If this occurs, these can usually be removed with the forceps.

Occasionally retained tick parts cause a foreign body reaction and require removal with a punch biopsy. This link demonstrates manual tick removal: https://youtu.

be/27McsguL2Og. If manual removal is not possible another alternative is to apply a small amount of undiluted dish soap over the tick and gently rub over the tick in a circular direction for 30 seconds. This can stimulate the intact tick to detach.[64] This is demonstrated in this link: https://www.jaad.org/article/S0190-9622(19)30974-0/fulltext#appsec1. After removal, the tick should be examined to ensure that it has been removed intact. It can either be placed in a container of alcohol for later identification (if necessary) or safely placed in the garbage after securing it in the adhesive tape. Applying commercially available tick-removal products, petroleum jelly, nail polish, alcohol, or any other caustic chemicals have not been studied to be safe or effective and should be avoided.[63]

Alpha-Gal Allergy

Aside from causing infections, recent studies in the United States and other countries suggest that ticks may play a role in causing an allergy to mammalian meat (alpha-gal allergy). An alpha-gal allergy is an allergy to the alpha-gal sugar molecule. Allergic reactions typically occur after people eat meat from mammals that have alpha-gal or are exposure to products made from mammals.[65] Clinically the symptoms include urticaria, angioedema, gastroenteritis, and anaphylaxis within hours after ingesting red meat.[66] Ticks have been implicated as a vector in alpha-gal allergy. In America, the tick culprit implicated is *Amblyomma americanum*. Table 14-9 lists species of ticks implicated in mammalian meat allergy internationally.[66.] When patients present with unexplained recurrent urticaria, angioedema or anaphylaxis with a history of tick exposure, alpha-gal allergy should be considered in the differential diagnosis. The CDC is working with healthcare providers and researchers to see if tick bites are indeed the cause.[65]

Clinical Course and Prognosis

Most cases of Lyme disease can be cured with a 2–4 week course of appropriate oral antibiotics but some patients

Table 14-9. Tick species implicated in mammalian meat allergies globally[66]

Region	Suspected tick species
United States	Amblyomma americanum
Panama	Amblyomma cajennense
Australia	Amblyomma sculptum
Australia	Ixodes holocyclus
Europe (France, Germany, Spain, Sweden, Switzerland, Norway, Italy)	Ixodes Ricinus
Japan	Haemaphysalis longicornis

can have symptoms of pain, fatigue, or difficulty thinking that can last for more than 6 months after treatment. This condition is called post-Treatment Lyme Disease Syndrome and though the cause is unknown, some have proposed a *Borrelia burgdorferi-* triggered "auto-immune response." Patients with Post-Treatment Lyme Disease Syndrome usually get better over time, but it can take many months to be completely symptom free and no definitive treatment has been established. NIH-funded studies have found that long-term outcomes are no better for patients who received additional prolonged antibiotic treatment that for patients who received placebo.[67]

Indications for Consultation

Chronic Lyme disease is different than late Lyme disease and less consistently defined and patients' symptoms generally fall into one of three categories.

1. Persistent symptoms after confirmed, appropriately treated Lyme (persistent post-treatment Lyme disease syndrome).
2. Atypical symptoms in the setting of positive serology, which may be due to asymptomatic past infections.
3. Symptoms attributable to borreliosis, but with negative, equivocal, or inconsistent serology results.[48] This diagnosis is controversial and when considered, should prompt a rheumatologic or infectious disease consult before therapy is initiated.[67]

Patient Information

- Centers for Disease Control and Prevention: Ticks. Extensive information for patients and clinicians including: Information on tick avoidance and symptom discussion. https://www.cdc.gov/ticks/avoid/index.html
- Minnesota Department of Health: Ticks. Broad information on Tickborne and other vector borne-disease. https://www.health.state.mn.us/diseases/tickborne/ticks.html

- Lyme disease. Mayo Clinic. https://www.mayoclinic.org/diseases-conditions/lyme-disease/symptoms-causes/syc-20374651

BED BUGS

Introduction

Table Key Points for Bed Bugs

√ Adult bed bugs (*Cimex lectularius*) are blood sucking, parasitic arthropods which are brown, oval, wingless and about the size of an apple seed.

√ Clinical manifestations vary from no reaction to typical appearing insect bites to papular urticaria or bullous reactions.

√ Bites usually appear on the waist, axillae and those areas that are typically exposed while sleeping such as the scalp, face, neck, and arms.

√ Once an infestation is established, bed bugs are extremely difficult to eradicate without the assistance of a pest management professional.

The obligate parasite, *Cimex lectularius*, better known as the common bedbug and its tropical cousin *Cimex hemipterus*, have coexisted with humans for centuries, dating back to the ancient Egyptians, 3,500 years ago.[68] Through the mid-20th century nearly one-third of U.S. households were infested with bedbugs.[69] Developed countries experienced a near 50 year hiatus from this pest, when it was almost removed from North America as a result of mass treatments with insecticides. In the past two decades, bed bugs have re-emerged worldwide for several possible reasons, including increased international travel, changes in pest control practices, and insecticide resistance.[70] Bed bugs can be found in settings from four-star hotels to homeless shelters. Anyone is a potential target.

Pathogenesis

Adult bed bugs are brown, oval, wingless somewhat flat insects about the size of an apple seed (Figure 14-17). As they feed, they grow in length from about 5–9 mm and change from brown to purple red. Young bugs are smaller and nearly colorless. Bed bugs usually hide during the day and feed at night. They are attracted to heat and carbon dioxide and feed on exposed skin. They then move back to their hiding places, typically mattress and box spring seams (Figure 14-18), bed frames, or bedroom furniture, although they can hide almost anywhere.[71] It is in these hiding places where the wary traveler can find evidence of a bed bug infestation, by the presence of dead bugs, feces, and molted skin casings.

Bed bugs are resilient; they can survive up to a year without a blood meal. Since bed bugs extract blood from

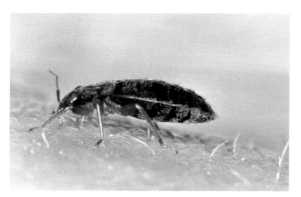

▲ Figure14-17. Cimex Lectularius (bed bug). This image depicts a left lateral view of a common bed bug, *Cimex lectularius*, which was photographed as it was perched atop the skin of its human host. Reproduced with permission from Centers for Disease Control and Prevention. PHIL Collection ID# 6283. Donated by the World Health Organization.

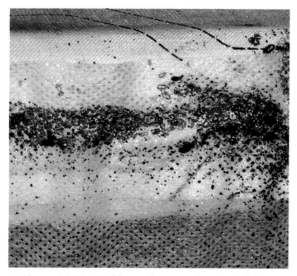

▲ Figure14-18. Bed bugs, feces, and molted skin casings on mattress box spring. Reproduced with permission from Stephen Kells PhD.

hosts, they could theoretically act as disease vectors. At least 45 know pathogens have been isolated from *Cimex* species, including hepatitis B, HIV, *Trypanosoma cruzi*, and methicillin-resistant *Staphylococcus aureus*.[72] To date any evidence for disease transmission is equivocal and their significance as disease vectors has yet to be established.[71]

Clinical Presentation

▶ History

While anyone can be a victim of bed bug bites, a suggestive history might include living in a known infested environment, recent acquisition of a used mattress or couch or travel to a potentially infested destination. The pest control company, Terminix compiles an annual list of the Top 50 Most Bed Bug Infested U.S. Cities. In 2019, the top five were: Philadelphia, PA; New York City, NY; Dallas-Fort Worth, TX; Indianapolis, IN; and Cincinnati, OH.[73] https://www.terminix.com/blog/whats-buzzing/top-bed-bug-cities/

▶ Physical Examination

Clinical manifestations vary from no reaction to typical appearing insect bites to papular urticaria or bullous reactions. While the bite appearance is not specific, bite distribution is often suggestive of bed bugs. Most commonly involved areas are the waist, axillae, and those areas that are typically exposed while sleeping such as the scalp, face, neck, and arms[74]. The timing between possible exposure and the development of the bites is not always diagnostic and depending on prior exposure and an individual's immune response, can be immediate (minutes) or even delayed by days, with a reaction that ranges from mild to intense.[74] Occasionally patients present with dermatitis or secondary infection at the bite sites. A few studies have suggested bed bug bites may cause systemic reactions such as asthma, generalized urticaria and anaphylaxis.[71]

▶ Laboratory Findings

Lab results are nonspecific, although severe and persistent bed bug infestation has been implicated in the development of iron deficiency anemia.[75]

Diagnosis

The appearance of the insect bite does little to assist in identifying the culprit insect; a mosquito bite looks like a flea bite which looks like a bed bug bite. Bites organized in linear or clustered groups of three (breakfast, lunch, and dinner) have been suggested as implicating a flea or bed bug, but this is far from diagnostic (Figure 14-19). Having a high index of suspicion is important. The nonspecific presentation of bed bug bites can lead to delays in diagnosis and significant distress for the patient. Delayed diagnosis also creates an opportunity for bedbug infestations to spread to other people and locations.

▶ Differential Diagnosis

Bed bug bites have been misdiagnosed as drug eruptions, food allergies, dermatitis herpetiformis,

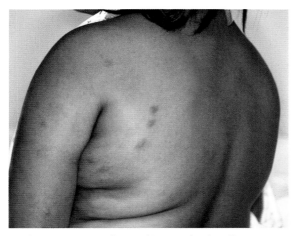

△ **Figure14-19.** Bed Bugs bites on back in linear distribution.

staphylococcal, or varicella infections and scabies.[76] Common considerations include:

✓ Other arthropod bites: May be indistinguishable from bed bug bites.

✓ Urticaria: The individual lesions last less than 24 hours.

✓ Delusions of parasitosis: Can present with similar symptoms, but patients with bed bug infestations often struggle with psychopathology secondary to their infestation, so true infestation should be ruled out.

Management

Managing bed bugs requires treating the patient's symptoms, definitively identifying bed bugs as the culprit, and eradicating the infestation at its source.

The patient should be treated symptomatically with oral antihistamines and topical corticosteroids and with topical or oral antibiotics if the bites are infected.

To identify bed bugs, it helps to know where to look. Most bed bugs are found within 8 feet of a person's resting place. As the infestation grows, bed bugs will spread further. Instruct patients to look in the mattress creases, box springs, bed frames, and bedding, in the cracks and crevices of furniture, behind peeling wall, or anything hanging on the wall, in the curtains, in cracks in hardwood floors under carpeting, behind electrical outlets or switch plates. Look for bug casings or dead bugs or run tape along surfaces in an effort to catch bugs (which move very quickly!).[77] Commercially available "bed bug traps" can be set at night in an attempt to catch and identify culprit bugs. Trained dogs have been demonstrated to detect bed bug infestations with 95–98% accuracy.[78]

Once an infestation is established, bed bugs are extremely difficult to eradicate. Patients should be instructed NOT to use pesticides for garden or agricultural use and NOT to use homemade or custom-formulated products purchased from questionable sources, both of which have the potential to cause more harm to patients than the bed bugs themselves.[77] The best option is to hire a pest management professional with experience in the treatment of bed bug infested environments. Bed bugs are susceptible to both freezing and heating and while frozen carbon dioxide sprays and heat remediation systems are available to treat infestations, both require special equipment and expert monitoring.

Exposure to heat of at least 48°C/118.4°F is effective in at killing bed bugs in all life stages.[79] Conversely, exposure to temperatures below -13°C/8.6°F will result in 100% mortality in all life stages of bed bugs.[80] The exact temperatures required to kill bed bugs depends on the exposure time.[81] The Environmental Protection Agency has registered over 300 chemicals to treat bed bugs.[82]

The best advice is to prevent a bed bug infestation before it occurs by being proactive and avoid bringing them home. Avoid buying used furniture, especially mattresses. Avoid potentially infested environments. Be cognizant when traveling and practice "universal bed bug precautions." Suggestions include checking hotel rooms before unpacking, especially bed sheets, linens and mattress seams, and the luggage rack for signs of bed bugs.[83] Bed bugs are attracted to the smell of humans; store dirty clothes in plastic bags. Hang items if possible, close and zip suitcases and bags, especially at night and if possible, store them off the floor, away from the bed, in plastic bags, or in the bathtub or shower.

If exposure or infestation is suspected, once home, clothing and luggage should be carefully examined and sealed in plastic until it can be cleaned. Suitcases and bags should be vacuumed, with vacuum bag sealed in a plastic bag and discarded.[83] Bed bugs in potentially infested clothing can be killed by drying items in the dryer on high heat for 30 minutes.[84] Putting infested items in a freezer can also kill bedbugs, if the internal temperature of the item being frozen reaches −18°C/0°F for at least 4 days.[85] The University of Minnesota publishes a step-by-step instruction sheet on how to safely freeze household items suspected of bed bug infestation (see Patient Information).

Clinical Course and Prognosis

Bed bug bites are simply bug bites. The symptoms generally resolve with no or symptomatic treatment only and no residual physical sequelae. The mental anguish of continued exposure and a personal environmental infestation can be devastating, however, and should not be underestimated.

Indications for Consultation

A dermatologist might be consulted if the diagnosis is in question or if a suspicious bug needs identification. Occasionally, a mental healthcare professional might be needed to help with the psychosocial aspects. If a patient's home is truly infested with bed bugs, the most important consultation will be that of a pest management professional.

Patient Information

- JAMA Patient Page: Bed bugs. http://jama.ama-assn. org/content/301/13/1398.full.pdf
- University of Minnesota Department of Entomology: Let's Beat the Bedbug! www.bedbugs.umn.edu
- Using Freezing Conditions to Kill Bed Bugs. Let's Beat the Bug! University of Minnesota. https://www.bed-bugs.umn.edu/sites/bedbugs.umn.edu/files/y2014m05d23_using_freezing_conditions_to_kill_bed_bugs.pdf
- Laundering Items to Kill Bed Bugs. Let's Beat the Bug! https://www.bedbugs.umn.edu/sites/bedbugs.umn.edu/files/y2014m05d22_laundering_items_to_kill_bed_bugs.pdf

REFERENCES

1. Chosidow O. Clinical practices. Scabies. *N Engl J Med.* 2006;354 (16):1718–1727.
2. Chosidow O. Seminar: scabies and pediculosis. *Lancet.* 2000;355(6206):819–826.
3. Walter B, Heukelback J, Fengler G et al. Comparison of dermoscopy, skin scraping, and the adhesive tape test for the diagnosis of scabies in a resource-poor setting. *Arch Dermatol.* 2011;147(4):468–473.
4. Chandler D, Fuller L. A review of scabies: an infestation more than skin deep. *Dermatology* 2019;235(2):79–90.
5. Engelman D, Fuller L, Steer A. International Alliance for the Control of Scabies Delphi Panel. Consensus criteria for the diagnosis of scabies: a Delphi study of international experts. *PLos Negl Trop Dis.* 2018; 24;12(5): e0006549.
6. Scabicides. Centers for Disease Control. https://www.cdc.gov/parasites/scabies/health_professionals/meds.html. Accessed 07.12.2020.
7. Hoffman J, Mobner R, Schon M. Lipper U. Topical Scabies therapy with permethrin is effective and well tolerated in infants younger than two months. *J Dtsch Dermatol Des.* 2019;17(6):5970600.
8. Benzyl Benzoate (Topical Route) https://www.mayoclinic.org. Accessed 07.122.2020.
9. Sharquie KE, Al-Rawi JR, Noaimi AA, Al-Hassany HM. Treatment of scabies using 8% and 10% topical sulfur ointment in different regimens of application. *J Drugs Dermatol.* 2012; 11(3):357-64.
10. Jannic A, Bernigaud C, Brenaut E, Chosidow A. Scabies Itch. *Dermatol Clin.* 2018;36(3):301-308.
11. Rosumeck S, Nast A, Dressler. Ivermectin and permethrin for treating scabies. *Cochrane Database Syst Rev.* 2018; 2;4(4):CD012994.
12. Rosumeck, S, Nast A, Dressler C. Evaluation of ivermectin vs permethrin for treating scabies-summary of a Cochrane review. *JAMA Dermatol.* 2019; 1;155(6):730-732.
13. Currie B and McCarthy J. Permethrin and ivermectin for scabies. *N Eng J Med.* 2010;362(8):717-725.
14. Khalil S, Abbas O, Kibbi A, Kurban M. Scabies in the age of increasing drug resistance. *PLoS Negl Trop Dis.* 2017; .30;11(11):e0004920.
15. Gopinath H, Aishwarya M, Karthikeyan K. Tackling scabies: novel agents for a neglected disease. *Int J Dermatol.* 2018; ;57(11):1293-1298.
16. Strong M, Johnstone P. Interventions for treating scabies. *Cochrane Database Syst Rev.* 2007 Jul 18;2007(3):CD000320. doi: 10.1002/14651858.CD000320.pub2.
17. Scabies Treatment. ttps://www.cdc.gov/parasites/scabies/treatment.html. Accessed 07.12.2020.
18. Pearson ML, Selby JV, Katz KA,et.al., ; Unexplained Dermopathy Study Team. Clinical, epidemiologic, histopathologic and molecular features of an unexplained dermopathy. *PLoS One.* 2012;7(1):e29908. doi: 10.1371/journal.pone.0029908. Epub 2012 Jan 25.
19. Middelveen MJ, Stricker RB. Morgellons disease: a filamentous borrelial dermatitis. *Int J Gen Med.* 2016; 14;9:349-354.
20. Burkhart CN, Burkhart CG. Head lice scientific assessment of the nit sheath with clinical ramifications and therapeutic options. *J Am Acad Dermatol.* 2005;53(1):129-33.
21. Ko CJ, Elston DM. Pediculosis. *J Am Acad Dermatol.* 2004;50(1):1-12. PMID:14699358.
22. Frankowski B and Bocchini J. Clinical Report-Head Lice. *Pediatrics.* 2010;126(2):392-403.
23. Jahnke C, Bauer E, Hengge U, Feldmeier H. Accuracy of diagnosis of pediculosis capitis: visual inspection vs. wet combing. *Arch Dermatol.* 2009;145(3):309-313.
24. Parasites-Lice. Centers for Disease Control. http://www.cdc.gov/parasites/lice/. Accessed 07.04.2020.
25. Dourmishev AL, Dourmishev LA, Schwartz RA. Ivermectin: pharmacology and application in dermatology. *Int J Dermat.* 2005;44(12):981-988
26. Ulesfia® Highlights of Prescribing Information. www.https://accessdata.fda.gov. Accessed 07.04.2020.
27. Spinosad®Highlights of Prescribing Information. www.https://spinosadrx.com. Accessed 07.04.2020.
28. Stough D, Shellabarger S Quiring J, Gabrielsen A. Efficacy and safety of spinosad and permethrin crème rinses for pediculosis capitis (head lice). *Pediatrics.* 2009;124(4):e389-e394.
29. Koch E, Clark J, Cohen B, Meinking T, Ryan W, Stevenson A, Yetman R, Yoon K. Management of Health Louse Infestations in the United States-A Literature Review. *Pediatric Dermatol.* 2016;33(5):466-472.
30. Sklice (ivermectin lotion, .05%). www.https://sklice.com. Accessed 07.04.2020.
31. Product calculator. https://www.ridlice.com/en/rid-lice-products/lice-killing-shampoo/. Accessed 07.04.2020.
32. Burgess IF. The mode of action of dimeticone 4% lotion against head lice, *Pediculus capitis. BMC Pharmacol.* 2009; 20;9:3.
33. Burgess IF, Brunton ER, Burgess NA. Single application of 4% dimeticone liquid gel versus two applications of 1% permethrin creme rinse for treatment of head louse infestation: a randomised controlled trial. *BMC Dermatol.* 2013; 1;13:5.
34. Candy K, Nicolas P, Andriantsoanirina V, Izri A, Durand R. In vitro efficacy of five essential oils against Pediculus humanus capitis. *Parasitol Res.* 2018;117:603–609.

35. Yones D, Bakir H, Baroumi S. Chemical composition and efficacy of some selected plant oils against Pediculus humanus capitis in vitro. *Parasitol Res.* 2016;115:3209–3218.

36. Waldman N. Seizure caused by dermal application of over-the-counter eucalyptus oil head lice preparation. *Clin Toxicol.* 2011;49(8):750–1.

37. Mozelsio NB, Harris KE, McGrath KG, Grammer LC. Immediate systemic hypersensitivity reaction associated with topical application of Australian tea tree oil. *Allergy Asthma Proc.* 2003;24(1):73–5.

38. Toloza A, Laguna M, Ortega-Insaurralde I, Vassena D, Risau-Gusman S. Insights about health live transmission from field data and mathematical modeling. *J Med Entomol.* 2018;55(4):929–937.

39. Lyme and other tickborne diseases increasing. https://www.cdc.gov/media/dpk/diseases-and-conditions/lyme-disease/index.html. Accessed 07.04.2020.

40. Lyme Disease. https://www.cdc.gov/lyme/. Accessed 07.05.2020.

41. Borrelia mayonii. https://www.cdc.gov/lyme/mayonii/index.html

42. Bacon RM, Kuleler KJ, Mead PS. Surveillance for Lyme disease—United States, 1192-2006. *MMWR Surveill Summ.* 2008; 57(10):1–9.

43. Eisen R, Eisen L, Beard C. County-Scale Distribution of Ixodes scapularis and Ixodes pacificus (Acari: Ixodidae) in the Continental United States. *J Med Entomol* ;2017;53(2):349–386. Doi: 10.1093/jme/tjv237.

44. Bhate C, Schwartz RA. Lyme disease: Part 1 Advances and perspectives. *J Am Acad Dermatol*; 2011. 64(4):619–39.

45. Ticks. Minnesota Department of Health. https://www.health.state.mn.us/diseases/tickborne/ticks.html. Accessed 07.04.2020.

46. Lyme Disease: Reported cases of Lyme disease by state or locality, 2009-2018. https://www.cdc.gov/lyme/stats/tables.html. Accessed 07.05.2020.

47. Lyme Disease (Borrelia burgdorferi) 2017 Case Definition. Centers for Disease Control and Prevention. https://wwwn.cdc.gov/nndss/conditions/lyme-disease/case-definition/2017/. Accessed 07.05.2020.

48. Ross Russell AL, Dryden MS, Pinto AA, Lovett JK. Lyme disease: diagnosis and management. *Pract Neurol.* 2018.;18(6):455–464.

49. Lyme Disease Signs and Symptoms: Centers for Disease Control and Prevention. https://www.cdc.gov/lyme/signs_symptoms/index.html. Accessed July 5, 2020.

50. Hansen K, Crone C, Kristoferitch W. Lyme neuroborreliosis. In: Said G, Krarup C, ed. *Handbook of Clinical Neurology.* Elsevier, 2013.

51. Morbidity and Mortality Weekly Report (MMWR) Updated CDC Recommendation for Serologic Testing. *Weekly*/August 16, 2019/68(32);703. https://www.cdc.gov/mmwr/volumes/68/wr/mm6832a4.htm?s_cid=mm6832a4_w. Accessed 07.12.2020.

52. Lyme Disease Diagnosis and Testing. Centers for Disease Control. https://www.cdc.gov/lyme/diagnosistesting/index.html. Accessed 07.12.2020.

53. Talagrand-Reboul E, Raffetin A, Zachary P, Jaulhac B, Eldin C. Immunoserological Diagnosis of Human Borrelioses: Current Knowledge and Perspectives. *Front Cell Infect Microbiol.* 2020; 19;10:241.

54. Steen CJ, Carbonaro PA, Schwartz RA. Arthropods in Dermatology. *J Am Acad Dermatol* 2004;50(6):819–842.

55. Tick Bite Prophylaxis. Centers for Disease Control. https://www.cdc.gov/lyme/treatment/index.html. Accessed 07.12.2020.

56. Lyme Disease Treatment. Centers for Disease Control. https://www.cdc.gov/lyme/treatment/index.html. Accessed 07.12.2020.

57. Stupica D, Lusa L, Ruzić-Sabljić E, Cerar T, Strle F. Treatment of erythema migrans with doxycycline for 10 days versus 15 days. *Clin Infect Dis.* 2012;55(3):343–50.

58. Lyme Disease. Centers for Disease Control. https://www.cdc.gov/lyme/treatment/index.html. Accessed 09.06.2021.

59. Research on doxycycline and tooth staining. Rocky Mountain Spotted Fever. Centers for Disease Control. https://www.cdc.gov/rmsf/doxycycline/index.html. Accessed 07.15.2020.

60. Todd SR, Dahlgren FS, Traeger MS, Beltrán-Aguilar ED, Marianos DW, Hamilton C, McQuiston JH, Regan JJ. No visible dental staining in children treated with doxycycline for suspected Rocky Mountain Spotted Fever. *J Pediatr.* 2015;166(5):1246–51.

61. Hu LT. Lyme Disease. *Ann Intern Med.* 201 ;3;164(9):ITC65–ITC80

62. Sanchez E, Vannier E, Wormser GP, Hu LT. Diagnosis, Treatment, and Prevention of Lyme Disease, Human Granulocytic Anaplasmosis, and Babesiosis: A Review. *JAMA.* 2016; 26;315(16):1767–77.

63. Gammons M, Salam G. Tick removal. *Am Fam Physician.* 2002; 15;66(4):643–5.

64. Tkachenko E, Blankenship K, Goldberg D, Scharf MJ, Weedon S, Levin NA. Dish soap for complete tick detachment. *J Am Acad Dermatol.* 2019; 13:S0190-9622(19)30974-0.

65. Alpha-Gal allergy. Ticks. Centers for Disease Control and Prevention. https://www.cdc.gov/ticks/alpha-gal/index.html. Accessed 07.18.2020.

66. Wong XL, Sebaratnam DF. Mammalian meat allergy. Int J Dermatol. 2018;57(12):1433–1436.

67. Post-treatment Lyme disease syndrome. Lyme Disease. Centers for Disease Control and Prevention. https://www.cdc.gov/lyme/postlds/index.html. Accessed 07.18.2020.

68. Krause-Parello CA, Sciscione P. Bedbugs: an equal opportunist and cosmopolitan creature. *J Sch Nurs.* 2009 Apr;25(2):126–32.

69. Sfeir M, Munoz-Price LS. Scabies and bedbugs in hospital outbreaks. *Curr Infect Dis Rep.* 2014;16(8):412.

70. Romero A, Potter MF, Potter DA, Haynes KF. Insecticide resistance in the bed bug: a factor in the pest's sudden resurgence? *J Med Entomol.* 2007 Mar;44(2):175–8.

71. Goddard J and deShazo R. Bed Bugs (Cimex lectularius) and Clinical Consequences of Their Bites. *JAMA.* 2009;301(13):1358–1366.

72. Doggett SL, Dwyer DE, Peñas PF, Russell RC. Bed bugs: clinical relevance and control options. *Clin Microbiol Rev.* 2012; 25(1):164-92.1128/CMR.05015-11.

73. Terminex 2019 Top 50 Bed Bug Cities in the U.S. https://www.terminix.com/blog/whats-buzzing/top-bed-bug-cities/.

74. Ibrahim O, Syed UM, Tomecki KJ. Bedbugs: Helping your patient through an infestation. *Cleve Clin J Med.* 2017;84(3):207–211.

75. Pritchard MJ and Hwang SW. Severe anemia from bedbugs. *CMAJ*, 2009;181(5):287–288.

76. Doggett SL, Russell R. Bed bugs - What the GP needs to know. *Aust Fam Physician.* 2009;38(11):880–4. PMID: 19893834.

77. Pfiester M, Koehler PG, Pereira RM. Ability of bed bug-detecting canines to locate live bed bugs and viable bed bug eggs. *J Econ Entomol.* 2008;101(4):1389–96.

78. Bed Bug Control in Residences. Let's Beat the Bug! University of Minnesota. https://www.bedbugs.umn.edu/bed-bug-control-in-residences. Accessed 07.18.2020.

79. Kells SA, Goblirsch MJ. Temperature and Time Requirements for Controlling Bed Bugs (Cimex lectularius) under Commercial Heat Treatment Conditions. Insects. 2011 Aug 29;2(3):412–22.

80. Olson JF, Eaton M, Kells SA, Morin V, Wang C. Cold tolerance of bed bugs and practical recommendations for control. *J Econ Entomol.* 2013;106(6):2433–41.

81. Understanding Bed Bug Treatments. Let's Beat the Bug! University of Minnesota. https://www.bedbugs.umn.edu/homeowners-and-tenants/understanding-treatments. Accessed 07.18.2020.

82. Pesticides to Control Bed Bugs. United States Environmental Protection Agency. https://www.epa.gov/bedbugs/pesticides-control-bed-bugs. Accessed 07.18.2020.

83. Inspecting Your Hotel Room for Bed Bugs. Let's Beat the Bug. University of Minnesota. https://www.bedbugs.umn.edu/travelers/inspecting-your-hotel-room-for-bed-bugs. Accessed 07.18.2020.

84. Laundering Items to Kill Bed Bugs. Let's Beat the Bed Bug! https://www.bedbugs.umn.edu/bed-bug-control-in-residences/laundering. Accessed 07.18.2020/

85. Using Freezing Conditions to Kill Bed Bugs. Let's Beat the Bed Bug! University of Minnesota. https://www.bedbugs.umn.edu/bed-bug-control-in-residences/freezing. Accessed 07.18.2020.

Skin Signs of Systemic Disease

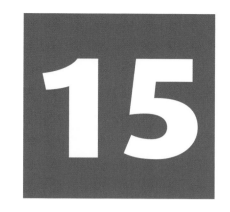

David R. Pearson

INTRODUCTION TO CHAPTER

The skin is immunologically and metabolically dynamic, highly vascular, and directly interfaces with the environment. It also plays a critical role in maintenance of homeostasis, protection, and sensation. As such, cutaneous pathology is a window to many systemic disease processes. A careful history and thorough physical examination of the skin, hair, nails, and mucosal surfaces, paying particular attention to morphology, distribution, and other subtle clinical clues, may result in critical diagnostic, prognostic, and therapeutic benefit that is acquired at the bedside. For example, recognition of nailfold capillary abnormalities may distinguish the hand rash seen in dermatomyositis from that observed in eczema and lead to a diagnosis of interstitial lung disease, or underlying hepatitis C viral infection may be uncovered through identification of oral erosive lichen planus.

The following sections will discuss important skin signs in systemic diseases, with particular focus on *autoimmune connective tissue disorders* and diseases of the *endocrine, gastrointestinal, hepatic, pulmonary,* and *renal* organ systems.

AUTOIMMUNE CONNECTIVE TISSUE DISORDERS

Autoimmune connective tissue disorders are a heterogeneous group of immunologically complex diseases. Diagnosis may be challenging because manifestations are often protean and overlap conditions are frequent. The clinical presentation ranges from mild and skin-limited to severe, life-threatening multisystem disease, and patients may require broad-spectrum systemic immunosuppressants to adequately control symptoms and progression. Due to their diverse symptomatology, a multi-disciplinary approach may often provide the best care for patients. In the following sections, lupus erythematosus, dermatomyositis, systemic sclerosis, and vasculitis will be discussed. Important cutaneous manifestations of other autoimmune connective tissue disorders will also be briefly reviewed.

LUPUS ERYTHEMATOSUS

Introduction

Lupus erythematosus (LE) is a complex autoimmune disorder that affects multiple organ systems and has a wide variety of clinical and immunologic manifestations. Cutaneous involvement is particularly common and may lead to substantial morbidity or disfigurement, profound impact on quality of life, and serve as a marker for underlying systemic disease. We will focus this discussion on lupus-specific phenotypes including *acute* cutaneous lupus erythematosus (ACLE), *subacute* cutaneous lupus erythematosus (SCLE), and *discoid* lupus erythematosus (DLE); the most common form of chronic cutaneous lupus erythematosus (CCLE). A brief discussion of several less common lupus-specific presentations and lupus-nonspecific cutaneous disease will follow. It is common for patients to

demonstrate multiple cutaneous phenotypes, particularly if there is underlying systemic lupus erythematosus (SLE).

In North America, SLE has a prevalence of about 240 per 100,000 people.[1] Cutaneous lupus erythematosus is at least as prevalent as the systemic variant according to population-based studies.[2,3] Risk is highly dependent on demographic factors, most prominently sex and ethnicity, though there is variation between different phenotypes. Overall women are affected at 5–6 times the rate of men, and African Americans are more likely to have LE, and more severe disease, than White or Asian Americans.[1]

Pathogenesis

LE, like other autoimmune connective tissue disorders, results from complex interactions between inherent genetic and epigenetic risk factors and environmental triggers including ultraviolet (UV) light, medications (Table 15-1), tobacco use, and viruses. Keratinocytes, dendritic cells, and endothelial cells are activated, and type I interferon-regulated cytokines and chemokines are released, which stimulate both the innate and adaptive immune response and result in the characteristic CD4- and CD8-mediated interface dermatitis.[4] Pathological feedback loops may be due in part to persistent reactivation of innate immunopathology through effector pathways of the adaptive immune response.[4] Further variations in immunoregulation, including those controlling apoptosis, antibody production, antigen presentation, and other pathways, are contributory.[4]

Acute Cutaneous Lupus Erythematosus (ACLE)

History and Physical Examination

Acute cutaneous lupus erythematosus is characterized by the rapid onset of symptoms, often following UV exposure,

Table 15-1. Common culprits of drug-induced lupus and dermatomyositis.[40–42]

	Clinical presentation	Common culprit drugs	Special considerations
SLE	Constitutional symptoms, arthralgias, myalgias, serositis, photosensitivity. Typical malar rash, renal, and CNS involvement are rare (except TNF-α inhibitors related).	Procainamide, hydralazine, isoniazid, penicillamine, minocycline, TNF-α inhibitors.	• Procainamide: pulmonary involvement. • Hydralazine: glomerulonephritis. • Minocycline: autoimmune hepatitis • TNF-α inhibitors: more likely to see malar rash, renal, and CNS. involvement, and anti-dsDNA autoantibodies.
SCLE	Erythematous scaly annular to nummular patches and plaques on the trunk and extremities.	Terbinafine, TNF-α inhibitors, PPIs, hydrochlorothiazide, CCB, ACE inhibitors.	More likely to be widespread than idiopathic SCLE.
DM	May be identical to idiopathic DM.	Statins, penicillamine, hydroxyurea, TNF-α inhibitors, PPI.	• Hydroxyurea: clinically amyopathic, associated with malignancy. • Hydroxychloroquine: paradoxical reaction (see text).

ACE, angiotensin converting enzyme; CCB, calcium channel blocker; CNS, central nervous system; DM, dermatomyositis; PPI, proton pump inhibitor, SCLE, subacute cutaneous lupus erythematosus; SLE, systemic lupus erythematosus.

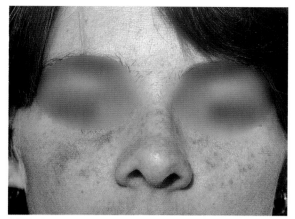

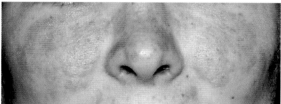

▲ **Figure 15-1.** A and B. Malar rash of acute cutaneous lupus erythematosus. A. There is photodistributed erythema and edema of the nose and medial cheeks; note characteristic sparing of the nasolabial fold. B. This eruption is more robust, yet the nasolabial fold remains notably spared.

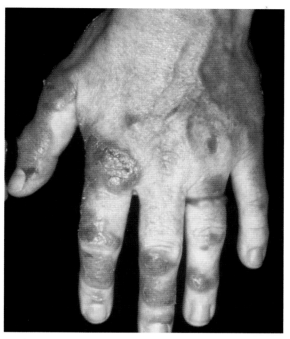

▲ **Figure 15-2.** Acute cutaneous lupus erythematosus. Bright red, edematous plaques on the hands, with relative sparing of the knuckles.

and may precede, occur simultaneously with, or follow systemic symptoms such as fatigue or malaise, fevers, chills, weight loss, arthralgias or inflammatory arthritis, myalgias, headaches, nonscarring alopecia, oral ulcerations, and internal involvement including nephritis, pericarditis, pleuritis, and cerebritis. Virtually all patients with ACLE have underlying SLE.

The characteristic cutaneous presentation for limited ACLE is the *malar* or *butterfly* rash, with symmetric erythema, edema, and fine scaling over the bridge of the nose and medial cheeks, classically sparing the nasolabial folds (Figures 15-1A and 15-1B). Poikiloderma (erythema, dyspigmentation, and atrophy) is common. The forehead, upper cutaneous lip, and chin may be involved, and erosions and hyperkeratotic scaling may be observed in more severe or longstanding cases. *Generalized* involvement with widespread, typically photodistributed erythema, edema, and fine scaling of the neck, trunk, and extremities may occur. When the hands are affected, the knuckles are often relatively spared (Figure 15-2). The rash may sting, burn, or become pruritic. Larger areas of involvement and blistering are often exquisitely painful and may require hospitalization in a burn unit for management. Typically, ACLE does

not lead to scarring, but post-inflammatory dyspigmentation may be long lasting.

There are several rare forms of ACLE that result in blistering but are important to recognize as they may require rapid escalation of care. *Toxic epidermolytic necrolysis* (TEN)-like ACLE results from a profound inflammatory response that leads to diffuse vesiculation or frank skin sloughing, mimicking drug-induced TEN. Mucosal involvement may be absent or minimal. In *bullous LE*, a rare variant characterized by autoantibodies directed against type VII collagen, tense blisters and erosions develop on photodistributed inflamed or non-inflamed skin (Figure 15-3). This form may be the first manifestation of SLE.

Lupus nephritis is a leading cause of morbidity and mortality among lupus patients and affects African Americans more often and more aggressively than White Americans, even after accounting for socioeconomic factors.[5] Up to 10% of patients with lupus nephritis will develop end-stage renal disease.[5] Clinical manifestations may not be apparent, so periodic screening of kidney function and urine composition is necessary. Proteinuria, hematuria, elevated creatinine, and hypertension may be observed. Histologic findings are associated with outcome; endocapillary or mesangial proliferative changes carry a worse prognosis.

Pleuritis, which may lead to pleural effusion, is among the most common pulmonary manifestations in SLE.

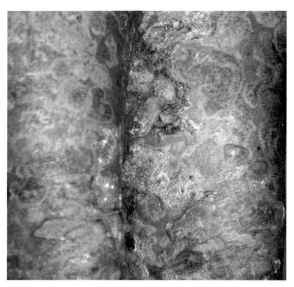

▲ **Figure 15-3.** Bullous lupus. Denuded tense blisters and erosions arising from inflamed skin on the legs.

Interstitial lung disease (ILD), pulmonary embolism (in the setting of antiphospholipid antibody syndrome), pneumonitis, pulmonary hypertension, and diffuse alveolar hemorrhage may be observed.[6] Shrinking lung syndrome is a rare complication.

▶ Laboratory Findings

A positive anti-nuclear antibody (ANA) is seen in >95% of patients but is not universal. With widespread or systemic involvement, nonspecific inflammatory markers such as the erythrocyte sedimentation rate (ESR) and C-reactive protein (CRP) are commonly elevated. Blood counts and complement levels may be depressed and liver enzymes elevated in an acute flare. Creatinine may be elevated and both proteinuria and hematuria may be measured. Specific autoantibodies are associated with distinct clinical phenotypes (Table 15-2).

Skin biopsy demonstrates a subtle interface dermatitis with basal vacuolization and increased dermal mucin. Findings may overlap with other forms of cutaneous lupus, although basement membrane thickening and perivascular and periadnexal lymphocytic infiltration is less marked.

Table 15-2. Select autoantibodies and clinical associations.

Autoantibody	Estimated prevalence	Clinical association	Special considerations
ANA	>95% ACLE 50% SCLE 20% DLE 50% DM 95% SSc	Nonspecific.	Low titers (≤1:80) seen in >15% of general population.
dsDNA	60% SLE	Lupus nephritis.	Highly specific; correlates with disease activity.
Sm	30% SLE	Lupus nephritis.	Highly specific.
SSA (Ro)	50% SLE >75% SCLE >95% NLE 20% DM 60% SjS	SCLE, NLE, SjS, photosensitivity.	52 kDa SSA more specific for myositis and PBC.
SSB (La)	20% SLE 30% SCLE 30% SjS	SjS, SCLE.	Usually observed with anti-SSA autoantibodies.
U1-RNP	50% SLE 100% MCTD 10% DM	Nonspecific.	Required for diagnosis of MCTD.
Cardiolipin	50% SLE	Hypercoagulability.	May be associated with livedo reticularis.
Histone	40% SLE 40% SSc	Non-specific.	May be seen in idiopathic and drug induced SLE.
Mi-2	20% DM	Classic DM with characteristic skin involvement.	Typically responds well to immunosuppressants.
MDA-5	10–20% DM	Clinically amyopathic, rapidly progressive ILD.	More commonly reported in Asia.

(continued)

Table 15-2. Select autoantibodies and clinical associations. (Continued)

Autoantibody	Estimated prevalence	Clinical association	Special considerations
TIF-1γ	20–40% DM	Malignancy, less severe myositis.	
NXP-2	10% DM	Adults: malignancy, calcinosis; juveniles: calcinosis, myositis.	
Jo-1, PL-7, or PL-12	20% DM	Anti-synthetase syndrome.	Mechanic's hands, ILD, arthritis, myositis, Raynaud phenomenon.
Topoisomerase I (Scl-70)	60% dcSSc Occasional lcSSc	dcSSc ILD, SRC.	
Centromere	70% lcSSc Occasional dcSSc	lcSSc with pulmonary hypertension.	Immunofluorescence pattern observed on ANA test.
RNA polymerase III	30–40% dcSSc	Rapid progression, SRC.	May have malignancy association.
c-ANCA (PR-3)	90% GPA	GPA.	May be seen in levamisole vasculopathy.
p-ANCA (MPO)	40% EGPA 60% MPA Occasional GPA Occasional cPAN	MPA, EGPA, cPAN.	May be seen in levamisole vasculopathy.

ACLE, acute cutaneous lupus erythematosus; cPAN, cutaneous polyarteritis nodosa; dcSSc, diffuse cutaneous systemic sclerosis; DLE, discoid lupus erythematosus; DM, dermatomyositis; EGPA, eosinophilic granulomatosis with polyangiitis (Churg-Strauss); GPA, granulomatosis with polyangiitis; ILD, interstitial lung disease; kDa, kilodalton; lcSSc, limited cutaneous systemic sclerosis; MCTD, mixed connective tissue disease; MPA, microscopic polyangiitis; NLE, neonatal lupus erythematosus; PBC, primary biliary cirrhosis; SCLE, subacute cutaneous lupus erythematosus; SjS, Sjögren syndrome; SLE, systemic lupus erythematosus; SRC, scleroderma renal crisis; SSc, systemic sclerosis

Subacute Cutaneous Lupus Erythematosus (SCLE)

Medications are a frequent trigger for SCLE and are attributed with about one-quarter to one-third of cases (Table 15-1).

▶ History and Physical Examination

Patients with SCLE are highly photosensitive. In contrast to other forms of cutaneous lupus, the skin lesions of SCLE predominate on the trunk and extensor surfaces of the proximal extremities. The upper back, V of the chest, and upper arms are most commonly affected, while the central face is generally spared. Two primary subtypes exist. The *annular* or *polycyclic* variant demonstrates erythematous, scaly papules and plaques that coalesce into ring-shaped and curvilinear lesions with relative central clearing (Figure 15-4). The *papulosquamous* variant may resemble psoriasis or an eczematous dermatitis with nummular erythema and scaling.

Approximately 30–50% of SCLE patients meet criteria for SLE and overlap with Sjögren syndrome is common.[7] Cytopenias and joint symptoms, as well as sicca and xerophthalmia, may be observed, but severe internal manifestations of SLE such as nephritis or cerebritis are uncommon.

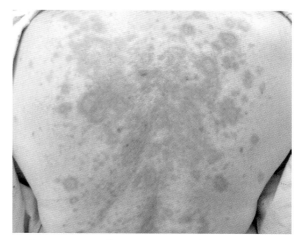

▲ **Figure 15-4.** Subacute cutaneous lupus erythematosus. Annular, erythematous, and scaly plaques on the upper torso.

Rowell syndrome, a rare variant of SCLE, demonstrates acrofacially predominant erythema multiforme (EM)-like targetoid, dusky papules which may evolve into blisters. Mucosal erosions are often observed. This diagnosis remains controversial and may be classified as a variant of acute cutaneous lupus by some experts.

▶ Laboratory Findings

About half of patients with SCLE have a positive ANA; anti-SSA (Ro) autoantibodies are observed in over three-quarters of patients (Table 15-2). Workup may reveal cytopenias, elevated inflammatory markers, and other findings in cases of coexistent SLE, and periodic laboratory monitoring is recommended.

A skin biopsy often demonstrates a more pronounced interface dermatitis, subtle basement membrane thickening, and epidermal atrophy, between the spectrum from acute cutaneous lupus to DLE. Increased dermal mucin, a mild to moderate perivascular and periadnexal lymphocytic infiltrate, hyperkeratosis, and follicular plugging may be detected.

Discoid Lupus Erythematosus (DLE)

Discoid lupus erythematosus is the most common form of chronic cutaneous lupus. Only 5–20% of DLE patients will progress to SLE, but up to one-quarter of SLE patients will have discoid lesions at some point during their disease.[8] Risk is higher for generalized DLE, patients with a positive ANA, and those with systemic symptoms such as arthralgias or nephritis.

▶ History and Physical Examination

Classic or *localized* DLE presents as an edematous or indurated, erythematous to violaceous expanding papule or plaque, though lesions are rarely caught at this stage. As the lesion matures, intense inflammation leads to profound scarring and dyspigmentation (Figures 15-5 and 15-6). Lesions are often hypo- to depigmented centrally and

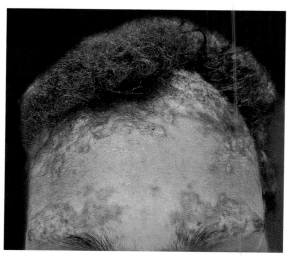

▲ **Figure 15-6.** Discoid lupus erythematosus. Scattered facial and scalp plaques demonstrating atrophic scarring, erythema, and scaling.

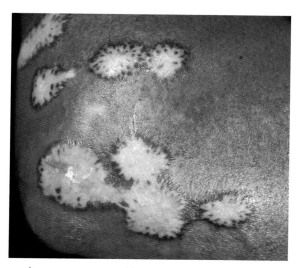

▲ **Figure 15-5.** Discoid lupus erythematosus. Pink, atrophic plaques resulting in profound dyspigmentation.

hyperpigmented peripherally, with overlying hyperkeratosis. Dyspigmentation may be more difficult to observe in lighter-skinned patients. Itching and burning are common early symptoms. These symptoms may persist in late-stage discoid lesions and be accompanied by pain and disfigurement due to scarring. Lesions have a strong predilection for the head and neck, and involvement of the conchal bowl is a diagnostic clue (Figure 15-7). They may also present in a pattern reminiscent of the malar rash of acute cutaneous lupus, including sparing of the nasolabial folds. When it involves hair-bearing areas, DLE leads to scarring alopecia. Although lesions may be induced by sun exposure, this form of cutaneous lupus is less photosensitive than acute or subacute cutaneous lupus.

Generalized DLE demonstrates discoid lesions below the head and neck region (Figure 15-8); it is uncommon to have disease involving the trunk and extremities that spares the head and neck. *Hypertrophic* DLE is an uncommon variant characterized by markedly hyperkeratotic plaques, usually on the extremities. More classic DLE lesions are often observed elsewhere. The uncommon *mucosal* variant may present with plaques present on the orogenital mucosae. Longstanding insufficiently treated discoid lesions may give rise to squamous cell carcinomas.

▶ Laboratory Findings

Only a minority of patients with DLE have a positive ANA. Like other forms of cutaneous lupus, workup should be undertaken to evaluate for coexistent SLE and repeated periodically during follow up.

A skin biopsy shows a more mature interface dermatitis with a thickened basement membrane. Follicular plugging

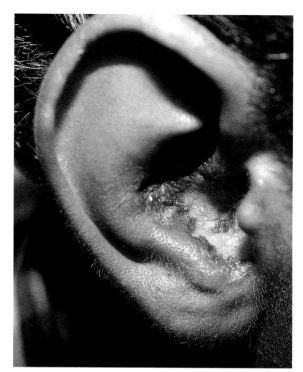

▲ **Figure 15-7.** Discoid lupus erythematosus. Involvement of the conchal bowl is a clue to the diagnosis.

and hyperkeratosis are common. In the dermis, a lymphocytic perivascular and periadnexal infiltrate is usually observed, as is increased mucin. Scarred lesions may have significant fibrosis, particularly when sampled in hair-bearing regions.

Less Common Forms of Cutaneous Lupus Erythematosus

Tumid Lupus Erythematosus

Tumid lupus erythematosus (TLE) is an uncommon form of chronic cutaneous lupus erythematosus which presents as itchy to burning erythematous papules and nodules photodistributed on the cheeks, upper chest, back, and upper arms. There is no overlying scale and these lesions may resemble urticaria, though do not migrate. Serologic abnormalities are absent. TLE rarely progresses to SLE, but patients with other forms of cutaneous lupus may demonstrate tumid lesions.

Lupus Panniculitis

Lupus panniculitis results from intense inflammation in the subcuticular fat, leading to disfiguring atrophic plaques

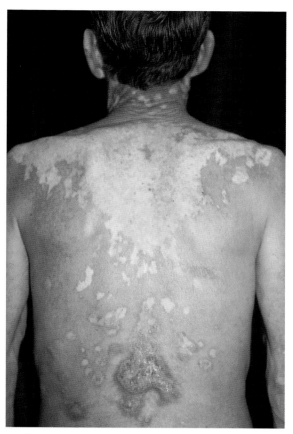

▲ **Figure 15-8.** Generalized discoid lupus erythematosus, demonstrating involvement of the trunk in addition to involvement on the neck. This patient also had involvement of his upper extremities. Note depigmentation in areas of inactive disease on the upper back.

characteristically distributed on the cheeks, proximal upper and lower extremities, breasts, and buttocks. If DLE is present superficially, this full-thickness lesion is often referred to as *lupus profundus*. Lupus panniculitis does not typically progress to SLE and serologic abnormalities are absent.

Chilblain Lupus Erythematosus

Chilblain LE resembles idiopathic pernio, with erythematous, violaceous, or dusky subcutaneous papules most commonly on the toes and fingers. Lesions may become scaly or eroded, and may be tender, itch, or burn. Onset is triggered by cold, moist environments, but unlike idiopathic pernio, disease may persist in warmer climates. Chilblain LE is often observed with discoid lesions elsewhere, and up to 20% of patients develop systemic disease.[9]

Neonatal Lupus Erythematosus

Neonatal LE is caused by transplacental transfer of maternal anti-SSA autoantibodies, rather than inherent neonatal autoimmunity. The eruption is characterized by annular to nummular erythematous or hyperpigmented patches and thin plaques that preferentially occur in a periorbital distribution, but may arise elsewhere, and may be present at birth. Neonatal LE is the most common cause of congenital heart block, which may be permanent and complicated by cardiomyopathy.[10] Hepatobiliary involvement and cytopenias may also occur. Clearance of maternal antibodies by 6–8 months ultimately leads to resolution of the rash.

Nonspecific Cutaneous Manifestations of Lupus Erythematosus

Cutaneous Vascular Lesions: *Raynaud phenomenon* demonstrates triphasic color change with initial blanching and bluish-purple vascular congestion, followed by rubrous hyperemia, in response to cold exposure (Figure 15-9). *Livedo reticularis*, which may also be triggered by exposure to cold, presents as lacy to net-like erythematous patches most often localized to the extremities. *Cutaneous infarcts* from micro- or macro- thromboses may occur and should raise suspicion for underlying *antiphospholipid antibody syndrome* (Figure 15-10). *Vasculitis*, including cutaneous small vessel vasculitis (CSVV), urticarial vasculitis, and polyarteritis nodosa (PAN), may be seen in LE patients.

Nonscarring Alopecia: Several different forms of nonscarring hair loss may be observed in LE. Patchy to diffuse alopecia is correlated with underlying LE activity; skin biopsy demonstrates interface dermatitis. *Telogen effluvium* is common due to systemic stressors. *Lupus hair*, short, fragile hair long the frontal hairline, may be seen in patients with chronically active LE.[11]

Overlap Conditions: Some patients may demonstrate features of LE along with features of other autoimmune

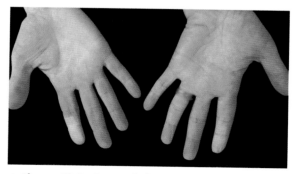

▲ **Figure 15-9.** Raynaud phenomenon. Note sharply demarcated blanching of the index finger and dusky discoloration of several digits.

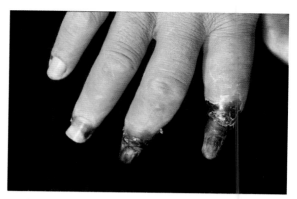

▲ **Figure 15-10.** Digital necrosis in a patient with antiphospholipid antibody syndrome and underlying systemic lupus erythematosus.

connective tissue disorders, such as dermatomyositis, systemic sclerosis (SSc), or morphea. *Mixed connective tissue disease* (MCTD), a distinct clinical entity characterized by elevated anti-U1-RNP autoantibodies, has features of LE, SSc, myositis, and rheumatoid arthritis (RA). Raynaud phenomenon is nearly universal and pulmonary involvement may result in interstitial lung disease or pulmonary hypertension. In contrast, patients diagnosed with *undifferentiated connective tissue disease* do not meet criteria for a defined autoimmune connective tissue disorder, and may demonstrate nonspecific symptoms including Raynaud phenomenon, photosensitivity, arthralgias, and/or other findings.

Diagnosis

In addition to historical and physical examination findings, initial workup should assess for SLE with the following:

- Complete blood count (CBC) with differential.
- Comprehensive metabolic panel (CMP), ESR, CRP, urinalysis.
- ANA in most CLE patients.
- Complement levels and more specific autoantibodies should be assessed if appropriate.
- A skin biopsy may be particularly useful in confirmation of the diagnosis and exclusion of mimickers, and direct immunofluorescence (DIF) usually demonstrates a positive lupus band.

In SLE patients, ongoing monitoring of laboratory parameters is important to monitor disease activity. Flares of disease may result in depressed complements and/or elevated dsDNA autoantibodies in some phenotypes. Periodic monitoring of labs in cutaneous LE patients is also important to monitor for progression to systemic disease.

▶ Differential diagnosis

✓ Seborrheic dermatitis and erythematotelangiectatic rosacea may be confused for the malar rash. Look for sparing of the nasolabial fold, poikiloderma, absence of pustules, and underlying systemic symptoms, such as fatigue, arthralgias, oral ulcers, and nonscarring alopecia.

✓ Tinea corporis may resemble annular SCLE but has a positive KOH examination and typically responds to topical antifungals.

✓ Psoriasis may resemble papulosquamous SCLE but can be distinguished by skin biopsy.

✓ Distinguishing idiopathic and drug induced SCLE is challenging, and cessation of potentially causative agents, when present, is advised.

✓ Early lesions of DLE may be mistaken for acute cutaneous LE, seborrheic dermatitis, or psoriasis.

✓ Hyperkeratotic DLE lesions may mimic prurigo nodularis or squamous cell carcinomas.

Management

Behavioral interventions for LE are critical. Given the role UV light plays in triggering and exacerbating disease, sun protection and sun avoidance strategies are a cornerstone to avoid flares. High sun protection factor (SPF) sunscreens containing a physical blocker, such as zinc oxide or titanium dioxide, are preferred. Tinted sunscreens containing iron oxides may offer additional protection against provocative visible wavelengths and be more cosmetically acceptable to patients with darker pigmentation.[12] Sun protective clothing and wide-brimmed hats confer added protection. These precautions, along with demographic factors, increase the risk of vitamin D deficiency; thus, LE patients should have periodic monitoring of vitamin D and be started on supplementation if indicated. Tobacco cessation is important, as cigarette smoking has been shown to both exacerbate LE and interfere with the effectiveness of systemic treatments.[13]

Initial pharmacologic management of cutaneous LE is skin-directed. Topical corticosteroids (usually ointments and creams) are a mainstay of treatment; low potency (class V–VII) topical corticosteroids are preferred for the face, groin, and other intertriginous areas. Medium potency (class III–IV) topical corticosteroids may be used on the trunk and extremities. High potency (class I–II) topical corticosteroids should be reserved for severe or refractory disease. Long-term use of topical corticosteroids may result in permanent cutaneous atrophy and should occur under the supervision of an experienced clinician. Topical calcineurin inhibitors (tacrolimus ointment or pimecrolimus cream) are an alternative to topical corticosteroids that do

not result in cutaneous atrophy. Intralesional corticosteroid injections (e.g., triamcinolone acetonide suspension 2.5–20 mg/mL) are a useful adjunctive therapy in persistent or hyperkeratotic DLE.

In cases where topical therapies do not adequately treat cutaneous LE or if there is coexistent SLE, patients should be referred for specialty care. Oral anti-malarials are the preferred first-line systemic treatment. Hydroxychloroquine is utilized most commonly and is generally well-tolerated. Unless otherwise contraindicated, all patients with lupus nephritis should be placed on hydroxychloroquine. Retinopathy is a chief concern with this medication, but appropriate dosing (maximum 5 mg/kg real body weight per day) as well as baseline and annual screening eye exams by a provider familiar with hydroxychloroquine-associated retinopathy decreases this risk.[14] Chloroquine is an alternative but has a less favorable side-effect profile and lower dosing recommendation (2.3 mg/kg real body weight per day).[14] Quinacrine, if available, can be added to either hydroxychloroquine or chloroquine for additional benefit without increased ocular toxicity.

Methotrexate and mycophenolate mofetil are next line agents for persistent disease. These agents are immunosuppressive and require surveillance laboratory monitoring. Methotrexate may be more helpful in treating concomitant joint symptoms; however, if nephritis is present, mycophenolate mofetil is preferred.[15] Dapsone is the treatment of choice for bullous lupus. In severe disease resistant to multiple treatments, lenalidomide, a thalidomide derivative, should be considered, but birth control is essential as it is teratogenic. Systemic corticosteroids may be crucial for rapid symptom relief in severe flares but are not preferred for long-term or repeated short-term management. High-dose systemic corticosteroids with either mycophenolate mofetil or cyclophosphamide is the treatment of choice for patients with active inflammatory lupus nephritis, while those with chronic or sclerotic disease may benefit most from renoprotective measures to reduce proteinuria.[5]

Belimumab, a monoclonal antibody directed against B-cell activating factor (BAFF; also known as B-lymphocyte stimulator [BLyS]) and rituximab, a monoclonal antibody directed against CD-20, have demonstrated benefit in SLE but their performance in treating cutaneous LE has been inconsistent, and their future role requires further study. Emerging treatments for cutaneous and systemic LE focus on other pathogenic inflammatory pathways, including plasmacytoid dendritic cells and type I interferon signaling.

Clinical Course and Prognosis

Lupus erythematosus follows a relapsing and remitting course. Flares are more common following the known environmental exposures such as UV light, but stressors – both physical and psychosocial – are well known to cause exacerbations. The rate of progression to SLE varies based on cutaneous LE subtype; nearly all patients with acute cutaneous LE have SLE while patients with SCLE and DLE are much less likely to have systemic disease. It is important to periodically monitor brocheolar lavage or patients for progression because this may necessitate more aggressive treatment directed at internal disease. Prognosis is tied to underlying systemic involvement.

Indications for Consultation

Most patients with LE benefit from multidisciplinary care by a dermatologist and rheumatologist. Management of lupus nephritis should involve a nephrologist. Further care coordination is dependent on systemic manifestations and may include psychological support due to its impact on patients' quality of life.

Patient Information

- Lupus Foundation of America, Inc. www.lupus.org
- American Academy of Dermatology https://www.aad.org/public/diseases/a-z/lupus-overview
- National Institute of Arthritis and Musculoskeletal and Skin Diseases. www. niams.nih.gov/health-topics/lupus
- Lupus Research Alliance www.lupusresearch.org

▼ DERMATOMYOSITIS

▷ Introduction

Dermatomyositis is an uncommon autoimmune connective tissue disorder characterized by involvement of three primary organ systems: skin, muscles, and lungs. Like lupus erythematosus, there is considerable clinical variation, and some patients may have disease limited to only one or two of these organ systems. Joint involvement is common. Patients with *clinically amyopathic* dermatomyositis have skin-predominant disease, while those with *classic* dermatomyositis display involvement of both skin and muscles. *Anti-synthetase syndrome*, which demonstrates considerable overlap with dermatomyositis and is considered to be a variant by some experts, is typified by interstitial lung disease (ILD), myositis, inflammatory arthritis, and mechanic's hands, hyperkeratosis and fissuring in the first web spaces of the hands that often extends onto the pulp of the digits. *Juvenile* dermatomyositis affects children and young adults and is associated with calcinosis cutis. *Drug-induced* dermatomyositis may be triggered by medications (Table 15-1). Dermatomyositis may be particularly challenging to diagnose and delays in recognition and treatment are common. Since dermatomyositis may be a paraneoplastic condition (caused by underlying malignancy), and some variants demonstrate rapidly progressive ILD, prompt recognition and appropriate screening is crucial to prevent morbidity or mortality.

Dermatomyositis has an estimated prevalence of 1–6 per 100,000.[16] Estimates of the relative proportions of clinically amyopathic versus classic dermatomyositis patients vary, but at least 20% are clinically amyopathic.[17] Pulmonary involvement is estimated to occur in 10–45% of patients.[18] 10–25% of patients have underlying malignancy, though risk is correlated strongly with patient age.[18,19]

Pathogenesis

Environmental triggers may cause dermatomyositis in genetically susceptible individuals. Like lupus erythematosus, UV light, drugs, and viruses, as well as pollutants, have been reported as inciting factors.[16,18] These exogenous stimuli may perpetuate activation of innate and adaptive immune responses through type I interferons and other cytokines and chemokines, leading to the development of T- and B-cell-mediated immunopathology and autoantibody production. There is evidence that initiation of the classical complement cascade, leading to activation of the membrane attack complex, results in microvascular inflammation, injury, and infarction, and ultimately leads to myositis; similar findings have been demonstrated in skin microvasculature.[16,18]

Clinical Presentation

▷ History and Physical Examination

The skin eruption of dermatomyositis is erythematous, but may appear deep red or violaceous, and demonstrates fine scaling and poikiloderma. Photodistributed involvement on the face is common, but in contrast to cutaneous LE, the nasolabial folds may not be spared. Erythema and swelling of the upper eyelids (*heliotrope rash*) is an important sign (Figure 15-11). *Gottron sign* is characterized by a rash over the extensor surfaces of the joints of the hands, feet, and extremities. *Gottron's papules*, small, flat-topped papules that may demonstrate scale, can arise from Gottron sign, most often overlying the metacarpophalangeal joints and interphalangeal joints of the fingers (Figure 15-12). The *shawl sign*, rash on the posterior neck, shoulders, and V of the chest, may be observed (Figure 15-13). The lateral thighs are often involved (*holster sign*). *Nailfold changes*

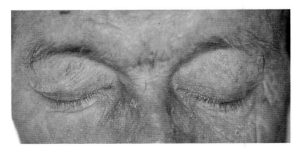

▲ **Figure 15-11.** Dermatomyositis. Facial erythema and the heliotrope rash, demonstrating faint pink/violaceous discoloration on the superior eyelid, with lesser involvement along the inferomedial eyelid.

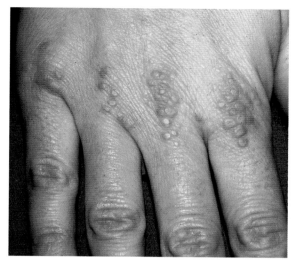

▲ **Figure 15-12.** Gottron's papules in dermatomyositis. Flat-topped pink papules overlying the metacarpophalangeal joints.

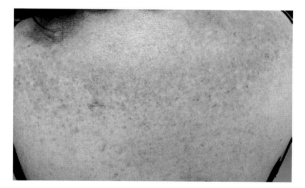

▲ **Figure 15-13.** Shawl sign in dermatomyositis. Violaceous poikiloderma with scaling on the posterior neck and upper back, extending toward the shoulders.

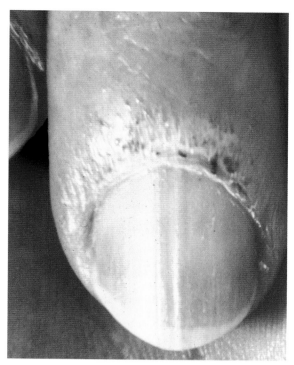

▲ **Figure 15-14.** Dermatomyositis. Nailfold changes with capillary dropout and dilation, cuticular hemorrhage, and ragged overgrowth of the cuticles. Similar changes may be observed in systemic sclerosis.

including capillary dropout, dilation, and hemorrhage, and ragged cuticular overgrowth (Samitz sign) are common (Figure 15-14). *Mechanic's hands*, typical of anti-synthetase syndrome, may occur in other variants of dermatomyositis and classically describe hyperkeratosis and fissuring in the first web spaces of the hands, often extending on the pulp of the digits. Scalp erythema and scaling are common. Skin involvement with dermatomyositis can be intensely pruritic and may significantly impair quality of life. Calcinosis cutis may develop in areas of involvement but is more common in juvenile dermatomyositis.

Myositis most often manifests as proximal, symmetric muscle weakness of the extremities; however, axial involvement is also common. Myalgias and inflammatory arthritis may be present. Fatigue, dyspnea, and musculoskeletal symptoms contribute to difficulties rising from a chair, ascending stairs, combing one's hair, or impede other activities of daily living (ADLs). Weakness may be distal or involve the diaphragm, pharynx, or larynx in some cases. Pulmonary disease in dermatomyositis is characterized by ILD; bibasilar crackles may be indicative. Pneumomediastinum or pneumothorax may occur in the absence of ILD.[20] These patients tend to be amyopathic but may suffer from cutaneous ulcerations and inflammatory arthritis. ILD or diaphragmatic involvement may become rapidly progressive and require hospitalization and mechanical ventilation and may result in death.

Weight loss, fever, chills, or other unexplained symptoms are concerning for underlying malignancy. Dermatomyositis is not associated with a specific underlying malignancy. When it is present, malignancy is most often diagnosed within 2–5 years of the onset of dermatomyositis symptoms.[19]

► Laboratory Findings

There is no single laboratory test that can confirm or refute a diagnosis of dermatomyositis. Minimum laboratory workup should include CBC, CMP, and objective assessment for muscle damage by creatinine kinase (CK), aldolase, lactate dehydrogenase (LDH), and/or alanine and aspartate aminotransferases (ALT and AST, respectively). ESR and CRP may be elevated. Periodic monitoring of these parameters is important to assess disease activity. Skin biopsy demonstrates a subtle interface dermatitis with basal vacuolization and increased dermal mucin that may be indistinguishable from cutaneous LE.

Autoantibody testing is more variable in dermatomyositis than in LE. ANA is positive in about half of patients. Other autoantibodies (U1-RNP, SSA, SSB, and others) are variably positive. There has been significant interest in studying the relationship between myositis-specific and myositis-associated autoantibodies and clinical phenotype, and some autoantibodies demonstrate strong correlation (Table 15-2). However, the absence of myositis-specific or myositis-associated autoantibodies does not exclude a diagnosis of dermatomyositis.

Systemic workup should be symptom-directed. Performing pulmonary function testing (PFTs) with assessment of the diffusing capacity for carbon monoxide (DLCO) is a reasonable, noninvasive screening approach for pulmonary involvement. In a patient with symptoms or signs concerning for ILD, high resolution chest computed tomography (CT) is warranted. In patients with muscle symptoms, evaluation for myositis may include muscle biopsy, electromyography, or magnetic resonance imaging of large muscle groups (e.g., the thighs). An electrocardiogram or endoscopy may also be appropriate in patients with myositis.

Guidelines for malignancy screening in dermatomyositis are not well-established. CT imaging of the chest, abdomen, and pelvis and colonoscopy should be strongly considered. In female patients, mammography, Papanicolaou smear, serum CA125, and transvaginal ultrasound are recommended. In male patients, serum prostate-specific antigen (PSA) should be measured. Additional malignancy workup should be directed by symptoms and signs. No clear consensus exists about the need for ongoing malignancy screening, but in most cases, malignancy develops 2–5 years before or after the diagnosis of dermatomyositis.[19]

Diagnosis

Like other autoimmune connective tissue disorders, diagnosis relies on the integration of clinical, histopathologic, and laboratory evidence. Assessment for pulmonary involvement and myositis is important as therapeutic strategies diverge. Adult patients should be screened for underlying malignancy; this association is much weaker in juvenile and young adult patients.

▶ ### Differential diagnosis

✓ The rash of dermatomyositis may be misdiagnosed as psoriasis, cutaneous LE, eczema, or allergic contact dermatitis. Poikiloderma and the distribution of the eruption are important clues to the correct diagnosis.

✓ Hand dermatitis can be confused with mechanic's hands; the latter is often less responsive to steroids and may be accompanied by nailfold changes or other cutaneous signs of dermatomyositis.

✓ Seborrheic dermatitis and scalp psoriasis are important differential diagnoses for scalp involvement.

Management

Therapy for dermatomyositis depends upon clinical presentation. Systemic corticosteroids (e.g., prednisone 1 mg/kg/day) often lead to early improvement in skin and muscle symptoms, but prolonged tapers are required to avoid relapse or rebound and cutaneous disease may be refractory even after myositis is controlled. For persistent cutaneous or systemic disease, many providers start antimalarials first-line due to their favorable side effect profile. However, up to 20% of patients may experience paradoxical exacerbation of skin disease from hydroxychloroquine.[21] Methotrexate and mycophenolate mofetil are additional first-line alternatives; mycophenolate mofetil is preferred in patients with ILD.[22] Azathioprine may be more beneficial for myositis and inflammatory arthritis than skin involvement. Tofacitinib, a Janus kinase (JAK) inhibitor targeting JAK1 and JAK3, is emerging as a promising treatment option.

In patients with refractory or severe disease, intravenous immunoglobulin (IVIg) or rituximab may be appropriate, although the latter has less consistent benefit for skin disease. Oral tacrolimus or cyclophosphamide may be beneficial in case of severe pulmonary involvement. TNF-α inhibitors should be used with caution due to the risk of precipitating or exacerbating disease. A variety of other agents have reported benefit in case reports or small studies.

Topical or intralesional corticosteroids, with potency or concentration appropriately selected in regard body location, and topical calcineurin inhibitors may serve as adjunctive therapy for skin involvement, though may not be sufficient to control disease without concomitant systemic treatment. Hyperkeratotic areas may be amenable to treatment with topical retinoids. Sun avoidance and sun protective behaviors are important to avoid UV light-related flares. Physical and occupational therapy are important for maintaining and improving function.

In cases of malignancy-associated dermatomyositis, treatment of the underlying cancer is critical. However, dermatomyositis may persist even after remission of malignancy.

Clinical Course and Prognosis

Dermatomyositis is a chronic disease that follows a relapsing-remitting course. While some patients achieve clinical remission, many patients will require ongoing pharmacotherapy to control disease. Cutaneous scalp and hand symptoms may be more difficult to control than skin disease elsewhere. Longstanding myositis or corticosteroid-induced myopathy from long-term use of systemic corticosteroids may result in persistent weakness that may be difficult to discriminate from active disease. Overall mortality may approach 25% at 5 years and most often attributed to ILD, underlying malignancy, or myositis of critical muscles such as the diaphragm.[23]

Indications for Consultation

Patients with dermatomyositis should be managed with a multidisciplinary team, depending upon the clinical manifestations. Dermatologists and rheumatologists care for most patients. Neurologists may be involved if myositis predominates, and pulmonologists should be consulted if ILD is present. When paraneoplastic, oncologists should be involved in care of the underlying malignancy. Physical and occupational therapists play an important role in preserving and improving function.

Patient Information

- The Myositis Foundation www.myositis.org
- National Institute of Neurological Disorders and Stroke https://www.ninds.nih.gov/disorders/all-disorders/dermatomyositis-information-page
- Genetic and Rare Diseases Information Center https://rarediseases.info.nih.gov/diseases/6263/dermatomyositis

SYSTEMIC SCLEROSIS

Introduction

Systemic sclerosis (SSc) is a rare autoimmune disorder characterized by cutaneous sclerosis, or thickening of the skin, but the lungs, kidneys, gastrointestinal tract, and musculoskeletal system may also be involved. Early recognition and treatment are crucial because cutaneous sclerosis, which most often precedes internal involvement, may lead to joint contractures and loss of function, skin ulceration and infection, digital autoamputation, thoracic and abdominal restriction, pain, and itch. Internal manifestations are associated with morbidity and mortality. Two primary variants exist: *diffuse cutaneous* systemic sclerosis (dcSSc) and *limited cutaneous* systemic sclerosis (lcSSc). Limited cutaneous systemic sclerosis is defined as skin thickening distal to the elbows and knees, with or without facial involvement, whereas diffuse cutaneous systemic sclerosis demonstrates sclerosis distally as well as on the proximal extremities and trunk. Due to differences in clinical presentation and prognosis related to skin and internal organ involvement, distinction between these variants is important. Additionally, "systemic sclerosis" is preferred over "scleroderma," to distinguish this disease from *morphea*, historically called

"localized scleroderma." While these diseases are related, they do not exist on a continuum and the preferred terminology highlights the important prognostic implications of internal organ involvement in systemic sclerosis. *Limited cutaneous systemic sclerosis* is preferred over "CREST" syndrome (Calcinosis, Raynaud phenomenon, Esophageal dysmotility, Sclerodactyly, and Telangiectasias) since not all patients display every clinical manifestation.

Systemic sclerosis has a prevalence of up to 34 per 100,000 people.[24] The male-to-female ratio is nearly 9:1, although males have a higher risk of the diffuse subtype, pulmonary hypertension, and digital ulcers.[24,25] African Americans are affected nearly twice as often as White Americans, and even after controlling for sex, disease variant, antibody status, and socioeconomic factors, have earlier onset, more severe disease, and higher mortality.[25]

Pathogenesis

The pathogenesis of systemic sclerosis is a complex interplay between micro- and macrovascular dysregulation, extracellular matrix deposition, and immunopathology. Environmental factors, such as drugs, pollutants, or other physiologic stressors, may trigger disease in genetically susceptible individuals. Microvasculopathy and hypoxia-mediated tissue damage stimulate myofibroblast differentiation, resulting in fibrosis and sclerosis.[26] Activation of both the innate and adaptive immune response with autoantibody production further perpetuates inflammatory-mediated extracellular matrix deposition. Microvasculopathy may be the inciting factor behind the ischemia, fibrosis, and eventual sclerosis in the skin and internal organs.[26]

Clinical Presentation

History and Physical Examination

Raynaud phenomenon is often the presenting sign and may be accompanied by nailfold changes and digital ulcers. *Nailfold changes* include capillary dropout, dilation, and hemorrhage, and ragged cuticular overgrowth. Punctate or larger *digital ulcers* are often on the distal pulp but may be present on the dorsal surfaces or more proximally (Figure 15-15).

Cutaneous sclerosis spreads proximally from acrofacial sites (hands, feet, and face) (Figure 15-16). Early *sclerodactyly*, sclerosis of the digits, may resemble nonpitting edema of the fingers, but skin becomes thickened and bound down to deeper structures. Left untreated, sclerodactyly progresses to sclerotic and then atrophic phases over several years (Figure 15-17). Joint contractures and bony resorption may result in digital autoamputation, and digital ulcers or gangrene may result. Mask-like facies, microstomia, and loss of dynamic and static rhytides resulting in an artificially youthful appearance may occur with facial involvement (Figure 15-18). Perioral involvement may lead to restriction of the oral aperture. As cutaneous sclerosis progresses proximally in diffuse cutaneous systemic

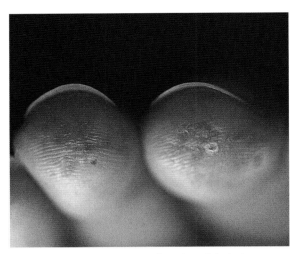

▲ **Figure 15-15.** Systemic sclerosis. Digital ulcers on the distal digital pulps

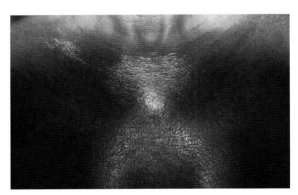

▲ **Figure 15-16.** Cutaneous sclerosis and hyperpigmentation on chest of a patient with diffuse cutaneous systemic sclerosis.

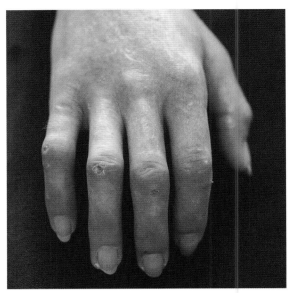

▲ **Figure 15-17.** Sclerodactyly in systemic sclerosis. There is cutaneous sclerosis of the fingers, resulting in joint contractures and a claw-like appearance to the digits. Digital ulcers are present on the dorsal surfaces, as well as scarring from past ulcerations.

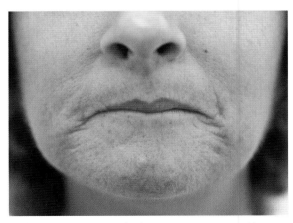

▲ **Figure 15-18.** Facial sclerosis in a patient with limited cutaneous systemic sclerosis, resulting in a mask-like facies with nasal beaking and microstomia. There are numerous mat-like telangiectasias.

sclerosis, contractures of larger joints such as the wrists, ankles, elbows, and knees may occur, and be accompanied by intense pruritus or pain.

Calcinosis cutis is common and may present as pale, rock-hard subcutaneous nodules, but consistency can vary to a thick paste or even liquid. These are most often located on the hands but may be present in other areas of cutaneous sclerosis. Spontaneous drainage of superficial lesions is common. *Onychodystrophy* resulting in changes in nails size, shape, and texture may occur. Mat-like *telangiectasias* are most often observed in limited cutaneous systemic sclerosis on the hands and face but may be widespread.

Pulmonary involvement is the leading cause of mortality for systemic sclerosis patients. Diffuse cutaneous systemic sclerosis demonstrates a higher rate of ILD and pulmonary hypertension is more often observed in limited cutaneous systemic sclerosis, but overlap exists. Dyspnea and a dry cough are the most prevalent symptoms, and heart failure may develop. Auscultation of the chest may demonstrate bibasilar crackles. Scleroderma renal crisis (SRC) affects up to one in six patients with diffuse cutaneous systemic sclerosis, with onset within the first 5 years after non-Raynaud symptoms; it may be precipitated by systemic corticosteroids.[27] Symptoms may be subtle, and include significantly elevated blood pressures, rapidly declining kidney function, and oliguria. Esophageal involvement manifesting as gastroesophageal reflux and/or dysmotility may be observed in both variants. Tendon friction rubs, joint contractures, and inflammatory arthritis are more common in diffuse cutaneous systemic sclerosis but may be present in limited cutaneous systemic sclerosis. Auscultation or palpation near joints may be demonstrative.

Overlap syndromes may manifest with inflammatory myositis or cutaneous eruptions similar to cutaneous lupus or dermatomyositis.

▶ Laboratory Findings

Laboratory workup should include evaluation of potentially affected organs and autoantibodies. CBC, CMP, urinalysis, and N-terminal pro-B-type natriuretic peptide should be assessed. Most patients with SSc have a positive ANA. Other autoantibodies are correlated with disease phenotype (Table 15-2), though overlap exists.

Skin biopsy demonstrates thickened, hyalinized collagen in the dermis with "trapping" and atrophy of adnexal structures as well as loss of subcutaneous fat. Occasionally a sparse perivascular lymphocytic infiltrate may be observed.

A transthoracic echocardiogram (TTE) and complete pulmonary function testing (PFTs), including diffusing capacity for carbon monoxide (DLCO), should be obtained and periodically repeated to evaluate for pulmonary hypertension and ILD. High-resolution chest CT imaging should be performed if there is suspicion for ILD, and endoscopy or manometry considered if esophageal symptoms are present. For patients with renal involvement, close monitoring of blood pressure is important.

Diagnosis

Diagnosis is dependent on clinical, histopathologic, and laboratory features. Important clues include the presence of Raynaud phenomenon, nailfold changes or the early, edematous phase of sclerodactyly, and a positive ANA. Patients require workup and ongoing monitoring for cardiopulmonary, renal, musculoskeletal, and gastrointestinal involvement.

▶ Differential Diagnosis

✓ Morphea is important to distinguish, since systemic sclerosis carries substantial risk of internal organ involvement that may result in substantial morbidity or mortality (Figure 15-19). Generalized forms of morphea almost universally spare the digits. While arthralgias may be observed, cardiopulmonary, gastrointestinal, and renal involvement should be absent in morphea.

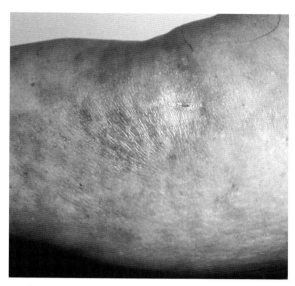

▲ **Figure 15-19.** Morphea. A circumscribed, lilac-colored firm plaque on the extremity. Morphea almost universally spares the digits when the distal extremities are involved.

✓ Sclerodermoid graft-versus-host disease is distinguished by clinical history.

Management

Treatment of systemic sclerosis is challenging and usually requires a multi-modal approach based on clinical presentation.

Mild Raynaud phenomenon may be managed with behavioral interventions such as avoidance of cold, moist environments, and keeping both the peripheral and core body temperatures elevated. Smoking cessation is generally recommended. More severe disease should be managed with calcium channel blockers (nifedipine or amlodipine) or phosphodiesterase-5 (PDE-5) inhibitors (sildenafil or tadalafil). Recalcitrant disease and those with persistent digital ulcers may require more aggressive management with endothelin-1 receptor antagonists (bosentan) or intravenous prostanoids (iloprost). Topical nitroglycerin formulations and digital or palmar botulinum toxin injections may also be beneficial.

First-line treatment for cutaneous sclerosis is methotrexate, although mycophenolate mofetil may be preferred when ILD predominates. Psoralens plus UVA (PUVA) or UVA1 phototherapy may soften areas of sclerosis. IVIG and rituximab may be appropriate for refractory disease and hematopoietic stem cell transplantation may lead to improvement in severe cases. Physical and occupational therapy are particularly important for maintaining and improving functional outcomes. Systemic corticosteroids should be avoided because they may precipitate scleroderma renal crisis in susceptible individuals.

Treatment of pulmonary hypertension overlaps with that for severe Raynaud phenomenon, and includes PDE-5 inhibitors, endothelin-1 receptor antagonists, and prostanoids. ILD may be treated with immunosuppressives including mycophenolate mofetil, cyclophosphamide, and oral tacrolimus alone or in combination with antifibrotic agents such as nintedanib. Lung transplantation may be performed if patients do not respond to the treatment. Angiotensin-converting enzyme (ACE) inhibitors are first-line treatment for renal involvement, and demonstrated to reduce morbidity and mortality. Renal transplantation may be necessary in severe or refractory cases. Proton pump inhibitors (PPIs) are preferred over histamine type-2 (H2) receptor antagonists for treatment of gastroesophageal reflux.

Clinical Course and Prognosis

Systemic sclerosis may be gradually progressive or follow a relapsing-remitting course. Prognosis is linked to both cutaneous activity as well as internal organ manifestations, which may be predicted based on clinical phenotype. Sclerodactyly and joint contractures may lead to severe functional impairments. Mortality among patients with severe pulmonary or renal disease remains high.

Indications for Consultation

Nearly all patients with systemic sclerosis should be managed in partnership with a dermatologist, rheumatologist, and, if pulmonary disease exists, a pulmonologist. Patients with renal involvement, particularly those with scleroderma renal crisis, should be managed with a nephrologist. Physical or occupational therapy should be consulted early to avoid functional limitations due to sclerodactyly or joint contractures. Systemic sclerosis may have a profound impact on quality of life, and psychosocial support may be needed.

Patient Information

- Scleroderma Foundation www.scleroderma.org
- Scleroderma Research Foundation https://srfcure.org/
- American Academy of Dermatology https://www.aad.org/public/diseases/a-z/scleroderma-treatment
- National Institute of Arthritis and Musculoskeletal and Skin Diseases https://www.niams.nih.gov/health-topics/scleroderma

▼ VASCULITIS

Introduction

Vasculitis refers to inflammation of blood vessels. Vasculitides are a heterogeneous group of disorders that may be classified by the size of the blood vessel involved: small (arterioles, capillaries, and post-capillary venules), medium (small arteries and veins), and large vessels (the aorta and other named vessels).

Vasculitides commonly affect the skin, and cutaneous involvement may occur primary to the skin or secondary due to underlying systemic diseases. Cutaneous features are dependent on the size of the blood vessel involved. Idiopathic vasculitides are rare diseases but prevalence, incidence rates, and demographics are distinct by subtype. In general, women are affected more often than men, and adults more often than children.

- *Small vessel* vasculitides (cutaneous small vessel vasculitis [CSVV], IgA vasculitis, and others) affect blood vessels in the superficial to mid dermis and result in dependently-distributed macular to papular petechiae and purpura. Some lesions may be targetoid, urticarial, or vesicular.
- *Medium vessel* vasculitides, such as polyarteritis nodosa (PAN), involve deep dermal and subcuticular blood vessels. Livedo racemosa, nodules, retiform purpura, or frank necrosis may result.
- *Small and medium vessel* vasculitides, characterized by the antineutrophil cytoplasmic antibody (ANCA)-associated vasculitides, may have features of both.
- *Large vessel* vasculitides, including temporal arteritis, may have prominent systemic symptoms. In comparison to medium vessel vasculitides, more exaggerated nodules or necrosis may be present.

Pathogenesis

The pathogenesis is generally divided into immune complex-mediated vasculitides (CSVV, cryoglobulinemic vasculitis, PAN) and pauci-immune-mediated vasculitides (ANCA-associated vasculitis).

▶ Immune Complex-Mediated Vasculitis

Medications, infection, or other environmental stimuli, or endogenous factors such as autoimmunity or malignancy, may trigger immune complex formation against various antigens. Complement fixation results in a mast cell activation, C3a and C5a anaphylatoxin generation, and neutrophil chemotaxis, leading to neutrophil-mediated vascular destruction and the characteristic clinical and histopathologic findings.[28]

▶ Pauci-Immune-Mediated Vasculitis

Like immune complex-mediated vasculitis, an exogenous trigger, such as an upper respiratory infection, activates neutrophils and leads to upregulation of proinflammatory cytokines, adhesion molecules, and activation of endothelial cells.[29] This stimulates cell surface expression of ANCA autoantigens; circulating ANCAs further stimulate neutrophil chemotaxis and immune-mediated vascular destruction.[29]

Clinical Presentation

▶ Cutaneous Small Vessel Vasculitis

Cutaneous small vessel vasculitis is the most common cutaneous vasculitis. The annual incidence is about 40 per million person-years.[30] In about half of cases, the trigger for cutaneous small vessel vasculitis is unknown. Bacterial and viral infections, underlying inflammatory conditions (including autoimmune connective tissue disorders and inflammatory bowel disease [IBD]), and drug exposure account for most of the remainder, while underlying malignancy, usually hematologic, causes a minority of cases.

History and Physical Examination

Macular to papular petechiae and purpura are distributed on dependent body surfaces and in areas where clothing is tight (Figure 15-20). Koebner's isomorphic response, the spread of new lesions into areas of trauma, may be observed. In cutaneous small vessel vasculitis, lesions may appear targetoid, urticarial, or vesicular. The eruption may be asymptomatic or associated with burning, itching, or pain. Arthralgias are common, but hematuria, proteinuria, and abdominal pain raise the concern for systemic involvement, including glomerulonephritis and gastrointestinal disease. Postinflammatory dyspigmentation is commonly observed and may persist long after resolution of inflammation.

IgA vasculitis (including *Henoch-Schonlein purpura*) is an IgA-predominant vasculitis that confers a higher risk of systemic involvement and may be complicated by persistent renal involvement (Figure 15-21). In children it is more common following an upper respiratory infection. Arthralgias, colicky abdominal pain and

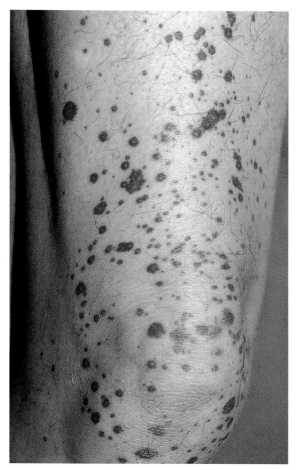

▲ **Figure 15-21.** IgA vasculitis. Purpuric macules and papules on the leg; the cutaneous findings are clinically indistinguishable from the more common IgG-mediated cutaneous small vessel vasculitis, although the IgA variant confers an increased risk of systemic involvement.

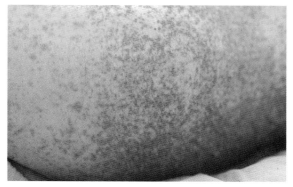

▲ **Figure 15-20.** Petechiae are purpuric macules indicative of extravasated erythrocytes. In cutaneous small vessel vasculitis, they may precede or appear concurrent with the better-known "palpable purpura."

gastrointestinal bleeding, and microscopic hematuria and proteinuria are commonly observed. Intussusception may be a complication.

Urticarial vasculitis may be associated with underlying SLE and systemic symptoms. Urticarial lesions persist >24 hours, distinguishing them from spontaneous urticaria (Figure 15-22). In addition to greater risk of arthritis and renal involvement, patients with *hypocomplementemic urticarial vasculitis syndrome*, characterized by urticarial vasculitis with depressed complement levels, show increased risk of chronic obstructive pulmonary disease (COPD) and ocular symptoms.

Cryoglobulinemic vasculitis is reviewed later in this chapter. *Erythema elevatum diutinum* is rare, sclerosing

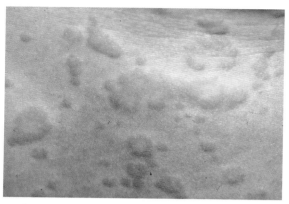

▲ **Figure 15-22.** Urticarial vasculitis. Urticarial papules and plaques with persist >24 hours and are associated with an underlying cutaneous small vessel vasculitis.

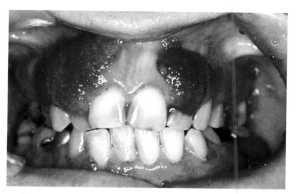

▲ **Figure 15-23.** Strawberry gums. Friable, hyperplastic gingival tissue pathognomonic for granulomatosis with polyangiitis.

small vessel vasculitis that may be associated with infection, IBD, or IgA monoclonal gammopathy.

Laboratory Findings

Patients should be evaluated for systemic involvement with a CBC, CMP, and urinalysis with microscopy to assess for renal dysfunction, hematuria, proteinuria, and red cell casts. Further workup may be directed by severity of symptoms or suspicion for underlying disease, and include ESR, CRP, 24-hour urine protein and creatinine clearance, stool guaiac, ANA, rheumatoid factor (RF), cryoglobulins, complement levels (for urticarial vasculitis), serum protein electrophoresis (SPEP), and hepatitis B and C serologies.

Skin biopsy demonstrates leukocytoclastic vasculitis in the superficial to mid dermis with perivascular and trans-mural neutrophils, nuclear karyorrhexis and leukocytocla-sia, fibrinoid necrosis of vessel walls, and extravasation of erythrocytes are observed. Perilesional direct immunofluo-rescence is important prognostically; perivascular IgA pre-dominance informs a diagnosis of IgA vasculitis.

▶ ANCA-associated vasculitides

ANCA-associated vasculitides are rare, with a combined prevalence of about 40 per 100,000.[31] Granulomatosis with polyangiitis (GPA) and microscopic polyangiitis (MPA) are more common than eosinophilic granuloma-tosis with polyangiitis (EGPA; Churg-Strauss syndrome). Constitutional symptoms, including fever, weight loss, and arthritis, are common.

Granulomatosis with Polyangiitis

Granulomatosis with polyangiitis is a necrotizing granu-lomatous systemic vasculitis, which most often affects the upper and lower respiratory tracts and results in a pauci-immune glomerulonephritis. Epistaxis, dyspnea,

hemoptysis, pleuritis, and cavitary lung lesions may be present. Ocular symptoms, including scleritis and episcle-ritis, are common. Mucocutaneous involvement includes palpable purpura, subcutaneous nodules, retiform pur-pura, and cutaneous ulcers. "Saddle nose" deformity, oral ulcers, and friable, hyperplastic gingival tissue ("strawberry gums") may be seen (Figure 15-23).

Laboratory workup demonstrates positive cytoplas-mic (c)-ANCA directed against proteinase-3 (PR-3) in over 90% of patients, but perinuclear (p)-ANCA targeting myeloperoxidase (MPO) may also be seen.[32] ESR and CRP are usually elevated. Chest imaging (plain films and CT) may demonstrate infiltrates or nodularity and diffuse alve-olar hemorrhage (DAH) may be demonstrated by brocheo-lar lavage (BAL). CT of the sinuses should be considered. Renal involvement may demonstrate impaired renal func-tion, proteinuria, hematuria, and red cell casts. Skin biopsy demonstrates leukocytoclastic vasculitis with perivascular and extravascular granulomas, which may involve vessels of the deep dermis or subcutis.

Eosinophilic Granulomatosis with Polyangiitis

Eosinophilic granulomatosis with polyangiitis is a necro-tizing granulomatous systemic vasculitis characterized by asthma and eosinophilia. Asthma and nasal polyps typically precede eosinophilia and subsequent development of vas-culitis. Peripheral neurological (mononeuritis multiplex) and cardiac (cardiomyopathy and pericarditis) involve-ment is more common than in granulomatosis with poly-angiitis, while renal manifestations are less frequent. Skin disease demonstrates features of both small and medium vessel vasculitis.

On laboratory evaluation, anti-MPO autoantibodies are present in approximately 40% of patients and confer a more severe course with systemic involvement.[32] Eosinophilia and elevated IgE levels are anticipated. Workup should include neurological and cardiac evaluation, particularly if anti-MPO autoantibodies are present. Skin biopsy demonstrates leukocytoclastic vasculitis with perivascular and extravascular granulomas. Eosinophils are conspicuous. Some nodules may show palisaded eosinophilic granulomas.

Microscopic Polyangiitis

Microscopic polyangiitis is a necrotizing systemic vasculitis which demonstrates nearly universal pauci-immune glomerulonephritis and cutaneous involvement. The lower respiratory tract is affected more often than the upper respiratory tract, resulting in dyspnea, and neurologic symptoms (peripheral neuropathy and mononeuritis multiplex) may result. Skin involvement most often manifests as palpable purpura, but signs of medium vessel vasculitis may be present.

Anti-MPO autoantibodies are seen in 60% of patients.[32] Impaired renal function, proteinuria, hematuria, and red cell casts may be observed. Chest imaging may show signs of involvement and diffuse alveolar hemorrhage (DAH) may be demonstrated by brocheolar lavage (BAL). Skin biopsy shows segmental necrotizing leukocytoclasic vasculitis which may affect vessels in the superficial to deep dermis and subcutis.

▷ Polyarteritis Nodosa

Polyarteritis nodosa has a prevalence of approximately 3 per 100,000; with reduction in the number of patients with hepatitis B infection, the annual incidence has decreased over time to around 1.5 per million.[33]

History and Physical Examination

Typical features of medium vessel vasculitis are present, including livedo reticularis, livedo racemosa, subcutaneous nodules, retiform purpura, or peripheral gangrene (Figures 15-24 and 15-25). Cutaneous ulcers may develop. Urticarial lesions may be observed in some patients.

Classic polyarteritis nodosa involves internal organs and may demonstrate constitutional symptoms, arthritis, myopathy (including cardiomyopathy), abdominal pain from gastrointestinal involvement, and hypertension from renovascular involvement. Peripheral neurologic signs include mononeuritis multiplex. Orchitis may be present. *Cutaneous* polyarteritis nodosa has skin-limited disease and a more benign course.

Laboratory Findings

Classic polyarteritis nodosa may be associated with underlying hepatitis B infection, while cutaneous polyarteritis nodosa may demonstrate p-ANCA positivity in a minority of cases. ESR and CRP may be elevated and leukocytosis may be observed. Renal function should be assessed with creatinine, blood urea nitrogen (BUN), and urinalysis, although red cell casts are not anticipated. Further workup

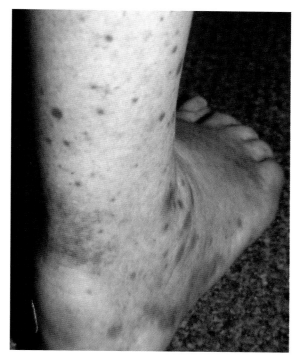

▲ **Figure 15-24.** Polyarteritis nodosa. Purpuric papules and plaques on the lower leg

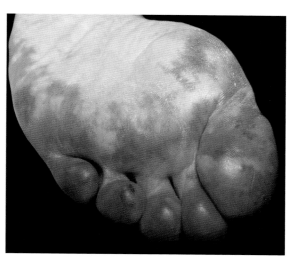

▲ **Figure 15-25.** Retiform purpura. Angulated, stellate purpuric, and dusky plaques on the foot.

should be directed by systemic symptoms, and may include chest or abdominal imaging, neurologic assessment, and echocardiography. Renovascular manifestation may be confirmed by angiography.

Temporal arteritis

Temporal arteritis (also known as giant cell arteritis) results from segmental necrotizing vasculitis of cranial arteries. Headache, jaw claudication, visual disturbances (including blindness) may be observed. *Polymyalgia rheumatica*, demonstrating fatigue and proximal and axial myalgias, is commonly associated. Tender, palpable temporal arteries with rare progression to ulceration of the temples or tongue may result. Elevated ESR and CRP are usually observed. Biopsy of the temporal or imaging (ultrasonographic or magnetic resonance imaging) are diagnostic.

Diagnosis

Diagnosis of vasculitis is based on clinical, laboratory, and histopathologic signs and symptoms. The skin examination is particularly useful for narrowing the differential diagnosis based on the size of affected blood vessels. Workup should be targeted to assess for systemic involvement as this carries prognostic implications. Skin biopsy with direct immunofluorescence can be particularly useful in establishment of the correct diagnosis.

Differential Diagnosis

Cutaneous Small Vessel Vasculitis

The most common mimicker is cutaneous vasculopathy, caused by hemorrhage or thrombosis resulting in petechiae or purpura. Hemorrhage into dependent areas of morbilliform eruptions due to hydrostatic pressure should be distinguished from cutaneous small vessel vasculitis by the presence of more characteristic rash on the trunk. Individual lesions in typical urticaria last <24 hours, in comparison to urticarial vasculitis, and pruritus is more commonly observed than pain or burning.

ANCA-Associated Vasculitides

ANCA-associated vasculitides may mimic one another; systemic signs and symptoms and skin biopsies are useful in diagnosis. The presence of glomerulonephritis can distinguish these vasculitides from polyarteritis nodosa. Cocaine-associated vasculopathy, which notably may demonstrate c- or p-ANCA positivity, can be easily screened for with urine or serum toxicology.

Polyarteritis Nodosa

Noninflammatory cutaneous or systemic vasculopathies are the primary differential diagnoses and can be evaluated by skin biopsy and coagulation workup. ANCA-associated vasculitides develop different systemic manifestations.

Management

Aggressiveness of treatment of vasculitis is dependent upon systemic involvement and disease severity. The discussion below will focus on cutaneous therapies; additional interventions may be required depending on extracutaneous manifestations.

Cutaneous Small Vessel Vasculitis

The majority of cases of skin-limited small vessel vasculitis will resolve spontaneously without treatment over a period of weeks. Symptomatic disease may be managed with rest, elevation, non-steroidal anti-inflammatory drugs (NSAIDs), or mid-potency topical corticosteroids. Colchicine or dapsone may be used for refractory cutaneous disease, but are less effective for internal involvement. The use of systemic corticosteroids remains controversial for IgA vasculitis/Henoch-Schonlein purpura, but may be used if the kidneys are involved. Methotrexate and hydroxychloroquine have been used for long-term control of recalcitrant symptoms.

ANCA-Associated Vasculitides

High-dose systemic corticosteroids in combination with cyclophosphamide or rituximab are used for induction therapy. Maintenance treatment with methotrexate, mycophenolate mofetil, or azathioprine is usually required. IVIg and plasma exchange have been used in refractory cases.

Polyarteritis Nodosa

Initial control of classic polyarteritis nodosa is typically achieved with systemic corticosteroids (1 mg/kg/day) with or without cyclophosphamide or rituximab, followed by transition to methotrexate, mycophenolate mofetil, or azathioprine for maintenance treatment. If there is concomitant hepatitis B infection, it should be treated. Cutaneous polyarteritis nodosa may be treated with medium- to high-potency topical or intralesional corticosteroids. Colchicine and dapsone may be beneficial for more widespread but skin-limited disease. If refractory, systemic corticosteroids, hydroxychloroquine, methotrexate, or mycophenolate mofetil may be used.

Clinical Course and Prognosis

Cutaneous small vessel vasculitis typically resolves over a period of weeks, but in cases where it persists, it may become chronic. Most renal involvement is mild but may require ongoing therapy. ANCA-associated vasculitides and classic polyarteritis nodosa should be managed aggressively to prevent morbidity and mortality. Cutaneous polyarteritis nodosa generally follows a protracted but benign course.

Indications for Consultation

Patients with skin-limited vasculitis should be managed by a dermatologist. Those with systemic involvement should be treated by a multidisciplinary team including a dermatologist and rheumatologist, and may include experts in cardiology, gastroenterology, nephrology, neurology, otorhinolaryngology, and pulmonology, depending upon signs and symptoms. Hospitalization may be required in severe cases.

Patient Information

OTHER AUTOIMMUNE CONNECTIVE TISSUE DISORDERS

Introduction

Several other autoimmune connective tissue disorders may have characteristic cutaneous findings. Below, skin changes associated with *rheumatoid arthritis, Sjögren syndrome, relapsing polychondritis, juvenile idiopathic arthritis*, and *adult-onset Still disease* will be reviewed.

Rheumatoid Arthritis (RA)

Rheumatoid arthritis is a common chronic, symmetric, inflammatory, and erosive polyarthritis that affects approximately 1.5 million patients in the United States.[34] Women are affected at approximately two times the rate of men, and onset is usually in the sixth decade. *Rheumatoid nodules* are the most common cutaneous manifestation and appear in 10–30% of patients.[34] Look for subcutaneous nodules over pressure points and periarticular areas that are usually asymptomatic but may be tender. *Reactive granulomatous dermatitis*, a term that encompasses palisaded and neutrophilic granulomatous dermatitis (PNGD) and interstitial granulomatous dermatitis (IGD), presents with erythematous papules, nodules, and plaques, sometimes with overlying crust, on the extremities or trunk.[35] These may adopt a linear conformation on truncal locations. *Pyoderma gangrenosum* (PG; reviewed later in this chapter) may occur secondary to RA. Pretibial ulcers, splenomegaly, and granulocytopenia characterize *Felty syndrome*; these patients are at increased risk of hematologic malignancy. *Rheumatoid vasculitis* is uncommon in the era of modern RA treatments. While classically described as a medium vessel vasculitis, smaller blood vessels may be affected. Its appearance is typical of these entities. Treatment is directed at the underlying RA, although surgical excision can be effective for persistent rheumatoid nodules. Adjunctive immunosuppression above that used in the treatment of RA may be necessary for pyoderma gangrenosum and rheumatoid vasculitis.

Sjögren Syndrome

Secretory glands are the primary targets of the autoimmune response in Sjögren syndrome, one of the most common systemic autoimmune diseases. Females are affected nearly 10:1 compared to males.[36] Sjögren syndrome may occur as a primary disease or in association with other autoimmune connective tissue disorders such as SLE or RA. The most prominent features are *sicca* symptoms, xerophthalmia, and xerostomia, but xerosis of other mucocutaneous sites (vaginal mucosa, skin) may develop. Corneal ulceration, thrush, and dental caries may be complications. Sjögren syndrome carries an increased risk of cutaneous small vessel vasculitis. *Annular erythema*, which resembles subacute cutaneous LE or tumid LE, may present on the face or other body sites. Anti-SSA and anti-SSB autoantibodies are expected. Sjögren syndrome patients should be assessed for the development of extranodal B-cell lymphomas, which may occur at 6–19 times the rate of the general population.[36]

Relapsing Polychondritis

Relapsing polychondritis is a rare, multisystem autoimmune disease typified by inflammation in cartilaginous tissues and proteoglycan-rich structures. Patients present with recurrent episodes of chondritis that may lead to cartilage destruction and disfigurement or loss of function. *Auricular chondritis*, characterized by bright erythema and swelling of the cartilaginous portions of the external ear with sparing of the cartilage-free lobule, affects 90% of patients and may be the presenting symptom in 20% (Figure 15-26).[37] *Nasal chondritis* is also common but may

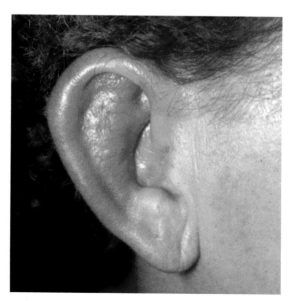

▲ **Figure 15-26.** Auricular chondritis in relapsing polychondritis. Note sparing of the cartilage-free lobule. Reproduced with permission from Knoop KJ, Stack LB, Storrow AB, et al: The Atlas of Emergency Medicine, 5th ed. New York, NY: McGraw Hill; 2021. Photo contributor: Lawrence B. Stack, MD.

be less clinically evident until permanent cartilage loss has led to a "saddle nose" deformity. Laryngeal involvement may lead to laryngomalacia and hoarseness; lower tracheobronchial involvement may result in airway collapse and is the leading cause of mortality.[37] Arthropathy is usually an asymmetric, nonerosive poly- or oligoarthritis. Episcleritis, scleritis, and conjunctivitis are seen frequently, and valvular heart disease or other cardiovascular manifestations are the second leading cause of death.[37] When found with aphthous ulcers, occasionally the term *MAGIC* syndrome is used (Mouth And Genital ulcers with Inflamed Cartilage). Diagnosis is clinical, but other associated autoimmune diseases such as rheumatoid arthritis are common. Mild cases may be treated with anti-neutrophilic agents such as colchicine or dapsone, while more severe disease may require systemic corticosteroids for flares and steroid-sparing agents such as methotrexate, azathioprine, cyclosporine, cyclophosphamide, or TNF-α inhibitors for long-term therapy.

Juvenile Idiopathic Arthritis and Adult-Onset Still Disease

These autoinflammatory syndromes are characterized by periodic fevers with associated transient erythematous eruptions, markedly elevated inflammatory markers, and risk for progression to macrophage activation syndrome or hemophagocytic lymphohistiocytosis.

▶ Juvenile Idiopathic Arthritis

Juvenile idiopathic arthritis (JIA) is a broad category of idiopathic inflammatory arthritis that affects children. Only systemic juvenile idiopathic arthritis (sJIA; Still disease) will be considered here since it is the primary variant with cutaneous involvement. This presentation is characterized by daily high fevers, widespread lymphadenopathy, symmetric oligo- to polyarthritis, and hepatosplenomegaly. An asymptomatic, erythematous, evanescent eruption occurs with fevers (Figure 15-27). Laboratory findings are not specific, but elevated ESR, CRP, and ferritin are expected. Leukocytosis, thrombocytosis, and elevated liver enzymes are also common. Macrophage activation syndrome, an overwhelming inflammatory response (cytokine storm) is a potentially fatal complication from multiorgan failure. Systemic corticosteroids are historically first-line therapy, but IL-1 antagonists (anakinra, canakinumab, rilonacept) and tocilizumab (anti-IL-6 monoclonal antibody) are emerging treatment alternatives.[38]

▶ Adult-Onset Still Disease

Adult-onset Still disease shares many clinical features with systemic juvenile idiopathic arthritis. Daily fevers, arthritis characteristically affecting the carpal joints, and hepatomegaly are typical. A transient, salmon-colored exanthem accompanies fever; it may be macular or urticarial. Elevated

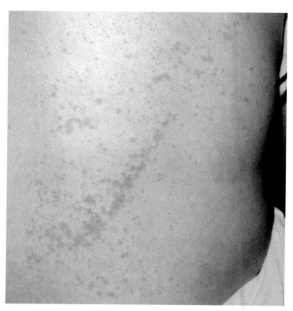

▲ **Figure 15-27.** Systemic juvenile idiopathic arthritis (Still disease). Evanescent pink eruption on the torso in febrile patient.

ESR, CRP, and markedly increased ferritin (>4000 mg/mL) may be observed, along with leukocytosis and elevated liver enzymes. Severe and potentially lethal complications include hemophagocytic lymphohistiocytosis, which may exist on a spectrum with macrophage activation syndrome, disseminated intravascular coagulopathy, and thrombotic thrombocytopenic purpura. Systemic corticosteroids remain first-line treatment. Methotrexate is the most commonly used second-line therapy.[39] Anakinra, canakinumab, rilonacept, and tocilizumab demonstrate promising therapeutic effectiveness for refractory disease.

ENDOCRINE DISEASES

Endocrinologic diseases have diverse mucocutaneous findings related to the underlying disease. These manifestations may offer clues to diagnosing the underlying disorder. In the following sections, cutaneous findings associated with *diabetes mellitus, thyroid disease, polycystic ovarian syndrome,* and *other endocrine and metabolic diseases* will be discussed.

▼ DIABETES MELLITUS

Introduction

Diabetes mellitus is a heterogeneous group of diseases characterized by hyperglycemia and resulting in effects on all organ systems, including the skin. Type I diabetes mellitus accounts for 5–10% of cases and results from immune-mediated destruction of pancreatic β islet cells.[43] Type II diabetes mellitus is caused by end-organ insulin resistance, ultimately resulting in decreased production, and accounts for 80% of cases.[43] The remainder are less common subtypes.

Cutaneous findings are seen in 30–97% of patients with diabetes.[43,44] Skin manifestations may precede other markers for metabolic dysfunction and allow for earlier recognition of prediabetic states, overt diabetes, or complications of the disease.

Pathogenesis

Many of the cutaneous findings in diabetes result from hyperglycemia and hyperinsulinemia. Elevated insulin levels further stimulate the insulin-like growth factor 1 (IGF-1) pathway in keratinocytes and fibroblasts, leading to common findings such as acanthosis nigricans and acrochordons.[45] Hyperglycemia-mediated microangiopathy may also play a role in the development of some skin lesions.

Clinical Presentation

▶ History and Physical Examination

More Specific Findings

- *Necrobiosis lipoidica* presents with yello-brown, erythematous, atrophic plaques with a red to purple margins and central telangiectasias (Figure 15-28). The plaques are typically well-demarcated and most often occur over the shins; ulceration may result. Historically, necrobiosis lipoidica was closely associated with diabetes: 60% of patients had diabetes and an additional 20% had impaired glucose tolerance.[44,46] More recent estimates have not demonstrated the same strength of association. Only 0.3–1.6% of diabetics, more often type I, have necrobiosis lipoidica.[44,46]

- *Generalized granuloma annulare* (but not other, more localized variants) has been associated with diabetes. Patients present with diffuse, symmetrically-distributed red-brown papules without overlying scale that coalesce into larger plaques (Figure 15-29). As they expand outward, plaques may become annular in shape, but non-annular variants are also common. Generalized granuloma annulare is found in only 0.3% of diabetics, but 21–77% of patients with the disease have diabetes, most often type II.[44]

- *Diabetic dermopathy* is among the most commonly observed cutaneous findings in diabetes, found in 40–70% of patients, and consists of irregular tan macules and slightly depressed, atrophic papules on the shins (Figure15-30).[44,45] Lesions are typically asymptomatic, but scarring may result.

- *Scleredema diabeticorum* is characterized by ill-defined, impressively thickened, indurated skin on the upper back, posterior shoulders, and posterior neck, though it

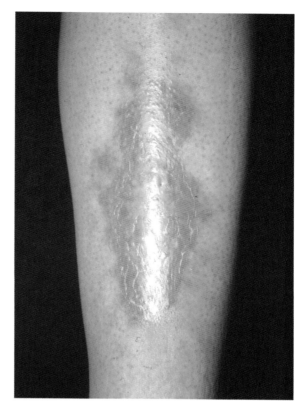

▲ **Figure 15-28.** Necrobiosis lipoidica. Yellow-brown to pink atrophic plaque on the shin.

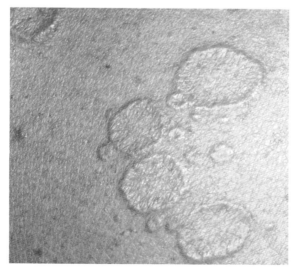

▲ **Figure 15-29.** Generalized granuloma annulare. Erythematous, annular papules, and plaques scattered on the torso.

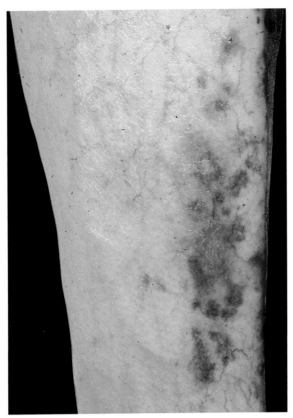

Figure 15-30. Diabetic dermopathy. Irregular tan macules and depressed atrophic papules on the shin, which may lead to scarring. Reproduced with permission from Charles E. Crutchfield III, MD.

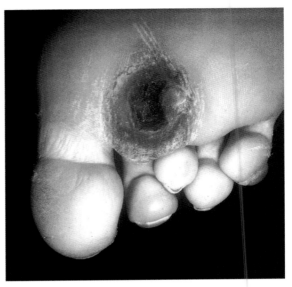

Figure 15-31. Neuropathic ulcer. Breakdown of thickened calluses over pressure points on the feet is likely the result of neuropathy, microangiopathy, and mechanical factors.

may spread elsewhere. Lesions are generally asymptomatic, though the involved areas may become stiff and range of motion limited. Poorly controlled, male type II diabetics are most often affected. Thickened skin over the dorsal hands, distinct from scleredema diabeticorum, is common among diabetics and may affect over 30% of patients.[44] It may result in *diabetic cheiroarthropathy*, inability to appose the palms (prayer sign). Numerous indurated micropapules over the dorsal digits and periungual, known as *Huntley papules*, are also observed in about 75% of patients.[44]

- *Diabetic bullae* are non-inflammatory, rapidly enlarging blisters that appear on the lower extremities of type I and insulin-dependent type II diabetics and may follow hypoglycemic episodes. While initially tense and filled with clear serous fluid, they become flaccid as they enlarge and may become secondarily hemorrhagic or infected. The upper extremities are less often affected.
- *Neuropathic ulcers* result from a combination of motor and sensory neuropathy, microangiopathy, and

mechanical factors in patients with longstanding or poorly controlled diabetes. A thickened callus, typically localized to the plantar forefoot at the metatarsal heads, breaks down into a deep, ragged ulcer (Figure 15-31). Lesions may be insensate, even when enlarging or secondarily infected.

Less Specific Findings

- *Acanthosis nigricans* is characterized by velvety, hyperpigmented plaques on the posterior and lateral neck, axillae, groin, or abdominal folds (Figure 15-32). Adults and children may develop acanthosis nigricans. Hispanics and African Americans are disproportionately affected.
- *Acrochordons* (skin tags) are commonly observed in a similar distribution along the neckline as well as intertriginous areas such as the axillae, groin, and inframammary and abdominal folds. Both acanthosis nigricans and acrochordons are more common among type II diabetics.
- Yellowish discoloration of the skin and nails, as well as facial erythema (*rubeosis*) due to microvascular changes, are seen frequently.
- *Eruptive xanthomas*, itchy to tender yellow-red papules on the extensor extremities and buttocks due to hypertriglyceridemia from insulin deficiency (Figure 15-33), and *acquired perforating disorders* (Kyrle's disease), hyperkeratotic papules on the extremities and trunk, are reviewed later in this chapter.

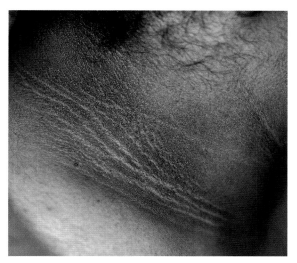

▲ **Figure 15-32.** Acanthosis nigricans. Velvety, hyperpigmented plaque on the lateral neck in a patient with diabetes mellitus.

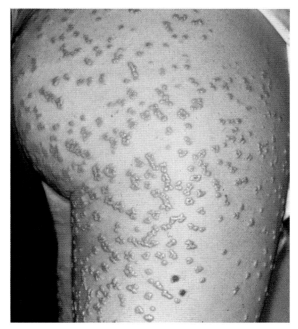

▲ **Figure 15-33.** Eruptive xanthomas. Itchy, pink to yellowish papules on lateral buttocks and thighs.

▶ Laboratory Findings

Elevated fasting serum glucose and hemoglobin A1c are anticipated, particularly in poorly-controlled diabetics. An oral glucose tolerance test (GTT) may be useful in prediabetics. Elevated triglycerides are seen in the context of eruptive xanthomas.

Diagnosis

Cutaneous manifestations of diabetes are diagnosed based on their characteristic clinical appearance or by skin biopsy. Screening lipids and a serum protein electrophoresis may be appropriate for patients with cutaneous xanthomas.

▶ Differential Diagnosis

✓ Early lesions of necrobiosis lipoidica may resemble nummular dermatitis or psoriasis.

✓ Generalized granuloma annulare should be distinguished from eczematous reactions and tinea corporis; lack of scale is characteristic.

✓ Scleredema diabeticorum has a different distribution and systemic manifestations than systemic sclerosis.

Management, Clinical Course, and Prognosis

Improved control of diabetes (both hyper- and hypoglycemia) is a goal for all patients, and may improve or prevent worsening of many associated cutaneous findings. Lifestyle interventions such as diet and activity level modifications are recommended.

Medium- to high-potency topical and intralesional corticosteroids are first-line therapy for necrobiosis lipoidica and generalized granuloma annulare. Narrowband UVB (nbUVB), PUVA, and UVA1 phototherapy may be helpful in refractory cases. Pentoxifylline has been used with some success in necrobiosis lipoidica. Systemic immunosuppressants such as methotrexate or mycophenolate mofetil, may work in both diseases. Refractory generalized granuloma annulare may respond to TNF-α inhibitors such as adalimumab or infliximab. The clinical course of both diseases may be protracted.

There are no consistently effective therapies reported for scleredema diabeticorum; a chronic course is expected. Topical and intralesional corticosteroids as well as PUVA and UVA1 phototherapy have demonstrated success in some cases. Pentoxifylline may be effective. Glycemic control does not treat scleredema, but may be preventative.

Neuropathic ulcers require diligent wound care and healing times are prolonged. Gangrene and osteomyelitis are frequent complicating factors, and amputation may be required.

Indications for Consultation

Poorly controlled or brittle diabetics may require a team-based approach with an endocrinologist. Refractory necrobiosis lipoidica, generalized granuloma annulare, and scleredema diabeticorum are most often managed by a dermatologist. Neuropathic ulcers require multidisciplinary care; a wound care specialist should be involved in care for these patients.

Patient Information

American Diabetes Association https://www.diabetes.org/

THYROID DISEASE

Introduction

Thyroid disease is very common; worldwide, the leading cause is iodine deficiency. In the United States, autoimmune thyroid disease is the leading cause of both hyperthyroidism (Graves disease) as well as hypothyroidism (Hashimoto thyroiditis). Cutaneous findings are present in the majority of patients, but may be nonspecific. Autoimmune thyroid disease also carries an association with other autoimmune skin diseases such as alopecia areata, vitiligo, and LE.

Pathogenesis

Graves disease is an autoimmune disease characterized by circulating anti-thyroid-stimulating-hormone (TSH) receptor autoantibodies, resulting in thyrotoxicosis. Specific manifestations of Graves disease, including *thyroid ophthalmopathy, thyroid dermopathy* (pretibial myxedema), and *thyroid acropachy*, are attributed to autoimmune-mediated cytokine stimulation of fibroblasts leading to glycosaminoglycan accumulation, rather than excess thyroid hormone levels.[47,48] In contrast, the clinical presentation of other causes of hyperthyroidism, such as multinodular toxic goiter or overtreatment of hypothyroidism, are primarily mediated by thyroid hormone levels.

Hashimoto thyroiditis (chronic lymphocytic thyroiditis) is caused by an autoimmune attack against the thyroid gland, most often due to anti-thyroglobulin or anti-thyroid peroxidase autoantibodies.[47] This results in the decreased secretion of thyroid hormone and the clinical presentation. Other causes of hypothyroidism include iodine deficiency, treatment of hyperthyroidism, localized radiation (e.g., in the treatment of lymphoma) or other iatrogenic insult, or postpartum thyroiditis. *Myxedema*, distinct from thyroid dermopathy, is caused by mucopolysaccharide accumulation in the skin. Congenital hypothyroidism is caused by thyroid hormone deficiency *in utero*.

Clinical Presentation

History and Physical Examination

Hyperthyroidism

Nonspecific cutaneous findings of hyperthyroidism include warm, moist, smooth skin, flushing, hyperhidrosis, and nail changes, including softening and onycholysis. Hair changes include diffuse, nonscarring alopecia and soft, fine, down-like texture. Hyperpigmentation and generalized pruritus may be observed. Patients with hyperthyroidism may also demonstrate weight loss, heat intolerance, agitation, palpitations, tachycardia or arrhythmia, weakness, oligomenorrhea, and loose stools (Table 15-3).

Graves disease may result in specific cutaneous findings. *Thyroid ophthalmopathy*, found in 20-50% of patients, may present with irritation, blurred vision, or diplopia. Periorbital erythema, exophthalmos, and excessive tearing are noted on examination (Figure 15-34).[49,50] *Thyroid dermopathy* (pretibial myxedema) is found in about 5% of Graves patients but as many as 15% of those with thyroid ophthalmopathy; it presents with a waxy, non-pitting edema, erythema, and induration typically localized to the shins and dorsal feet, but more widespread involvement may occur (Figure 15-35).[50,51] A *peau d'orange* appearance due to hair follicles is common, and as lesions

Table 15-3. Comparison of common, nonspecific symptoms of hyper- and hypothyroidism. Thyroid ophthalmopathy, thyroid dermopathy, and thyroid acropachy are all specific to Graves disease (see text).

Location	Hyperthyroidism	Hypothyroidism
Skin	Warm, moist, smooth, flushing, hyperhidrosis, hyperpigmentation.	Cool, dry, coarse, mottled, yellowish discoloration, myxedema.
Hair	Soft, fine, downy with diffuse nonscarring alopecia.	Dull, brittle, slow-growing, loss of lateral 1/3 of eyebrows.
Nails	Nail softening, onycholysis.	Brittle, striated.
General	Weight loss, heat intolerance, weakness.	Weight gain, cold intolerance, weakness.
Cardiac	Palpitations, tachycardia, arrhythmia.	Bradycardia, pericardial effusions.
Gastroenterological	Loose stools.	Constipation.
Genitourinary	Oligomenorrhea.	Menorrhagia.
Neurologic	Agitation, generalized pruritus.	Psychomotor slowing.

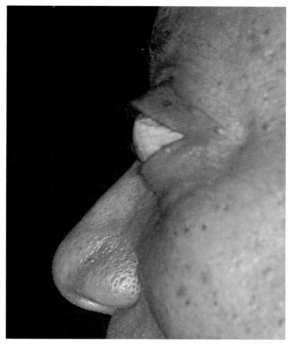

▲ **Figure 15-34.** Thyroid ophthalmopathy associated with Graves disease. Exophthalmos may be most apparent when viewed from the side. Reproduced with permission from Charles E. Crutchfield III, MD.

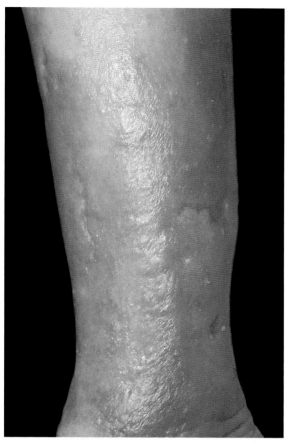

▲ **Figure 15-35.** Thyroid dermopathy associated with Graves disease. Erythematous, indurated plaques on the shins with characteristic *peau d'orange* appearance due to hair follicles.

progress, they may become progressively nodular or verrucous. There may be associated hyperhidrosis or hypertrichosis. *Thyroid acropachy* is rarely seen outside of patients with thyroid dermopathy. It is characterized by soft tissue swelling and periosteal bone formation of the fingers, toes, metacarpals, and metatarsals.

Hypothyroidism

Nonspecific cutaneous findings of hypothyroidism include cool, dry, coarse skin, mottling of skin, yellowish discoloration due to carotenemia, and brittle, striated nails. Hair changes include dull, brittle, slow-growing hair. Patients with hypothyroidism may additionally experience weight gain, cold intolerance, psychomotor slowing, bradycardia, pericardial effusions, weakness, menorrhagia, and constipation. *Myxedema,* distinct from thyroid dermopathy, presents as diffuse, non-pitting edema, a "doughy" texture to the skin, and facial changes including a broad nose, macroglossia, periorbital edema, and thickened lips. Loss of the lateral third of the eyebrows may be observed (Table 15-3).

In addition to typical findings of chronic hypothyroidism, *congenital hypothyroidism* may additionally present with intellectual disability, hypertelorism, an enlarged abdomen with an umbilical hernia, and delayed growth.[45]

▶ Laboratory Findings

Screening TSH as well as free thyroxine (FT4) is recommended in patients suspected of thyroid disease.

Patients with hyperthyroidism typically demonstrate elevated FT4 and appropriately depressed TSH. Radionuclide scanning shows increased radioactive iodine uptake in the thyroid gland. In Graves disease, MRI of the orbits can delineate extraocular muscle enlargement found in thyroid ophthalmopathy. Skin biopsy of thyroid dermopathy demonstrates full thickness dermal infiltration of abundant mucin, reducing normal collagen fibrils to thin wisps.

Patients with hypothyroidism demonstrate depressed FT4 levels; elevated TSH is expected in hypothyroidism due to thyroid gland dysfunction (autoimmune or otherwise), while a low TSH is observed in pituitary disease (central hypothyroidism). Subclinical hypothyroidism may demonstrate an elevated TSH but normal FT4, and may precede overt hypothyroidism. Hashimoto thyroiditis most often demonstrates anti-thyroglobulin and/or anti-thyroid peroxidase autoantibodies, but in some cases more obscure autoantibodies may be present.

Diagnosis

Diagnosis of thyroid disease follows clinical presentation and laboratory evaluation. Many of the clinical manifestations of both hyper- and hypothyroidism are individually nonspecific, thus a careful review of systems is necessary. Skin biopsy and imaging may be additionally useful in Graves disease.

▷ Differential Diagnosis

✓ Thyroid ophthalmopathy is usually distinctive, but other causes of exophthalmos should be explored, particularly if the presentation is asymmetric.

✓ Thyroid dermopathy can be confused with stasis dermatitis, lipodermatosclerosis, or cellulitis.

✓ Clubbing due to hypoxia may mimic thyroid acropachy, but the presence of thyroid dermopathy, thyroid ophthalmopathy, and thyrotoxicosis should lead to the correct diagnosis.

Management

Treatment of most cutaneous features of thyroid disease is by normalization of thyroid function. In hyperthyroidism, this may be through pharmacotherapy, most often methimazole or propylthiouracil, radioiodine ablation, or surgical thyroidectomy. Hypothyroid patients may be treated with synthetic levothyroxine.

The specific, immune-mediated findings of Graves disease are typically refractory to thyroid hormone normalization, and treatment is difficult. Thyroid ophthalmopathy is typically managed with systemic immunosuppressives; corticosteroids, IVIg, TNF-α inhibitors, tocilizumab, and rituximab have been used with variable success. Teprotumumab, a monoclonal antibody directed against IGF-1 receptor, was recently FDA-approved for the treatment of thyroid ophthalmopathy. Treatment of thyroid dermopathy is disappointing. High-potency topical and intralesional corticosteroids are first-line, often in combination with compression. Pentoxifylline and octreotide have been reported to be beneficial. Systemic immunosuppressants have also been used. There are no specific therapies for thyroid acropachy.

Clinical Course and Prognosis

With appropriate normalization of thyroid hormone, most symptoms associated with thyroid disease will resolve. Left uncorrected, hyperthyroidism may precipitate "thyroid storm," resulting in confusion, dehydration, fever, and death. Untreated, severe hypothyroidism may result in "myxedema coma," which may also be fatal.

Thyroid ophthalmopathy, thyroid dermopathy, and thyroid acropachy may be refractory to treatment.

Indications for Consultation

Patients with difficult to control symptoms of thyroid disease, or those requiring fine control of thyroid hormone, may be best managed by an endocrinologist. Thyroid ophthalmopathy should be treated in partnership with an ophthalmologist, and thyroid dermopathy with a dermatologist.

Patient Information

American Thyroid Association https://www.thyroid.org

 POLYCYSTIC OVARIAN SYNDROME

Introduction

Polycystic ovarian syndrome (PCOS; Stein-Leventhal syndrome) is characterized by chronic oligo- or anovulation, hyperandrogenism, and evidence of polycystic ovaries by ultrasound, although not all patients demonstrate all three findings. It is the most common cause of hyperandrogenism and one of the most common endocrinologic disorders of premenopausal women, occurring in 6–10% of the population.[52,53] Cutaneous manifestations of this multisystem disorder may be particularly distressing to patients and offer clues to proper diagnosis.

Pathogenesis

The pathogenesis of PCOS is complex and incompletely understood. Increased pulsatility of gonadotropin-releasing hormone (GnRH) by the hypothalamus leads to preferential upregulation of luteinizing hormone (LH) over follicle-stimulating hormone (FSH) from the anterior pituitary, ultimately increasing ovarian androgen secretion.[52,53] Insulin further stimulates ovarian androgen production and inhibits hepatic synthesis of sex hormone-binding globulin (SHBG), elevating circulating free testosterone.[52] Circulating androgens and insulin lead to the characteristic clinical manifestations.

Anovulation and further conversion of androgens to estrogens are attributable for the increased risk of endometrial cancer observed in PCOS patients.

Clinical Presentation

▷ History and Physical Examination

The cutaneous presentation of PCOS may be subdivided into signs and symptoms of hyperandrogenism and of insulin resistance.

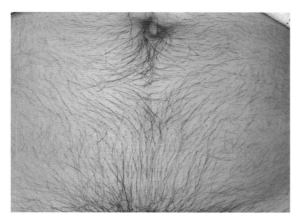

▲ **Figure 15-36.** Hirsutism is defined by excess terminal hair growth in a male pattern, as observed on the abdomen of this young woman. Reproduced with permission from Hoffman BL, Schorge JO, Halvorson LM, et al: *Williams Gynecology,* 4th ed. New York, NY: McGraw Hill; 2020.

Hyperandrogenism

Hirsutism is excess growth of terminal hair in a male pattern, most often on the upper cutaneous lip and beard distribution, areolae, lower back and abdomen, and superomedial thighs (Figure 15-36). It may be observed in 60% of PCOS patients, with variation by ethnicity.[52] Due to increased androgen-mediated sebum production, both *acne* and *seborrhea* may be observed. Acne in PCOS typically affects the lower face, neck, and upper trunk and tends toward moderate to severe and inflammatory. It may be refractory to typical therapies. Male-pattern *androgenetic alopecia* is less common, but presents with non-inflammatory hair loss affecting the crown and biparietal scalp. Signs of *virilization* are rare in PCOS, but may be observed. These include a deepened voice, increased muscle mass, reduction of breast size, and cliteromegaly.

Insulin Resistance

Acanthosis nigricans and acrochordons (see subsection on Diabetes Mellitus) are commonly observed in PCOS. *HAIR-AN syndrome* (HyperAndrogenism, Insulin Resistance, and Acanthosis Nigricans) is a subset of PCOS patients who demonstrate increased rates of virilization. Obesity and metabolic syndrome are prevalent in PCOS with associated risk of cardiovascular disease, non-alcoholic fatty liver disease (NAFLD), and non-alcoholic steatohepatitis (NASH).

Oligo- or anovulation is anticipated in PCOS, and patients have difficulty conceiving. Patients with PCOS also have higher rates of obstructive sleep apnea and endometrial cancer.

▶ Laboratory Findings

An elevated LH:FSH ratio greater than 2-3:1 is anticipated, but not universal. Dehydroepiandrosterone sulfate (DHEAS) levels are typically elevated but should be below 700 µg/dL. Serum total and free testosterone, and the corresponding free androgen index (FAI) (ratio of free testosterone to SHBG), may be elevated, but many patients with PCOS have normal circulating levels of androgens and likely have increased sensitivity at the level of the androgen receptor. A pelvic ultrasound may demonstrate characteristic polycystic ovaries.

Further evaluation for insulin resistance, including fasting serum glucose and a glucose tolerance test (GTT) should be considered.

Diagnosis

Diagnosis is clinical. The presence of menstrual irregularities and hyperandrogenism should raise suspicion for PCOS and prompt further workup.

▶ Differential Diagnosis

Exclusion of ovarian or adrenal causes of hyperandrogenism is important. Virilizing tumors of the ovary or adrenals result in greater elevations of testosterone (>200 ng/dL) and DHEAS (>700 µg/dL). Hyperprolactinemia and hypothyroidism may result in oligo- or anovulation but typically demonstrate different systemic features. Serum prolactin and thyroid hormone studies, respectively, allow differentiation.

Acne vulgaris and female pattern androgenetic alopecia are common among premenopausal females and may not be associated with PCOS. It is important to understand that physiologic ethnic variation in body and facial hair patterns observed in patients of Mediterranean or South Asian descent is not hirsutism.

Management

Behavioral modifications to diet and activity levels are recommended in most patients, as these beneficially affect the fertility and metabolic manifestations of PCOS though their effects on hirsutism and acne are minimal.

Hirsutism may be treated through physical or chemical *depilation,* the removal of the visible portion of the hair shaft (e.g., shaving). This process does not stimulate more rapid hair growth or conversion of vellus to terminal hairs. *Epilation,* complete removal of the hair shaft, may occur through physical (e.g., plucking, threading) or light-based (e.g., laser) modalities. Laser hair removal is only effective for pigmented hair. Electrolysis is an alternative. Eflornithine cream, which slows hair growth through inhibition of ornithine decarboxylase, is an effective topical treatment for hirsutism.

Like other forms of acne, topical therapies should be utilized in most patients with PCOS-associated acne (see Chapter 10). Treatment for androgenetic alopecia may involve use of topical minoxidil 5% foam or solution. Care should be taken to apply this to areas of hair loss only, or unintended terminal hair growth may result.

Antiandrogenic combined oral contraceptive pills are the first-line systemic pharmacotherapy and demonstrate beneficial effects on menstrual irregularities, hirsutism, and acne. Spironolactone, an antiandrogen, is typically added for patients with refractory hirsutism, acne, and/or androgenetic alopecia at a starting dose of 50 mg daily. Other antiandrogens, such as flutamide or finasteride, are not routinely used for the treatment of hirsutism or acne in PCOS. Refractory acne vulgaris may be managed with additional oral antibiotics or isotretinoin.

Metformin is the preferred agent for insulin resistance in PCOS. It may demonstrate beneficial effects on hirsutism, acne, and acanthosis nigricans.[54]

Clinical Course and Prognosis

Lifestyle modifications and pharmacotherapy may reduce the risk of associated diseases, including metabolic syndrome, cardiovascular disease, obstructive sleep apnea, non-alcoholic liver disease, and endometrial cancer. Unfortunately many of the therapies directed at hirsutism and acne do not demonstrate therapeutic durability; recurrence of hair growth and acne is expected upon cessation of treatment.

Indications for Consultation

Patients with PCOS should be managed in partnership with an endocrinologist, dermatologist, and gynecologist, depending upon their clinical manifestations. Due to reduced fertility, those wishing to conceive should be referred to a reproductive endocrinologist or fertility specialist.

Patient Information

- The American College of Obstetricians and Gynecologists https://www.acog.org/patient-resources/faqs/gynecologic-problems/polycystic-ovary-syndrome
- PCOS Awareness Association https://www.pcosaa.org/pcos-home
- The National Polycystic Ovarian Syndrome Association https://pcoschallenge.org/

OTHER ENDOCRINE AND METABOLIC DISEASES

Acromegaly and Gigantism

Acromegaly and gigantism are due to growth hormone (GH) excess, most often from a pituitary adenoma. If growth hormone excess occurs before closure of the epiphyseal growth plates, gigantism may result; if excess occurs afterwards, it manifests clinically as acromegaly. Skin thickening due to glycosaminoglycan deposition and thickened collagen fibrils may lead to coarse facial features, including enlargement of the brows, nose, lips, tongue, and chin, with frontal bossing and increased size of the hands and feet. *Cutis verticis gyrata*, furrowing of the scalp and posterior neck, may be observed. Increased sebaceous and sweat gland activity may lead to oily skin and hyperhidrosis. Treatment involves removal of the adenoma with adjunctive somatostatin analogs (octreotide).

Adrenal Dysfunction

▶ Cushing Syndrome

Cushing syndrome results from hypercortisolemia, which may be due to increased secretion of adrenocorticotropic hormone (ACTH) by the pituitary (Cushing disease) or other tumor, increased secretion of cortisol from the adrenal glands, or exogenous systemic corticosteroid administration. The most conspicuous manifestation is the Cushingoid body habitus, demonstrating enlargement of fat pads on the cheeks (moon facies), dorsocervical area (buffalo hump), and supraclavicular area. Central obesity and thinning of the extremities due to loss of muscle mass is observed. Other cutaneous signs include broad, dark purple *striae* (in contrast to the thin, pale to pink striae typically observed due to pregnancy, weight gain, or rapid growth spurts), delayed wound healing, and acneiform eruptions. Diabetes, hypertension, and osteoporosis may be complicating factors. Surgical removal of the tumor, or in iatrogenic case, gradual taper of systemic corticosteroids, is warranted.

▶ Addison Disease

Addison disease is due to adrenal insufficiency, most often due to autoimmune or infection-mediated destruction of the adrenal glands. Decreased cortisol production results in loss of feedback inhibition on the hypothalamic-pituitary axis, resulting in increased secretion of corticotropin releasing hormone (CRH). Production of proopiomelanocortin, the precursor to ACTH as well as melanocyte-stimulating hormone (MSH), is increased. Cutaneous hyperpigmentation most often distributed on sun exposed sites, as well as the palmar creases, hair, nails, and on mucosal surfaces, results from increased MSH.[45] Decreased axillary and genital hair may occur in female patients due to loss of adrenal androgen production.[45] Associated mineralocorticoid deficiencies resulting in hyponatremia, hyperkalemia, and metabolic acidosis, may be life-threatening. Treatment requires exogenous corticosteroid and mineralocorticoid supplementation.

Xanthomas

Xanthomas result from dermal collections of lipid-laden macrophages, or occasionally, extracellular lipid deposition in the dermis.[55] They occur most often in the setting

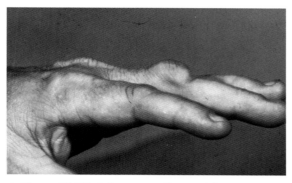

▲ **Figure 15-37.** Tuberous xanthoma. A large subcutaneous nodule overlying the third proximal interphalangeal joint of the hand.

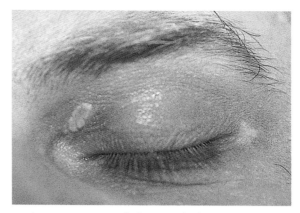

▲ **Figure 15-38.** Xanthelasma palpebrarum. Thin, yellowish plaques on the periocular areas. While in may be associated with hyperlipidemia, half of patients have normal lipid levels and should be evaluated for monoclonal gammopathy.

of primary or secondary hyperlipidemia and may signify increased risk of cardiovascular disease.

Eruptive xanthomas are itchy to tender, erythematous to yellowish papules that rapidly appear on the extensor extremities and buttocks due to highly elevated triglyceride levels; pancreatitis due to hypertriglyceridemia may occur (Figure 15-33). They may be observed in diabetes mellitus and typically respond promptly to triglyceride-lowering therapies. *Tuberous xanthomas* are larger, yellowish, subcutaneous papules and nodules that appear in a similar distribution but are due to hypercholesterolemia or hypertriglyceridemia (Figure 15-37). *Tendinous xanthomas* manifest as subcutaneous papules and nodules on the Achilles tendon, as well as extensor tendons of other areas of the extremities. They may be persistent even after correction of hyperlipidemia.

Plane xanthomas are thin, yellowish papules, and plaques that may occur at many body sites. While they are typically associated with hyperlipidemia, plane xanthomas may be associated with monoclonal gammopathies. In *xanthelasma palpebrarum*, thin plaques are located in the periocular area, most commonly on the upper medial eyelid (Figure 15-38).[56] It is associated with hyperlipidemia, diabetes mellitus, and thyroid disease; however, half of patients are normolipemic. *Xanthoma striatum palmare* describes plane xanthomas localized to the palmar creases; it is nearly diagnostic for familial dysbetalipoproteinemia due to apolipoprotein E mutation. Intertriginous and webspace xanthomas, in contrast, and essentially pathognomonic for homozygous familial hypercholesterolemia. The presence of xanthoma striatum palmare or intertriginous xanthomas should prompt cardiovascular evaluation given the associated increased risk of atherosclerotic heart disease.

GASTROINTESTINAL DISEASES

Diseases of the gastrointestinal (GI) tract may result in cutaneous pathology. Disorders associated with *inflammatory bowel disease* and *other gastrointestinal disorders* will be reviewed in the following section.

INFLAMMATORY BOWEL DISEASE

Introduction

The majority of patients with inflammatory bowel disease (IBD) have Crohn's disease (CD) or ulcerative colitis (UC). These autoimmune diseases predominantly affect the alimentary tract but have a variety of extraintestinal manifestations. Mucocutaneous involvement is common (Table 15-4). UC universally involves the rectum and progresses proximally in a contiguous fashion, while CD, in contrast, may involve any portion of the GI tract and is typified by discontinuous "skip" areas of involvement from the oral mucosa to the anus.

Table 15-4. Mucocutaneous findings and relative associations with Crohn's disease and ulcerative colitis.

Condition	IBD association
Perianal fissures, fistulae, skin tags	CD
Knife-cut ulcers	CD
Metastatic CD	CD
Indurated swelling of genitals	CD
Oral cobblestoning, granulomatous cheilitis	CD
Aphthous ulcers	CD > UC
Erythema nodosum	CD, UC
Pyoderma gangrenosum	UC > CD
Pyostomatitis vegetans	UC > CD

CD, Crohn's disease. IBD, inflammatory bowel disease; UC, ulcerative colitis.

Annual incidence rates are similar; UC is slightly more common than CD (7.3 per 100,000 versus 5.8 per 100,000, respectively).[57] Young adults are most often affected. Cutaneous disease is observed in approximately 10–25% of patients with IBD.[57,58]

Pathogenesis

Direct involvement of mucocutaneous surfaces may be observed in CD; the pathogenesis is identical to the granulomatous tissue response observed in the GI tract. Mucocutaneous disease does not occur in UC due to the nature of GI tract involvement. Both UC and CD may result in reactive lesions, caused by distinct pathology that may be due in part to antigenic cross-reactivity and immune stimulation.[57]

Clinical Presentation

▶ History and Physical Examination

Specific Findings

- *Perianal fissures, fistulae,* and *skin tags* are present in over one-third of CD patients and may represent direct extension of colonic disease or extraintestinal disease.[57,58] They are more common among patients with colonic involvement of CD. Linearly-oriented, deep fissures in the perineal or perianal areas may be referred to as "knife-cut ulcers."

- Granulomatous inflammation may occur in the oral mucosa and lips, resulting in *oral cobblestoning* and *granulomatous cheilitis* (painless, indurated swelling of the lips), respectively. *Metastatic* CD results in granulomas discontinuous with the GI tract.

- Painful, indurated swelling of the labia majora, scrotum, or perianal areas, as well as lesions on the trunk or extremities, may develop.

Reactive Conditions

- *Erythema nodosum* is a nonspecific, reactive septal panniculitis that may be triggered by infections, medications, pregnancy, or other causes. It is the most common nonspecific cutaneous manifestation of IBD and occurs in approximately 5% of cases.[57] Tender, erythematous to hyperpigmented subcutaneous nodules are usually localized to the shins but may be present elsewhere on the extremities (Figure 15-39). Oral and genital *aphthous ulcers* are commonly observed in both UC and CD.

- *Pyoderma gangrenosum* (PG) is a reactive neutrophilic dermatosis that presents with exquisitely painful, ragged or cribriform ulcers that have a grayish to violaceous, undermined border (Figure 15-40). IBD is the leading cause of PG and accounts for 20-50% of cases, with UC more commonly implicated than CD.[57,58] Lesions begin as a pustule, ulcerate, and rapidly enlarge. Deep

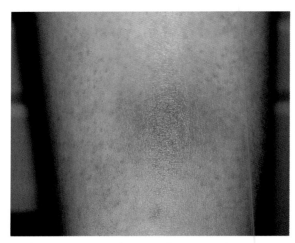

▲ **Figure 15-39.** Erythema nodosum. Tender, erythematous to hyperpigmented nodules most often located on the shins. This reactive condition may be triggered by inflammatory diseases (e.g., connective tissue disorders, inflammatory bowel disease, sarcoidosis), infection (e.g., hepatitis B or C viral infection, tuberculosis), medications, pregnancy, and other causes.

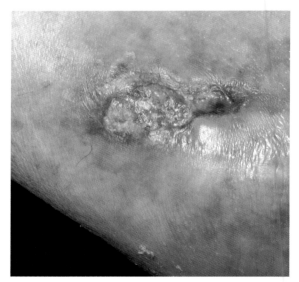

▲ **Figure 15-40.** Pyoderma gangrenosum. Deep, ragged, painful ulcers with a grayish-purple, undermined border. The shin is the most common location.

involvement with exposure of the subcutis, tendons, and skeletal muscle is common. Pathergy, induction of new lesions from trauma to the skin, is common but not universal. The most common site of involvement is the lower legs, but involvement of the peristomal skin is frequently observed. *Pyostomatitis vegetans* (PV) likely represents a variant of PG confined to the lips and oral mucosa that is strongly associated with IBD. Friable pustules develop into serpiginous erosions on the gingival, buccal, and labial mucosae, while crusting and vegetative plaques may develop on the lips. Pain is variable, even with extensive involvement.

▶ Laboratory Findings

Nonspecific inflammatory markers may be elevated. Eosinophilia is strongly associated with pyostomatitis vegetans. Histopathology of specific cutaneous findings demonstrates noncaseating granulomas in the dermis with a mixed inflammatory infiltrate composed of multinucleated giant cells, lymphocytes, plasma cells, and eosinophils. Endoscopic/colonoscopic findings and histopathology are diagnostic of GI tract disease.

The biopsy of PG is nonspecific. Histopathology demonstrates a dense neutrophilic infiltrate and may show underlying vasculitis. Microbial stains are negative.

Diagnosis

Patients with IBD often present with abdominal pain, diarrhea, and pain on defecation. Hematochezia and tenesmus are more common in UC, while weight loss, strictures, and extraintestinal symptoms are more common in CD. Diagnosis of extraintestinal CD is based on clinical presentation and diagnostic skin biopsy.

PG is a diagnosis of exclusion, and it is critical to rule out infection before initiation of treatment. In addition to skin biopsy, tissue cultures for aerobic and anaerobic bacteria, mycobacteria, and fungus should be performed. Additional recommended workup includes CBC, CMP, ANA, serum and urine protein electrophoresis, and ANCAs.

▶ Differential Diagnosis

✓ Specific mucocutaneous findings are typically distinctive. Other causes of perineal and perianal edema should be ruled out.

✓ Workup for erythema nodosum should exclude other causes, including infection, medication, and pregnancy.

✓ Aphthae may resemble herpetic infection, but are isolated to the mucosae rather than cutaneous surfaces.

✓ Mycobacterial, fungal, or other acute bacterial infections may be confused with PG. Other mimickers include venous stasis ulcers, arterial ulcers, and cutaneous squamous cell carcinoma.

Management

Management of the cutaneous manifestations of IBD parallels treatment of the underlying disease. Topically-directed therapies are generally disappointing for extraintestinal CD, but intralesional triamcinolone injections may have a role in limited disease. Systemic immunomodulatory and immunosuppressive agents for IBD are the cornerstone of therapy.

Systemic corticosteroids (0.5–1 mg/kg per day with prolonged taper) are the first-line treatment for PG. TNF-α inhibitors such as infliximab and adalimumab may be safer for long-term use and also benefit underlying IBD. Other steroid-sparing agents such as mycophenolate mofetil, azathioprine, and methotrexate have been used. Mild or limited disease may be managed with high-potency topical corticosteroids, intralesional triamcinolone injections, or anti-neutrophilic systemic agents such as dapsone or colchicine. Treatment of PV is similar; topical antiseptic mouthwashes are often utilized as adjunctive treatment.

Clinical Course and Prognosis

IBD follows a chronic, relapsing, and remitting course. Successful treatment of underlying IBD often leads to improvement in cutaneous symptoms; however, the severity of PG may be independent of intestinal disease. PG and PV frequently recur after successful treatment, often in the same location. PG usually leads to extensive scarring. Inappropriate serial, surgical debridements of PG can lead to permanent, disfiguring scarring and may profoundly impact function and quality of life.

Patients with IBD on long-term immunosuppressive regimens demonstrate an increased risk of skin cancer, and routine surveillance by a dermatologist is recommended.

Indications for Consultation

Patients with IBD should be managed in cooperation with a gastroenterologist. A dermatologist should be involved with significant skin involvement.

▶ Patient Information

- Crohn's & Colitis Foundation https://www.crohnscolitisfoundation.org
- National Organization of Rare Diseases https://rarediseases.org/rare-diseases/pyoderma-gangrenosum

▼ OTHER GASTROINTESTINAL DISORDERS

Introduction

Both *dermatitis herpetiformis* and systemic sclerosis are autoimmune diseases that may be associated with pathology of the alimentary tract.

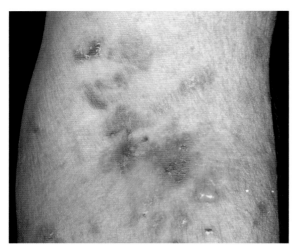

▲ **Figure 15-41.** Dermatitis herpetiformis. Intensely pruritic vesicles and erosions most often located on the extensor extremities and buttocks.

Dermatitis Herpetiformis

Dermatitis herpetiformis (DH) is an autoimmune immunobullous disease characterized by intensely pruritic papules, vesicles, and erosions most often located on the elbows, knees, and buttocks (Figure 15-41). The vast majority of patients with DH demonstrate villous atrophy consistent with gluten-sensitive enteropathy (celiac disease) on small bowel biopsy, but only about 25% of patients have symptoms of celiac disease.[57,59] Gluten-free diet is the mainstay of treatment for both celiac disease and DH; however, unlike the rapid improvement expected for bowel symptoms, skin symptoms may take months to years to improve.[57,60] Skin symptoms respond rapidly to dapsone, and relief of pruritus may be noted in as early as 24–48 hours. Chapter 19 contains more information on dermatitis herpetiformis.

Systemic Sclerosis

Between 40–80% of patients with systemic sclerosis have esophageal dysfunction, which manifests as gastroesophageal reflux or dysmotility.[61] Esophageal strictures and Barrett's esophagus may result. Proton pump inhibitors (PPIs) are the preferred treatment for reflux. Prokinetic agents such as domperidone or metoclopromide may benefit patients with dysmotility.

HEPATIC DISEASES

Cutaneous manifestations of hepatic diseases are common. In the following section, *cutaneous findings in chronic liver disease*, *cutaneous findings in viral hepatitis*, and *cutaneous manifestations of other hepatic disorders* will be reviewed.

CUTANEOUS FINDINGS IN CHRONIC LIVER DISEASE

Introduction

Chronic liver disease is particularly common and may be due to a variety of causes including toxic-metabolic insults, infection, and inflammatory disease. Many skin signs of liver disease are nonspecific to the etiology of hepatic dysfunction. In some cases, correction of liver disease may result in the improvement of cutaneous findings, while some changes may be persistent. Evaluation should include assessment of the liver's synthetic function and liver enzymes with a CMP and coagulation studies, viral hepatitis screening, and in select circumstances, autoimmune panels, and abdominal imaging. Treatment is generally directed at the underlying cause of liver dysfunction.

General Findings

- Hepatic *pruritus* is the most commonly observed cutaneous manifestation in patients with chronic liver disease and can have a profound negative impact on patient's quality of life, sleep, and daily function.[62,63] In some cases, this may be due to cholestasis resulting in elevated bile acid levels, but many patients with pruritus do not have elevated bile acids or respond to bile acid-lowering treatments. Cholestyramine has been used to treat bile acid-related pruritus. Other antipruritic agents such as gabapentin, naltrexone or naloxone, and antidepressants (selective serotonin reuptake inhibitors [SSRIs], serotonin-norepinephrine inhibitors [SNRIs], and tricyclic antidepressants [TCAs]) should be used with caution in patients with in chronic liver disease. Topically-directed therapy and narrowband UVB phototherapy (nbUVB) may be beneficial in some patients.

- *Jaundice* and *scleral icterus* is yellow to brown dyspigmentation due to hyperbilirubinemia >2.5 mg/dL.[63] Higher bilirubin levels generally correspond to more yellow-brown dyspigmentation, but the background level of each patient's natural skin pigmentation must be taken into account.

- *Spider angiomas* and *telangiectasias* may be observed in the general population, but multiple or numerous lesions should prompt evaluation for liver disease. Spider angiomas are composed of a centrally-located feeding arteriole and outwardly branching fine capillaries, resembling a spider or starburst (Figure 15-42), while telangiectasias are a network of superficially located capillaries. Both blanch with pressure and are attributed in part to hyperestrogenemia and increased circulating angiogenic cytokines.[63] *Palmar erythema*, also due in part to elevated estrogen levels, may be present diffusely and on the soles, but is most common on the thenar and hypothenar eminences. Portal

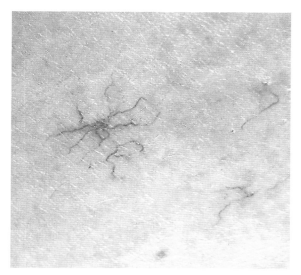

▲ **Figure 15-42.** Spider angiomas in patient with jaundice. These may also occur sporadically outside of liver disease.

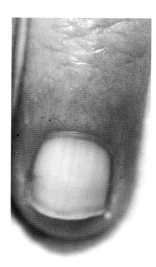

▲ **Figure 15-43.** Terry's nails (two-thirds nails). Apparent leukonychia of all but the most distal 1–2 mm of the nail bed.

hypertension may result in *caput medusae*, dilated and ectatic blood vessels visible on the periumbilical abdomen. Bruising may occur more easily and bleeding may become more prolonged with platelet sequestration and dysfunction of liver-derived clotting factors.

- Increased circulating estrogens may also result in *gynecomastia* and *testicular atrophy* in male patients. Body hair, especially in the genital and axillary areas, may become more sparse. Striae and a Cushingoid body habitus may develop in cirrhosis.

- *Terry's nails* (*two-thirds nails*) results in apparent leukonychia of all but the most distal 1–2 mm of the nail bed (Figure 15-43). Application of pressure resolves the leukonychia. *Muehrcke's nails*, attributed to hypoalbuminemia of various causes, including chronic liver disease, result in multiple transversely oriented bands of apparent leukonychia (Figure 15-44). Nail brittleness is common but nonspecific.

PORPHYRIA CUTANEA TARDA

Introduction

Porphyrias are a group of primarily hereditary disorders characterized by defects in heme biosynthesis. *Porphyria cutanea tarda* (PCT) is the most common porphyria and has a prevalence of about 1 in 25,000 in the United States.[64] The acquired form carries a strong association with hepatitis C infection.

Pathogenesis

Porphyria cutanea tarda results from inhibition of hepatic uroporphyrinogen decarboxylase (UROD) that is more

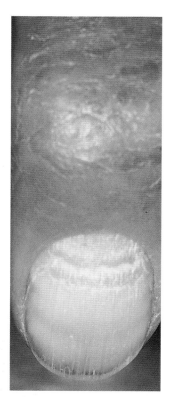

▲ **Figure 15-44.** Muehrcke's nails. Multiple transversely oriented bands of apparent leukonychia due to hypoalbuminemia of various causes, including chronic liver disease.

often acquired (80%) than due to an autosomal dominant mutation (20%); it is the only acquired porphyria.[64] Hepatitis C infection, alcohol and tobacco use, elevated estrogen, and iron overload in the setting of hemochromatosis are triggers for sporadic porphyria cutanea tarda. UROD dysfunction ultimately results in increased levels of circulating uroporphyrin and highly carboxylated porphyrins, which generate free radicals and are immunostimulatory when exposed to sunlight; characteristic skin findings are due to resulting inflammation and damage.[64]

Clinical Presentation

▶ History and Physical Examination

Patients present with skin fragility, erosions, and blistering on sun-exposed skin (Figure 15-45). Itch and burning are common symptoms. The dorsal hands, temples and superior cheeks, posterior neck, and forearms are most often involved. Milia, hypertrichosis, and chronic, sclerotic skin changes may be present in long standing cases. Other stigmata of chronic liver disease may be present.

▶ Laboratory Findings

Urinary porphyrins are elevated in porphyria cutaneous tarda. Serum and stool porphyrin levels may be normal or modestly elevated. When fractionated, elevated levels of uroporphyrin, hepta-, hexa-, and pentacarboxyl porphyrins are found. Up to 80% of patients with porphyria cutaneous tarda may have hepatitis C.[64] Elevated liver enzymes or evidence of decreased synthetic function is common.

Skin biopsy demonstrates pauci- or noninflammatory subepidermal blisters with festooning of the dermal

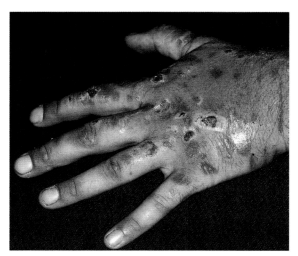

▲ Figure 15-45. Porphyria cutanea tarda. Note erosions, crusting, and scarring on the photoexposed dorsal hand.

papillae into the blister cavity. Hyalinized superficial dermal vessels and caterpillar bodies, composed of basement membrane material, are characteristic but not specific.

Periodic abdominal imaging should assess for the presence of cirrhosis or hepatocellular carcinoma (HCC), which may complicate the disease course.

Diagnosis

Diagnosis of porphyria cutanea tarda is dependent on clinical appearance, skin biopsy, and compatible porphyrin laboratory findings. Patients should be screened for hepatitis C and have iron levels evaluated.

▶ Differential Diagnosis:

✓ Pseudoporphyria may have identical clinical manifestations and is most often attributed to NSAID use or sulfa-containing diuretics. Porphyrin abnormalities in the urine, blood, and stool are absent.

✓ Idiopathic and drug-induced photosensitive disorders differ by histopathology and abnormal porphyrin laboratory findings.

Management

Treatment by reduction of iron stores through phlebotomy or low-dose hydroxychloroquine is effective for both acquired and hereditary porphyria cutanea tarda. The goal of phlebotomy is to keep ferritin levels <20 ng/mL, close to the lower limit of normal, which is most often accomplished through removal of 450 mL of blood every other week.[64] The dose of hydroxychloroquine is 100–200 mg twice weekly. In sporadic porphyria cutanea tarda, treatment should also be directed at the underlying cause. Photoprotection is important in the prevention of flares. Medium- to high-potency topical corticosteroids may serve as adjunctive treatment.

Clinical Course and Prognosis

Within several months, both phlebotomy and low-dose hydroxychloroquine lead to high remission rates. Urinary porphyrins should be followed during treatment, and therapy stopped when levels have normalized. Both cirrhosis and hepatocellular carcinoma may complicate the course of porphyria cutaneous tarda, and patients should be screened for with periodic abdominal imaging (typically ultrasound).

Indications for Consultation

Patients with underlying chronic liver disease should be cared for in partnership with a hepatologist or, in some circumstances when hepatitis C is attributed, an infectious disease specialist. Refractory cutaneous disease should be managed by a dermatologist.

Patient Information

National Institute of Health Genetic and Rare Diseases Information Center
https://rarediseases.info.nih.gov/diseases/7433/porphyria-cutanea-tarda

CUTANEOUS FINDINGS OF VIRAL HEPATITIS

Introduction

Hepatitis B and hepatitis C viral infections may result in more specific cutaneous findings than those observed above (Table 15-5). Due to their association with viral hepatitis, patients who present with the conditions outlined below should be screened for viral hepatitis and treated for infection. Additional skin-directed or systemic therapies may be necessary to achieve control of symptoms.

Vasculitis

Serum sickness-like reaction (SSLR) is associated with the acute, prodromal phase of hepatitis B infection and may occur in 10–30% of patients.[65,66] SSLR is caused by immune complex deposition. Patients present with diffuse urticaria, angioedema, and arthralgias. Hematuria and proteinuria may be observed. Skin biopsy demonstrates small vessel leukocytoclastic vasculitis. Treatment is primarily supportive, as SSLR will resolve as antibody levels rise.[66]

Classic *polyarteritis nodosa* (PAN) is an immune complex-mediated disease that occurs in approximately 5% of patients with chronic hepatitis B infection, but over 30% of patients with classic PAN may have hepatitis B.[63,66] When it involves the skin, classic PAN presents as a medium vessel vasculitis. Hypertension, abdominal pain, and neurologic symptoms may be observed.

Cryoglobulins are immune complexes that precipitate below 37°C. Type I cryoglobulins are composed of monoclonal IgM and occur in the setting of plasma cell dyscrasias; they result in microvascular occlusion rather than true vasculitis. Types II and III cryoglobulinemia may result in *mixed cryoglobulinemic vasculitis*, a small vessel vasculitis strongly associated with hepatitis C infection. Hepatitis B infection is a rare cause. Type II cryoglobulins are composed of monoclonal IgM directed against polyclonal IgG, while type III cryoglobulins consist of polyclonal IgM directed against polyclonal IgG. While up to half of patients with hepatitis C have circulating mixed cryoglobulins, only about 10–15% of these patients develop vasculitis.[65,66] Patients present with typical findings of small vessel vasculitis. Arthralgias are particularly common. Neurologic symptoms, gastrointestinal involvement, and glomerulonephritis may be associated. Diagnosis may be rendered through measurement of serum cryoglobulins and skin biopsy. Most patients are rheumatoid factor positive. Treatment of the infection leads to improvement, but immunosuppression may be necessary to control symptoms.

Lichen Planus

Lichen planus (LP) is an immune-mediated eruption that presents on mucocutaneous surfaces and has been associated with infections, medications, and environmental exposures. Oral LP has a strong association with hepatitis C infection, and over 25% of patients may carry the virus.[66] Papules, reticular or atrophic plaques, erosions, and frank bullae may develop. Oral erosive disease is often exquisitely painful, and symptoms may interfere with eating, drinking, and speech. Cutaneous LP tends to be less persistent than oral disease and less consistently associated with viral hepatitis. It most often presents as pruritic, flat-topped, shiny papules and confluent plaques on the ventral wrist and dorsal ankle (Figure 15-46), though more widespread

Table 15-5. Reactive cutaneous findings and relative associations with hepatitis B and C infections.

Finding	Viral hepatitis association
Serum sickness-like reaction	HBV
Polyarteritis nodosa	HBV
Papular acrodermatitis of childhood (Gianotti-Crosti)	HBV
Erythema nodosum	HBV > HCV
Mixed cryoglobulinemic vasculitis	HCV > HBV
Porphyria cutanea tarda	HCV
Lichen planus (especially oral erosive variant)	HCV
Necrolytic acral erythema	HCV

HBV, hepatitis B virus infection; HCV, hepatitis C virus infection

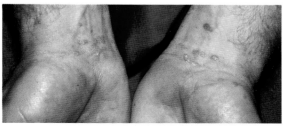

▲ **Figure 15-46.** Cutaneous lichen planus. Pruritic, flat-topped, shiny papules, and confluent plaques on the ventral wrist.

involvement may occur; profound postinflammatory dyspigmentation is common. Therapy for hepatitis C-related LP should involve treatment of the underlying infection, in addition to skin-directed or systemic treatment options (see Chapter 9).

Other Cutaneous Findings in Viral Hepatitis

Papular acrodermatitis of childhood (Gianotti-Crosti syndrome), which may present in acute hepatitis B infection, is rarely observed in the United States but is more common in Europe and Asia. Other viral infections such as Epstein-Barr virus (EBV) or respiratory syncytial virus (RSV) may be causative. Patients are rarely over 10 years of age and present with symmetric, relatively monomorphic, nonpruritic, erythematous papules on the face, extremities, and buttocks. Lymphadenopathy may be present. Treatment is primarily supportive as the eruption spontaneously resolves in 2–3 weeks.[66]

Necrolytic acral erythema (NAC) is strongly associated with hepatitis C infection and presents with itchy, scaly, deep red to purple plaques on the hands and feet. Hyperkeratosis, blistering, and erosions are common. The differential diagnosis includes necrolytic migratory erythema (glucagonoma syndrome) and zinc deficiency, but glucagon and zinc levels are normal. Treatment of viral infection leads to improvement.

Both hepatitis B and hepatitis C have been associated with erythema nodosum, a reactive septal panniculitis that demonstrates tender, erythematous to hyperpigmented subcutaneous nodules on the shins.

CUTANEOUS MANIFESTATIONS OF OTHER HEPATIC DISORDERS

Hemochromatosis

Primary hemochromatosis is an inherited disorder of iron transport resulting in iron overload. Grayish to bronze hyperpigmentation is the characteristic cutaneous finding (Figure 15-47), and it is often associated with chronic liver disease and diabetes, leading to the moniker, "bronze diabetes." Arthropathy and cardiac conduction defects may result, and iron may be deposited in the pancreas and pituitary, leading to widespread systemic manifestations.

Wilson Disease

Wilson disease (hepatolenticular degeneration) is an inherited disorder of copper transport resulting in tissue accumulation. Cutaneous manifestations are rare, but Kayser-Fleischer rings, greenish to brownish deposits along the periphery of the cornea, may be observed. Neurologic and hepatic disease are progressive without treatment.

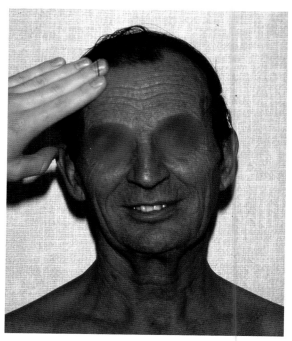

▲ **Figure 15-47.** Grayish-bronze hyperpigmentation from hemochromatosis. Note the dramatic difference in pigmentation of the patient's face and neck as compared to the photographer's hand.

PULMONARY DISEASES

Skin findings associated with pulmonary disease may share a common pathogenesis or be a secondary phenomenon. The following sections will focus on *sarcoidosis, pulmonary disease in autoimmune connective tissue disorders*, and select *digital and nail manifestations of pulmonary disease*.

SARCOIDOSIS

Introduction

Sarcoidosis is a chronic inflammatory disease characterized by noncaseating granulomas that can affect nearly any organ system. Pulmonary involvement occurs in over 90% of patients; over 30% have mucocutaneous involvement.[67–71] There are a wide variety of dermatologic manifestations of sarcoidosis, leading to its nickname as one of medicine's "great imitators."

Incidence rates vary by demographic factors. Females are affected about twice as often as males, and adults more than children.[70] In the United States, African Americans have a threefold higher incidence than White Americans (35.5 per 100,000 versus 10.9 per 100,000, respectively).[71]

Pathogenesis

The complex pathogenesis of sarcoidosis is not completely understood. Genetic risk factors, including various HLA and immune-related polymorphisms, confer increased risk, but no single gene mutation is solely responsible.[71] Various exogenous triggers are thought to lead to a dysregulated Th1 immune response with increased expression of TNF-α, IFN-γ, transforming growth factor (TGF)-β, and other cytokines, leading to granuloma formation.[67,69] TNF-α in particular is a critical cytokine for the maintenance of granulomas, driving interest in the use of TNF-α inhibitors as treatment. Foreign materials from occupational or environmental exposures, such as silicates, are occasionally implicated as polarizable material may be found in some sarcoidal granulomas. When present in old scars or tattoos, external trauma may be causative. Some cases of sarcoidosis may be triggered by infectious agents such as *Mycobacterium tuberculosis* or *Cutibacterium acnes*.

Clinical Presentation

▶ History and Physical Examination

Cutaneous sarcoidosis most commonly presents as symmetrically distributed red-brown to violaceous papules, plaques, and nodules with a preference for periorificial sites on the face as well as the rest of the head, neck, and upper trunk over the extremities (Figure 15-48). Most cutaneous lesions are asymptomatic or minimally symptomatic. Pruritus or tenderness are uncommon. Like other granulomatous diseases, lesions may appear yellow-brown (apple jelly) under diascopy (applying pressure with a glass slide against the lesion). *Lupus pernio* is characterized by centrofacial involvement, particularly on the nose, with disfiguring plaques and is associated with high rates of upper and lower respiratory tract involvement (Figure 15-49). Onychodystrophy is uncommonly observed. Less common forms of cutaneous sarcoidosis include lichenoid,

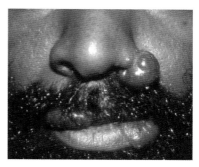

▲ **Figure 15-49.** Lupus pernio, cutaneous sarcoidosis. Erythematous to brownish firm papules and nodules located around the nares and mouth.

psoriasiform, atrophic, mucosal, and erythrodermic presentations. The *Darier-Roussy* variant is characterized by subcutaneous nodules on the extremities.

Erythema nodosum, a reactive septal panniculitis characterized by tender, erythematous to hyperpigmented nodules on the shins, is very commonly observed in patients with sarcoidosis (Figure 15-39). *Löfgren syndrome* presents with erythema nodosum, hilar adenopathy, arthritis, and fever. Bell's palsy due to facial nerve involvement is the most common presentation of central nervous system disease. Hepatomegaly may be observed.

Pulmonary symptoms may include cough, dyspnea, wheezing, and chest pain or tightness. Visual changes or eye pain may result from ophthalmologic involvement, most commonly anterior uveitis.

▶ Laboratory Findings

Angiotensin-converting enzyme (ACE) levels may be elevated in approximately 60% of patients, but are not specific.[68] Hypercalciuria, or less commonly hypercalcemia, may be observed due to conversion of 25-hydroxyvitamin D to 1,25-dihydroxyvitamin D by activated macrophages, stimulating intestinal absorption and urinary excretion of calcium. Hepatic or thyroid dysfunction is rare but may be noted on screening CMP and thyroid studies. Additional screening laboratory testing during workup should include a CBC, urinalysis, 24-hour urinary calcium, and vitamin D level. Plain films of the chest demonstrate abnormalities in 90% of patients; hilar or mediastinal adenopathy is most common but pulmonary infiltrates may be observed.[68] Pulmonary function tests (PFTs) may demonstrate restrictive or obstructive patterns, or hint at interstitial lung disease or pulmonary hypertension.[68,71] ECG may demonstrate heart block or other arrhythmias in cardiac sarcoidosis.

Noncaseating granulomas composed of epithelioid histiocytes with only sparse lymphocytic infiltrate are observed on histopathology. Microbial stains are negative, but occasionally polarizable material may be seen at the center of granulomas.

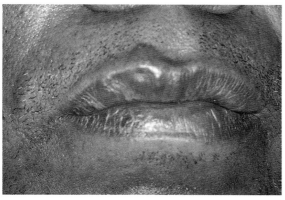

▲ **Figure 15-48.** Cutaneous sarcoidosis. A red-brown, indurated papules of cutaneous sarcoidosis on the lips.

Diagnosis

Diagnosis requires exclusion of other causes and is confirmed by the characteristic clinical presentation in combination with consistent histopathologic findings. Skin disease may precede systemic involvement, so all patients should undergo broad screening. Further workup should be directed toward signs and symptoms. Histopathologic specimens are most easily acquired by skin biopsy, but similar findings may be observed from other affected organs.

▶ Differential Diagnosis

✓ Exclusion of infectious granulomatous diseases that may demonstrate cutaneous and pulmonary manifestations (tuberculosis, atypical mycobacterial infections, and fungal infections) is critical.

✓ Skin-limited granulomatous processes such as granuloma annulare, necrobiosis lipoidica, and foreign body reactions may mimic sarcoidosis and must be excluded.

Management

Medium- to high-potency topical corticosteroids and intralesional triamcinolone are first-line treatments for cutaneous sarcoidosis; topical calcineurin inhibitors do not carry risk of skin atrophy but are generally less effective. Systemic corticosteroids may be indicated for rapid control of acute, severe internal disease, but are not safe for long-term use. Various steroid-sparing agents have demonstrated effectiveness in sarcoidosis. Hydroxychloroquine and methotrexate are first-line agents. Mycophenolate mofetil is an alternative. Severe or recalcitrant disease may be best managed with TNF-α inhibitors. Both adalimumab and infliximab have demonstrated benefit in sarcoidosis, but paradoxic induction of cutaneous disease has also been reported. Other immunomodulatory therapies such as doxycycline, minocycline, pentoxifylline, and apremilast have been used with mixed success.

Clinical Course and Prognosis

Most patients with sarcoidosis experience spontaneous remission in 2–5 years, but prognosis is dependent on demographic factors and disease subtype.[67] African American patients are more likely to experience chronic cutaneous disease more often than White American patients. Löfgren syndrome carries a favorable prognosis and may resolve more rapidly, whereas lupus pernio tends to be recalcitrant and may result in disfiguring scarring. Even when cutaneous granulomas resolve, persistent fibrosis may result. While most patients with pulmonary involvement have a good prognosis, pulmonary hypertension is the leading cause of death. Cardiac and neurosarcoidosis may also lead to significant morbidity or mortality.

Indications for Consultation

Most patients with sarcoidosis should be managed in partnership with a pulmonologist, and if skin disease is present, a dermatologist. Initial ophthalmologic screening is warranted since uveitis may be asymptomatic. Depending upon systemic manifestations, a neurologist, cardiologist, hepatologist, or rheumatologist may be helpful in treating patients with sarcoidosis.

Patient Information

- American Lung Association (https://www.lung.org/lung-health-diseases/lung-disease-lookup/sarcoidosis/learn-about-sarcoidosis)
- Foundation for Sarcoidosis Research https://www.stopsarcoidosis.org/
- Sarcoidosis Online Sites (S.O.S.) http://www.sarcoidosisonlinesites.com/

▼ DIGITAL AND NAIL MANIFESTATIONS OF PULMONARY DISEASE

Cyanosis

Cyanosis is bluish discoloration of the skin or mucous membranes, and most commonly observed on the distal digits, nose, and ears, although more extensive involvement may occur. It is nonspecific, but when associated with underlying hypoxia or digital clubbing, evaluation for an underlying cardiopulmonary etiology should be done.

Digital Clubbing

Digital clubbing (acropachy) is defined by transverse and longitudinal overcurvature of the nails with underlying soft tissue hypertrophy (Figure 15-50). Examination

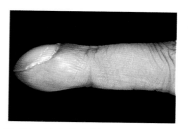

▲ **Figure 15-50.** Digital clubbing. Overcurvature of the nails and enlargement of the distal digit. clubbing is most often acquired from cardiopulmonary diseases. Reproduced with permission from Charles E. Crutchfield III, MD.

demonstrates an increase in Lovibond's angle, the angle formed by the proximal nailfold and nail plate, to more than 180° (normally 160°). Loss of the small diamond-shaped space formed when the dorsal surfaces of two nail plates are opposed (Schamroth sign) is anticipated. Most cases of digital clubbing are acquired and attributed in part to tissue hypoxia in the setting of cardiopulmonary disease.[72] Bronchiectasis, infections (including abscesses, tuberculosis, and pneumonia), COPD, pulmonary fibrosis, and thoracic and pulmonary tumors may be causative. Hereditary and idiopathic cases account for a minority. Inflammatory bowel disease or hepatic disease may also cause digital clubbing. Patients should be screened with a plain film of the chest and undergo further workup and management by a pulmonologist or cardiologist.

Yellow Nail Syndrome

Yellow nail syndrome is defined by the presence of thickened yellow to greenish discoloration of all 20 nails, lymphedema, and respiratory symptoms, though these manifestations may not be simultaneous (Figure 15-51).[73] The nails become opaque, overcurved, thickened, and demonstrate loss of the cuticle. Chronic cough, pleural effusions, bronchiectasis, and sinusitis are commonly observed.

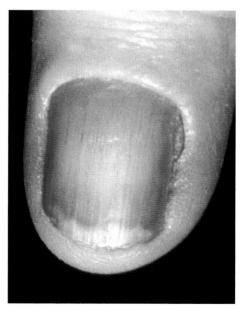

▲ **Figure 15-51.** Yellow nail syndrome. Thickened yellow nail plates which may be associated with lymphedema and respiratory symptoms.

Cutaneous findings are often present in renal disease and may offer clues for diagnosis and prognosis. *Calciphylaxis*, various *cutaneous manifestations of renal failure*, and *renal disease in autoimmune connective tissue disorders* will be reviewed in the following sections.

CALCIPHYLAXIS

Introduction

Calciphylaxis (calcific uremic arteriolopathy) is a rare, life-threatening calcifying vasculopathy that most often affects blood vessels in the dermis and subcutaneous tissue in patients with end-stage renal disease (ESRD). *Nonuremic calciphylaxis* affects patients without renal disease or those in earlier stages of chronic kidney disease (CKD), and is less commonly encountered.

The estimated annual incidence rate is 35 per 10,000 patients undergoing dialysis.[74] Females, White Americans, obese patients, and those with dialysis or undergoing renal replacement therapy (RRT) are more often affected.[75] Warfarin use is an additional risk factor.

Pathogenesis

The pathogenesis of calciphylaxis is not completely understood but results from two primary pathologies. (1) *Microvascular calcification* may be due to dysregulated inhibition of calcium-phosphate metabolism in the setting of low-level chronic inflammation, an elevated calcium-phosphate product or hyperparathyroidism due to renal disease, or other genetic or exogenous factors.[74,75] Adipocytes may become procalcific when exposed to high phosphate levels, perhaps accounting in part for the prevalent distribution overlying areas of adipose tissue.[74] (2) *Thrombosis* from endothelial dysfunction and calcification ultimately leads to the clinical manifestations.[74,75]

Clinical Presentation

▶ History and Physical Examination

Early lesions of calciphylaxis present with exquisitely tender to painful, ill-defined erythematous to violaceous plaques and nodules which may occur on a background of livedo reticularis or livedo racemosa (Figure 15-52). They are most often centrally located on the trunk or thighs. Progression to retiform purpura, bulla formation, or dusky discoloration may signal impending ulceration. Resultant stellate ulcers with black eschars are exceptionally painful and frequently become secondarily infected. Peripherally located lesions are less common and may be located on the digits or penis. Vascular calcification in other organs, including muscle, viscera, and the central nervous system, may occur.

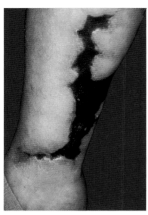

▲ **Figure 15-52.** Calciphylaxis. Extremely painful, deep ulcers with adherent black eschars on the lower leg. Reproduced with permission from Charles E. Crutchfield III, MD.

Laboratory Findings

Laboratory findings may be nonspecific. Elevated calcium-phosphate product and parathyroid hormone may be observed but are often normal even in patients with CKD or ESRD.[76] Elevated creatinine and blood urea nitrogen, with reduced glomerular filtration rate, are expected in patients with CKD or ESRD. Additional workup should include coagulation studies (INR, PT, PTT, factor V Leiden, protein C and S, antithrombin III, and antiphospholipid antibodies), CMP, CBC, and inflammatory markers. Vitamin D levels have not been shown to reliably correlate with disease.

Though there may be concern for exacerbation of the ulceration, skin biopsy is essential for diagnosis. A telescoping punch biopsy or incisional biopsy is preferred to improve diagnostic yield.[75,76] A telescoping punch biopsy, sometimes referred to as a "double punch biopsy," is performed by using a larger diameter punch biopsy (commonly 6 mm) to sample the epidermis, dermis, and superficial subcutaneous tissue. A smaller diameter punch biopsy (commonly 3–4 mm) is then used to sample deeper subcutaneous tissue from the initial defect. Microvascular fibrointimal hyperplasia, medial calcification, and thromboses are characteristic features. A mixed inflammatory response, epidermal necrosis, and panniculitis are commonly associated and extravascular calcification may be observed.

Imaging, particularly advanced modalities such as CT and nuclear bone scans, may demonstrate extracutaneous and cutaneous calcification.

Diagnosis

Diagnosis is based on the clinical presentation, exclusion of competing diagnoses, and skin biopsy findings. A high index of clinical suspicion is required. Pain out of proportion to exam findings may be an important early diagnostic clue.

▷ Differential Diagnosis

✓ Other causes of vascular occlusion that result in retiform purpura, including thrombotic and embolic processes and medium vessel vasculitides, are important diagnoses to consider. Clinical history and histopathologic findings aid in the correct diagnosis. Warfarin-induced skin necrosis may overlap. Purpura fulminans is important to rule out.

Management

Treatment of calciphylaxis is challenging and requires a multidisciplinary approach. Achievement of adequate analgesia and meticulous wound care is essential. Debridement of devitalized tissue may be required; in extensive cases, surgical debridement under general anesthesia may be indicated. Hyperbaric oxygen may be employed for wound healing.

If present, normalization of the elevated calcium-phosphate product is indicated. Cinacalcet and parathyroidectomy have been used in select cases. Patients on RRT may benefit from increased frequency or duration of dialysis, use of a low calcium dialysate, phosphate binders, and a low phosphate diet.[76] Calcium and vitamin D supplementation should be avoided.

Intravenous sodium thiosulfate is frequently used as a treatment. In patients on renal replacement therapy, this can be administered during hemodialysis. Anticoagulation may be indicated; however, warfarin should be avoided and there are concerns that subcutaneous anticoagulants may induce calciphylaxis lesions at the sites of injection, which should be rotated.[76] Other agents, including bisphosphonates, pentoxifylline, and vitamin K supplementation have been used but require additional study.

Clinical Course and Prognosis

The clinical course may be prolonged and prognosis is poor. Response to treatment is variable. Most patients require hospitalization and mortality is 45–80%.[74–76] The most common cause of death is sepsis.

Indications for Consultation

Patients with calciphylaxis should be managed in partnership with a nephrologist, dermatologist, and wound care specialist. Pain management specialists may be required to assist with achieving adequate analgesia. A surgeon experienced with cutaneous debridement may be needed if there is extensive involvement. An infectious disease specialist may be needed to manage secondary infections.

Patient Information

CUTANEOUS MANIFESTATIONS OF RENAL FAILURE

Introduction

Patients with CKD and ESRD may present with a variety of cutaneous findings due to metabolic derangement. In some cases, these symptoms may be alleviated by renal replacement therapy such as hemodialysis, while others resolve with renal transplantation.

Pruritus

Diffuse pruritus, often without apparent rash, is observed in half of patients with ESRD, and very common among CKD patients.[77] It may interfere with both sleep and daily function and may significantly impair patients' quality of life. The pathophysiology is poorly understood but likely due to a combination of subclinical or overt uremia, low-level systemic inflammation, xerosis, and/or upregulation of μ-opioid receptors.[77] Treatment is challenging and requires a multi-modal approach. Adequate moisturization is a cornerstone of therapy. Narrowband UVB phototherapy (nbUVB) has demonstrated success. Medium- to high-potency topical corticosteroids may be useful in areas of lichenification. Gabapentin may be effective in refractory patients.

Other Cutaneous Findings

Half-and-half nails (*Lindsay nails*) are commonly observed in patients with CKD or those on dialysis. It describes apparent white discoloration (leukonychia) of the proximal portion of the nail plate, with non-blanching reddish-brown discoloration distally. *Muehrcke's nails*, attributed to hypoalbuminemia of various causes including nephrotic syndrome, may result (Figure 15-44). In the setting of anemia of chronic disease associated with CKD, both *koilonychia* and *pallor* may be observed. Koilonychia is characterized by concave, "spoon-shaped" nails that are centrally indented and peripherally everted.

Acquired perforating dermatosis (Kyrle's disease) (Figure 15-53) results from transepidermal elimination of collagen, elastic fibers, or keratin in patients with CKD or other metabolic diseases, including diabetes mellitus. Patients present with itchy, erythematous to hyperpigmented, hyperkeratotic papules with central keratinaceous plugs most often located on the extremities or trunk. Topical corticosteroids, topical and systemic retinoids, and nbUVB phototherapy have been used with variable success. *Uremic frost* is a complication of highly elevated urea concentrations in the blood; it is rare due to use of renal replacement therapy. Urea is excreted by eccrine sweat glands and

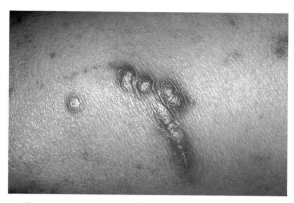

▲ **Figure 15-53.** Acquired perforating dermatosis (Kyrle's disease). Hyperpigmented, hyperkeratotic papules resulting from transepidermal elimination of collagen, elastic fibers, or keratin. Reproduced with permission from Charles E. Crutchfield III, MD.

precipitates on the skin with water evaporation, resulting in fine, powdery, white to yellowish crystals over the face, trunk, and extremities.[78]

REFERENCES

1. Rees F, Doherty M, Grainge MJ, Lanyon P, Zhang W. The worldwide incidence and prevalence of systemic lupus erythematosus: a systematic review of epidemiological studies. *Rheumatology (Oxford)*. 2017;56:1945-1961.
2. Durosaro O, Davis MD, Reed KB, Rohlinger AL. Incidence of cutaneous lupus erythematosus, 1965–2005: a population-based study. *Arch Dermatol*. 2009;145:249–53.
3. Grönhagen CM, Fored CM, Granath F, Nyberg F. Cutaneous lupus erythematosus and the association with systemic lupus erythematosus: a population-based cohort of 1088 patients in Sweden. *Br J Dermatol*. 2011;164:1335–41.
4. Wenzel J. Cutaneous lupus erythematosus: new insights into pathogenesis and therapeutic strategies. *Nat Rev Rheumatol*. 2019;15:519-532.
5. Almaani S, Meara A, Rovin BH. Update on lupus nephritis. *Clin J Am Soc Nephrol*. 2017;12:825-835.
6. Tselios K, Urowitz MB. Cardiovascular and pulmonary manifestations of systemic lupus erythematosus. *Curr Rheumatol Rev*. 2017;13:206-218.
7. Black DR, Hornung CA, Schneider PD, Callen JP. Frequency and severity of systemic disease in patients with subacute cutaneous lupus erythematosus. *Arch Dermatol*. 2002;138:1175-8.
8. O'Brien JC, Chong BF. Not just skin deep: systemic disease involvement in patients with cutaneous lupus. *J Investig Dermatol Symp Proc*. 2017;18:S69-S74.
9. Hedrich CM, Fiebig B, Hauck FH, et al. Chilblain lupus erythematosus--a review of literature. *Clin Rheumatol*. 2008;27:949-54.
10. Vanoni F, Lava SAG, Fossali EF, et al. Neonatal systemic lupus erythematosus syndrome: a comprehensive review. *Clin Rev Allergy Immunol*. 2017;53:469-476.

11. Concha JSS, Werth VP. Alopecias in lupus erythematosus. *Lupus Sci Med*. 2018;5:e000291.

12. Lyons AB, Trullas C, Kohli I, Hamzavi IH, Lim HW. Photoprotection beyond ultraviolet radiation: A review of tinted sunscreens. *J Am Acad Dermatol*. 2020:S0190-9622(20)30694-0..

13. Rahman P, Gladman DD, Urowitz MB. Smoking interferes with efficacy of antimalarial therapy in cutaneous lupus. *J Rheumatol*. 1998;25:1716-9.

14. Marmor MF, Kellner U, Lai TY, Melles RB, Mieler WF; American Academy of Ophthalmology. Recommendations on screening for chloroquine and hydroxychloroquine retinopathy (2016 Revision). *Ophthalmology*. 2016;123:1386-94.

15. Muangchan C, van Vollenhoven RF, Bernatsky SR, et al. Treatment algorithms in systemic lupus erythematosus. *Arthritis Care Res (Hoboken)*. 2015; 67: 1237-1245.

16. DeWane ME, Waldman R, Lu J. Dermatomyositis: Clinical features and pathogenesis. *J Am Acad Dermatol*. 2020;82: 267-281.

17. Bendewald MJ, Wetter DA, Li X, Davis MDP. Incidence of dermatomyositis and clinically amyopathic dermatomyositis: a population-based study in Olmsted County, Minnesota. *Arch Dermatol*. 2010;146:26-30.

18. Bogdanov I, Kazandjieva J, Darlenski R, Tsankov N. Dermatomyositis: Current concepts. *Clin Dermatol*. 2018;36:450-458.

19. Bowerman K, Pearson DR, Okawa J, Werth VP. Malignancy in dermatomyositis: A retrospective study of 201 patients seen at the University of Pennsylvania. *J Am Acad Dermatol*. 2020;83:117-122..

20. Tartar DM, Chung L, Fiorentino DF. Clinical significance of autoantibodies in dermatomyositis and systemic sclerosis. *Clin Dermatol*. 2018;36:508-524

21. Wolstencroft PW, Casciola-Rosen L, Fiorentino DF. Association between autoantibody phenotype and cutaneous adverse reactions to hydroxychloroquine in dermatomyositis. *JAMA Dermatol*. 2018;154:1199-1203.

22. Long K, Danoff SK. Interstitial lung disease in polymyositis and dermatomyositis. *Clin Chest Med*. 2019; 40: 561-572..

23. Marie I. Morbidity and mortality in adult polymyositis and dermatomyositis. *Curr Rheumatol Rep*. 2012;14:275-85.

24. Ingegnoli F, Ughi N, Mihai C. Update on the epidemiology, risk factors, and disease outcomes of systemic sclerosis. *Best Pract Res Clin Rheumatol*. 2018;32:223-240.

25. Pearson DR, Werth VP, Pappas-Taffer L. Systemic sclerosis: Current concepts of skin and systemic manifestations. *Clin Dermatol*. 2018;36:459-474.

26. Cutolo M, Soldano S, Smith V. Pathophysiology of systemic sclerosis: current understanding and new insights. *Expert Rev Clin Immunol*. 2019;15:753-764.

27. Woodworth TG, Suliman YA, Li W, Furst DE, Clements P. Scleroderma renal crisis and renal involvement in systemic sclerosis. *Nat Rev Nephrol*. 2016;12:678-691

28. Salama AD. Genetics and pathogenesis of small-vessel vasculitis. *Best Pract Res Clin Rheumatol*. 2018;32:21-30. doi: 10.1016/j.berh.2018.10.002.

29. Brilland B, Garnier AS, Chevailler A, et al. Complement alternative pathway in ANCA-associated vasculitis: Two decades from bench to bedside. *Autoimmun Rev*. 2020;19:102424.

30. Arora A, Wetter DA, Gonzalez-Santiago TM, Davis MD, Lohse CM. Incidence of leukocytoclastic vasculitis, 1996 to 2010: a population-based study in Olmsted County, Minnesota. *Mayo Clin Proc*. 2014;89:1515-24.

31. Berti A, Dejaco C. Update on the epidemiology, risk factors, and outcomes of systemic vasculitides. *Best Pract Res Clin Rheumatol*. 2018;32:271-294.

32. Pagnoux C. Updates in ANCA-associated vasculitis. *Eur J Rheumatol*. 2016;3(3):122-133.

33. Hernández-Rodríguez J, Alba MA, Prieto-González S, Cid MC. Diagnosis and classification of polyarteritis nodosa. *J Autoimmun*. 2014;48-49:84-9

34. Tilstra JS, Lienesch DW. Rheumatoid nodules. *Dermatol Clin*. 2015;33:361-71.

35. Rosenbach M, English JC. Reactive granulomatous dermatitis: a review of palisaded neutrophilic and granulomatous dermatitis, interstitial granulomatous dermatitis, interstitial granulomatous drug reaction, and a proposed reclassification. *Dermatol Clin*. 2015;33:373-87.

36. Parisis D, Chivasso C, Perret J, Soyfoo MS, Delporte C. Current State of Knowledge on Primary Sjögren's Syndrome, an Autoimmune Exocrinopathy. *J Clin Med*. 2020;9:E2299.

37. Borgia F, Giuffrida R, Guarneri F, Cannavò SP. Relapsing polychondritis: an updated review. *Biomedicines*. 2018;6:84.

38. Lee JJY, Schneider R. Systemic juvenile idiopathic arthritis. *Pediatr Clin North Am*. 2018;65:691-709.

39. Giacomelli R, Ruscitti P, Shoenfeld Y. A comprehensive review on adult onset Still's disease. *J Autoimmun*. 2018;93:24-36.

40. He Y, Sawalha AH. Drug-induced lupus erythematosus: an update on drugs and mechanisms. Curr Opin Rheumatol. 2018;30:490-497.

41. Vaglio A, Grayson PC, Fenaroli P, et al. Drug-induced lupus: Traditional and new concepts. Autoimmun Rev. 2018;17: 912-918.

42. Guicciardi F, Atzori L, Marzano AV, et al. Are there distinct clinical and pathological features distinguishing idiopathic from drug-induced subacute cutaneous lupus erythematosus? A European retrospective multicenter study. J Am Acad Dermatol. 2019;81:403-411

43. Karadag AS, Ozlu E, Lavery MJ. Cutaneous manifestations of diabetes mellitus and the metabolic syndrome. *Clin Dermatol*. 2018;36:89-93.

44. Murphy-Chutorian B, Han G, Cohen SR. Dermatologic manifestations of diabetes mellitus: a review. *Endocrinol Metab Clin North Am*. 2013;42:869-98.

45. Lause M, Kamboj A, Fernandez Faith E. Dermatologic manifestations of endocrine disorders. *Transl Pediatr*. 2017;6:300-312..

46. Perez MI, Kohn SR. Cutaneous manifestations of diabetes mellitus. *J Am Acad Dermatol*. 1994;30:519-31.

47. Burman KD, McKinley-Grant L. Dermatologic aspects of thyroid disease. *Clin Dermatol*. 2006;24:247-55.

48. Kraus CN, Sodha P, Vaidyanathan P, Kirkorian AY. Thyroid dermopathy and acropachy in pediatric patients. *Pediatr Dermatol*. 2018;35:e371-e374.

49. Fatourechi V. Thyroid dermopathy and acropachy. *Best Pract Res Clin Endocrinol Metab*. 2012;26:553-65.

50. Antonelli A, Fallahi P, Elia G, et al. Graves' disease: Clinical manifestations, immune pathogenesis (cytokines and chemokines) and therapy. *Best Pract Res Clin Endocrinol Metab*. 2020;34:101388.

51. Ai J, Leonhardt JM, Heymann WR. Autoimmune thyroid diseases: etiology, pathogenesis, and dermatologic manifestations. *J Am Acad Dermatol*. 2003;48:641-59; quiz 660-2.

52. Housman E, Reynolds RV. Polycystic ovary syndrome: a review for dermatologists: Part I. Diagnosis and manifestations. *J Am Acad Dermatol*. 2014;71:847.e1-847.e10; quiz 857-8.

53. Bozdag G, Mumusoglu S, Zengin D, Karabulut E, Yildiz BO. The prevalence and phenotypic features of polycystic ovary syndrome: a systematic review and meta-analysis. *Hum Reprod.* 2016;31:2841-2855.

54. Buzney E, Sheu J, Buzney C, Reynolds RV. Polycystic ovary syndrome: a review for dermatologists: Part II. Treatment. *J Am Acad Dermatol.* 2014;71:859.e1-859.e15; quiz 873-4..

55. Shenoy C, Shenoy MM, Rao GK. Dyslipidemia in dermatological disorders. *N Am J Med Sci.* 2015;7:421-8.

56. Nair PA, Singhal R. Xanthelasma palpebrarum - a brief review. *Clin Cosmet Investig Dermatol.* 2017;11:1-5.

57. Thrash B, Patel M, Shah KR, Boland CR, Menter A. Cutaneous manifestations of gastrointestinal disease: part II. *J Am Acad Dermatol.* 2013;68:211.e1-33.

58. Ungureanu L, Cosgarea R, Alexandru Badea MA, et al. Cutaneous manifestations in inflammatory bowel disease. *Exp Ther Med.* 2020;20:31-37.

59. Bolotin D, Petronic-Rosic V. Dermatitis herpetiformis. Part I. Epidemiology, pathogenesis, and clinical presentation. *J Am Acad Dermatol.* 2011;64:1017-24.

60. Bolotin D, Petronic-Rosic V. Dermatitis herpetiformis. Part II. Diagnosis, management, and prognosis. *J Am Acad Dermatol.* 2011;64:1027-33.

61. Denaxas K, Ladas SD, Karamanolis GP. Evaluation and management of esophageal manifestations in systemic sclerosis. *Ann Gastroenterol.* 2018;31:165-170.

62. Dogra S, Jindal R. Cutaneous manifestations of common liver diseases. *J Clin Exp Hepatol.* 2011;1:177-84.

63. Patel AD, Katz K, Gordon KB. Cutaneous manifestations of chronic liver disease. *Clin Liver Dis.* 2020;24:351-360.

64. Singal AK. Porphyria cutanea tarda: recent update. *Mol Genet Metab.* 2019;128:271-281.

65. Jones AM, Warken K, Tyring SK. The cutaneous manifestations of viral hepatitis. *Dermatol Clin.* 2002;20:233-47.

66. Akhter A, Said A. Cutaneous manifestations of viral hepatitis. *Curr Infect Dis Rep.* 2015;17:452.

67. Haimovic A, Sanchez M, Judson MA, Prystowsky S. Sarcoidosis: a comprehensive review and update for the dermatologist: part I. Cutaneous disease. *J Am Acad Dermatol.* 2012;66:699.e1-18.

68. Haimovic A, Sanchez M, Judson MA, Prystowsky S. Sarcoidosis: a comprehensive review and update for the dermatologist: part II. Extracutaneous disease. *J Am Acad Dermatol.* 2012;66:719.e1-10.

69. Wanat KA, Rosenbach M. Cutaneous sarcoidosis. *Clin Chest Med.* 2015;36:685-702. doi:

70. Noe MH, Misha Rosenbach M. Cutaneous sarcoidosis. *Curr Opin Pulm Med.* 2017;23:482-486.

71. Llanos O, Hamzeh N. Sarcoidosis. *Med Clin North Am.* 2019;103:527-534

72. Dubrey S, Pal S, Sarneet Singh S, Karagiannis G. Digital clubbing: forms, associations and pathophysiology. *Br J Hosp Med (Lond).* 2016;77:403-8.

73. Vignes S, Baran R. Yellow nail syndrome: a review. *Orphanet J Rare Dis.* 2017;12:42.

74. Nigwekar SU, Thadhani R, Brandenburg VM. Calciphylaxis. *N Engl J Med.* 2018;378:1704-1714.

75. Baby D, Upadhyay M, Joseph MD, et al. Calciphylaxis and its diagnosis: A review. *J Family Med Prim Care.* 2019; 8:2763-2767.

76. Nigwekar SU, Kroshinsky D, Nazarian RM, et al. Calciphylaxis: risk factors, diagnosis, and treatment. *Am J Kidney Dis.* 2015; 66:133-46.

77. Simonsen E, Komenda P, Lerner B, et al. Treatment of uremic pruritus: a systematic review. *Am J Kidney Dis.* 2017; 70:638-655.

78. Mathur M, D'Souza AVL, Malhotra V, Agarwal D, Beniwal P. Uremic frost. *Clin Kidney J.* 2014; 7:418-9.

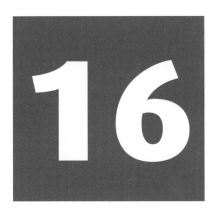

Urticaria

Caleb Creswell

INTRODUCTION TO CHAPTER

Urticaria (hives) is defined by the rapid appearance of lesions called wheals, which consist of dermal swelling presenting as pruritic papules or plaques with or without surrounding erythema. Wheals are smooth with no surface changes. Individual wheals last for 1–24 hours. Wheals form when mast cells release histamine in response to various stimuli. Urticaria is divided into acute (duration less than 6 weeks) and chronic (duration greater than 6 weeks) forms. Chronic urticaria can occur spontaneously or as a result of physical stimuli.

ACUTE URTICARIA

Introduction

Key Points

- ✓ Individual lesions of urticaria last for less than 24 hours.
- ✓ Urticaria may persist beyond 6 weeks in 20% of patients.
- ✓ Angioedema is often present in conjunction with urticaria.
- ✓ H_1 non-sedating antihistamines are the first line of therapy for urticaria.

Acute spontaneous urticaria is the most common form of urticaria. Acute spontaneous urticaria is defined as spontaneous urticaria of less than 6 weeks duration, whereas chronic spontaneous urticaria lasts more than 6 weeks. The majority of patients with spontaneous urticaria will fall in this category. The lifetime prevalence of urticaria is estimated to be approximately 9–20% and it can present in patients ranging in age from infants to the elderly.[1] Associated angioedema can sometimes be seen in patients with urticaria. It is defined as swelling of the deeper dermis and subcutaneous tissue lasting up to 72 hours. Angioedema is seen in conjunction with classic wheals in 30–40% of patients with urticaria.[1] When angioedema is seen without wheals this is frequently the result of drug therapy as with angiotensin-converting enzyme (ACE) inhibitors.

Pathogenesis

The underlying event leading to urticaria is mast cell degranulation, with release of histamine and other pro-inflammatory molecules including cytokines, prostaglandins, leukotrienes, and arachidonic acid metabolites causing rapid vasodilation and swelling of the surrounding tissue with plasma and activation of local itch sensory nerves.[1,2] There are numerous stimuli that can lead to mast cell activation through various pathways. More than 50% of acute spontaneous urticaria is idiopathic.

Among cases with a known cause, the most common cause is viral infections, particularly in children.[3] Drugs including beta-lactams, nonsteroidal anti-inflammatory drugs (NSAIDs), and ACE-inhibitors are another frequent cause[1,2] (Table 16-1). Food-induced type I hypersensitivity reactions are a rare cause of acute urticaria in adults, but

Table 16-1. Common Causes of Acute Urticaria

- **INFECTIONS:** Viral respiratory, especially rhinovirus and rotavirus (cause in 80% of children), *Heilobacter pylori*, mycoplasma, hepatitis, mononucleosis, parasitic helminths.
- **DRUGS and IV PRODUCTS:** Beta-lactams antibiotics, non-steroidal anti-inflammatory drugs (NSAIDS), aspirin, ACE-inhibitors, diuretics, opiates, contrast media, blood transfusion.
- **FOODS:** In adults' shellfish, freshwater fish, berries, nuts, peanuts, pork, chocolate, tomatoes, spices, food additives, and alcohol. In children milk and other dairy products, eggs, wheat, citrus.
- **INHALANTS:** Pollens, molds, dust mites, animal dander.
- **EMOTIONAL STRESS**
- **SYSTEMIC DISEASES:** Lupus erythematosus, Still's disease, thyroid disease, cryoglobulinemia, mastocytosis, carcinomas.

are a more common cause in children. In type I hypersensitivity reactions (food and latex allergies), antigen specific immunoglobulin IgE causes a cross linking of the high-affinity (Ig)E receptors leading to mast cell degranulation.[1] The exact mechanism leading to mast cell degranulation in non-type I forms of acute urticaria appears to be multifactorial and is less well-defined.

Clinical Presentation

History

A thorough history is important to establishing the diagnosis of urticaria because the wheals may have disappeared by the time of the office visit. Additionally, a detailed history is the most effective way to reveal an underlying cause of urticaria. It is important to inquire about the location, associated pruritus, and especially the duration of the lesions. Any lesions that last for longer than 24 hours should raise suspicion of an alternative diagnosis. Any symptoms that point to an anaphylaxis-type reaction or to swelling of the throat are important as these are rare, but life-threatening complications. To determine the underlying cause of urticaria, one should inquire about associated overall health, including signs of upper respiratory infection, sinus infection, auto-immune disease, and *Helicobacter pylori* infection. Medications and foods can be triggers for urticaria which usually appears 1–2 hours after ingestion. Finally, it is important to ask about any physical stimuli such as pressure, cold, or heat that may be causing the urticaria.

Physical Examination

The hallmark lesions of urticaria are wheals, which exhibit the following features:

- Central dermal swellings of various sizes and configurations with or without surrounding erythema (Figure 16-1 and 16-2).
- Pruritus or occasional burning sensations.
- Skin returning to normal appearance, usually within 1–24 hours.

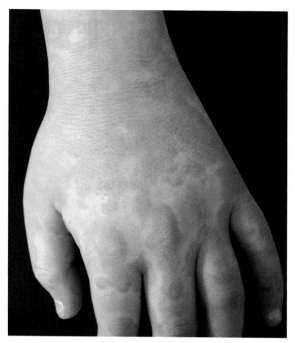

▲ **Figure 16-1.** Urticaria on hand: uniform pink wheals with smooth surface.

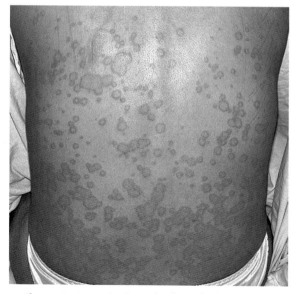

▲ **Figure 16-2.** Urticaria on back: multiple annular wheals with central clearing.

Angioedema occurs with wheals in approximately 40% of cases of urticaria and possibly more frequently in food-induced urticaria. It is defined as

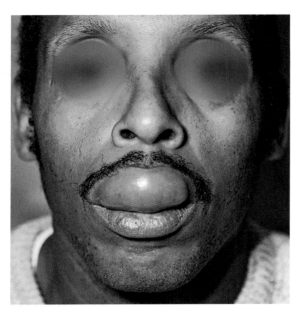

▲ **Figure 16-3.** Angioedema of upper lip induced by ACE inhibitor. Reproduced with permission from Knoop KJ, Stack LB, Storrow AB, et al: The Atlas of Emergency Medicine, 5th ed. New York, NY: McGraw Hill; 2021. Photo contributor: Lawrence B. Stack, MD.

- Abrupt swelling of the lower dermis and subcutis (Figure 16-3).
- Occasional pain instead of pruritus.
- Commonly involving the lips, cheeks, periorbital area, tongue, and may even involve the larynx and pharynx.
- Skin returning to normal appearance, usually within 72 hours.

  Angioedema without wheals often has differing underlying causes, therefore it is important to determine if primary lesions are wheals, angioedema, or both. Hoarseness can be a sign of laryngeal edema which can be a life-threatening complication due to airway compromise. Dyspnea, wheezing, abdominal pain, dizziness, and hypotension are clues to an anaphylaxis-like reaction.

▶ Laboratory Findings

Unless indicated by history, laboratory examination for acute spontaneous urticaria is not helpful. For patients with angioedema without wheals who are not on ACE inhibitors or nonsteroidal anti-inflammatory (NSAIDs), a C4 level can screen for acquired or hereditary complement deficiency.[4]

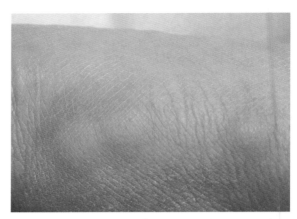

▲ **Figure 16-4.** Mosquito bites presenting as papular urticaria: group of 3 bites with central blanched center.

Diagnosis

The finding of wheals with or without angioedema is highly suggestive of urticaria. The most important distinction to make is between urticaria and anaphylaxis-like reaction with urticaria which requires emergent management. Signs such as dyspnea, wheezing, abdominal pain, dizziness, and hypotension are clues to an anaphylaxis-like reaction.

▶ Differential Diagnosis

✓ Viral exanthems: May present with urticarial lesions, which can fade quickly, but still typically last for more than 24 hours.

✓ Drug reactions: Fixed drug eruption, Stevens-Johnson syndrome, drug hypersensitivity syndrome, and simple morbilliform eruptions can sometimes be mistaken for urticaria; however, these diseases have distinguishing features and the lesions last for more than 24 hours.

✓ Insect bites: The papular urticarial lesions of insect bites usually have a blanched center and may have a central crust or puncta at the site of the bite (Figure 16-4). The lesions usually last longer than 24 hours.

✓ Mastocytosis: The rust-colored papules of mastocytosis do temporarily form wheals when rubbed or stimulated.

✓ Prebullous pemphigoid: This phase of pemphigoid may present with pruritic plaques that have an urticarial appearance, but lesions persist longer than 24 hours.

Table 17-2. Classic Type IV hypersensitivity cutaneous adverse drug reactions.

Cutaneous reaction	History and clinical findings	Treatment	Common offending agents
Simple Morbilliform Drug Eruption	Morbilliform eruption typically sparing the face and mucosal surfaces; absence of systemic findings or end-organ damage.	Discontinuation of medication. Topical steroids and antihistamines for pruritus.	Antibiotics (penicillins, sulfonamides, cephalosporins). Anticonvulsants. Calcium channel blockers. NSAIDs.
Drug-induced hypersensitivity syndrome (DIHS); also known as DRESS	Morbilliform eruption, classically involving face; spares mucosal surfaces; presence of systemic symptoms (including fevers). Transaminitis, acute kidney injury. Post-DIHS thyroiditis. Hypersensitivity myocarditis.	Discontinuation of medication. Prednisone 1–2 mg/kg daily orally for 3–6 months.	Abacavir Allopurinol. Antiepileptic drugs (carbamazepine, phenytoin, lamotrigine). Minocycline. Nevirapine. NSAIDs. Sulfa-based antimicrobials (trimethoprim/sulfamethoxazole, sulfasalazine).
Acute generalized exanthematous pustulosis (AGEP)	Pustular eruption favoring intertriginous areas; +/- systemic symptoms. Typically, no end-organ damage.	Discontinuation of medication. Topical steroids usually sufficient. Severe cases may require prednisone with quicker taper.	Antibiotics (penicillin and derivatives, macrolides, others). Antimalarials. Dialysate. Calcium channel blockers. Radiocontrast dye.
Fixed drug eruption	Sharply demarcated oval, dusky, violaceous patches which appear usually within a few hours after medication exposure. Oral and genital mucosa are common areas of involvement. Rare, severe generalized bullous form.	Avoidance of offending agent. Topical steroids and antihistamines for pruritus. Systemic steroids in severe cases.	Laxatives. NSAIDs Pseudoephedrine. Tetracycline antibiotics. Trimethoprim-sulfamethoxazole.
SJS/TEN	Tender, painful macular eruption with non-blanching targetoid lesions; may develop into bullae and formation and widespread epidermal sloughing. Mucosal involvement is characteristic. Systemic symptoms common, including multiorgan involvement and high risk for sepsis.	Avoidance of culprit medication. Transfer to burn center. Multidisciplinary involvement (Dermatology, wound care, Ophthalmology, Urology and/or OB/GYN, ENT). Treatment with cyclosporine and/or IVIG. TNF-alpha inhibitors.	Allopurinol. Antibiotics (particularly sulfonamides). Anticonvulsants. Nevirapine. NSAIDs.

AGEP, acute generalized exanthematous pustulosis; DIHS, drug-induced hypersensitivity syndrome; DRESS, drug reaction with eosinophilia and systemic symptoms; FDE, fixed drug eruption; OB/GYN, obstetrics/gynecology; SJS, Stevens–Johnson syndrome; TEN, toxic epidermal necrolysis; TNF, tumor necrosis factor.

that occurs each time with various antibiotics to lower pain and fever).

There needs to be a clear separation between a real and potentially life-threatening reaction from multiple intolerances and allergies reported by patients. Real intolerance reactions, sometimes also called "pseudoallergies," can include chemically unrelated drugs with common pathway of action such as inhibition of cyclooxygenase (with sometimes life-threatening angioedema and urticaria to NSAIDs or ACE inhibitors). These have to be clearly separated from non-specific intolerances that could be based on an underlying chronic idiopathic urticaria or non-specific, diffuse psychosomatic symptoms that are sometimes linked to depression and anxiety. Chronic, idiopathic urticaria can be aggravated by certain drugs. For example, opioids are known destabilizers of mast cells with release of histamine and this can aggravate an underlying chronic urticaria. Other symptoms may include very non-specific symptoms such as bloating, hypertension, headaches, drug fevers, among many others.[15,16]

Real and clinically relevant drug allergies/intolerances are not always identified correctly, nor always distinguished from falsely diagnosed drug reactions. This can greatly limit choice of medications a clinician is willing to prescribe which directly impacts costs, morbidity and mortality for the patient. Optimal treatments may be replaced by alternatives with more side effects and poorer efficacy. In particular this is a difficult problem in the hospital setting. Referral to Allergy should be done if there is any doubt about the nature of the drug reaction. Currently, the gold standard methods to determine drug allergy are in-vivo testing methods, which include drug prick, intradermal and patch testing with immediate (20 minute) or delayed readings (2–4 days), and finally, if necessary, by oral provocation testing.[17] The goal of a drug allergy evaluation is to prove or discard a possible allergy and to evaluate and test possible alternative treatments. It is up to the clinician whether to pursue in-vivo drug testing to determine if a reaction is truly drug allergy or drug intolerance. Of note, these in-vivo tests are not without risk and in-vitro testing methods are being currently developed and performed in certain laboratory settings. These in-vitro tests may include looking at cell surface markers, cytokine expression, and analysis of T-cell population in response to a drug exposure, which may also help distinguish between different types of drug rashes or exclude drug-intolerance reactions. Although there is enormous potential for these types of tests, they are still not standardized and not regularly performed in clinical practice due to cost, technical demand, and lack of well-controlled studies.[18]

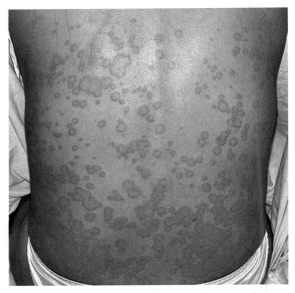

▲ **Figure 17-1.** Urticaria on back: multiple annular wheals with central clearing.

DRUG HYPERSENSITIVITY

Immediate-Type Hypersensitivity Reaction

The clinical spectrum of immediate-type hypersensitivity reactions classically includes urticarial eruptions, angioedema, or anaphylaxis with respiratory symptoms, hypotonia, and/or syncope. These reactions present with an acute onset of pruritic and less commonly, painful lesions within minutes to hours after ingestion of the medication. Classic medications include antibiotics (particularly penicillins and cephalosporins) NSAIDs, opiates, and contrast media though there are multiple causes. Urticaria presents with wheals (dermal swelling with or without associated erythema) and the individual wheals resolve within 24 hours (Figure 17-1). Angioedema presents as deeper, sometimes painful swelling, of the mucous membranes (Figure 17-2). The swelling resolves within 72 hours. Hoarseness can be a sign of laryngeal edema, which can be a life-threatening complication due to airway compromise. Dyspnea, wheezing, abdominal pain, dizziness, and hypotension are clues to an anaphylaxis-like reaction.

Besides avoidance of medication, it is essential to diagnose and triage the patient appropriately. Patients with perioral or airway involvement must be monitored closely, and some may warrant observation in the intensive care unit (ICU). Epinephrine injection (usually given intramuscularly) should be given for airway compromise or cardiovascular involvement, which may include

symptoms of hypotonia, syncope, dizziness, tachycardia, and hypotension. In addition, a combination of high dose oral non-sedating H1 antihistamines (e.g., 2 tablets of 10 mg cetirizine or 2 tablets of 180 mg fexofenadine) with 100 mg prednisone for a one-time dose, in adults should also be used in severe reactions, and be first line in hypersensitivity reactions without airway/cardiovascular compromise.[19]

Proper diagnoses of the culprit drugs are important. To diagnose allergic reactions, skin prick and intradermal tests with readings after 20 minutes are important to identify the culprit (particularly in patients treated with different drugs). For intradermal tests, sterile injectable drugs are necessary. Blood tests (e.g., specific IgE or Cellular Antigen stimulation test (CAST)) are usually not very sensitive and can give false negative results.[20] Skin tests also allow for evaluation of possible cross-reactions (e.g., penicillins and cephalosporins), to test alternative treatments, and to rule out immediate type reactions to additives (e.g., carboxymethylcellulose, latex or chlorhexidine).[21]

Delayed T-Cell Mediated Hypersensitivity Reactions

▶ A. Simple Morbilliform Drug Eruption

Morbilliform drug eruptions are the most common type of drug reaction and account for approximately 95% of skin reactions.[8] This type of hypersensitivity eruption presents insidiously approximately 4–14 days after starting the offending agent.[22] The rash is characterized by small pink,

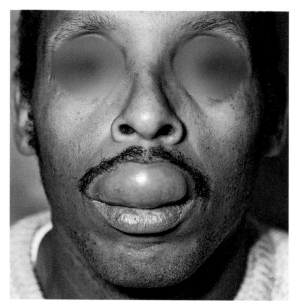

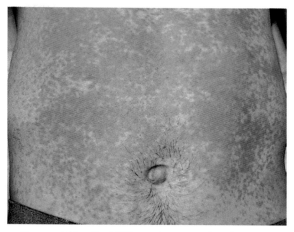

▲ Figure 17-3. Morbilliform drug eruption due to thiazide diuretic. Discrete and confluent pink macules and papules on trunk.

▲ Figure 17-2. Angioedema of upper lip induced by ACE inhibitor. Reproduced with permission from Knoop KJ, Stack LB, Storrow AB, et al: The Atlas of Emergency Medicine, 5th ed. New York, NY: McGraw Hill; 2021. Photo contributor: Lawrence B. Stack, MD.

pruritic, macules, and papules (Figure 17-3) which start on the trunk and pressure-bearing areas, spreading to other areas of the body, and sometimes becoming confluent. There is significant clinical overlap in morphology between these drug eruptions, viral exanthems, and acute graft versus host reaction disease (GVHD). A careful medication timeline and appropriate systemic laboratory workup are needed to help distinguish between these causes, yet it may still be difficult.

Generally, morbilliform drug eruptions are more prominent in areas of pressure or dependent areas and should spare the face. Facial involvement and systemic symptoms should prompt consideration for drug induced hypersensitivity syndrome (see below). Typically, it is enough to discontinue the medication and use topical steroids and oral antihistamines for pruritus; however, if a culprit medication is absolutely essential, the clinician at times may wish to treat through the rash and closely monitor for worsening if there is no evidence of systemic involvement (e.g., drug-induced hypersensitivity syndrome) or painful blisters.[22] However, identification of the culprit drug with possible cross-reactions in the aftermath of the rash is important with correct documentation in the drug allergy reporting system. To diagnose properly, a precise medication history with timing and doses of all medications used several days before onset of the rash is required. The clinical suspicions based on history can be confirmed by in-vivo testing using patch and intradermal tests with delayed readings after 2 and 4 days.[1]

▶ B. Drug-Induced Hypersensitivity Syndrome

Drug-induced hypersensitivity syndrome also known as drug reaction with eosinophilia and systemic symptoms (DRESS) is a severe adverse drug reaction. The eruption typically starts 2–6 weeks after the triggering medication; overall there is a longer latency period than with a simple morbilliform drug eruption. Clinically, drug-induced hypersensitivity syndrome resembles a simple morbilliform drug eruption, but distinguishing features are rash involving the face with underlying edema (Figure 17-4).[23] Furthermore, patients often have systemic findings, which may include fevers, lymphadenopathy, and organ involvement (particularly the liver and kidneys). Drug-induced hypersensitivity syndrome can be potentially fatal (especially in the case of drug-induced hypersensitivity syndrome triggered eosinophilic myocarditis). Eosinophilia may also be present but not a required diagnostic criterion. Drug-induced hypersensitivity syndrome requires close laboratory monitoring to detect these clues and to assess for organ damage, which may be suggested by elevated liver function tests or elevated creatinine. A punch biopsy of the rash may be helpful in determining that this may be a drug eruption; however, the biopsy cannot distinguish drug-induced hypersensitivity syndrome from a simple

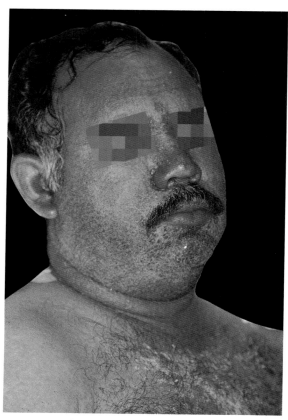

▲ **Figure 17-4.** Drug-induced hypersensitive syndrome due to carbamazepine. Facial edema with erythema and crusting with pustules on chest.

morbilliform drug eruption or viral exanthem (though presence of eosinophils may be helpful toward a drug-induced etiology). The differential diagnosis is similar to the one listed for simple morbilliform drug eruption.

It is important to distinguish drug-induced hypersensitivity syndrome from other cutaneous adverse reactions, as therapy differs significantly. Drug-induced hypersensitivity syndrome often requires treatment with prolonged course of oral steroids (1–2 mg/kg/day); dose depending on severity of the case.[23] The taper should be quite slow over several months, given risk for rebound associated with quicker tapers. Along with all prolonged courses of steroids, the patient should have recommended calcium and vitamin D for bone health, periodic monitoring of their blood sugars, and *Pneumocystis carinii* pneumonia prophylaxis. Diagnostic testing with intradermal tests and patch testing can be done after the rash is resolved, ideally, 6 months after onset of the rash. Diagnostic testing can be performed earlier in cases where a faster diagnosis is crucial, but there is a higher incidence of false positive results because the remaining hypersensitivity can induce non-specific local reactions.

▶ C. Acute Generalized Exanthematous Pustulosis

Acute generalized exanthematous pustulosis (AGEP) is a clinically distinct drug eruption that typically occurs within 1–3 days of medication exposure. It is characterized by a morbilliform eruption that develops innumerable pinpoint pustules that favor intertriginous areas (Figure 17-5 A and B). Patients may also develop fevers, and leukocytosis with neutrophilia; however, other organ involvement is not typically seen. A punch biopsy of a pustule should show a characteristic subcorneal pustule, spongiosis of the epidermis, and admixed neutrophils and eosinophils. The differential diagnosis depends on the stage of the eruption. If early, and still having morbilliform morphology, simple morbilliform drug eruption, drug-induced hypersensitivity syndrome, or any of the aforementioned differential diagnoses can be considered. If the clinician sees a pustular eruption, then pustular psoriasis, candidiasis, and certain rare bullous eruptions, such as IgA pemphigus or subcorneal pustular dermatoses may be considered.[24]

Similarly to all severe cutaneous drug reactions, withdrawal of the causative medication is of primary importance. Often, this may be enough in acute generalized exanthematous pustulosis, as resolution of the eruption is typically fast. Topical steroids may be utilized, and in severe cases, oral corticosteroids or retinoids can be considered.[24] Proper diagnosis and reporting with possible cross-reactions should be made based on the patient's history and delayed readings of patch and intradermal tests with suspected medications. In-vivo tests in the setting of acute generalized exanthematous pustulosis will usually produce localized pustular reactions.

▶ D. Fixed Drug Eruption

Fixed drug eruptions present as a solitary dusky erythematous plaque that can at times be edematous and even bullous (Figure 17-6). The lesions develop within hours of ingestion of the medication and usually recur at the same sites. Common sites include the lips, genitals, and extremities. Occasionally multiple lesions may be present. Typically, there is residual hyperpigmentation after the lesion regresses. A severe generalized bullous variant which has a course similar to Stevens–Johnson syndrome/toxic epidermal necrolysis, may occur rarely. In this variant, there is increased risk for secondary infection, as well as an increase in morbidity and mortality.[25] It may be enough to diagnose fixed drug eruptions clinically, however a punch biopsy can certainly aid in the diagnosis in atypical cases. Topical steroids and antihistamines for pruritus are generally used, though systemic steroids can be considered in severe cases, particularly for the generalized variant. Testing of fixed drug eruptions should be done by delayed readings of intradermal and patch tests performed on the location of an old lesion of the fixed drug eruptions. Testing

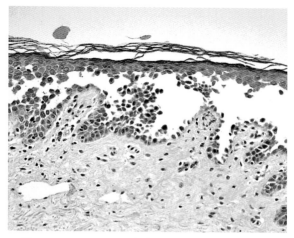

Figure 19-9. Histopathology of pemphigus. Suprabasilar bulla with acantholysis (disassociation of keratinocytes) and minimal inflammation.

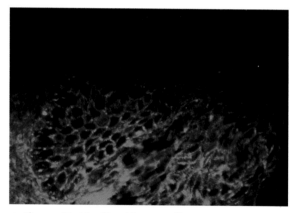

Figure 19-10. Direct immunofluorescence microscopy of perilesional skin in pemphigus. Intercellular IgG deposition.

Differential Diagnosis

Because the blister is superficial, other eroding diseases must be considered.

✓ Staphylococcal scalded skin syndrome (SSSS): Patients have sheets of exfoliating skin related to a staph-producing toxin. This is most often seen in children or dialysis patients.

✓ Stevens–Johnson syndrome/toxic epidermolysis (SJS/TEN): Clinically, ill patients with significant crusting of the lips, nose, and eyes.

✓ Mycoplasma-induced rash and mucositis: Usually seen in children. Patients present with hemorrhagic crusting of lips and nonspecific cutaneous eruption after prodrome of upper respiratory symptoms.

✓ Erythema multiforme: Patients present with "targetoid" lesions on acral surfaces +/- mucosal involvement. Classically associated with herpetic infection.

✓ Other: herpetic eruptions, bullous impetigo, vasculitis.

✓ Other immunobullous conditions (Table 19-1): dermatitis herpetiformis, epidermolyis bullosa acquista, IgA pemphigus.

When prominent oral involvement is present, consider:

✓ Aphthous ulcers.

✓ Herpetic gingivostomatitis.

✓ Lichen planus.

Management

If pemphigus vulgaris is suspected, a skin biopsy for routine histopathology should be done from the edge of a blister and a skin biopsy for direct immunofluorescence should be done from perilesional skin near a blister. Blood should be sent for indirect immunofluorescence and ELISA. Eroded areas should be covered with white petrolatum and non-stick dressings. Culture as appropriate for superinfection.

Treatment for pemphigus is dependent on the severity of the disease. For mild disease, topical corticosteroids may be utilized. Gel-based topical steroids or swish and spit solutions can be good options for mucosal surfaces. For moderate to severe disease, systemic corticosteroids are the initial drug of choice. Recently, rituximab plus short-term oral corticosteroid use has emerged as first-line treatment.[13] Other non-steroid sparing agents that can be used include azathioprine, mycophenolate mofetil, methotrexate, cyclophosphamide, intravenous immunoglobulin (IVIG), and plasmapheresis. Long-term monitoring of medications is usually required.

Clinical Course and Prognosis

Prior to the development of glucocorticoids, pemphigus vulgaris was frequently fatal. Mortality is still higher than the general population, with a standardized mortality ratio of 1.67 in France.[14] However, with advances in treatment, mortality in pemphigus vulgaris has improved over the years, with the age-adjusted mortality rate in the United States decreasing from 0.033 deaths per 100,000 per decade in the United States in 1979–1982 to 0.0066 in 1999–2002.[15] More recently, with the emergence of rituximab therapy, long-term remission is now common.

Indications for Consultation

All patients with pemphigus vulgaris must be referred to dermatology immediately. If the patient has widespread disease, is unable to eat or drink, or has signs of superinfection, patients should be hospitalized preferably in a burn unit. All patients should be screened for mucosal involvement and appropriate consultation with other services should be obtained as needed including ophthalmology, otolaryngology, urology, or gynecology.

Patient Information

- International Pemphigus and Pemphigoid Foundation: https://www.pemphigus.org/pemphigus/
- American Academy of Dermatology: https://www.aad.org/public/diseases/a-z/pemphigus-overview
- British Association of Dermatologists: www.bad.org.uk/shared/get-file.ashx?id=1984&itemtype=document
- Mayo Clinic: www.mayoclinic.org/diseases-conditions/pemphigus/symptoms-causes/syc-20350404
- NIH: https://www.niams.nih.gov/health-topics/pemphigus
- NORD: https://rarediseases.org/rare-diseases/pemphigus/

▼ DERMATITIS HERPETIFORMIS

Introduction

Dermatitis herpetiformis (DH) is an autoimmune blistering disease, which can occur in a younger subset of patients when compared to pemphigus vulgaris and bullous pemphigoid. The typical age of onset is between 30 and 40 years of age, with men affected more often than women. It is more common in those with Northern European ancestry. There seems to be strong genetic factors at play, as a genetic predilection is found in families and dermatitis herpetiformis is associated with HLA-DQ2 and HLA-DQ8.[16]

Patients with dermatitis herpetiformis are at higher risk for autoimmune diseases, most commonly hypothyroidism, as well as non-Hodgkin lymphoma.[16]

Pathogenesis

Dermatitis herpetiformis is a skin manifestation of gluten sensitivity. It is strongly associated with gluten-sensitive enteropathy or celiac disease, although the patient may not be symptomatic. IgA autoantibodies are found in both dermatitis herpetiformis and celiac disease, but IgG autoantibodies can also be seen especially in those with IgA deficiency. In dermatitis herpetiformis, epidermal transglutaminase is the main antigen.[16] In celiac disease, the main antigen is tissue transglutaminase. In the skin, transglutaminase is found in the dermal capillaries and the basal cells of the epidermis.

Transglutaminase is a cytoplasmic, calcium-dependent enzyme which catalyzes crosslinks between glutamine and lysine and serves many functions. As it relates to dermatitis herpetiformis and celiac disease, transglutaminase modifies the gliadin portion of gluten and makes it an autoantigen.

Protein-to-protein crosslinking between transglutaminase and gliadin complexes causes an intense autoantibody response. Due to the inflammation in the skin, a blister is formed in the basement membrane zone between the epidermis and dermis.

Clinical Presentation

▶ History

Patients will usually present with excoriations and complaints of intense pruritus. They may have gastrointestinal symptoms such as diarrhea and abdominal cramping.

▶ Physical Examination

Excoriations and crusted erosions are commonly present (Figure 19-11). Patients rarely present with intact blisters due scratching related to the intense nature of the pruritus. If blisters were present, they would be expected to be tense as the blister is forming between the dermis and the epidermis. The eruption is classically symmetric with a distribution on the extensor surfaces of the extremities, elbows, knees, buttocks, scalp, and neck. The face and groin may also be involved, but rarely the mucosa.[16]

▶ Laboratory Findings

Patients may have some or all of the following findings:

- Histopathology of a skin biopsy from an intact blister/vesicle (if it can be found) will show a subepidermal blister with neutrophils and some eosinophils in the tips of the dermal papillae (Figure 19-12).[17]
- Direct immunofluorescence of a skin biopsy from perilesional skin will show granular deposits of IgA at the tips of the dermal papillae (Figure 19-13).[17]

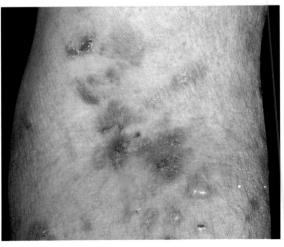

▲ **Figure 19-11.** Dermatitis herpetiformis. Vesicle and excoriated erosions on forearm.

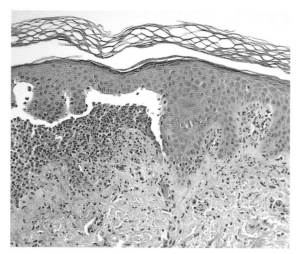

Figure 19-12. Histopathology of dermatitis herpetiformis. Subepidermal bulla with neutrophils and eosinophils in the tips of the dermal papillae.

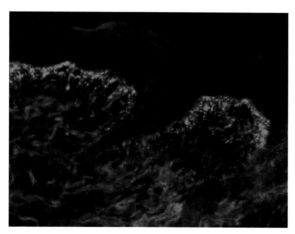

Figure 19-13. Direct immunofluorescence microscopy of perilesional skin in dermatitis herpetiformis. Granular deposits of IgA at the tips of the dermal papillae.

- Indirect immunofluorescence of the blood can identify anti-endomysial antibodies, which are specific for dermatitis herpetiformis.[17]
- ELISA for IgA anti-tissue transglutaminase and when available, ELISA for IgA anti-epidermal transglutaminase, can be elevated.[17]

Of note, a total IgA level should be done before any other serological tests as selective IgA deficiency is more common in celiac patients and needs to be considered in working up the dermatitis herpetiformis patient. If patients have IgA deficiency, their screening tests above may be falsely negative.[17]

Diagnosis

As other conditions can mimic dermatitis herpetiformis clinically, diagnosis of dermatitis herpetiformis is made based on histopathology, direct and indirect immunofluorescence patterns, and the presence of circulating antibodies. The key examination findings of dermatitis herpetiformis are erosions and excoriated papules on the extensor surfaces of the extremities, elbows, knees, buttocks, scalp, and neck.

▶ Differential Diagnosis

✓ Scabies: Presents as pruritic papules on elbows, knees, body folds, volar wrists, and finger web spaces. Linear burrows are pathognomonic. Mites are often seen in skin scrapings.

✓ Bullous pemphigoid: Tense bullae in a bilateral symmetric distribution.

✓ Other: Linear IgA bullous dermatosis, bullous pemphigoid, epidermolysis bullosa acquisita, atopic dermatitis, urticaria

Management

If dermatitis herpetiformis is suspected, a skin biopsy for routine histopathology should be done from the edge of a blister and a skin biopsy for direct immunofluorescence should be done from perilesional skin in the general area of the rash, but not right next to a blister. Blood should be sent for IgA levels, indirect immunofluorescence, and ELISA. Genetic testing for HLA-DQ2 and HLA-DQ8 can be considered in equivocal cases.

A strict gluten-free diet is a mainstay of therapy and consultation with a dietician is important as this diet is difficult to maintain. Even with a strict gluten-free diet, the skin lesions are slow to respond.[18] Dapsone and sulphapyridine rapidly control the skin lesions.[17] Long-term monitoring of these medications is required. Importantly, dapsone does not treat the gastrointestinal involvement associated with dermatitis herpetiformis and all patients should continue their gluten-free diet.[17] Systemic corticosteroids are not helpful in this disease. Antihistamines may help with pruritus.

Dermatitis herpetiformis is associated with other immune-mediated conditions and screening studies for thyroid disease, diabetes, and connective tissue disease should be considered.[16,17,19] If clinical signs of gastrointestinal disease or non-Hodgkin lymphoma are present, evaluation must be obtained as these diseases are associated with dermatitis herpetiformis. Patients with gastrointestinal disease are at risk for splenic atrophy and a blood smear should be done to evaluate for splenic dysfunction. Screening of family members can also be considered.

Clinical Course and Prognosis

Dermatitis herpetiformis is a chronic condition but can be well-controlled on a gluten-free diet or with medical management. Spontaneous remission has been reported.[20]

Indications for Consultation

Dermatitis herpetiformis is a complex blistering disorder that can be difficult to diagnosis. Patients should be referred to dermatology for diagnosis and management. Patients who have gastrointestinal disease or symptoms of non-Hodgkin lymphoma should be referred to the appropriate specialist.

Patient Information

- Celiac Disease Foundation
  www.celiac.org

- British Association of Dermatologists
  www.bad.org.uk/shared/get-file.ashx?id=77&item type=document

NON-IMMUNOBULLOUS BLISTERING CONDITIONS

More commonly, primary care providers will see blisters caused by non-immunobullous conditions. These can be caused by infections, metabolic disorders, inflammatory conditions, non-inflammatory conditions, and drug eruptions. Additionally, some diseases can produce such intense inflammation that they lead to a bullous presentation such as lichen planus, vasculitis, lupus, and erythema multiforme. Clues to diagnosis can be in the number and location of lesions, distribution, and presence or absence of surrounding inflammation. A summary of common conditions is in Table 19-2.

Table 19.2. Differential diagnosis of non-immunobullous conditions.

Disease	Etiology and exam	Diagnosis and treatment
Infectious		
Bullous impetigo	Toxins produced by *Staphylococcus aureus* lead to disruption of normal cell adhesion. Most common in children. Exam: honey-colored crusts or bullae.	Diagnosis with skin swab for bacterial culture showing *Staphylococcus aureus*. Treat with anti-staphylococcal antibiotics - Topicals for localized infection. - Oral antibiotics for more disseminated infection.
Herpes simplex	Caused by HSV-1, HSV-2. Most commonly oral or genital involvement but can occur anywhere. Primary infection often most severe. Exam: clustered vesicles on erythematous base.	Diagnosis with PCR for HSV-1 or HSV-2. Treat with oral antivirals.
Varicella (chickenpox)	Caused by VZV (primary infection). Exam: successive crops of lesions that progress from macules → papules → vesicles with red base → pustules → crusts. Eruption starts on head and spreads to trunk.	Diagnosis with PCR for VZV. Can treat symptomatically. If there are risks for more severe disease, treat with oral antivirals.

(continued)

Table 19.2. Differential diagnosis of non-immunobullous conditions. (Continued)

Disease	Etiology and exam	Diagnosis and treatment
Herpes zoster (shingles)	Caused by VZV (reactivation of latent disease). Exam: clustered vesicles on erythematous base in dermatomal distribution.	Diagnosis with PCR for VZV. Treat with oral antivirals. Vaccination is recommended for all adults ages 50 years and older, even with history of shingles.
Bullous tinea	Caused by dermatophyte infections. Exam: vesicles and bullae on plantar surface, especially instep of foot. Look for evidence of tinea elsewhere. Can develop "id" response with vesicles on palms and soles.	Diagnosis with KOH or fungal culture. Be sure to unroof bullae prior to scraping. Treat with topical anti-fungals, may need oral therapy.
Inflammatory		
Allergic contact dermatitis	Caused by type IV hypersensitivity reaction. When acute, exam with papules and vesicles on erythematous base. When chronic, exam with lichenified plaques. Unusual distributions and geometric or linear shapes due to contact with external allergen can be clue to diagnosis.	Diagnosis based on clinical history. Biopsy may be needed. Patch testing to determine allergen. Treatment with topical corticosteroids. For severe cases, may need oral corticosteroids.
Dyshidrotic dermatitis	Unclear etiology Can worsen with sweating and stress. Exam: "tapioca-like" vesicles on lateral fingers, palms, insteps, and borders of feet.	Diagnosis based on clinical history. KOH may be needed to rule out tinea infection. Treatment with topical corticosteroids, reduction of sweating.
Arthropod bite	Can be caused by any biting insect. Exam: scattered erythematous papules or vesicles on exposed surfaces (e.g., face, neck, arms, legs). Distribution sometimes linear or clustered together.	Diagnosis based on exam. Treat symptomatically with topical corticosteroids and oral antihistamines. Can have exaggerated response in immunocompromised patients (e.g., CLL, HIV); consider appropriate screening.

(continued)

Table 19.2. Differential diagnosis of non-immunobullous conditions. (Continued)

Disease	Etiology and exam	Diagnosis and treatment
Metabolic		
Porphyria cutanea tarda.	Caused by abnormalities in heme biosynthesis pathways. Associated with smoking, liver disease, alcohol use, hepatitis C, estrogen use. Exam: skin fragility and tense bullae on sun-exposed skin. Background of scarring common. Can have associated hypertrichosis and hyperpigmentation.	Diagnosis made with measurement of total plasma and urine porphyrins. Skin biopsy would be supportive. Treatment with phlebotomy, hydroxychloroquine. Avoid triggers.
Non-inflammatory		
Edema/stasis bullae	Develops in setting of edema. Exam: tense, non-inflammatory bullae and background edematous skin. Occurs in dependent areas (e.g., lower extremities).	Diagnosis based on exam. Treat underlying edema.
Coma blister	Develops in setting of prolonged pressure (e.g., coma). Exam: tense, non-inflammatory bullae on normal skin.	Diagnosis based on exam and history. To treat, relieve pressure. Will resolve spontaneously.
Friction blister	Develops in setting of friction, often on feet. Exam: tense bullae on normal skin.	Diagnosis based on exam and history. No treatment required, will resolve spontaneously.
Bullous diabeticorum	Unclear etiology. Associated with diabetes mellitus. Exam: tense, non-inflammatory bullae on normal skin. Often on lower extremities, develop abruptly.	Diagnosis based on exam and history. No treatment required, will resolve spontaneously in several weeks.

(continued)

Table 19.2. Differential diagnosis of non-immunobullous conditions. (Continued)

Disease	Etiology and exam	Diagnosis and treatment
Drug eruptions		
Stevens-Johnson syndrome/ Toxic epidermal necrolysis	Medication reaction, commonly antibiotics and anticonvulsants. Exam: widespread macules or patches that develop blisters and erode. Mucosal involvement frequent with significant crusting of lips, nose and eyes. Patient appears ill. Nikolsky sign is positive.	Diagnosis based on history and biopsy. Histopathology shows apoptotic (dead) keratinocytes and later subepidermal blister with epidermal necrosis. Immunofluorescence negative. Treatment is supportive. Discontinue offending agent.
Pseudoporphyria	Medication reaction, commonly NSAIDs. Exam: findings similar to porphyria cutanea tarda.	Diagnosis based on skin biopsy. Urine and plasma porphyrins will be normal. Stop offending agent.

CLL, chronic lymphocytic leukemia; HIV, human immunodeficiency virus; HSV, herpes simplex virus; NSAIDs, non-steroidal anti-inflammatory drugs; PCR, polymerase chain reaction; VZV, varicella zoster virus.

REFERENCES

1. Chee SN, Murrell DF. Pemphigus and quality of life. *Dermatol Clin.* 2011;29:521-5.
2. Alpsoy E, Akman-Karakas A, Uzun S. Geographic variations in epidemiology of two autoimmune bullous diseases: pemphigus and bullous pemphigoid. *Arch Dermatol Res.* 2015;307:291-8.
3. Langan SM, Groves RW, West J. The relationship between neurological disease and bullous pemphigoid: a population-based case-control study. *J Invest Dermatol.* 2011;131:631-6.
4. Persson MSM, Harman KE, Vinogradova Y, Langan SM, Hippisley-Cox J, Thomas KS et al. Incidence, prevalence and mortality of bullous pemphigoid in England. 1998-2017: a population-based cohort study. *Br J Dermatol.* 2021; 184(1):68-77.
5. Schmidt E, della Torre R, Borradori L. Clinical features and practical diagnosis of bullous pemphigoid. *Dermatol Clin.* 2011;29:427-38, viii-ix.
6. Lin L, Hwang BJ, Culton DA, Li N, Burette S, Koller BH et al. Eosinophils mediate tissue injury in the autoimmune skin disease bullous pemphigoid. *J Invest Dermatol.* 2018;138: 1032-43.
7. Liu SD, Chen WT, Chi CC. Association between medication use and bullous pemphigoid: a systematic review and meta-analysis. *JAMA Dermatol.* 2020;156:891-900.
8. Schmidt E, Zillikens D. Modern diagnosis of autoimmune blistering skin diseases. *Autoimmun Rev.* 2010;10:84-9.
9. Pohla-Gubo G, Hintner H. Direct and indirect immunofluorescence for the diagnosis of bullous autoimmune diseases. *Dermatol Clin.* 2011;29:365-72, vii.
10. Meijer JM, Diercks GFH, de Lang EWG, Pas HH, Jonkman MF. Assessment of diagnostic strategy for early recognition of bullous and nonbullous variants of pemphigoid. *JAMA Dermatol.* 2019;155:158-65.
11. Langan SM, Smeeth L, Hubbard R, Fleming KM, Smith CJ, West J. Bullous pemphigoid and pemphigus vulgaris--incidence and mortality in the UK: population based cohort study. *BMJ.* 2008;337:a180.
12. Venugopal SS, Murrell DF. Diagnosis and clinical features of pemphigus vulgaris. *Dermatol Clin.* 2011;29:373-80.
13. Joly P, Maho-Vaillant M, Prost-Squarcioni C, Hebert V, Houivet E, Calbo S et al. First-line rituximab combined with short-term prednisone versus prednisone alone for the treatment of pemphigus (Ritux 3): a prospective, multicentre, parallel-group, open-label randomised trial. *Lancet.* 2017;389:2031-40.
14. Jelti L, Cordel N, Gillibert A, Lacour JP, Uthurriague C, Doutre MS et al. Incidence and Mortality of Pemphigus in France. *J Invest Dermatol.* 2019;139:469-73.
15. Risser J, Lewis K, Weinstock MA. Mortality of bullous skin disorders from 1979 through 2002 in the United States. *Arch Dermatol.* 2009;145:1005-8.
16. Bolotin D, Petronic-Rosic V. Dermatitis herpetiformis. Part I. Epidemiology, pathogenesis, and clinical presentation. *J Am Acad Dermatol.* 2011;64:1017-24.
17. Bolotin D, Petronic-Rosic V. Dermatitis herpetiformis. Part II. Diagnosis, management, and prognosis. *J Am Acad Dermatol.* 2011;64:1027-33.
18. Nino M, Ciacci C, Delfino M. A long-term gluten-free diet as an alternative treatment in severe forms of dermatitis herpetiformis. *J Dermatolog Treat.* 2007;18:10-2.
19. Kárpáti S. Dermatitis herpetiformis. *Clin Dermatol.* 2012;30:56-9.
20. Paek SY, Steinberg SM, Katz SI. Remission in dermatitis herpetiformis: a cohort study. *Arch Dermatol.* 2011;147:301-5.

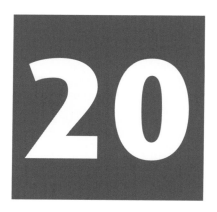

20

Benign Tumors and Vascular Birthmarks

Adam Mattox
Lindsey M. Voller
Sheilagh Maguiness

INTRODUCTION TO CHAPTER

Quick recognition and a clear understanding of the most common benign tumors are advantageous for clinicians. Confident reassurance helps to alleviate the concern of a patient but identifying a possible malignant lesion is crucial to further evaluation or referral. Knowledge of benign lesions will allow the clinician to first screen and differentiate those with simple or no required treatment from those that are of true concern.

The first section of this chapter covers benign tumors that are usually seen in adults. The second section of this chapter covers vascular tumors and vascular malformations in infants and children.

SEBORRHEIC KERATOSIS

Introduction

Incredibly common, one or more seborrheic keratosis is present in approximately 50% of adults. They are more common in lighter skin types, with some patients having hundreds scattered throughout their skin. Seborrheic keratoses occur on almost any skin surface, except for the palms and soles.[1] The pathogenesis is unknown, but they are more common in areas of sun exposure.

Clinical Presentation

History

Many patients with seborrheic keratoses present with the concern of a changing pigmented "mole" with fear that it may be melanoma or skin cancer. Seborrheic keratoses can arise de novo or start as a macule (used to be flat, but now it's raised). Patients may complain of pain and pruritus if the seborrheic keratosis is irritated by clothing. Seborrheic keratosis appears to be stuck on such that some patients will report scratching off the papule only to have it recur.

▶ Physical Examination

A classic seborrheic keratosis has a predilection for the trunk and presents as a well-defined hyperpigmented, ovoid papule, or plaque with a waxy texture and scaly surface. Multiple lesions are more common than a solitary one. Sizes range from a few millimeters to several centimeters in diameter (Figure 20-1). They are often oval with the long axis parallel to relaxed skin tension lines nearby. The astute clinician can quickly recognize these common lesions averting a biopsy, but occasionally the classic features of a seborrheic keratosis are obscured, and a biopsy is prudent. One morphologic variant is a macular seborrheic keratosis, common on the back, face, and scalp which presents as a macule or minimally elevated velvety plaque. The lack of a classic waxy texture allows for misdiagnosis of a solar lentigo or worse, melanoma. A facial variant is dermatosis papulosa nigra (DPN) which presents primarily in African American individuals as small dark papules scattered on the cheeks (Figure 20-2). Stucco keratosis is another variant that presents as multiple small,

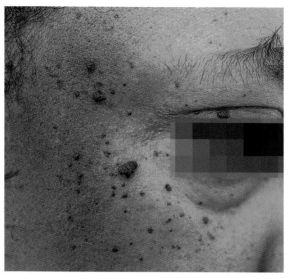

▲ **Figure 20-2.** Dermatosis papularis nigra. Variant of seborrheic keratosis commonly seen on the face in darker skin types.

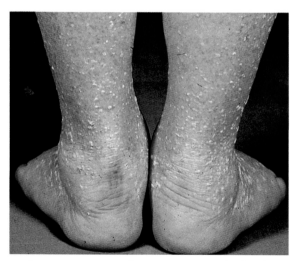

▲ **Figure 20-3.** Stucco keratosis. Variant of seborrheic keratosis seen on legs and feet. Presents with multiple small white hyperkeratotic papules.

lightly pigmented, or white keratotic papules on the distal lower extremities resembling the texture of a stucco wall (Figure 20-3).

▶ Laboratory

Histopathology of all variants of seborrheic keratoses demonstrate thickening of the epidermis (dermis unaffected) with trapping of keratin in elongated tracks called pseudo horn

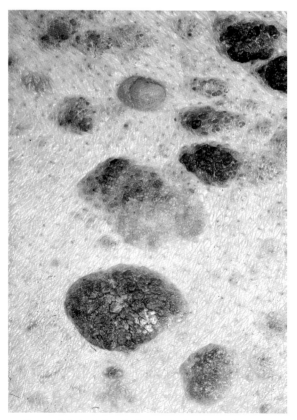

▲ **Figure 20-1.** Seborrheic keratosis. Tan to brown stuck on appearing papules and plaques with a waxy hyperkeratotic surface.

cysts. Pseudo horn cysts can be seen with a dermatoscope or magnifying glass and resemble milia-like cysts or crypts.

▶ Differential Diagnosis

✓ Lentigo: Macule with even hyperpigmentation and a smooth scalloped border, most commonly on sun exposed areas of face, neck, shoulders, chest, and hands.

✓ Nevus: Tan to black macules or papules; surface is not hyperkeratotic or waxy.

✓ Melanoma: Hyperpigmented macule/papule with asymmetry, irregular border, and multiple colors.

✓ Warts: Verrucous papules containing thrombosed capillaries visible as dark speckles.

✓ Squamous cell carcinoma and basal cell carcinoma: Eroded or bleeding papule that lacks the stuck on appearance and milia-like cysts.

Management

No specific treatment is required other than differentiating seborrheic keratoses from with malignant potential. For irritated or disfiguring lesions destruction with cryotherapy can be beneficial (see Chapter 7). Care must be taken to avoid overtreatment which can lead to scarring. Patients must be warned that persistent hypopigmentation may occur with any treatment. Alternative treatments include electrocautery or desiccation with or without curettage.

Clinical Course and Prognosis

Lesions can appear at any age in adulthood. They are often long-lived and accumulate over time. The prognosis is largely excellent. Collision nevi with a separate malignancy arising within and seborrheic keratosis and the exceedingly rare Sign of Leser-Trélat (sudden onset of numerous seborrheic keratoses associated with internal malignancy) are the exceptions.

Indications for Consultation

Lesions that cannot be clearly defined as benign.

Patient Information

• American Academy of Dermatology: https://www.aad.org/public/diseases/a-z/seborrheic-keratoses-overview

• DermNet New Zealand: https://dermnetnz.org/topics/seborrhoeic-keratosis/

▼ LENTIGO

Introduction

A hallmark of photo-aged skin, lentigines is common benign hyperplasias of melanocytes in areas of chronic sun exposure. They are usually acquired and appear in the third decade of life. Less commonly they can be congenital, as part of a syndrome like LEOPARD (Noonan) syndrome and Peutz-Jeghers syndrome.

Pathogenesis

Chronic repetitive exposure to sun and ultraviolet light induces mutations leading to enhanced melanin production and pigment retention by keratinocytes. Though not dangerous, they are a sign of significant sun exposure and indicate an increased risk of ultraviolet (UV) induced malignancy.

Clinical Presentation

▶ History

Commonly known as "liver spots" lentigines are persistent, hyperpigmented, and flat spots appearing after significant sun exposure and damage. Degree of pigmentation may be reported to fluctuate seasonally, darkening with sun exposure. Patients rarely bring lentigines to medical attention except in the context of "unsightly" age spots or concern for melanoma.[1] Common mutations may allow them to evolve into seborrheic keratosis or become benign lichenoid keratosis with inflammation.

▶ Physical Examination

Lentigines present as light or dark brown macules with sharp borders on sun exposed skin, especially dorsal hands (Figure 20-4), forearms, and shoulders. They may also occur on mucous membranes and the nail bed. Lentigo simplex occurs without ultraviolet exposure and can develop early as the first decade of life. These present as sharply marginated monochromatic light- or dark-brown

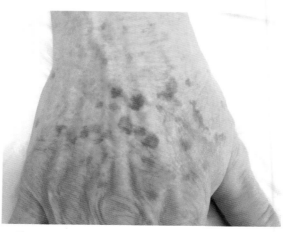

▲ **Figure 20-4.** Lentigines. Multiple brown macules scattered on sun exposed skin.

macules. They may also be accompanied by hypopigmented macules, actinic purpura, and gritty scale on the surface of actinic keratosis.

Laboratory Findings

Histopathology shows club-shaped rete ridges containing an increased number of melanocytes in contact with the basal cell layer of the epidermis. Characteristic features may be described as "dirty feet."

Differential Diagnosis

- Lentigo maligna: Macular hyperpigmentation, in a similar distribution, but with variations in color and irregular border, typically in older adults.
- Labial, penile, and vulvar melanosis: Usually light brown, but may be dark and irregularly bordered macules. May or may not have ultraviolet light exposure history

Management

Lentigines do not have a medical indication for removal. Prevention is the best approach to solar lentigines with the regular use of sunscreens. Common cosmetic management techniques include bleaching creams (e.g., hydroquinone), cryotherapy, and laser treatment. However, without strict sun protection macules will recur despite treatment.[2]

Clinical Course and Prognosis

The natural history of lentigines is to persist over time and darken with age and sunlight exposure.

Indications for Consultation

Cosmetically bothersome lentigines can be referred for laser and intense pulsed light treatment (monochromatic non-coherent light visible light).

Patient Information

DermNet New Zealand: https://dermnetnz.org/topics/solar-lentigo/

DERMATOFIBROMA (FIBROUS HISTIOCYTOMA)

Introduction

Dermatofibroma is a common lesion occurring in middle-aged adults, but seldom seen in children. It varies in presentation on visual inspection but has a consistent and characteristic firm texture on palpation. The pathogenesis is not certain but is thought to follow minor trauma as the result of an error in the healing process leading to scar formation of dermal fibroblasts. The mechanism is debated, a reactive or neoplastic origin.[3]

Clinical Presentation

History

Although most dermatofibromas are asymptomatic, itching, and pain may be reported. Most patients present with concern over a now symptomatic or more raised "mole." The classic dermatofibroma is a papule occurring on the leg of a woman which is traumatized by shaving.

Physical Examination

Usually a solitary papule, multiple dermatofibromas are not uncommon. They present as a firm, 3–10 mm papule or nodule on the distal lower extremities or proximal upper extremities. It may have an associated increase in pigmentation. The pigmentation of these lesions is symmetrical often with a lighter central area and a collaret of darker pigmentation (Figure 20-5A). Horizontal compression,

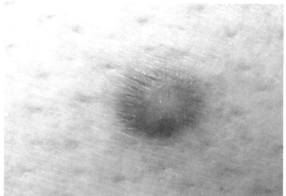

A

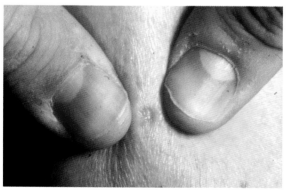

B

▲ **Figure 20-5.** A,B. Dermatofibroma. A. Tan to pink firm papule. B. Dimple sign with compression

or pinching of the lesion, leads to dimpling (dimple sign) due to deep collagen connection (Figure 20-5B). Dermatofibromas can entrap nerves within the scar leading to sensations of itch or sensitivity.

Laboratory Findings

Histopathology shows a spindle cell proliferation of fibroblasts in the dermis. This proliferation is not well circumscribed and infiltrates adjacent structures surrounding individual collagen bundles described as "collagen trapping." The characteristic immunohistochemical staining is Factor XIIIa positive and CD34 negative.

Differential Diagnosis

- Nevus: Tan to dark brown soft macule or papule. Dimple sign is absent.
- Dermatofibrosarcoma protuberans: Firm nodule similar to a dermatofibroma, but larger in size (≥2–3 cm) and showing progression in size with time.
- Melanoma: Flat or raised lesion with variable pigment and irregular borders.

Management

Treatment options are limited. Intralesional triamcinolone injections can be used but carry risk of adjacent atrophy and have limited success. Reassurance of the benign nature of the lesions with no treatment is appropriate for small and asymptomatic lesions. Those lesions with prominent itch or tenderness can be surgically removed with the caveat that the patient is trading the round scar of a dermatofibroma for a linear scar of the excision. Unfortunately, lesions may recur even after excision. Involution may occur after many years if ignored.

Clinical Course and Prognosis

The course of a dermatofibroma is largely stable and benign. Large size, morphologic, or symptomatic changes are indications for biopsy or excision. Rarely, the histologic variant of cellular dermatofibroma can metastasize, thus is an indication for excision with clear margins. The development of multiple dermatofibromas can be associated with the following: systemic lupus erythematosus, treatment with prednisone or immunosuppressive drugs, chronic myelogenous leukemia, and human immunodeficiency virus (HIV). Screening is appropriate if history suggests dermatofibromas are secondary to these factors.

Indications for Consultation

Patients with lesions with continued growth, recurrent, poorly defined lesions, or multiple lesions should be referred to dermatology.

Patient Information

DermNet New Zealand https://dermnetnz.org/topics/dermatofibroma/

SKIN TAG (ACROCHORDON, CUTANEOUS PAPILLOMA)

Clinical Presentation

► History

Skin tags are very common, soft, pedunculated papillomas occurring on intertriginous sites. They tend to present in individuals in the mid-40's to late 60's in sites of friction such as the neck, axillae, and groin. Weight gain correlates with an increased incidence.[4] A few genetic syndromes present with numerous skin tags.[3]

► Physical Examination

They present as soft pedunculated skin-colored papules with a thin stalk (Figure 20-6). The stalk contains a central blood vessel.

► Laboratory Findings

Histopathology shows loose fibrous tissue in the dermis of a polyp with thin epidermis.

Differential Diagnosis

- Neurotized nevus: Very similar to skin tags but presents as a single lesion.
- Neurofibroma: May be polypoid, but typically are larger than skin tags, and may present within the context of a genetic syndrome.

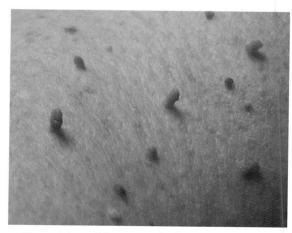

▲ **Figure 20-6.** Skin tags. Soft, skin colored to tan, polypoid papules.

- Dermatosis papulosa nigra: More commonly occurring on the face, smaller and has waxy, verrucous texture.

Management

Cryotherapy can be useful with numerous lesions, but success is limited to lesions that have a narrow stalk. Broad based lesions are best treated with thin shave excision. Electrodessication and removal with iris scissors can be used for smaller lesions. Any treatment often leaves behind a small hypopigmented macule.

Clinical Course and Prognosis

Increasing incidence and numbers of skin tags is noted during weight gain, pregnancy, or concurrent with insulin treatment and diabetes. Skin tags usually remain asymptomatic unless traumatized or twisted. Once inflamed, pain and necrosis may follow.

Indications for Consultation

Patients with numerous or symptomatic skin tags should be referred to dermatology.

Patient Information

DermNet New Zealand: https://dermnetnz.org/topics/skin-tag/

SEBACEOUS HYPERPLASIA

Introduction

Onset of sebaceous hyperplasia is usually in adults over age 40 years and lesions commonly accumulate with age. A variety of mechanisms contribute to pathogenesis including cyclosporine treatment, genetic syndromes (e.g., Muir-Torre), but most are associated with age-related hormonal environment. The result of these influences is enlargement of sebaceous glands caused by an increased number of sebocytes.[3]

Clinical Presentation

History

Patients usually complain of yellowish, skin-colored papules appearing in oily skin locations like the forehead, infraorbital cheeks, and temples. They can arise in other sites as well, the areolas, nipples, penis, neck, and chest. Patients with a history of basal cell carcinoma may mistake the similar clinical presentation of sebaceous hyperplasia as an early basal cell carcinoma. Sebaceous hyperplasia usually will not display continuous growth or bleeding common in basal cell carcinomas.

Physical Examination

Sebaceous hyperplasia present as 2–6 mm yellow to skin colored papule(s) on the central face and forehead

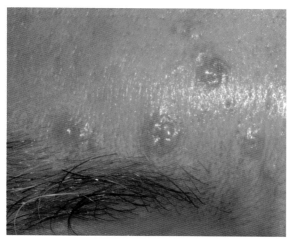

▲ **Figure 20-7.** Sebaceous hyperplasia. Pink to yellow papules with central depression above eyebrow.

(Figure 20-7). Dermoscopy or magnification will reveal a central depression surrounded by yellow lobules. Telangiectasias present in the papule can be reminiscent of basal cell carcinoma.

▶ Laboratory Findings

Histopathology shows hyperplasia of sebaceous glands.

Differential Diagnosis

- Milia: 1–2 mm white cyst with no central depression.
- Basal cell carcinoma: papules have a more shiny appearance without visible yellowish glands and the texture is more friable and tends to bleed.
- Acne: Transient erythematous inflammatory papules lasting less than 2 months.

Management

Lesions that are progressive or show symptoms of tenderness or bleeding should be biopsied to rule out basal cell carcinoma. Observation is sufficient for stable lesions. Cosmetically bothersome lesions can be treated with shave removal with or without electrodessication. Electrodessication on its own can be used as well for smaller lesions. A small scar is often left after treatment. Treatment with 1450-nm diode laser may require several treatments but delivers effective results with few adverse effects.

Clinical Course and Prognosis

Sebaceous hyperplasia is benign, but papules commonly accumulate with age. The papules are largely asymptomatic, and treatment is commonly considered cosmetic.

Indications for Consultation

Patients with progressive lesions or who want cosmetic treatment could be referred to dermatology.

Patient Information

DermNet New Zealand: https://dermnetnz.org/topics/sebaceous-hyperplasia/

▼ LIPOMA

Introduction

A lipoma is a benign localized overgrowth of fat cells in the subcutaneous tissue. Lipomas may occur as single or multiple tumors. Familial tendencies may be explained by chromosomal alterations in the tumor. Protease inhibitors used to treat HIV disease may result in systemic fat alteration ranging from lipoatrophy to angiolipomas and lipomas. Angiolipomas are diagnosed histologically, with adipose collections containing a proliferation of capillary-sized vessels. Erythrocytes and microthrombi may be present in the vessel lumens.

Clinical Presentation

▶ History

Patients may present with solitary or multiple lesions. There may be a family history. A number of syndromes present with multiple, numbering from a few to hundreds. Lipomas come in two main variants, classic and angiolipoma. The angiolipoma variant may be more painful but is otherwise clinically indistinguishable from the classic lipoma. The mechanism for pain is not known, but neurons that form with the vessels or microthrombi are thought to be contributors. Pain may be described as a deep aching sensation with minor pressure or trauma and can be quite distressing.

▶ Physical Examination

A lipoma usually presents as a subcutaneous rubbery nodule or tumor often occurring on the trunk, neck, arms, and axillae (Figure 20-8).

▶ Laboratory Findings

Histopathology shows a well-circumscribed adipose tumor with a thin capsule. Histologic variants include angiolipoma, spindle cell lipoma, fibrolipoma, pleomorphic lipoma, angiomyolipoma, and hibernoma.

Differential Diagnosis

- Liposarcoma: Similar presentation to a standard lipoma, but much more aggressive history of growth.
- Epidermal cyst: Firm cyst with a central puncta.

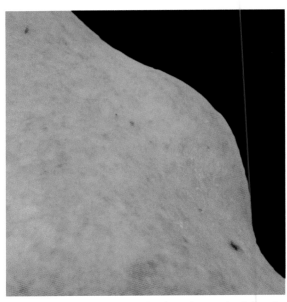

▲ **Figure 20-8.** Lipoma on back. Soft, poorly defined, subcutaneous nodule or tumor. Overlying skin appears normal.

- Neurofibroma: Exophytic skin colored papules or more rarely, a plexiform subcutaneous mass with a firm consistency.
- Lymphadenopathy: Located in common lymph node basins, tends to be deeper and denser.
- Cancer metastatic to skin: Present more superficial, firm tumor present in the dermis, history of malignancy.

Management

Options for management include observation or surgical removal.[5] During excision, the tissue that makes up the lipoma has a more dense and rubbery texture than normal adjacent adipose tissue. The tumor often has a lobulated but contiguous shape. Classic lipomas have a tendency to have a deeper yellow color than surrounding normal fat cells. Injected deoxycholic acid has been approved for the treatment of submental fat, but some clinicians will use it to treat lipomas off label. The efficacy of deoxycholic acid to dissolve a lipoma appears suboptimal compared to normal physiologic fat, requiring re-retreatment and likely high cost. Liposuction is another effective treatment for multiple or large lipomas to minimize scarring.

Clinical Course and Prognosis

Lipomas usually grow until attaining a certain size, and then persist as a constant size. For asymptomatic lipomas, the clinical course is largely indolent and benign, and no treatment is necessary. Surgery is reserved for symptomatic or bothersome tumors. Excision is often effective, but lipomas can occur.

Indications for Consultation

Symptomatic or large lesions may be referred for surgical treatment.

Patient Information

Cleveland Clinic: https://my.clevelandclinic.org/health/diseases/15008-lipomas

KELOID/HYPERTROPHIC SCAR

Introduction

The terms keloid and hypertrophic scar are often erroneously used synonymously. There is a key difference that has major clinical implications. A hypertrophic scar may be symptomatic and increase in firmness but will not extend beyond the border of the original injury. A keloid scar will grow beyond the borders of the original injury, often expanding with claw-like extensions at the periphery. The threshold for injury producing a keloid appears to be much lower than that for hypertrophic scarring. The pathogenesis of keloid formation is not known, but is initiated with skin injury and appears to be mediated by transforming growth factor-β.[6]

Clinical Presentation

History

Patients complain of a raised, firm, irregularly bordered, pink to tan scar that continues to grow. Keloid scars may be disfiguring or symptomatic (pain and pruritus). Common locations are the sternum, ears, neck, trunk, and extremities. The incidence is higher among individuals with darker skin types.[7]

Physical Examination

A hypertrophic scar is a firm pink-tan plaque occurring at the site of injury and remains limited by the borders (regular) of the original injury (Figure 20-9A). A keloid will form a thick firm fibrous plaque or tumor that grows into healthy skin beyond the immediate confines of the initial injury (Figure 20-9B).

Laboratory Findings

Histopathology is similar for keloids and hypertrophic scars. Keloid shows whorls of fibroblasts in the dermis. Histopathology of a keloid may show thicker bands of collagen in the dermis.

Differential Diagnosis

- Sclerotic basal cell carcinoma: Similar appearance, but with progressive growth and bleeding.

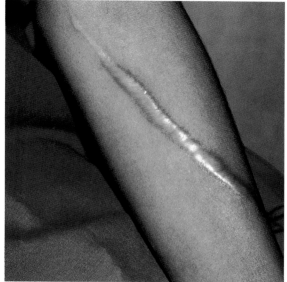

A

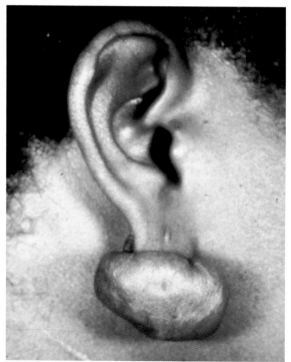

B

▲ **Figure 20-9.** A. Hypertrophic scar. Thick pink scar following laceration on arm. Scar does not extend beyond margins of the original laceration. B. Keloid at the site of ear piercing. Firm, smooth, skin-colored to tan, tumor outgrowing the original scar.

- Dermatofibrosarcoma protuberans: Firm tan nodule with progressive growth without injury history.
- Foreign body granuloma: Reactive process at site of injury or previous surgery. Firm nodule with red to brown hyperpigmentation.
- Sarcoidosis: Firm pink-tan sclerotic papules, central face affected (spared by keloid).
- Lobomycosis: Firm, smooth, dome-shaped papules occurring at the site of injury and wound contamination. Fungal infection endemic to tropical and subtropical climates.

Management

Hypertrophic scars will spontaneously become more supple over a period of years. Unfortunately, their original dimensions will persist. Softening can be expedited with intralesional triamcinolone injections.[8] It may take multiple sessions spaced 1–2 months apart to alleviate symptoms. Keloids can be treated similarly but often respond to treatment more slowly.[9] Keloids are also more likely to recur after therapy is discontinued. Injecting lesions with a mixture of 5-fluorouracil and triamcinolone can increase efficacy. Surgical correction of hypertrophic scars is often successful. However, attempts at keloid excision should be approached with caution. Often surgical excision leads to more extensive damage and larger keloid formation. Treatments adjuvant to surgery can include continuation of intralesional triamcinolone, radiation treatment, or application of imiquimod 5% cream.

Clinical Course and Prognosis

Hypertrophic scars may soften spontaneously with time. Keloids are extremely prone to recurrence and resistant to treatment. A multidisciplinary treatment plan is required for severe cases.

Indications for Consultation

Patients with lesions that fail to respond to intralesional steroid therapy should be referred to dermatology.

Patient Information

- American Academy of Dermatology: https://www.aad.org/public/diseases/a-z/keloids-overview
- Society for Pediatric Dermatology: https://pedsderm.net/site/assets/files/1028/spd_scars_color_web_1.pdf

EPIDERMAL (EPIDERMOID) CYST

Introduction

One of the most common benign tumors of the skin, the epidermal cyst is a capsule filled with keratin debris. They are sometimes called sebaceous cyst (a misnomer as they have no relationship to sebaceous glands). They can occur in adolescents through older adults and may be associated with an acne vulgaris history. Frequently, they are the result of plugging of follicular openings or epidermal implantation after surgery or trauma. Arising from the infundibulum of the hair follicle, the resulting capsule histology is similar to that of the epidermis and stratum corneum. Cells forming the cyst lining are constantly sloughed into the center of the cyst and undergo degradation leading to the soft keratin containing a necrotic center.[3]

Clinical Presentation

▶ History

Epiderma cysts can occur in almost any skin area but are most common on the central trunk and face. Patients may complain of a cyst "infection" which likely represents rupture of the cyst capsule allowing keratin contents into the dermis. Normally located in the stratum corneum, the keratin and cellular debris in the dermis triggers a robust foreign body inflammatory reaction with swelling (may double or triple in size), pain, and pus as its hallmark.

▶ Physical Examination

They present as asymptomatic, firm, skin colored, nodule, or cyst. There is often a rudimentary connection between the capsule and the epidermis creating an indentation overlying the center of the cyst (Figure 20-10). A central punctum is also common. This connection can be patent allowing visualization of the oxidized keratin (dark color) or even extrusion of cyst contents. A strong odor is usually associated with this soft "cheesy" material.

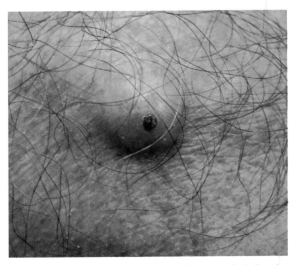

▲ Figure 20-10. Epidermoid cyst. Firm, well-defined, dermal papule, or nodule with central punctum.

Laboratory Findings

Histopathology shows a cyst in the dermis lined with stratified squamous epithelium (granular layer is present, analogous to the epidermis and stratum corneum) and filled with keratin flakes. If rupture has occurred, a brisk inflammatory reaction with foreign body giant cells will be present in the adjacent dermis.

Differential Diagnosis

- Pilar cyst: Similar to epidermal cyst, but with no central punctum, often located on scalp.
- Proliferating epidermoid cyst/proliferating pilar cyst: Similar presentation, but with carcinomatous changes on histology.
- Boil or acne cyst: More acute and inflammatory.
- Carbuncle: Multiple adjacent hair follicles inflamed and ruptured forming a contiguous abscess
- Lipoma: Malleable and more mobile (no epidermal connection) nodule.
- Neurofibroma: Soft pedunculated papule, may "buttonhole" when pushed into the dermis.
- Squamous cell carcinoma, metastatic cancer: Firm (less compressible) dome-shaped papule or nodule on sun-exposed skin.[10]

Management

Post rupture inflammatory reaction can lead to resolution in a limited number of cases. However, the cyst is likely to recur. If the cyst is inflamed at the time of presentation, excision is postponed a few weeks. Initial treatment is aimed at reducing inflammation by incision and drainage (I&D), 2 weeks of doxycycline (matrix metalloproteinase anti-inflammatory effect), or perilesional triamcinolone injections. Surgical removal of the entire capsule is the standard of care, and should be performed when the cyst is not inflamed.[11] To rule out any potentially dangerous conditions in the differential diagnosis, it is prudent to always submit the excised tissue for pathologic review.

Clinical Course and Prognosis

Cysts on the trunk may be asymptomatic, of no concern to the patient for decades. Their benign nature reserves treatment for those becoming symptomatic or in anticipation of pain and inflammation.

Indications for Consultation

High risk or complex location needing excision and multiple lesions.

Patient Information

DermNet New Zealand: https://dermnetnz.org/topics/epidermoid-cyst/

PILAR CYST

Introduction

Pilar cysts (also known as trichilemmal cysts) are relatively common, presenting in approximately 10% of the population. They arise from outer root sheath cells of the hair follicle. As in epidermoid cysts, the lining defines the cyst type and produces its contents. Cells lining the cyst continue to produce keratin, but without connection to a hair. The compact laminate keratin forms a hard sphere within the dermis.[3]

Clinical Presentation

History

Commonly presenting on the scalp, women over age 60 are predominantly affected. There may be a family history.

Physical Examination

Pilar cysts present as a dome-shaped nodule in the dermis or subcutis of the scalp, they do not have a punctum, and have a more firm texture than epidermoid cysts (Figure 20-11).

Laboratory Findings

On histology, the capsule is made of a stratified squamous epithelium, but lacks a granular layer, demonstrating abrupt trichilemmal keratinization. Cyst contents are dense homogenous densely packed keratin that may calcify.

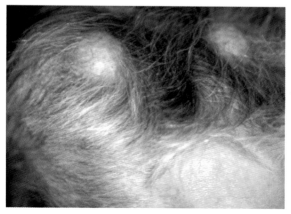

▲ **Figure 20-11.** Pilar cysts. Two pilar cysts visible on hair bearing scalp. Punctum is not present.

Differential Diagnosis

Differential is similar to that of epidermoid cysts, see above.

Management

Asymptomatic and smaller lesions are often observed as they may remain quiescent. Simple I&D, to remove the keratin sphere will likely recur. As in epidermal cysts, complete removal of the cyst lining is required for a durable cure.

Clinical Course and Prognosis

One or multiple cysts may occur. Typically they grow to a certain size and remain unchanged. Often cysts will remain asymptomatic for years and may be observed. Complete excision of the cyst capsule reduces the risk of recurrence.

Indications for Consultation

Tender enlarging lesions requiring surgical removal.

Patient Information

DermNet New Zealand: https://dermnetnz.org/topics/trichilemmal-cyst/

MILIA

Introduction

Milia represent a smaller variant of epidermal cyst.[12] They have similar pathology, derived from the infundibulum of vellus hair follicles. They occur in 50% of infants, but often resolve spontaneously. In adults, they are more likely to be persistent or recurrent. Primary milia are present congenitally, as multiple eruptive milia, and milia en plaque (plaque containing dense milia).[13] Secondary milia develop after recovery from inflammatory skin disease such as blistering skin disease, herpes zoster, polymorphous light eruption, systemic lupus erythematosus (SLE), Stevens–Johnson syndrome, and contact dermatitis.[3] Surgery and skin trauma may contribute to formation. Medications such as topical steroids, occlusive moisturizers, cyclosporine, and 5-fluorouracil can also be causes. Milia are also common in several genodermatoses such as Rombo, Brooke-Spiegler, Bazex, and pachyonychia congenita type two.

Clinical Presentation

▶ History

Milia have a bimodal incidence affecting infants and children and again in middle age. Most commonly papules occur around the eyes and on the upper face. Typically, they are not symptomatic, but patients may consider them unsightly.

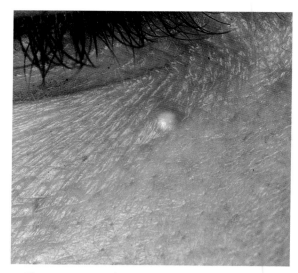

▲ **Figure 20-12.** Milia. Firm, 2-mm white papule below eye.

▶ Physical Examination

They present as small 1–4 mm white firm dome shaped papules which are most common around the eyes and on the upper face (Figure 20-12).

▶ Laboratory Findings

Histopathology shows the same findings as an epidermal cyst (capsule of stratified squamous epithelium with a granular layer present and keratin flake debris), but the diameter of the cyst is smaller.

Differential Diagnosis

- Closed comedones: More common in teenagers and adults with acne.
- Syringoma: Skin colored to clear papules, 1–3 mm in diameter primarily present on the lower eyelids.
- Trichoepithelioma: Multiple skin-colored papules that form most prominently in the area of the medial canthus, but may extend onto the eyelids and dorsal nose. Often associated with cylindromatosis (CYLD) gene mutation.
- Xanthelasma: Soft, yellow-orange, oblong plaques near medial canthi in middle-aged adults.
- Follicular mucinosis variant of cutaneous T-cell lymphoma: Flesh-colored follicular papules within hypopigmented or erythematous plaques and localized alopecia.

Management

Observation is often best, but tretinoin cream has been reported effective. Central contents can be extracted by simple incision overlying the lesion with a #11 blade. Avoid incising deeper than the keratin contents which is less than 1 mm. Careful removal of the cyst wall may be possible though the incision once the keratin contents have been extracted. Care should be taken not to cause undo trauma that will lead to scar formation.

Clinical Course and Prognosis

Milia are likely to stay small (1–4 mm) after appearance, but often persist for months. Once treated, they are not likely to recur. New secondary milia may occur if there is ongoing skin injury.

Indications for Consultation

Patients with multiple lesions, enlarging or recurrent lesions should be referred to dermatology.

Patient Information

DermNet New Zealand: https://dermnetnz.org/topics/milium/

▼ DIGITAL MUCOUS CYST

Introduction

Digital mucous cysts are pseudo-cysts as they do not have a cellular lining (true capsule). They represent an extrusion of mucinous contents from a local joint space into the surrounding dermis. As the mucin collection grows, it compacts cells in the dermis at the margin, mimicking a capsule. They are more prevalent in women, and in patients with osteoarthritis of the adjacent distal interphalangeal joint (DIP) joint.[3]

Clinical Presentation

▶ History

Patients complain of a shiny, translucent bump appearing within or adjacent to the nail unit of a digit. Usually occurring as a solitary asymptomatic papule, multiple digital mucous cysts can be associated with connective tissue disease (systemic sclerosis or juvenile rheumatoid arthritis).

▶ Physical Examination

They are most commonly present as a translucent skin-colored cyst papule on the distal aspect of a digit of the hand either overlying the proximal matrix of the nail or underlying the nail bed (Figure 20-13). They may cause distortion (longitudinal groove, increased transverse nail curvature,

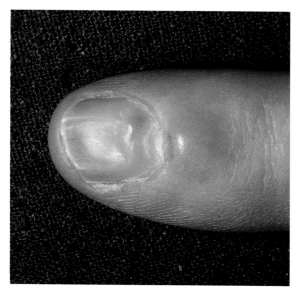

▲ **Figure 20-13.** Digital mucous cyst. Translucent dermal or subcutaneous papule compressing the proximal nail matrix producing a groove in the nail plate.

red or blue discoloration of the lunula, or longitudinal nail splitting) of nail formation due to pressure exerted on the nail matrix.[7] As the nail grows distally, it maintains the shape of the compressed matrix.

▶ Laboratory Findings

Histopathology shows a focal area of mucin in the dermis with densely packed dermal cells and structures at the margin. A true capsule is absent.

Differential Diagnosis

- Glomus tumor: Rare benign bluish colored neoplasm, usually solitary, around or often under the nail plate. One of the painful tumors of the skin. Pain triggered by cold.
- Osteoma: Solid, non-compressible nodule that most often develops in the site of previous trauma.
- Neuroma: pain can be disabling, may be the result of injury, and occurs closer to joints instead of the nail unit.

Management

Extrusion of cyst contents can alleviate pressure on the matrix and pain.[7] However, resolution after simple rupture is temporary, only to recur. Treatment of the connecting sinus tract with cautery or ligation serves to reduce the rate of recurrence.[14,15]

Clinical Course and Prognosis

Asymptomatic lesions may be observed. Symptomatic cysts or those causing nail dystrophy can be excised. During excision, care must be taken to avoid scarring the nail matrix, which would effectively trade one type of nail dystrophy for another.

Indications for Consultation

Patients with multiple lesions and recurrent lesions for surgical excision.

Patient Information

DermNet New Zealand: https://dermnetnz.org/topics/digital-myxoid-pseudocyst/

ACQUIRED VASCULAR LESIONS (CHERRY ANGIOMA, VENOUS LAKE, SPIDER ANGIOMA)

Introduction

These vascular lesions are given names according to their clinical or histological appearance. Cherry angiomas have a strong family tendency with initial presentation in individuals in the late 20s and increase in number through those in the 50s. Deeper in the skin, a venous lake represents dilation of the venules of sun exposed skin. Spider angiomas occur on the face and upper trunk in children and high estrogen states.[3]

Clinical Presentation

▶ History

Being low pressure and flow lesions, it is unusual for bleeding to be a complaint. Adult patients may express concern with the large number of asymptomatic bright red papules on the trunk, and can be reassured they are cherry angiomas. Eruptive lesions may occur after nitrogen mustard treatment. Dilation of venules deeper in sun-damaged skin causes a dark blue to purple spot which can be considered unsightly to patients. The dark coloration can be misdiagnosed as a pigmented lesion, causing concern for melanoma. Spider angiomas occur singly or in groups on the face and upper trunk in healthy children. They are more common in pregnant women and adults with end stage liver disease.

▶ Physical Examination

Cherry hemangiomas present as small, bright red, dome-shaped papules on the trunk (Figure 20-14).

A venous lake is a purple, deeper lesion usually localized to the lower lip (Figure 20-15).

Spider angiomas are small macular lesions on the face which present with a central, bright red feeder vessel and

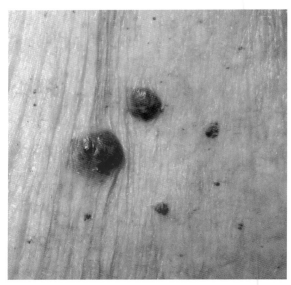

▲ **Figure 20-14.** Cherry angiomas. Multiple small asymptomatic bright red to purple dome-shaped papules.

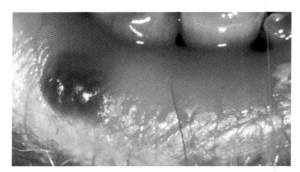

▲ **Figure 20-15.** Venous lake. Soft, compressible bluish purple, smooth papule on the lower lip mucosa.

peripheral dilated vessels (Figure 20-16). They will blanch with diascopy. (Pressure applied to the skin surface with a glass slide.)

▶ Laboratory Findings

Histopathology shows dilated capillaries in the dermis.

Differential Diagnosis

- Traumatic blister: Transient, resolves in days to weeks.
- Melanocytic lesion: A dark purple cherry angioma or venous lake may appear to be black and mimic nevi. However, their underlying color is revealed when pressed with a glass slide or with the use of dermoscopy.

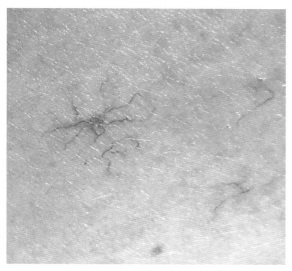

▲ **Figure 20-16.** Spider Angioma. Bright red central papule with radial telangiectasia.

- Amyloidosis: Should be considered if there is a purpuric halo around a cherry angioma.

Management

Once diagnosed, no treatment is required. However, some lesions may be treated either due to inadvertent trauma leading to bleeding or for cosmetic purposes. Pulsed dye laser (PDL) therapy can lead to resolution of most lesions. Larger lesions on the trunk respond better to shave removal with cautery of the underlying vessels. For lesions on the central face, PDL therapy or fine needle cautery of central feeder vessel will lead to resolution.[16]

Indications for Consultation

Lesions in frictional sites that sustain trauma leading to tenderness or bleeding. Cosmetic treatment.

Patient Information

DermNet New Zealand: https://dermnetnz.org/topics/cherry-angioma/
    https://dermnetnz.org/topics/venous-lake/
    https://dermnetnz.org/topics/spider-telangiectasis/

▼ PYOGENIC GRANULOMA

Introduction

Pyogenic granuloma is a lobular capillary hemangioma, which grows stretching the overlying epidermis, ultimately eroding and bleeding. The term pyogenic granuloma is a misnomer since the bleeding papule is not a granuloma

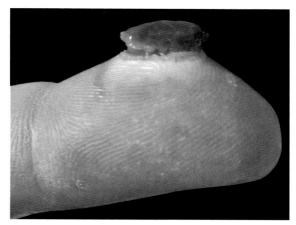

▲ **Figure 20-17.** Pyogenic granuloma. Exophytic bright red macerated or bleeding papule with collaret of thickened skin on finger.

nor is it an infection. Pyogenic granulomas can be seen in patients taking isotretinoin, capecitabine, or indinivir.[3]

Clinical Presentation

▶ History

Most often a pyogenic granuloma presents as a quickly growing, bleeding papule, or nodule. It tends to evolve rapidly from a small erythematous papule to an exophytic nodule up to 2 cm in diameter over a few weeks. Lesions most commonly arise in children, young adults, and during pregnancy. They will recur if only treated superficially. Recurrent pyogenic granulomas may have one or more satellite lesions.

▶ Physical Examination

Pyogenic granulomas present as a sessile red to purple exophytic papule that bleeds with minimal trauma (Figure 20-17). They are most common on the head, neck, and extremities. A subset also is present in the oral mucosa. The chronic ulceration is a rich environment for secondary staphylococcal colonization and resultant crust may be present.

▶ Laboratory Findings

Histopathology shows a proliferation of solidly packed capillary endothelial cells in the dermis. An epidermal collarette is common and the surface may be impetiginized.

▶ Differential Diagnosis

✓ Infantile hemangioma: See Table 20-1 of infantile vascular lesions for additional diagnoses.

Table 20-1. Differential diagnosis of common infantile vascular lesions.

Vascular lesion	Age at presentation	Identifying features	Growth characteristics
Nevus Simplex	Birth	Ill-defined, pink to bright red macule that may become more prominent with crying or vigorous activity.	Fades within 1–2 years of life; lesions on nape of neck may persist into adulthood.
Capillary Malformation (Port-Wine Stain)	Birth	Well-demarcated, irregular, dark pink to red patch or slightly raised plaque.	Grows in proportion to infant; progressively darkens and may become more nodular in quality with age.
Infantile Hemangioma	~4 weeks	*Superficial:* bright red to violaceous papules, plaques, or nodules without a subcutaneous component. *Deep:* subcutaneous tumor with a bluish or flesh-colored surface.	Rapid growth during first few months of life, followed by slower growth up to one year of age; involution may take years to fully occur.
Congenital Hemangioma	Birth	Red, violaceous, or bluish nodules or tumors with prominent superficial telangiectasias and a halo of vasoconstriction.	*Rapidly involuting* congenital hemangiomas involute around 12–15 months. *Non-involuting* congenital hemangiomas do not involute.

✓ Ulcerated melanoma, squamous cell carcinoma, metastatic carcinoma: May present as a similar growth in older adults but is not usually exophytic.

✓ Glomus tumor: Often a blue firm nodule for longer, only ulcerating in later phase, often painful.

Management

Surgical excision is indicated as these lesions have a high tendency for bleeding which is difficult to control. Shave removal with cautery of the base may be sufficient. Deeper excision may be required for recurrent lesions.

Clinical Course and Prognosis

Pyogenic granulomas are rapidly growing, friable, and usually bleed. Though benign, constant bleeding is bothersome. If treated insufficiently, recurrence is common.

Indications for Consultation

Surgical excision, recurrent lesions.

Patient Information

Society for Pediatric Dermatology: https://pedsderm.net/site/assets/files/1028/spd_pyogenic_granuloma_color_web.pdf

DermNet New Zealand: https://dermnetnz.org/topics/pyogenic-granuloma/

▼ VASCULAR BIRTHMARKS

Introduction

Over the last decade, many advances have been made in the field of vascular anomalies. This chapter will update primary care providers on the basic classification of vascular birthmarks in children, focusing on the most commonly presenting entities, namely infantile hemangiomas and capillary malformations. Vascular anomalies encompass a large number of diagnoses. These conditions are divided into *vascular tumors* or *vascular malformations* based on their biology and growth characteristics. The most complete classification is given by the International Society for the Study of Vascular Anomalies (ISSVA).[17] This section highlights common vascular lesions of infancy and childhood, including their typical morphology, natural history, and preliminary management with a focus on the *vascular tumors* of infantile hemangiomas and congenital hemangiomas and the *vascular malformations* of nevus simplex and capillary malformation (port-wine stain).

▼ INFANTILE HEMANGIOMAS

Introduction

Infantile hemangiomas, colloquially termed "strawberry marks," are the most common benign birthmarks observed in infants, affecting approximately 4% of newborns.[17,18] Infantile hemangiomas are distinct from vascular malformations owing to their proliferative phase during the first few months of life, followed by gradual involution and ultimate regression. The incidence of infantile hemangiomas is increased among female, White, and low birthweight infants, in addition to those with a history of placental anomalies.[19] Most infantile hemangiomas are benign and do not require intervention; however, in a minority of cases, complications such as ulceration, esthetic compromise, or underlying structural anomalies may be associated. In these cases, prompt referral to specialty care for work-up and treatment is needed.

Pathogenesis

The etiology of infantile hemangiomas remains poorly understood, though a somatic mutation within a known oncogenic pathway is suspected. Other theories include a pathogenic association with the glucose transporter protein, GLUT-1, which is expressed robustly in infantile hemangioma tissue. Tissue hypoxia and vasculogenesis/angiogenesis from aberrant proliferation of endothelial progenitor cells may also play a role.[20]

Clinical Presentation

▶ History and Physical Examination

Infantile hemangiomas are not evident at birth; precursor lesions may manifest as a faint red patch, localized pallor, duskiness, and/or telangiectasias.[21] Infantile hemangiomas can be classified based on their appearance during the proliferative phase:

- Superficial (bright red to violaceous, finely lobulated papules, plaques, or nodules without a subcutaneous component) (Figure 20-18).
- Deep (subcutaneous tumor with a bluish or flesh-colored surface).
- Mixed (superficial and deep infantile hemangioma) (Figure 20-19).[21]

These lesions may appear on any cutaneous or mucosal surface in localized, segmental, or multifocal distributions.

▶ Laboratory Findings

While not indicated for lesions clinically consistent with an infantile hemangioma, a biopsy may be performed in cases of diagnostic uncertainty. Histopathology demonstrates

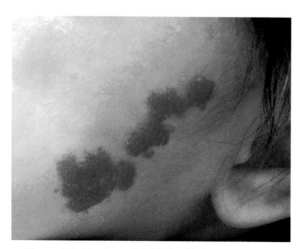

▲ **Figure 20-18.** Superficial infantile hemangioma on the left cheek of an infant.

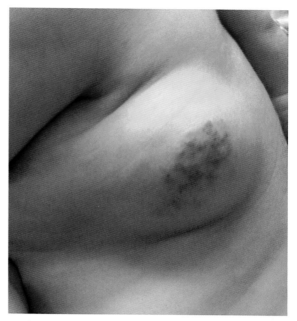

▲ **Figure 20-19.** Mixed superficial and deep infantile hemangioma on the left flank of an infant.

cellular hyperplasia and proliferation of endothelial cells in the dermis and/or subcutaneous region. Lesional cells stain positively for GLUT-1, which distinguishes infantile hemangiomas from congenital hemangiomas.[22]

Diagnosis

Diagnosis is often made clinically. If needed, Doppler ultrasonography can serve as a useful adjunct in confirming the high-flow vascular characteristics of an infantile hemangioma; magnetic resonance imaging (MRI) may be needed in rare cases, either to aid in the diagnosis of atypical appearing lesions or for further work-up if underlying structural anomalies are suspected.[23] Refer to Table 20-1 for a differential diagnosis.

Management

Although many infantile hemangiomas can be monitored for spontaneous regression, 5–10% of lesions require intervention to prevent complications.[24] Treatment should be individualized based on the location and size of the lesion. High-risk lesions, defined as those with potential for life-threatening complications, functional impairment, ulceration, structural anomalies, or permanent disfigurement warrant systemic therapy, of which oral propranolol has become the first-line.[25] Oral propranolol has revolutionized the treatment of infantile hemangiomas since its chance discovery for this use in 2008.[26] It is safe and highly efficacious when prescribed and monitored by a specialist

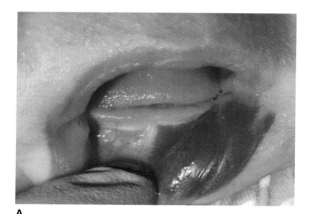

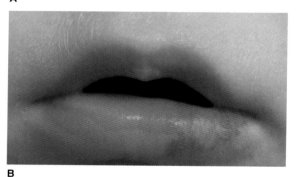

Figure 20-20. A, B. High risk infantile hemangioma treated with oral propranolol. A. Age one month before treatment. B. Age 6 months, status post propranolol with near resolution at 5 months after treatment.

(Figure 20-20 A, B). Careful monitoring is required for side effects including hypoglycemia (mitigated by administering with feedings), bradycardia, and hypotension. Topical timolol can be considered for smaller, more superficial infantile hemangiomas.[25] Oral corticosteroids and other systemic chemotherapeutic agents are no longer regularly employed in the management of complicated infantile hemangiomas.

Clinical Course and Prognosis

Infantile hemangiomas typically become apparent within the first 4 weeks of life and double their size by 2 months; peak growth of the superficial component is achieved between 5 and 7 weeks of age.[27] A period of slower growth follows thereafter, with proliferation continuing up to 12 months. Following proliferation, involution occurs with flattening, softening, and fading of coloration until complete regression around age 4 years.

Over half of untreated infantile hemangiomas may be associated with significant or even severe sequelae.[28]

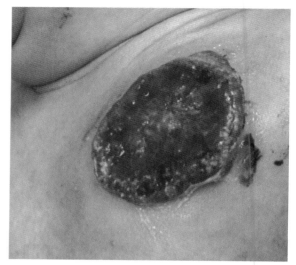

Figure 20-21. Ulcerated hemangioma.

Infantile hemangiomas of the face and scalp have a high risk of scarring, permanent disfigurement, and alopecia. Periocular infantile hemangiomas may cause astigmatism, proptosis, and amblyopia, potentially leading to permanent visual compromise.

Lesions arising in the mandibular distribution or anterior neck may also have concomitant airway involvement with risk for airway obstruction, while those involving the mouth and/or oral cavity may result in feeding impairment in the setting of rapid proliferation and ulceration. Segmental infantile hemangiomas on the lips, nasal columella, superior helix of the ear, gluteal cleft, perineum, and intertriginous regions are at especially high risk of ulceration (Figure 20-21). Furthermore, infants with at least five cutaneous infantile hemangiomas have increased likelihood of underlying hepatic hemangiomas, a minority of which are associated with high-output congestive heart failure and severe hypothyroidism.[25]

Indications for Consultation

Hemangioma specialists (often a pediatric dermatologist or pediatric hematologist/oncologist) should be consulted by 1 month of age, preferably as early as first identification, for management of high-risk lesions as defined earlier. In addition to important anatomic locations, structural anomalies warranting referral include a large (>5 cm), segmental infantile hemangioma of the face, neck, and/or scalp, which may indicate PHACE syndrome (posterior fossa anomalies, hemangioma, arterial lesions, cardiac abnormalities/coarctation of the aorta, and eye anomalies).[29] Similarly, LUMBAR syndrome (lower body infantile hemangioma and other skin defects, urogenital anomalies and ulceration, myelopathy, bony deformities, anorectal malformations and arterial anomalies, and renal anomalies) should be suspected with segmental lumbosacral or perineal infantile hemangiomas.[30]

Patient information

- Hemangioma Investigator Group: https://hemangiomaeducation.org
- The Society for Pediatric Dermatology: https://pedsderm.net

▼ CONGENITAL HEMANGIOMAS

Introduction

Congenital hemangiomas are rare, benign vascular tumors affecting <1% of both male and female newborns.[31] Unlike infantile hemangiomas, congenital hemangiomas are fully formed at birth. They have traditionally been subdivided into two primary categories based on their clinical behavior: *rapidly involuting congenital hemangiomas* and *non-involuting congenital hemangiomas*.[30] These lesions may be difficult to differentiate in the immediate newborn period; infants should be followed closely to ensure proper diagnosis and to assess their need for future treatment.

Pathogenesis

The exact pathogenesis of congenital hemangiomas is not well-understood; however, somatic activating mutations in *GNAQ* and *GNA11* have been identified in an increasing number of cases.[32,33] Similar to port-wine stains and Sturge-Weber syndrome, these mutations lead to upregulation of mitogen-activating protein kinase (MAPK) pathways and their downstream signaling.[23]

Clinical Presentation

▶ History and Physical Examination

Congenital hemangiomas are fully developed and therefore clinically apparent at birth. They have a predilection for the head, neck, and extremities. *Rapidly involuting congenital hemangiomas* have varied clinical presentations, including exophytic red, violaceous, or gray tumors with prominent peripheral vasculature, overlying telangiectasias, and/or infiltrative papules or nodules; blanching or a halo of pallor can also be seen (Figure 20-22).[34] *Non-involuting congenital hemangiomas* may present as an admixture of red, blue, and white patches with an atrophic surface or larger plaques/nodules with soft tissue swelling. Certain non-involuting congenital hemangiomas are warm to the touch and can be painful.[35]

▶ Laboratory Findings

Rapidly involuting congenital hemangiomas may be associated with transient thrombocytopenia that typically

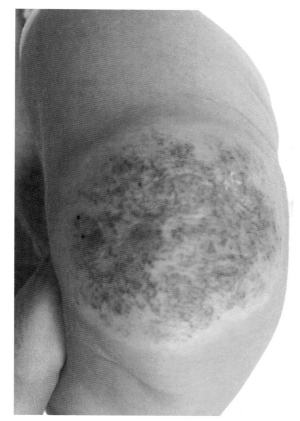

▲ **Figure 20-22.** Rapidly involuting congenital hemangioma on the thigh of a 6-week old infant

normalizes within the first few weeks of life.[36] Biopsy of *rapidly involuting congenital hemangiomas* reveals lobules of capillaries in the dermis and subcutaneous region with surrounding fibrous tissue; a central zone of advanced involution is often present. Histopathology of early *non-involuting congenital hemangiomas* demonstrates thin-walled, capillary lobules, and interlobular fibrous tissue; later in life, the majority of lesions consist of prominent interlobular arteries and veins. Importantly, congenital hemangiomas lack positivity to glucose transporter 1(GLUT-1) staining, differentiating them from infantile hemangiomas.[22]

Diagnosis

Occasionally, congenital hemangiomas may be diagnosed on prenatal imaging.[37] Similar to infantile hemangiomas, postnatal diagnosis is based on clinical appearance of the lesion, although skin biopsy, Doppler ultrasonography, and/or magnetic resonance imaging (MRI) may be indicated when the diagnosis is uncertain. A differential diagnosis is listed in Table 20-1.

Management

Treatment is based on the type, size, and associated complications of the congenital hemangioma. Most uncomplicated rapidly *involuting congenital hemangiomas* can be monitored clinically for involution; cases associated with bleeding, hemodynamic instability, or ulceration may require early excision. Surgical excision may also be performed for symptomatic *non-involuting congenital hemangiomas*, or for those located in cosmetically sensitive locations, later in childhood/early adolescence. Oral propranolol is generally ineffective.[23]

Clinical Course and Prognosis

Rapidly involuting congenital hemangiomas begin their regression prenatally and typically involute shortly after 1 year of age; however, dermal atrophy and/or telangiectasias may persist. Rarely, rapidly involuting congenital hemangiomas have been associated with severe bleeding and ulceration; this is a particular concern when located on the scalp.[34]

Non-involuting congenital hemangiomas, as the name implies, do not involute, and rather grow proportionately with the infant. Certain rapidly involuting congenital hemangiomas may involute incompletely and leave behind a residual lesion that appears indistinguishable from a *non-involuting congenital hemangioma*; such lesions have been termed partially involuting congenital hemangiomas.[38]

Indications for Consultation

Referral is indicated for complicated congenital hemangiomas and for those warranting surgical excision due to their anatomic location.

Patient Information

- Hemangioma Investigator Group: https://hemangiomaeducation.org
- The Society for Pediatric Dermatology: https://pedsderm.net

▼ NEVUS SIMPLEX

Introduction

Nevus simplex (also known as salmon patch or fading capillary stain) is the most common type of simple capillary malformation, occurring in up to 83% of newborns.[39] It affects males and females equally, as well as infants of all ethnicities.[40] Nevus simplex is typically a benign finding that can generally be monitored for spontaneous resolution.

Pathogenesis

Nevus simplex is thought to represent superficial dilatation of capillaries and/or postcapillary venules, arising from remnants of fetal blood circulation.[41]

Clinical Presentation

▶ History and Physical Examination

Typical clinical presentation is an ill-defined, pink to bright red macule or patch apparent at birth. It characteristically involves the midline (Figure 20-23). Commonly affected body sites include the forehead/glabella in a V-shaped distribution (angel's kiss), eyelid(s), nose, nape of neck (stork bite), occiput, and sacrum; the term "nevus simplex complex" is used for more extensive lesions extending beyond these sites.[42] The lesion blanches partially when compressed and may become more prominent with crying, activity, or changes in temperature. Eczematous dermatitis may develop over affected areas.[43]

▶ Laboratory Findings

Biopsy is not necessary for nevus simplex. Histopathology would show thin and ectatic vessels within the superficial dermis.[44]

Diagnosis

Most nevus simplex lesions can be diagnosed based on clinical history and physical examination alone, though

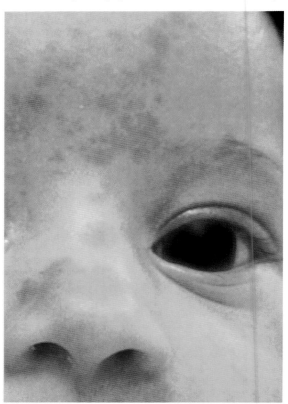

▲ **Figure 20-23.** Nevus simplex affecting the glabella, nasal bridge, and left upper eyelid of an infant.

occasionally they can be difficult to distinguish from a port-wine stain or hemangioma precursor.[45] A differential diagnosis for nevus simplex is listed in Table 20-1.

Management

Clinical monitoring of a nevus simplex is typically appropriate. For persistent lesions located in cosmetically-sensitive areas, several sessions of pulsed dye laser to lighten the coloration may be performed by an experienced specialist (e.g., pediatric dermatologist, plastic surgeon).

Clinical Course and Prognosis

The majority of nevus simplexes fade within the first 1–2 years of life; however, depending on location, some lesions persist into adulthood, particularly those located on the occiput or nape of the neck.

Indications for Consultation

While the vast majority of infants with nevus simplex exhibit no extracutaneous manifestations, several syndromes have been associated with prominent and persistent lesions, including Beckwith-Wiedemann syndrome. In addition to facial nevus simplex, features of Beckwith-Wiedemann syndrome facilitating its recognition consist of macroglossia, abdominal wall defects, lateralized overgrowth, predisposition to embryonal tumors, and hypoglycemia.[46] Specialist referral may also be warranted for lumbosacral nevus simplex occurring concomitantly with other local cutaneous findings (e.g., aplasia cutis, dermal sinus or pit, gluteal cleft deformity, hypertrichosis, or lipoma) to rule out underlying spinal dysraphism.[43] In general, consultation is not indicated for isolated lumbosacral nevus simplex.

Patient Information

- Hemangioma Investigator Group: https://hemangiomaeducation.org
- The Society for Pediatric Dermatology: https://pedsderm.net

CAPILLARY MALFORMATION (PORT-WINE STAIN)

Introduction

Capillary malformations, commonly referred to in the literature as port-wine stains, represent malformation and progressive dilatation of dermal capillaries. In contrast with nevus simplex, capillary malformations do not resolve spontaneously. Capillary malformations are also less common than nevus simplex, affecting <1% of newborns, without racial or gender predilection.[47] They may be associated with soft tissue overgrowth and genetic syndromes such as Sturge–Weber syndrome.

Pathogenesis

The pathogenesis of capillary malformations has been attributed to somatic activating *GNAQ* (encoding q class of G-protein alpha subunits) mutations, leading to dysregulation of downstream vascular MAPK pathways.[48] Signal dysregulation during embryonic development may cause impairment in differentiation of endothelial cells and progressive dilatation of venule-like vasculature.[49]

Clinical Presentation

▶ History and Physical Examination

The vast majority of capillary malformations are present at birth and persist throughout life.[50] Classically, the lesion is a well-demarcated, irregular, dark pink to red patch or slightly raised plaque that grows in proportion to the infant.[51] Capillary malformations tend to affect the head and neck, but they can occur throughout the body in a localized, segmental, or widespread distribution. Capillary malformations affecting the face often follow a dermatomal distribution along the trigeminal nerve, particularly the ophthalmic (V1) and maxillary (V2) branches.[52] Similar to nevus simplex, dermatitis may develop over sites affected by capillary malformations.

▶ Laboratory Findings

Rare, dilated capillaries may be seen on biopsy of capillary malformations in young children; haphazardly-arranged, ectatic dermal vessels in the papillary and reticular dermis are demonstrated with lesion progression.[22]

Diagnosis

Diagnosis of a capillary malformation is made based on clinical presentation. A differential diagnosis is listed in Table 20-1.

Management

Potential sequelae of untreated capillary malformations include permanent disfigurement, thickening and development of nodularity, and negative impact on quality of life.[53] Infants with capillary malformations should therefore be referred for specialist management. Early treatment with pulsed dye laser is the gold standard therapy and can be performed safely early in infancy under the care of an experienced dermatologist or pediatric dermatologist (Figure 20-24).[54] However, it should be noted that complete clearance with laser therapy is rare, and certain lesions are resistant to treatment; management of parental expectations is therefore important.[55]

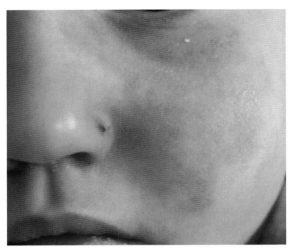

△ **Figure 20-24.** Capillary malformation of the left cheek following treatment with pulsed dye laser.

Clinical Course and Prognosis

Within the first few months of life, capillary malformations may lighten as fetal-type hemoglobin transitions to adult-type.[45] As the infant ages, capillary malformations may progressively darken to a deeper red to purple color and may become hyperkeratotic with a nodular, "cobblestone" quality later in adolescence and adulthood. Soft tissue overgrowth and bony hypertrophy can also occur, potentially distorting facial features (Figure 20-25).

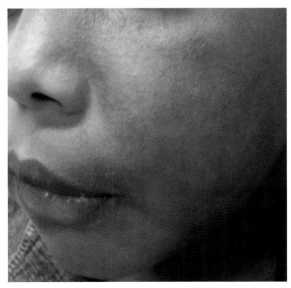

△ **Figure 20-25.** Capillary malformation of the left cheek associated with mild soft tissue overgrowth of the upper lip.

Indications for Consultation

Patients with capillary malformations in cosmetically sensitive areas should be referred for specialist management and consideration of pulsed dye laser. Infants with high-risk capillary malformation phenotypes should also be referred to rule out underlying syndromic associations. Sturge–Weber syndrome is a neurocutaneous disorder characterized by facial port-wine stain, leptomeningeal angiomatosis, and glaucoma. While the the V1 dermatome distribution was previously considered highest risk, hemifacial, and forehead distributions have since been deemed better predictors.[56,57] Early identification, referral (e.g., pediatric dermatology and neurology), and treatment of Sturge–Weber syndrome can help preserve visual function and improve neurodevelopmental outcomes.[58] Any infant with extensive capillary malformations, overgrowth of an extremity, or multifocal lesions should be referred for specialty care and management as several genetic syndromes may be considered in these settings.[59]

Patient Information

- Hemangioma Investigator Group: https://hemangiomaeducation.org
- The Society for Pediatric Dermatology: https://pedsderm.net

▼ REFERENCES

1. Wollina U. Seborrheic Keratoses – The Most Common Benign Skin Tumor of Humans. Clinical presentation and an update on pathogenesis and treatment options. *Open Access Maced J Med Sci.* 2018;6(11):2270-2275.
2. Stankiewicz K, Chuang G, Avram M. Lentigines, laser, and melanoma: A case series and discussion. *Lasers Surg Med.* 2012;44(2):112-116.
3. Kang S, Amagai M, Bruckner A, et al. *Fitzpatrick's Dermatology*, 9th ed. New York: McGraw-Hill Education. 2019.
4. Hirt PA, Castillo DE, Yosipovitch G, et al. Skin changes in the obese patient. *J Am Acad Dermatol.* 2019;81(5):1037-1057.
5. Salam GA. Lipoma excision. *Am Fam Physician.* 2002;65(5):901-904.
6. Potter K, Konda S, Ren VZ, et al. Techniques for optimizing surgical scars, Part 2: hypertrophic scars and keloids. *Skinmed.* 2017;15(6):451-456.
7. Ekstein SF, Wyles SP, Moran SL, et al. Keloids: a review of therapeutic management. *Int J Dermatol.* September 2020:ijd.15159.
8. Juckett G, Hartman-Adams H. Management of keloids and hypertrophic scars. *Am Fam Physician.* 2009;80(3):253-260.
9. Klifto KM, Asif M, Hultman CS. Laser management of hypertrophic burn scars: a comprehensive review. *Burn trauma.* 2020;8:tkz002.
10. Jaros J, Hunt S, Mose E, et al. Cutaneous metastases: A great imitator. *Clin Dermatol.* 2020;38(2):216-222.
11. Zuber TJ. Minimal excision technique for epidermoid (sebaceous) cysts. *Am Fam Physician.* 2002;65(7):1409-1412, 1417-1418, 1420.

12. Berk DR, Bayliss SJ. Milia: a review and classification. *J Am Acad Dermatol*. 2008;59(6):1050-1063.

13. Del Rosso JQ, Silverberg N, Zeichner JA. When acne is not acne. *Dermatol Clin*. 2016;34(2):225-228.

14. Jabbour S, Kechichian E, Haber R, et al. Management of digital mucous cysts: a systematic review and treatment algorithm. *Int J Dermatol*. 2017;56(7):701-708.

15. Zuber TJ. Office management of digital mucous cysts. *Am Fam Physician*. 2001;64(12):1987-1990.

16. Mlacker S, Shah V V, Aldahan AS, et al. Laser and light-based treatments of venous lakes: a literature review. *Lasers Med Sci*. 2016;31(7):1511-1519.

17. Wassef M, Blei F, Adams D, et al. Vascular anomalies classification: recommendations from the International Society for the Study of Vascular Anomalies. *Pediatrics*. 2015;136(1): e203-e214.

18. Munden A, Butschek R, Tom WL, et al. Prospective study of infantile haemangiomas: incidence, clinical characteristics and association with placental anomalies. *Br J Dermatol*. 2014;170(4):907-913.

19. Darrow DH, Greene AK, Mancini AJ, et al. Diagnosis and management of infantile hemangioma. *Pediatrics*. 2015;136(4):e1060-e1104.

20. Smith CJF, Friedlander SF, Guma M, et al. Infantile hemangiomas: an updated review on risk factors, pathogenesis, and treatment. *Birth defects Res*. 2017;109(11):809-815.

21. Harter N, Mancini AJ. Diagnosis and management of infantile hemangiomas in the neonate. *Pediatr Clin North Am*. 2019;66(2):437-459.

22. Miller DD, Gupta A. Histopathology of vascular anomalies: update based on the revised 2014 ISSVA classification. *Semin Cutan Med Surg*. 2016;35(3):137-146.

23. Haggstrom A, Garzon M. Infantile Hemangiomas. In: Bolognia J, Schaffer J, Cerroni L, eds. *Dermatology*. Fourth. Philadelphia, PA: Elsevier; 2018:1786-1804.

24. Hoeger PH, Harper JI, Baselga E, et al. Treatment of infantile haemangiomas: recommendations of a European expert group. *Eur J Pediatr*. 2015;174(7):855-865.

25. Krowchuk DP, Frieden IJ, Mancini AJ, et al. Clinical practice guideline for the management of infantile hemangiomas. *Pediatrics*. 2019;143(1):e20183475.

26. Léauté-Labrèze C, de la Roque ED, Hubiche T, et al. Propranolol for severe hemangiomas of infancy. *N Engl J Med*. 2008;358(24):2649-2651.

27. Macarthur K, Püttgen KM. Vascular Tumors. In: Kang S, Amagai M, Bruckner AL, et al., eds. *Fitzpatrick's Dermatology*, 9th ed. New York: McGraw-Hill Education. 2019.

28. Baselga E, Roe E, Coulie J, et al. Risk factors for degree and type of sequelae after involution of untreated hemangiomas of infancy. *JAMA Dermatology*. 2016;152(11):1239.

29. Garzon MC, Epstein LG, Heyer GL, et al. PHACE syndrome: consensus-derived diagnosis and care recommendations. *J Pediatr*. 2016;178:24-33.

30. Liang MG, Frieden IJ. Infantile and congenital hemangiomas. *Semin Pediatr Surg*. 2014;23(4):162-167.

31. Kanada KN, Merin MR, Munden A, et al. A prospective study of cutaneous findings in newborns in the united states: correlation with race, ethnicity, and gestational status using updated classification and nomenclature. *J Pediatr*. 2012;161(2):240-245.

32. Ayturk UM, Couto JA, Hann S, et al. Somatic activating mutations in GNAQ and GNA11 are associated with congenital hemangioma. *Am J Hum Genet*. 2016;98(4):789-795.

33. Smith RJ, Metry D, Deardorff MA, et al. Segmental congenital hemangiomas: Three cases of a rare entity. *Pediatr Dermatol*. 2020;37(3):548-553.

34. Haggstron AN, Chamlin SL. Infantile hemangiomas and other vascular tumors. In: Eichenfield L, Frieden I, Zaenglein E, Andrea M, eds. *Neonatal and Infant Dermatology*. Third. Philadelphia, PA: Elsevier; 2014:336-351.

35. Lee PW, Frieden IJ, Streicher JL, et al. Characteristics of non-involuting congenital hemangioma: A retrospective review. *J Am Acad Dermatol*. 2014;70(5):899-903.

36. Rangwala S, Wysong A, Tollefson MM, et al. Rapidly involuting congenital hemangioma associated with profound, transient thrombocytopenia. *Pediatr Dermatol*. 2014;31(3):402-404.

37. Feygin T, Khalek N, Moldenhauer JS. Fetal brain, head, and neck tumors: Prenatal imaging and management. *Prenat Diagn*. May 2020:Epub ahead of print.

38. Nasseri E, Piram M, McCuaig CC, et al. Partially involuting congenital hemangiomas: A report of 8 cases and review of the literature. *J Am Acad Dermatol*. 2014;70(1):75-79.

39. Ulbrecht M, Cleary GM. Common Newborn Dermatologic Conditions. In: Russell JJ, Ryan Jr. EF, eds. *Common Dermatologic Conditions in Primary Care*. Cham, Switzerland: Springer International Publishing; 2019:11-18.

40. Hunt R, Chang MW, Shah KN. Neonatal Dermatology. In: Kang S, Amagai M, Bruckner AL, et al., eds. *Fitzpatrick's Dermatology*, 9th ed. New York: McGraw-Hill Education. 2019.

41. Baselga E. Vascular Malformations. In: Bolognia J, Schaffer J, Cerroni L, eds. *Dermatology*. Fourth. Philadelphia, PA; 2018:1805-1827.

42. Schaffer J V. Facial involvement in genodermatoses. *Clin Dermatol*. 2014;32(6):772-783.

43. Rozas-Muñoz E, Frieden IJ, Roé E, et al. Vascular stains: proposal for a clinical classification to improve diagnosis and management. *Pediatr Dermatol*. 2016;33(6):570-584.

44. Stockman DL. Nevus Simplex. In: Stockman DL, ed. *Diagnostic Pathology: Vascular*. 1st ed. Philadelphia, PA: Elsevier; 2015:24-26.

45. Maguiness SM, Garzon MC. Vascular Malformations. In: Eichenfield L, Frieden I, Zaenglein E, Andrea M, eds. *Neonatal and Infant Dermatology*. Third. Philadelphia, PA: Elsevier; 2014:352-368.

46. Brioude F, Kalish JM, Mussa A, et al. Clinical and molecular diagnosis, screening and management of Beckwith–Wiedemann syndrome: an international consensus statement. *Nat Rev Endocrinol*. 2018;14(4):229-249.

47. Wójcicki P, Wójcicka K. Epidemiology, diagnostics and treatment of vascular tumours and malformations. *Adv Clin Exp Med*. 2014;23(3):475-484.

48. Tan W, Nadora DM, Gao L, et al. The somatic GNAQ mutation (R183Q) is primarily located within the blood vessels of port wine stains. *J Am Acad Dermatol*. 2016;74(2):380-383.

49. Nguyen V, Hochman M, Mihm MC, et al. The pathogenesis of port wine stain and sturge weber syndrome: complex interactions between genetic alterations and aberrant MAPK and PI3K Activation. *Int J Mol Sci*. 2019;20(9):2243.

50. Stephens MR, Putterman E, Yan AC, et al. Acquired port-wine stains in six pediatric patients. *Pediatr Dermatol*. 2020;37(1):93-97.

51. Happle R. Capillary malformations: a classification using specific names for specific skin disorders. *J Eur Acad Dermatology Venereol*. 2015;29(12):2295-2305.

52. Cox J, Bartlett E, Lee E. Vascular malformations: a review. *Semin Plast Surg.* 2014;28(2):58-63.

53. Hagen SL, Grey KR, Korta DZ, et al. Quality of life in adults with facial port-wine stains. *J Am Acad Dermatol.* 2017;76(4):695-702.

54. Updyke KM, Khachemoune A. Port-wine stains: a focused review on their management. *J Drugs Dermatol.* 2017;16(11):1145-1151.

55. Paller AS, Mancini AJ. Vascular Disorders of Infancy and Childhood. In: Paller AS, Mancini AJ, eds. *Hurwitz Clinical Pediatric Dermatology: A Textbook of Skin Disorders of Childhood and Adolescence.* 5th ed. New York, NY: Elsevier; 2016:279-316.

56. Waelchli R, Aylett SE, Robinson K, et al. New vascular classification of port-wine stains: improving prediction of Sturge–Weber risk. *Br J Dermatol.* 2014;171(4):861-867.

57. Boos MD, Bozarth XL, Sidbury R, et al. Forehead location and large segmental pattern of facial port-wine stains predict risk of Sturge-Weber syndrome. *J Am Acad Dermatol.* 2020;83(4):1110-1117.

58. Zallmann M, Leventer RJ, Mackay MT, et al. Screening for Sturge-Weber syndrome: A state-of-the-art review. *Pediatr Dermatol.* 2018;35(1):30-42.

59. Gupta D, Sidbury R. Cutaneous Congenital Defects. In: Gleason C, Juul S, eds. *Avery's Diseases of the Newborn.* 10th ed. Philadelphia, PA: Elsevier; 2017:1511-1535.

Actinic Keratosis, Basal Cell Carcinoma, and Squamous Cell Carcinoma

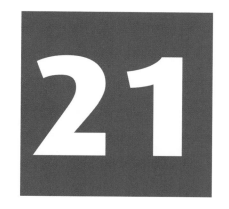

Adam Mattox

INTRODUCTION TO CHAPTER

Actinic keratoses (AKs) are one of the most common skin findings in dermatology. An AK is a neoplasm of the epidermis and considered as a precursor lesions to squamous cell carcinoma (SCC). Ultraviolet (UV) light exposure is the main cause of AKs. They are very common in sun-exposed skin, especially in the light skin type and, elderly patients. The presence of several AKs may be an indicator that the patient has incurred sufficient sun damage for increased risk of basal cell carcinoma and squamous cell carcinoma.

Basal cell carcinomas (BCCs) and squamous cell carcinomas (SCCs) are the most common types of skin cancers and the most common of all cancers in the United States.[3] Both are caused by UV light exposure and usually occur on sun-exposed skin. BCCs and SCCs are sometimes called "non-melanoma skin cancer (NMSC)" and are readily treatable if detected early. BCCs are the most common type of skin cancer in the immunocompetent individual and rarely metastasize. SCCs are the second most common skin cancer in the immunocompetent individual and can metastasize to regional lymph nodes if not treated early. Routine skin examinations are crucial to early detection. Sun avoidance and protection with proper habits, clothing, and sunscreen are important for the prevention of BCCs and SCCs.[4]

ACTINIC KERATOSIS

Introduction

Actinic keratoses are precancerous lesions of the keratinocytes and are very common in individuals over the age of 55 years with light skin types. They mostly develop in sun-exposed areas of the skin such as the head, neck, and distal extremities. Damage caused by UV light exposure is the predominant cause. Lighter skin type and genetic predisposition makes some patients especially susceptible. If untreated, a small percentage of AKs will transform into SCC. Appropriate treatment during the precancerous phase is less invasive and aimed at preventing transformation.[1]

Pathogenesis

AKs develop after intense or long-term exposure to UV light (natural or artificial). Chronic sun exposure may lead to p53 tumor suppressor gene mutation of individual keratinocytes in the epidermis.[2] The same genetic mutations are seen in AKs and SCCs. The mutations will lead to propagation of the abnormal keratinocytes leading to faster division of these cells and development of a clinically apparent lesion. If left untreated, approximately 10% of AKs may become SCCs.

Clinical Presentation

▶ History

Patients typically complain of persistent scaly rough lesions (several at once is common) on frequently sun-exposed areas such as the face, scalp, and ears. Dorsal hands and forearms in men and lower legs in women are also commonly affected areas. The lesions usually do not have any symptoms such as itching or pain. Patients often scratch off the overlying scale, only to have it recur.

▶ Physical Examination

Actinic keratoses can present as a solitary papule, a field of multiple papules, or a plaque (Figures 21-A,B). Solitary lesions often appear as an ill-defined, red macule, or papule (3–6 mm) with gritty scale. The lesions are ill-defined often easier to palpate than see and some are slightly tender. A solitary AK can be hypertrophic, presenting as a hyperkeratotic papule with a thick layer of compact stratum corneum adherent to its surface. A hypertrophic AK may resemble a cutaneous horn. UV damage often affects a broad area, leading to multiple lesions in a field. The plaque-type AKs may form from multiple lesions reaching confluence or a single lesion that grows over time. They also have rough gritty scale and can be associated with in situ SCC or sub-clinical SCC.

▶ Laboratory Findings

Histopathology of AK exhibits partial thickness cellular atypia affecting the epidermal basal layer. The abnormal keratinocytes may also extend deeper along adnexal structures of the skin such as hair follicles. These lesions are described histologically as "actinic keratoses with appendageal involvement" and may need more aggressive and deeper penetrating treatments to reach the involved structures.

Diagnosis

AKs typically present as hyperkeratotic papules or as a scaly red plaque(s) in chronically sun-exposed areas of the face, scalp, ears, dorsal hands, and arms. They have rough, gritty scale on the surface.

▶ Differential Diagnosis

✓ Seborrheic keratosis: A tan or brown well-defined papule or plaque with waxy texture.

✓ Viral wart: A hyperkeratotic papule containing thrombosed capillaries seen as black speckles.

✓ SCC: A firm papule with scale, and more consistently tender to palpation.

✓ Cutaneous horn: Not limited to AK, may overly a range of irritated benign or malignant lesions.

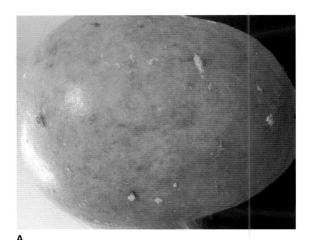

A

B

▲ **Figure 21-1.** A,B. Actinic keratosis. A. Multiple pink macules with rough, gritty scale scattered on the scalp. Some hypertrophic actinic keratoses (AK) are present with thick white scale. B. Close up view of AK and hypertrophic AK.

A skin biopsy may be necessary if the clinical exam is not diagnostic.

Management

There are many options for the treatment of AK. Treatment modalities can be combined or cycled through to improve efficacy.

- *Cryotherapy* is the most common treatment for AKs (see Chapter 7).[5] Liquid nitrogen is applied to the lesions using a spray dispenser or a cotton applicator until a 1–2 mm rim of frost develops at the periphery. This method may cause a blister in the lesion and skin surrounding the treated area, but blister formation is not necessary for effective treatment. If present, the blister heals and the roof desquamates with resolution of the AK. If no blister occurs, desquamation of the lesion may still occur in about 7 days.[6]

- *Field therapy* is used to treat diffuse and numerous AKs and can be effective in treating subclinical lesions. Several topical medications are available, and treatment is usually initiated and monitored by a dermatologist. Topical 5-Fluorouracil (5-FU) in a cream or liquid has been available for decades and is commonly used for field therapy.[7] 5-FU is a pyrimidine analog and incorporates into DNA and RNA of keratinocytes, leading to cell death and inflammation.[8] Applying the cream under occlusion (termed "Chemo Wraps") can enhance penetration and efficacy. However, the covered treated surface area should be limited to avoid side effects from absorption. Combination treatment with equal parts calcipotriene 0.005% ointment and 5-FU 5% cream has been shown to maintain efficacy while shortening the treatment duration to 4 days.[9] Another common topical treatment, imiquimod cream 5% works by stimulating T lymphocytes against the abnormal keratinocytes.[10] In 2012, ingenol mebutate gel 0.05% was approved for AK treatment. This medication causes necrosis of AKs within 2 to 3 days of use.[11] All topical field therapies caused intense inflammation in the treated sites (Figure 21-2).[12]

- *Photodynamic therapy (PDT)* is a field therapy traditionally performed in a dermatology clinic. It has gained greater popularity for treatment of AKs. For PDT, a photosensitizing chemical such as aminolevulinic acid (ALA) is applied to the field containing AKs for incubation and uptake by AK keratinocytes. Once exposed to the proper wavelength of light, ALA is converted into protoporphyrin IX, a powerful photosensitizer, inside the abnormal keratinocytes. An energy rich singlet oxygen species is generated causing membrane disruption and cell death.[13] Sunlight PDT is gaining popularity because it is less painful. Unfortunately, variance in weather makes it challenging to standardize treatment.

Clinical Course and Prognosis

The clinical prognosis of AKs is very good. In immunocompetent patients, upwards of 90% of AKs will be cleared by the immune system. High quality sun protection and sun avoidance help to optimize the cutaneous immune system. Unfortunately, a clinician cannot predict which AKs will evade the immune system and transition to an in situ SCC or SCC. None of the mentioned treatments are always completely effective, but a persistent or recurrent AK could be an indication for a biopsy to screen for malignancy.[1]

Indications for Consultation

Patients with a heavy burden or ongoing incidence of new AKs would benefit from field treatment and treatment of subclinical lesions. A primary care clinician may consider referring to dermatology for specialized field therapy or PDT.

Patient Information

- American Academy of Dermatology: https://www.aad.org/public/diseases/skin-cancer/actinic-keratosis-overview
- Skin Cancer Foundation: https://www.skincancer.org/skin-cancer-information/actinic-keratosis/

BASAL CELL CARCINOMA

Introduction

BCC is by far the most common type of cancer and skin cancer in the United States. It is estimated that there are 1.2–1.5 million new cases each year in the United States with incidence rising.[14] Fortunately, these are slow-growing, localized tumors with only rare metastatic potential. BCCs are more common in the elderly, lighter skin population, but can arise in patients in their 20s and 30s. Intense sun exposure or artificial UV light especially prior to age 18 is the primary cause of BCCs with family history and light-colored skin, hair, and eyes being important risk factors.[3] Although less common, BCC can occur patients with darker skin tones.[14]

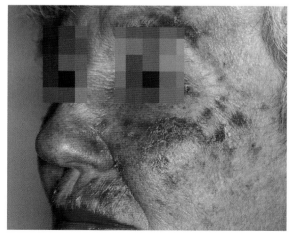

Figure 21- 2. Actinic keratosis after 4 weeks of treatment with 5-fluorouracil cream. Typical response to treatment with erythema, crust and erosions in the treated areas on the face.

Pathogenesis

BCCs are cancers of the epidermal keratinocytes of the hair follicles and the epidermis. They develop after intense or chronic UV light exposure.[15] Ionizing radiation from radiation treatment can also promote iatrogenic development of BCCs. Exposure to intense UV light leads to DNA mutation in the tumor suppressor genes of the sonic hedgehog pathway in keratinocytes. Mutations in the PTCH (patched) gene and in the tumor suppressor gene p53 gene are also implicated in the development of BCCs.[2] Patients with basal cell nevus syndrome (Gorlin's syndrome) develop hundreds of BCCs due to a genetic mutation in the sonic hedgehog pathway.

Clinical Presentation

BCCs most commonly occur on frequently sun-exposed areas such as the head and neck. There are several histologic subtypes of BCC, thus, history and clinical presentations vary depending upon the subtype.[16]

- *Nodular BCC* is the most common subtype. Patients often complain of a pimple-like papule that does not heal or has chronic intermittent bleeding. The lesions are often painful when manipulated. They typically appear as a translucent pearly papule with erythema, telangiectasia, and well-defined rolled borders most commonly on the head and neck region, especially the central face (Figure 21-3A and B). As the tumor grows, the center of the tumor often ulcerates creating a crater-like appearance. Neglected ulcerated lesions have been colloquially referred to as a "rodent ulcers." Infrequently, nodular BCCs are pigmented with an appearance reminiscent of a melanoma or dysplastic nevus (Figure 21-4).

- *Superficial BCC* is the second most common subtype. Patients often complain of a chronic area of "eczema." Like dermatitis, lesions may be pruritic or sensitive to touch but do not bleed like nodular BCC. Again like dermatitis, superficial BCC appears as an erythematous patch or flat topped plaque with well-defined borders on the trunk and extremities (Figure 21-5). It occurs commonly on the head and neck as well. If misdiagnosed and treated as eczema or psoriasis, it will not resolve. Unlike nodular, superficial BCCs lack the translucent and telangiectatic appearance, but can have a slightly raised, rolled border.

- *Infiltrative (also known as sclerotic or morpheaform) BCC* is the most elusive subtype with the highest risk of recurrence. Patients may complain of a "scar" without injury, or the lesion may go unnoticed for years. Clinically, they appear as a depressed scar-like plaque (Figure 21-6) that lacks features of nodular or superficial BCC. Owing to its subtle presentation, infiltrative BCC can grow to be a large and deep tumor before

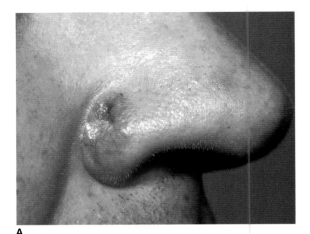

A

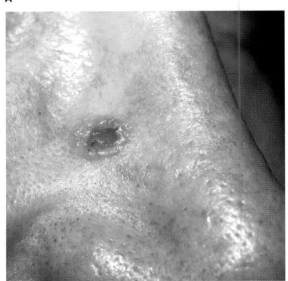

B

▲ **Figure 21-3.** A,B. Nodular basal cell carcinomas on nose. A. Papule with shiny, translucent, "pearly" surface, telangiectasia, and central ulcerative necrosis. B. Pink, pearly papule with well-defined "rolled appearing" borders and central ulcer.

detection. Morpheaform BCCs can be slightly erythematous, but often are lighter colored than the surrounding skin resembling a scar. The borders are very ill-defined making the diagnosis and treatment challenging. They typically affect the head and neck region, but can appear anywhere. Recurrent BCC may develop an infiltrative subtype.

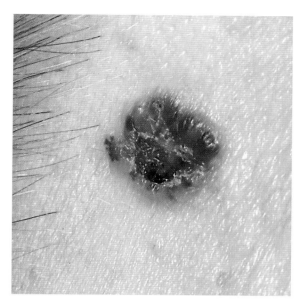

▲ **Figure 21-4.** Pigmented basal cell carcinoma. Gray-black papule with erosion giving the appearance of a melanocytic lesion.

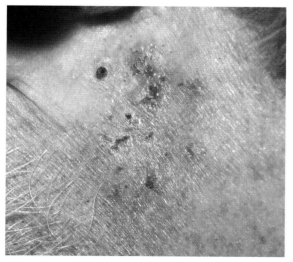

▲ **Figure 21- 5.** Superficial basal cell carcinoma. Erythematous poorly defined plaque with erosions and slightly raised, pearly border.

▷ Laboratory Findings

The histopathology of a BCC is a tumor of basophilic cells with hyperchromatic nuclei and peripheral palisade arrangement. Often tumor aggregates are outlined by

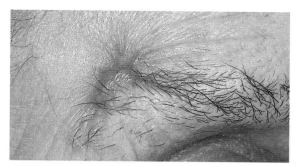

▲ **Figure 21-6.** Infiltrative (morpheaform or sclerotic) basal cell carcinoma. Scar-like plaque above eyebrow.

stromal retraction. A nodular BCC has tumor arranged in large round aggregates in the dermis; in superficial BCC the tumor aggregates are multifocal, and in contact with the basement membrane of the epidermis with limited dermal invasion. Infiltrative (sclerotic/morpheaform) BCCs have poorly differentiated and smaller tumor aggregates at the periphery, intercalating between the collagen of the dermis and extending relatively far from the primary lesion. A single tumor may have more than one subtype represented on histologic examination.

Diagnosis

The most common presentation of a nodular BCC is a pearly shiny papule with telangiectasia. A superficial BCC presents as an erythematous patch or plaque. An infiltrative BCC resembles a scar with ill-defined borders.

▷ Differential Diagnosis

For nodular BCC

✓ Intradermal nevus: A well circumscribed skin-colored papule without telangiectasia or pearly appearance.

✓ Inflamed seborrheic keratosis: A tan scaly papule that can be shiny with reddish halo, but lacks telangiectasia.

✓ SCC: Often a firm scaly red papule.

✓ Melanoma or dysplastic nevus: Pigmented BCCs may have dark pigmentation that mimics a melanocytic lesion.

For superficial BCC

✓ Large AK: Tends to have more gritty scale and is less contiguous.

✓ SCC in situ: Pink patch or plaque with profuse gritty scale.

✓ Dermatitis: Should respond to topical steroids.

For sclerotic/morpheaform BCC

✓ Scar: Scars have well-defined borders while a sclerotic BCC typically has ill-defined borders and no injury history.

Management

Treatment of BCCs can vary depending on multiple factors including the histologic subtype, location, previous treatment, size, and the patient's overall health.[4,17–19]

Standard Excision

A BCC can be excised in a fusiform or elliptical technique. The tumor is identified and excised with the recommended 4 mm margins to a depth of fat. The wound is repaired in a linear layered fashion. The specimen is submitted in formalin to pathology for processing and evaluation of margins. Standard of care vertical sectioning is performed, allowing for evaluation of about 1% of the surgical margin. The cure rate for standard excisions is 90–95% using 4 mm margins. This is a common and effective method for treatment of BCCs of the trunk and extremities where tissue sparing is not critical.[18]

Electrodessication and Curettage (ED&C)

In this procedure, the tumor is curetted with parallel strokes in three different directions followed by electrodessication of the entire surface ulcer. To achieve quoted cure rates, each cycle of curettage and electrodessication is repeated twice for a total of three times. This is effective for treatment of low risk BCC such as small nodular BCC or superficial subtype BCC of the trunk and extremities. The cure rate for ED&C treatment of BCC is near 90%. This technique is not recommended for treatment of sclerotic or morpheaform BCC.[19]

Mohs Micrographic Surgery

Mohs Micrographic Surgery (MMS) has the highest cure rate of any available treatment for BCC.

In MMS, the dermatologic surgeon acts as the surgeon and the pathologist. The tumor is excised with narrow (1–2 mm) margins, oriented with notches, and processed using the Mohs-specific horizontal (en face) frozen technique which allows for visualization of 100% of the deep and peripheral margin. The tissue is mounted on a glass slide and stained with hematoxylin and eosin. The slide is examined by the dermatologic surgeon for any evidence of tumor at the surgical margin. If no tumor is present at the margin this is the end of tissue excision (and histologic exam). If tumor is present, it is mapped and guides the Mohs surgeon to excise additional tissue in that location of the involved margin. The process is repeated on the specimen until the margins are clear. Once the tumor has been successfully removed, the defect can be reconstructed safely knowing that the margins are clear. This rapid and efficient method of tumor removal has a cure rate of nearly 99% for BCC. Mohs micrographic surgery is most commonly used for the indications as listed in Table 21-1. Additionally,

Table 21-1. Selected most common indications for Mohs micrographic surgery treatment of basal cell carcinoma (BCC) or squamous cell carcinoma (SCC).[20]

- Location at high risk for disfigurement or functional impairment (e.g., face, hand, genital).
- Aggressive histologic subtype (e.g., poorly differentiated SCC, infiltrative BCC).
- Tumors with perineural invasion.
- Large (>2 cm) tumors.
- Recurrent tumor.
- Immunocompromised patient.
- Genetic syndrome at increased risk of skin cancer.
- Incompletely excised tumors (e.g., excision attempted, but margins involved).
- Location in previously radiated skin, scar, chronic inflammation, osteomyelitis.
- Tumor with clinically indistinct margins.

the American Academy of Dermatology has created a free fast clinical decision-making tool, the Mohs AUC App for smartphones.[4, 20]

Topical Treatments

Topical treatments should largely be reserved for superficial BCC in low-risk sites below the neck. Efficacy rates decrease with increasing tumor depth seen in nodular and infiltrative BCC. In the United States, imiquimod cream and 5-fluorouracil solution or cream are approved for treatment of small superficial BCC below the neck. Recommended treatment durations are in the range of 6 weeks, so in the author's experience patients often choose an alternative.[18]

Photodynamic Therapy

PDT is approved for the treatment of BCC in Europe and Australia, but not in the United States. However, PDT is becoming more widely used for the treatment of superficial BCC on the trunk and extremities.[18]

Systemic Therapy

Oral vismodegib and sonidegib, are oral Hedgehog pathway inhibitors approved to treat metastatic and locally advanced BCC that is not amenable to surgery or radiation.[21,22] Though published cure rates are inferior to surgery, the data are collected from diverse populations. Dermatologists primarily use these medications to treat patients with basal cell nevus syndrome (tertiary prevention) and tumors that would cause significant morbidity if treated surgically (e.g., enucleation).

Clinical Course and Prognosis

The usual course of BCC is to grow in the skin becoming locally destructive to skin and adjacent tissue. Even if initially ignored, patients ultimately bring a burdensome bleeding papule or non-healing wound to their physician's attention for diagnosis and treatment. Depending on the location, BCC may take years to be locally destructive enough to reach critical anatomy and become fatal. However, continued growth may complicate treatment. Thus, early treatment is recommended. When diagnosed early, surgical treatment is well tolerated and safe for patients of all ages.

Prognosis for BCC is very good. When treated appropriately, recurrence rates are low. When recurrence does happen, the indolent nature of BCC often precludes significant morbidity and mortality until it can be treated again.

Indications for Consultation

The majority of BCC are treated by dermatologists and dermatologic surgeons in the United States. Many BCCs in low-risk sites can be managed with elliptical excision to the depth of fat. If surgical margins are not clear or the tumor recurs, the patient should be referred to an appropriate specialist for definitive treatment unless the primary care provider has previous experience and adequate knowledge of these tumors and treatments. BCC affecting high risk sites such as the face, scalp, or hands should be referred to a dermatologist or dermatologic surgeon. The American Academy of Dermatology has created a fast, free, clinical tool to assist with treatment decision making, the Mohs Appropriate Use Criteria (AUC) app for smartphones.[20]

Patient Information

- American Academy of Dermatology: https://www.aad. org/public/diseases/skin-cancer/types/common/bcc
- Skin Cancer Foundation: https://www.skincancer.org/ skin-cancer-information/#basal
- American College of Mohs Surgery: https://www.skin- cancermohssurgery.org/

▼ SQUAMOUS CELL CARCINOMA

Introduction

Cutaneous SCC is the second most common skin cancer after BCC with over 400,000 new cases annually in the United States. Generally, the incidence ratio of BCCs over SCCs is 4:1. However, this ratio is reversed in solid organ transplant patients where SCCs are more common than BCCs by a 4:1 ratio.[23] Unlike BCCs, SCCs have the potential for local and distant metastasis. UV exposure is the most common cause of SCC.[24]

Pathogenesis

SCCs are malignant tumors of epidermal keratinocytes. AKs are often (but not mandatory) precursor lesions for SCC. Intense UV exposure or cumulative UV DNA damage may lead to p53 tumor suppressor gene mutations and development of AKs and ultimately SCC.[24] Other factors that have been associated with SCC development include human papilloma virus (high risk HPV subtypes),

long-standing burns and scars, ionizing radiation, chronic inflammation, arsenic exposure, and tobacco use. Certain genetic syndromes can also promote SCC development, including xeroderma pigmentosum, oculocutaneous albinism, and dystrophic epidermolysis bullosa.[3]

Clinical Presentation

▶ History and Physical Examination

As with BCCs, patients may complain of a wart or pimple-like bump on sun-exposed skin that grows slowly with episodes of bleeding and pain. Since there can be a continuum of AK, in situ SCC, and SCC, presentations can vary as described in the following paragraphs. Most SCCs occur on sun-exposed areas such as the face, balding scalp, dorsal hands and forearms, and lower legs especially in women. SCCs commonly arise from an area of extensive photodamage, therefore, a lesion in a skin area or field with multiple AKs should elicit clinical suspicion. They typically present as papules with overlying scale that are tender to palpation and occasionally bleed.

There are several subtypes of SCC:[25]

Squamous cell carcinoma in situ (SCCIS) is limited to the epidermis (dermal invasion absent). Whereas an AK is defined as cellular atypia present in partial thickness epidermis, once full thickness cellular atypia is present in the epidermis the lesion is defined as SCCIS. A SCC in situ can be described as an intraepidermal carcinoma. SCCIS typically occurs on sun exposed areas with extensive photodamage. It appears as a rough, pink, scaly papule, or plaque resembling a hypertrophic AK. Differences can be subtle but SCCIS often has more induration or tenderness (Figure 21-7). SCCIS and AKs may be present on the same lesion with gradual transition from partial atypia to full thickness atypia.

Bowen's disease is an SCCIS presenting as a well-demarcated, erythematous plaque with minimal scale and is often located on the lower extremities particularly in women (Figure 21-8). This lesion may be clinically misdiagnosed as eczema, psoriasis, or even superficial BCC. Just as AK's can transition to SCCIS, SCCIS can transition to invasive SCC if not treated appropriately. Erythroplasia of Queyrat is an SCCIS on the penile shaft, usually in uncircumcised men. This lesion appears as a non-scaly, erythematous, thin plaque on the shaft or corona of the penis (Figure 21-9) that may be present for years and is often misdiagnosed as dermatitis or a candida infection.

Invasive Squamous Cell Carcinoma (SCC) is defined by tumor involvement (islands of atypical keratinocytes) of the dermis. The degree of histologic keratinocyte differentiation may also be described by grade (well, moderate, poor, and infiltrative). Clinically, invasive SCC appears as a solitary hyperkeratotic pink nodule or papule on sun-exposed areas (Figure 21-10). When diagnosed early, the metastatic potential for SCC remains low. However, the risk increases

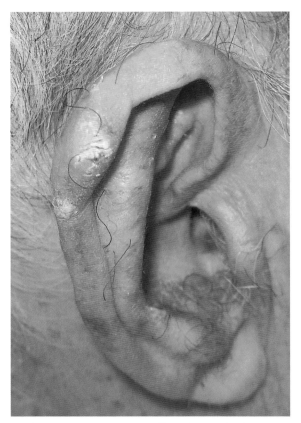

▲ **Figure 21-7.** Squamous cell carcinoma in situ. Hyperkeratotic plaque on the helix of the ear.

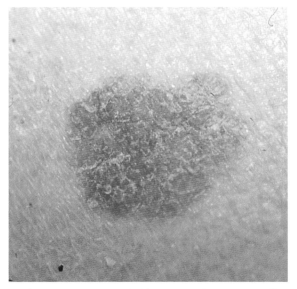

▲ **Figure 21-8.** Bowen's Disease. Erythematous well-demarcated plaque.

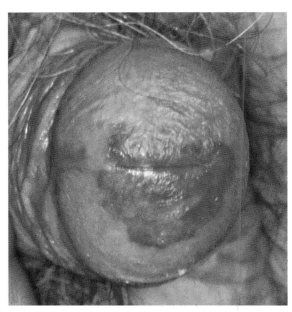

▲ **Figure 21-9.** Erythroplasia of Queyrat. Erythematous thin plaque around the urethral meatus.

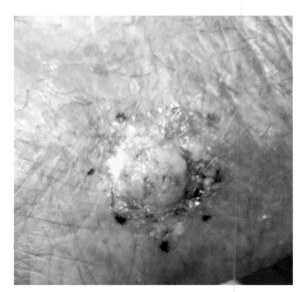

▲ **Figure 21-10.** Invasive squamous cell carcinoma. Macerated, crusted, hyperkeratotic nodule on the dorsal hand.

with accumulation of risk factors such as diameter ≥2 cm, poorly differentiated histology, perineural invasion, and tumor invading beyond subcutaneous fat.[26–28] Some skin locations are also more susceptible to metastasis such as lower lips and ears. Adjacent skin and regional lymph nodes are common locations for early metastasis; other

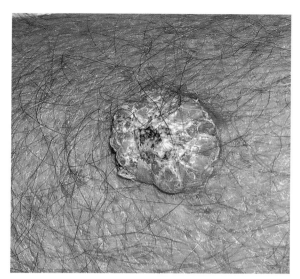

▲ Figure 21-11. Keratoacanthoma type of SCC. Erythematous nodule with a central hyperkeratotic core.

organ tissue affected by metastasis occurs later. A compromised immune system, such as in solid organ transplant recipients, can also allow SCC to metastasize at an earlier stage and increase the incidence of local recurrence.

Keratoacanthoma type SCC is an invasive SCC with a unique clinical history and presentation. It tends to grow quickly (centimeters) in a matter of weeks and may regrow after biopsy, before treatment. Keratoacanthoma-type SCC appears as a solitary symmetric smooth erythematous nodule with a central core of friable scale. It may look similar to a large molluscum contagiosum or irritated superficial cyst (Figure 21-11).

Verrucous carcinoma is an invasive SCC that presents as verrucous warty-like plaques usually on feet or on distal fingers. These long-standing lesions are often treated for years as common warts without resolution. Verrucous carcinomas are thought to arise from HPV-induced abnormal keratinocytes.

▷ Laboratory Findings

The histopathology of SCCIS shows abnormal keratinocytes involving the entire thickness of the epidermis. Invasive SCCs are graded based on degree of keratinocyte differentiation. Well-differentiated SCCs have a higher level of maturation, keratinization, and are more localized. Poorly differentiated SCCs have no or very limited maturation and structure. Poorly differentiated lesions may have a more spindle (long, narrow) cell appearance with higher risk of metastasis and local recurrence. When SCC tumor islands are histologically in contact with nerve bundles, the phenomenon of perineural invasion is present.[29] An

infiltrative SCC has a desmoplastic (firm, fibrous) scar-like appearance with single cell strands infiltrating the dermis and subcutis. Perineural invasion and desmoplastic SCC may involve deeper layers of the skin with wider subcutaneous extension than clinically expected. Typically these histologic findings are subtle and can be missed with routine hematoxylin and eosin (H&E) staining. Specialized immunohistochemical stains are more visually revealing.

Diagnosis

An SCC typically presents as a hyperkeratotic erythematous papule or plaque on sun damaged skin.

▷ Differential Diagnosis

✓ Viral wart: Presents as a hyperkeratotic papule with visible thrombosed (dark) capillaries and less redness.

✓ BCC: Often less scaly and shinier (pearly) surface with red telangiectasia.

✓ Seborrheic keratosis: Well defined with a stuck on tan waxy keratotic surface.

✓ Dermatitis: Improves with topical steroids and has a poorly defined border compared to SCC.

✓ Epidermoid cyst: Similar nodular or crateriform morphology, but more compressible and keratinaceous contents expressed.

✓ Cutaneous horn: acquired hyperkeratosis accumulates over a malignant or irritated benign papule.

Management

Biopsy techniques and pathology reports

Clinically suspicious lesions should be biopsied for confirmation of the diagnosis of SCC and identification of any high risk histologic features.[24] A shave biopsy to the depth of dermis (at a level where minimum pinpoint bleeding is observed) is often sufficient. If the papule or nodule has a thick cap of scale or crust, a scoop or "saucerization" technique with the bendable blade is helpful to achieve the necessary depth.

An invasive SCC cannot be diagnosed if the specimen is too superficial (i.e., does not contain dermis). If dermis is absent, the pathologist may only be able to diagnose SCCIS or AK but will often mention this limitation as "extending to the base of the specimen" in comments. A shave biopsy is rarely sufficient treatment for SCCs.

Some pathology reports of biopsies of SCC include comments on the margins which may be misunderstood. A shave biopsy report noting "the lesion appears excised in the margins examined" has a negative predictive value of 75%, and in general, the patient should not be considered treated.[12] A pathology report noting the lesion is "narrowly excised" or "approaches the margin" likely has a worse negative predictive value and will also need an excision or Mohs micrographic surgery. Additional work up and screening for a primary tumor may also be indicated if a pathology report states, "no epidermal connection is visualized, metastatic disease cannot be ruled out."

Management of squamous cell carcinoma

Most SCCs are treated surgically either by fusiform excision down to fat or Mohs micrographic surgery. For fusiform excision, typical margins range from 4 to 6 mm depending on size and the surgeon's confidence in identifying the clinical margin. Mohs micrographic surgery indications are listed in Table 21-1. The American Academy of Dermatology has created a treatment decision-making algorithm, the Mohs Appropriate Use Criteria (AUC) app for smartphones. It is simple, quick, and can be downloaded free of charge on most platforms.[20] For clinically advanced SCC or those with high-risk features and significant risk of metastasis, proper staging with sentinel lymph node biopsy or radiologic imaging may be indicated.[25, 30] Cure rates for radiation therapy, are lower than that of Mohs. Adjuvant radiation may be recommended following surgery for high-risk tumors or individuals. For non-metastatic SCC, radiation treatment alone is largely reserved for patients with palliative needs or who are unwilling to have surgery.

Management of in situ squamous cell carcinoma

By definition, SCCIS is lower risk than SCC. However, an SCCIS occurring on high risk skin locations (e.g., face, hands, genitals) or with a large clinical size would meet criteria for Mohs surgery or excision. For small tumors in low-risk locations, non-surgical options can be considered for SCCIS treatment. Destruction with electrodessication and curettage or off label topical treatments such as imiquimod cream 5% or 5-fluorouracil cream 5% have acceptable cure rates in the treatment of SCCIS. The clinician should avoid usage of non-invasive techniques in the treatment of SCC, due to the increased recurrence rate and metastatic potential.

Clinical Course and Prognosis

The prognosis for SCCIS and SCC diagnosed early is good, and unlikely to change a patient's life expectancy or health if treated appropriately. If neglected SCC can become metastatic, complicating treatment especially if the patient is immunocompromised or an allogeneic bone marrow recipient. Treatment with immune checkpoint inhibitors has provided medical oncologists with a more effective treatment for metastatic cutaneous SCC than traditional chemotherapy.[22,31] However, checkpoint inhibitor use is largely limited to the immunocompetent patient.

With appropriate treatment, recurrence rates are low. Unfortunately, the risk of developing additional future primary SCCIS or SCC remains relatively high. Although the United States Preventive Services Task Force (USPSTF) has no recommendations for skin cancer screening,[32] the risk of subsequent primary skin cancers supports the need for ongoing skin examinations. After treatment of local disease, common screening intervals are as follows: complete skin examination with regional lymph node examination every 3–12 months for 2 years, then every 6–12 months for 3 years, then annually for life. Risk factor modification is recommended for secondary prevention with sun protection and sun avoidance.

Indications for Consultation

Generally, a well-differentiated SCC or an SCCIS in a low-risk site is effectively treated with an elliptical excision down to fat by a surgically trained healthcare provider. Any malignancy in a high-risk area or an SCC with high-risk features on any skin site should be evaluated by a dermatologist and dermatologic surgeon for proper diagnosis, staging, and treatment.

Patient Information

- American Academy of Dermatology: https://www.aad.org/public/diseases/skin-cancer/types/common/scc
- Skin Cancer Foundation: www.skincancer.org/skin-cancer-information/squamous-cell-carcinoma
- American College of Mohs Surgery: https://www.skincancermohssurgery.org/

REFERENCES

1. de Oliveira ECV, da Motta VRV, Pantoja PC, Ilha CSD, Magalhaes RF, Galadari H et al. Actinic keratosis - review for clinical practice. *Int J Dermatol.* 2019;58:400-7.
2. Lebwohl M. Actinic Keratosis. *JAMA.* 2016;315:1394-5.
3. Kim RH, Armstrong AW. Nonmelanoma skin cancer. *Dermatol Clin.* 2012;30:125-39, ix.
4. Shelton ME, Adamson AS. Review and update on evidence-based surgical treatment recommendations for nonmelanoma skin cancer. *Dermatol Clin.* 2019;37:425-33.
5. de Berker D, McGregor JM, Hughes BR, Subcommittee BAoDTGaA. Guidelines for the management of actinic keratoses. *Br J Dermatol.* 2007;156:222-30.
6. Dianzani C, Conforti C, Giuffrida R, Corneli P, di Meo N, Farinazzo E et al. Current therapies for actinic keratosis. *Int J Dermatol.* 2020;59:677-84.
7. Cornejo CM, Jambusaria-Pahlajani A, Willenbrink TJ, Schmults CD, Arron ST, Ruiz ES. Field cancerization: Treatment. *J Am Acad Dermatol.* 2020;83:719-30.
8. Sachs DL, Kang S, Hammerberg C, Helfrich Y, Karimipour D, Orringer J et al. Topical fluorouracil for actinic keratoses and photoaging: a clinical and molecular analysis. *Arch Dermatol.* 2009;145:659-66.
9. Cunningham TJ, Tabacchi M, Eliane JP, Tuchayi SM, Manivasagam S, Mirzaalian H et al. Randomized trial of calcipotriol combined with 5-fluorouracil for skin cancer precursor immunotherapy. *J Clin Invest.* 2017;127:106-16.
10. Hashim PW, Chen T, Rigel D, Bhatia N, Kircik LH. Actinic Keratosis: current therapies and insights into new treatments. *J Drugs Dermatol.* 2019;18:s161-6.

11. Lebwohl M, Swanson N, Anderson LL, Melgaard A, Xu Z, Berman B. Ingenol mebutate gel for actinic keratosis. *N Engl J Med*. 2012;366:1010-9.

12. Grada A, Feldman SR, Bragazzi NL, Damiani G. Patient-reported outcomes of topical therapies in actinic keratosis: a systematic review. *Dermatol Ther*. 2021;e14833.

13. Lee Y, Baron ED. Photodynamic therapy: current evidence and applications in dermatology. *Semin Cutan Med Surg*. 2011;30:199-209.

14. Cameron MC, Lee E, Hibler BP, Barker CA, Mori S, Cordova M et al. Basal cell carcinoma Epidemiology; pathophysiology; clinical and histological subtypes; and disease associations. J *Am Acad Dermatol*. 2019;80:303-17.

15. Rubin AI, Chen EH, Ratner D. Basal-cell carcinoma. *N Engl J Med*. 2005;353:2262-9.

16. Kim DP, Kus KJB, Ruiz E. Basal cell carcinoma review. *Hematol Oncol Clin North Am*. 2019;33:13-24.

17. Renzi M, Schimmel J, Decker A, Lawrence N. Management of skin cancer in the elderly. *Dermatol Clin*. 2019;37:279-86.

18. Ceilley RI, Del Rosso JQ. Current modalities and new advances in the treatment of basal cell carcinoma. *Int J Dermatol*. 2006;45:489-98.

19. Kim JYS, Kozlow JH, Mittal B, Moyer J, Olencki T, Rodgers P et al. Guidelines of care for the management of basal cell carcinoma. *J Am Acad Dermatol*. 2018;78:540-59.

20. Connolly SM, Baker DR, Coldiron BM, Fazio MJ, Storrs PA, Vidimos AT et al. AAD/ACMS/ASDSA/ASMS 2012 appropriate use criteria for Mohs micrographic surgery: a report of the American Academy of Dermatology, American College of Mohs Surgery, American Society for Dermatologic Surgery Association, and the American Society for Mohs Surgery. *J Am Acad Dermatol*. 2012;67:531-50.

21. Jacobsen AA, Aldahan AS, Hughes OB, Shah VV, Strasswimmer J. Hedgehog pathway inhibitor therapy for locally advanced and metastatic basal cell carcinoma: A systematic review and pooled analysis of interventional studies. *JAMA Dermatol*. 2016;152:816-24.

22. Krišto M, Šitum M, Čeović R. Systemic therapies for advanced basal cell and cutaneous squamous cell carcinomas: novel targeted therapies and immunotherapies. Acta *Dermatovenerol Croat*. 2020;28:80-92.

23. Madan V, Lear JT, Szeimies RM. Non-melanoma skin cancer. Lancet 2010;375:673-85.

24. Combalia A, Carrera C. Squamous cell carcinoma: an update on diagnosis and treatment. *Dermatol Pract Concept*. 2020;10:e2020066.

25. Alam M, Ratner D. Cutaneous squamous-cell carcinoma. *N Engl J Med*. 2001;344:975-83.

26. Jambusaria-Pahlajani A, Kanetsky PA, Karia PS, Hwang WT, Gelfand JM, Whalen FM et al. Evaluation of AJCC tumor staging for cutaneous squamous cell carcinoma and a proposed alternative tumor staging system. *JAMA Dermatol*. 2013;149:402-10.

27. Karia PS, Jambusaria-Pahlajani A, Harrington DP, Murphy GF, Qureshi AA, Schmults CD. Evaluation of American Joint Committee on Cancer, International Union Against Cancer, and Brigham and Women's Hospital tumor staging for cutaneous squamous cell carcinoma. *J Clin Oncol*.2014;32:327-34.

28. Schmults CD, Karia PS, Carter JB, Han J, Qureshi AA. Factors predictive of recurrence and death from cutaneous squamous cell carcinoma: a 10-year, single-institution cohort study. *JAMA Dermatol*. 2013;149:541-7.

29. Que SKT, Zwald FO, Schmults CD. Cutaneous squamous cell carcinoma Incidence, risk factors, diagnosis, and staging. *J AmAcad Dermatol*. 2018;78:237-47.

30. Maher JM, Schmults CD, Murad F, Karia PS, Benson CB, Ruiz ES. Detection of subclinical disease with baseline and surveillance imaging in high-risk cutaneous squamous cell carcinomas. *J Am Acad Dermatol*. 2020;82:920-6.

31. Krausz AE, Ji-Xu A, Smile T, Koyfman S, Schmults CD, Ruiz ES. A Systematic review of primary, adjuvant, and salvage radiation therapy for cutaneous squamous cell carcinoma. *Dermatol Surg*. 2021.

32. Bibbins-Domingo K, Grossman DC, Curry SJ, Davidson KW, Ebell M, Epling JW et al. Screening for Skin Cancer: US preventive services task force recommendation statement. *JAMA*. 2016;316:429-35.

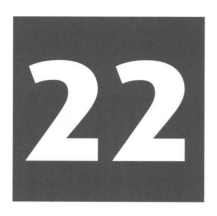

Nevi and Melanoma

Lori A. Fiessinger

INTRODUCTION TO CHAPTER

Melanocytic nevi (moles) are common benign skin tumors. In most people, these are primarily of cosmetic significance. However, nevi can occasionally become irritated or subjected to trauma and may need to be removed for this reason. Atypical nevi are considered benign, but they have some features that resemble melanoma and can be a marker for the increased risk of developing melanoma.

Melanoma is a potentially deadly cancer of melanocytes whose incidence is on the rise. It is unique among most serious cancers, because it can be detected by both patients and clinicians with a simple skin examination. When detected at early stages, melanoma is very treatable. Recognition of early melanomas by both patients and clinicians is key.

MELANOCYTIC NEVI

Introduction

Melanocytic nevi (moles) are among the most common benign tumors in humans. White individuals tend to have higher numbers of nevi than other populations. When nevi are present in Asian and Black individuals, they are more likely to be on the palms and soles. Interestingly, nevi are also less common in patients with light skin tones with the melanocortin-1 receptor (MC1-R) gene pigment variant (Fitzpatrick type I: red hair, fair skin, always burns, never tans skin type).[1]

Nevi begin to appear in early childhood, reach a maximum number in the 3rd to 4th decade of life, and then subsequently decline in number.[2] Genetic factors likely play a role in a person's potential for development of nevi and total nevi counts in adulthood. Nevi are more common on sun-exposed skin, as natural sunlight and artificial ultraviolet light are factors in their induction.

Melanocytic nevi can be subdivided into two major categories: congenital and acquired.

CONGENITAL MELANOCYTIC NEVI

Introduction

Key points for congenital melanocytic nevi

- ✓ Congenital melanocytic nevi are present in 1% of Caucasian infants at birth and have no gender predilection.
- ✓ They represent as tan, brown or black plaques usually ranging in size from <1 cm to >20 cm.
- ✓ The lifetime risk of developing melanoma in all sizes of congenital melanocytic nevi is estimated to be only 1-2%. However, in giant congenital melanocytic nevi with multiple smaller satellites, the risk is estimated to be as high as 10-15%.
- ✓ Patients with large and giant congenital nevi should be referred to dermatology for evaluation and long-term monitoring of their nevi.

Table 22-1. Categories and size of congenial nevi.

Category	Size in Adulthood	Risk of Melanoma
Small	<1.5 cm	Not increased compared to acquired melanocytic nevi.
Medium	1.5–19.9 cm	Not increased compared to acquired melanocytic nevi.
Large	20–40 cm	2% risk.
Giant	>40 cm	2% risk, risk increased when multiple CMN or satellites present.

CMN, congenital melanocytic nevus.

Our understanding of congenital melanocytic nevi has recently evolved and now two variants are recognized: those present at birth and those that develop before puberty. Congenital melanocytic nevi are present in 1% of White infants at birth and have no gender predilection. Congenital melanocytic nevi present at birth are highly variable in size and appearance, ranging from millimeters in size to occupying up to 80% of total body surface area. Giant congenital melanocytic nevi are very rare.

Congenital melanocytic nevi arising after birth but before puberty appear nearly identical to acquired melanocytic nevi by naked eye examination, but they differ in dermoscopic features, histopathology, and long-term evolution.

Congenital melanocytic nevi are traditionally classified by the projected size in adulthood (Table 22-1). Congenital melanocytic nevi are benign tumors, but they do have a small risk for developing melanoma that is proportional to size.

Pathogenesis

Mutations in the mitogen-activated protein kinase (MAPK) pathway have been implicated in the pathogenesis of congenital melanocytic nevi present at birth, most often NRAS.[1]

Clinical Presentation

History

When congenital melanocytic nevi are present at birth, they grow in proportion to the area of the body they reside on. They are usually asymptomatic, but often are visually disconcerting to the parents. There is risk of malignant transformation, so they do need to be monitored indefinitely for changes.

When congenital melanocytic nevi develop after birth but before puberty, they present as brown macules or papules. They appear very similar to the acquired melanocytic nevi by naked eye examination, but congenital melanocytic nevi will often show globular or cobblestone patterns on dermoscopy. They will have specific features on

histopathology, will progress to intradermal nevi later in life, and will typically persist for life. Acquired melanocytic nevi typically appear after puberty and regress in the 5th or 6th decades of life.[3]

Physical Examination

Congenital melanocytic nevi present at birth are shades of brown or black. They are usually palpable with well-defined borders, but they may have irregular contours. The surface can be smooth (Figure 22-1) but may also have a pebble-like surface. Lesions may also be cribriform, lobular, rugose, or bulbous. They commonly have dark terminal hairs.

Giant congenital melanocytic nevi are often surrounded by smaller satellite nevi. Giant congenital melanocytic nevi occasionally are distributed in areas that would be covered by a bathing suit, termed garment nevus (Figure 22-2). Dermoscopy of congenital melanocytic nevi is often challenging and requires advanced skills because they are often not perfectly uniform. Follow-up with sequential digital dermoscopy imaging can be helpful to monitor for changes. Giant congenital melanocytic nevi involving the scalp or midline can be associated with deep involvement including muscle, bone, dura mater, and leptomeninges.[4] The involvement of the congenital melanocytic nevi into the meninges or brain results in neurocutaneous melanocytosis. This can present with seizures, focal neurologic defects, or obstructive hydrocephalus. The prognosis is poor when neurological symptoms occur.

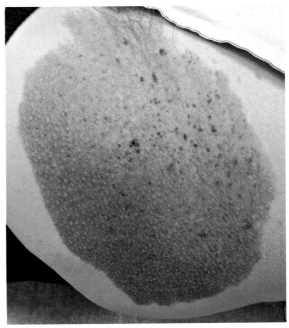

Figure 22-1. Congenital melanocytic nevus. Large 22-cm plaque with dark papules on lateral aspect of hip.

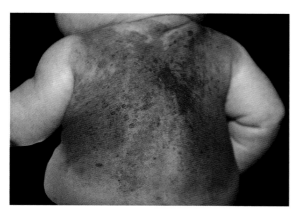

▲ **Figure 22-2.** Classic giant garment congenital melanocytic nevus in an infant, composed of brown plaque with brown and black papules within it.

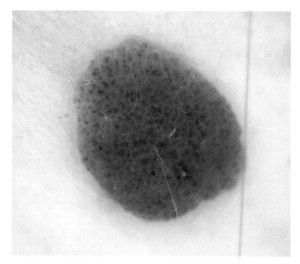

▲ **Figure 22-3.** Dermoscopy of a congenital melanocytic nevus showing globular/cobblestone pattern with terminal hairs. Reproduced with permission from Dr. Fiessinger.

Increased risk of malignant transformation to melanoma is associated with congenital melanocytic nevi of giant size with multiple satellite lesions and in patients with abnormal neurological screening tests. When cutaneous melanoma arises in a congenital melanocytic nevus, it more often develops in the deep dermis or subcutis rather than at the dermal–epidermal junction, making diagnosis by vision inspection difficult and resulting in more advanced disease at the time of diagnosis. Palpation of congenital melanocytic nevi for nodular areas is important when looking for malignant transformation. Other clinical features that should raise concern for the development of melanoma include ulceration, bleeding, or onset of new symptoms.

Congenital melanocytic nevi developing after birth but before puberty are usually brown macules or papules. They can range in size from a few millimeters to a few centimeters. On dermoscopy, globular or cobblestone patterns are often found (Figure 22-3). Over time, these congenital melanocytic nevi will transform into intradermal or compound nevi. These nevi typically persist for life. The risk of transformation to melanoma is very low, similar to that of acquired melanocytic nevi.

▷ Laboratory Findings

There are no features on histopathology that can absolutely determine if a nevus is congenital in origin, but there are some suggestive features.

The histopathological findings of congenital melanocytic nevi present at birth include benign features of junctional and dermal nevi and in some instances a "neural" component with neuroid tubes and corpuscles. There may also be melanocytic aggregates resembling blue nevi.

The histopathological findings of congenital melanocytic nevi not present at birth but developing before puberty include benign features of junctional and dermal

nevi with melanocytes within or aggregated about follicles, vessel walls, and nerves.

Diagnosis

Congenital melanocytic nevi are diagnosed with a combination of clinical information (presence before birth or after birth but before puberty), clinical features, histopathology features, and sometimes dermoscopic features.

▷ Differential Diagnosis

- ✓ Common acquired melanocytic nevi: Small congenital melanocytic nevi can be virtually indistinguishable clinically from common acquired nevi.
- ✓ Other melanocytic nevi: Congenital blue nevi have a deep blue color, nevus spilus presents with multiple 2–3 mm dark brown nevi on a large light-brown patch.
- ✓ Other pigmented congenital lesions: Becker's nevus, pigmented epidermal nevus, and café-au-lait spots.

Management

Congenital melanocytic nevi have a small risk of malignant transformation that is related to their size, so they need to be monitored for changes indefinitely. The highest risk of melanoma is in large/giant congenital melanocytic nevi. Half of the patients who develop melanomas in congenital nevi will develop the melanoma between the ages of 3 and 5 years. For this reason, some advocate for prophylactic staged excision of the large/giant congenital melanocytic nevi early in life.[5] However, the value of excision of congenital melanocytic nevi has been questioned because it is usually impossible to remove all the nevus, poor cosmetic results are common, and there are attendant medical and psychological risks to repeated large excisions.[4]

Clinical Course and Prognosis

Melanoma that develops in a large or giant congenital melanocytic nevus present from birth has a poor prognosis because it usually is detected late. The lifetime risk of developing melanoma in all sizes of congenital melanocytic nevi is estimated to be only 1–2%.[6] The risk of melanoma seems to be proportional to size and phenotype of the congenital melanocytic nevi. Large and giant congenital melanocytic nevi carry a 2% risk of malignant transformation.[7] The risk is highest for giant congenital melanocytic nevi with multiple smaller satellites, estimated to be as high as 10–15%.[6]

Indications for Consultation

Patients with large and giant congenital nevi should be referred to pediatric dermatology for evaluation and long-term monitoring of their nevi.

Patient Information

The Association for Large Nevi and Related Disorders: www.nevus.org

ACQUIRED MELANOCYTIC NEVI

Introduction

Key points for acquired melanocytic nevi

✓ Acquired melanocytic nevi are not present at birth and begin to regress in the 5th and 6th decades of life.

✓ They can present as well circumscribed macules, papules, or nodules (<1 cm in diameter) ranging in color from skin colored to pink, brown and blue/black.

✓ About one third of melanomas develop from a pre-existing nevus, so clinicians should take care in examining any moles that a patient notes have changed.

Common acquired melanocytic nevi are skin-colored papules or brown macules that develop during childhood or early adulthood. Having above average number of nevi is associated with the increased risk of melanoma. Nevi tend to be more numerous in light-skinned individuals. Nevi are usually more elevated around puberty and continue to develop through early adulthood. Acquired melanocytic nevi begin to regress in the 5th and 6th decades of life, resulting in lower nevi counts in the elderly.

Pathogenesis

Acquired melanocytic nevi are thought to be either benign hamartomas or benign proliferations of melanocytic nevus cells. They are thought to arise from cells delivered from the neural crest to the skin during embryologic development. The majority of acquired melanocytic nevi show activating mutations in BRAF.[1]

Clinical Presentation

▶ History

Acquired melanocytic nevi are usually asymptomatic. Patients may bring nevi to the attention of a clinician because of new onset, growth, symptoms of pain or itch, interference with activities of daily living, or alarming appearance. They may also bring them to attention because of a cosmetically undesirable appearance.

▶ Physical Examination

Acquired melanocytic nevi are small, circumscribed macules, papules, or nodules. They range in color from blue/black through brown, pink to skin-colored. Acquired melanocytic nevi are almost always less than 1 cm in diameter. Melanocytic lesions greater than 1 cm may be congenital nevi, atypical nevi, or melanoma. Nevi may occur anywhere on the body, but there is a predilection to sun-exposed skin.

- *Junctional nevi* arise at the skin dermal–epidermal junction; they are typically macular and brown in color (Figure 22-4 A,B). Dermoscopy will show a uniform pigmented network trailing off in the periphery.

- *Intradermal nevi* present with nevus cells confined to the dermis of the skin and are papular very light brown or skin toned (Figure 22-5 A, B). Dermoscopy will show only focal globular pigmentation or comma-shaped blood vessels.

- *Compound nevi* have both junctional and dermal components and are usually papular and pigmented. Dermoscopy will show features of both junctional and intradermal nevi, including cobblestone-like globular pattern and comma-shaped blood vessels (Figure 22-6).

Less common presentations of nevi are as follows:

- *Halo nevi (Sutton nevus)* are usually benign melanocytic nevi surrounded by a halo of depigmentation (Figure 22-7), which may be due to a direct cytotoxic effect of lymphocytes surrounding the nevus. The halo usually heralds involution of the nevus over months to years. Halo nevi most commonly occur in childhood and are thought to be inconsequential. Patients may have associated vitiligo. When halo nevi develop in adulthood, there is concern that melanoma can masquerade as a

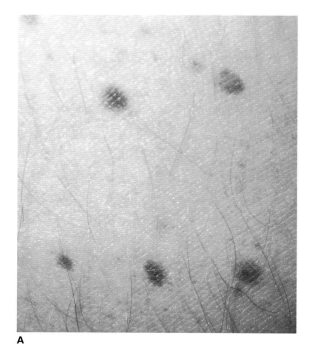

A

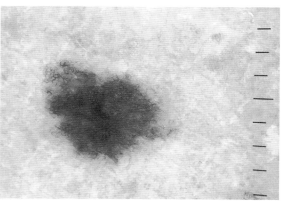

B

▲ **Figure 22-4 A, B.** Junctional nevi, clinically and dermoscopically. A. Tan macules with uniform colors and borders. B. Dermoscopy image of a junctional nevus shows reticular pattern, uniformly and evenly distributed. Reproduced with permission from Dr. Fiessinger.

halo nevus or that melanoma at another body site may precipitate the development of halo nevi elsewhere on the body. Many experts recommend full body skin, genital, and ophthalmologic examination for adults with new onset halo nevus. However, a recent retrospective study found only a 1% risk of development of melanoma within 1 year of diagnosis of halo nevus in

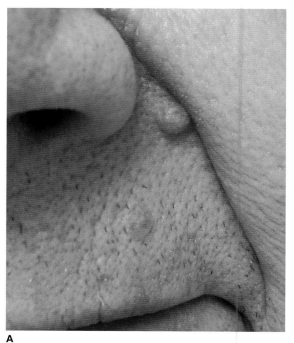

A

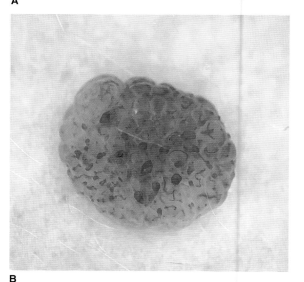

B

▲ **Figure 22-5 A, B.** Intradermal nevi clinically and dermoscopically. A. Skin-colored dome-shaped papules. B. Dermoscopy shows classic comma-shaped blood vessels. Reproduced with permission from Dr. Fiessinger.

adults.[8] Any atypical appearance or dermoscopy features of the nevus itself justify removal and histopathological examination.

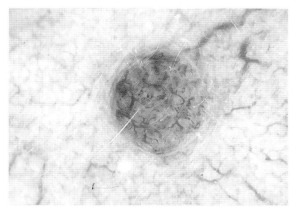

Figure 22-6. Dermoscopy photograph of a compound nevus. These can exhibit features of both junctional and intradermal nevi. This compound nevus has both comma shaped vessels and globules of pigment. Reproduced with permission from Dr. Fiessinger.

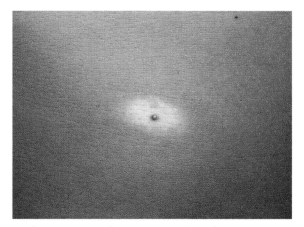

Figure 22-7. Halo nevus. Macule with hypopigmented halo.

- *Blue nevi* are acquired nevi that range in color from blue to black (Figure 22-8). The onset is usually in childhood, with predominance in Asian individuals. These nevi are benign, but melanoma, especially nodular melanoma and cutaneous metastases of melanoma may masquerade as blue nevi. Indications for biopsy include atypical features such as size >1 cm or irregular shape or color, late onset, or clinical changes to the lesion.
- *Spitz nevi* are small, typically pink or tan nevi that appear suddenly, primarily in children. They have characteristic dermoscopic (starburst pattern or symmetric pseudopods) and histopathological features but can easily be mistaken for melanoma clinically or on histopathology (Figure 22-9 A, B). Spitz nevi are unusual in patients

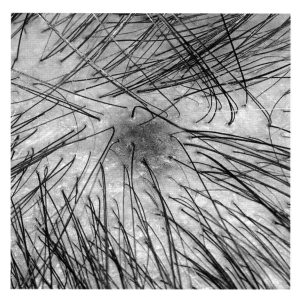

Figure 22-8. Blue nevus. Blue-gray papule on scalp.

over the age of 40; therefore, skin lesions with the dermoscopic features of Spitz nevi are best removed in this age group to exclude melanoma with Spitzoid features.

Laboratory Findings

The histopathologic findings of common acquired melanocytic nevi show mature melanocytes arranged as individual cells or in nests. The margin of the nevus is discrete.

Diagnosis

Common acquired melanocytic nevi present as tan, brown, or black macules or papules or skin-colored papules with uniform colors and borders. The adoption of dermoscopy has enhanced the ability of the clinician to differentiate normal nevi from atypical nevi and melanomas. The greatest limitation of dermoscopy is that it requires additional training. For this reason, we have dedicated chapter 4 to an introduction to dermoscopy.

Differential Diagnosis

Table 22-2 lists the differential diagnosis for common acquired nevi, which primarily includes other pigmented tumors.

Management

Nevi are usually asymptomatic. Indications for removal of a nevus include changes to the lesion, atypical features suspicious for melanoma, repeated irritation, or cosmetic concerns. About one-third of melanomas develop from a

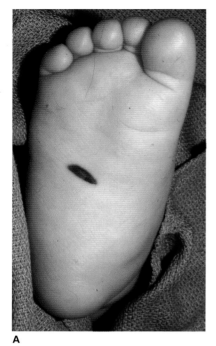

A

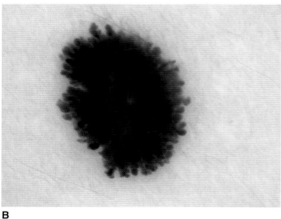

B

▲ **Figure 22-9 A, B. A.** Spitz nevus on child's foot. These can be pigmented or nonpigmented. **B.** Dermoscopy shows darkly pigmented spitz nevus with blue-gray globules centrally and pseudopods at the periphery.

pre-existing nevus, so clinicians should take care in examining any moles that the patient has noticed to be changed. Clinically suspicious lesions often have one or more of the following features of the **ABCDE** rule (Table 22-3). Melanocytic lesions are also suspicious for melanoma if they are painful or pruritic or if the lesion becomes eroded in the absence of trauma. Dermoscopy can aid in the evaluation of nevi and other cutaneous neoplasms.

Table 22-2. Differential diagnosis of pigmented lesions.

Pigmented lesion	Clinical findings
Benign nevus	Symmetric, uniform color and border, size usually <6 mm, resembles other nevi on a patient.
Atypical nevus	Size >6 mm, asymmetric, irregular color or border, appears different than other moles on a patient.
Congenital nevus	Two variants: Present at birth or present around puberty. Often greater than 1 cm in size by adulthood.
Melanoma	Features similar to atypical nevus. Changing or symptomatic lesion.
Lentigo	Evenly colored, sharply marginated, resembles other lentigos in sun-damaged skin.
Seborrheic keratosis	Warty, with typically a "stuck-on" appearance, sharp round border.
Pigmented basal cell cancer	May be indistinguishable from melanoma clinically, dermoscopy helpful to differentiate.
Dermatofibroma	Even color or lighter center, puckers when pinched.
Becker's nevus	Large unilateral brown patch on shoulder or chest, may have increased hair.

Table 22-3. ABCDE rule for features of melanoma.

A: Asymmetry
B: Border is irregular, notched, or blurred
C: Color is variable or irregularly distributed
D: Diameter is greater than 6 mm
E: Evolving or changing lesion.

While the United States Preventive Services Task Force (USPSTF) found that there was insufficient evidence to recommend routine skin cancer screening exams for individuals without a history of precancerous or cancerous skin lesions, the unique risk factors for melanoma of an individual should be considered.

Genetic factors increasing risk of melanoma include the following:[1]

- Family history of melanoma
- Fair skin with tendency to burn
- Red hair color
- Greater than 100 nevi
- At least five clinically atypical melanocytic nevi
- Multiple solar lentigines

Environmental factors include history of indoor tanning, chronic sun exposure, high intensity intermittent sun exposure, and immunosuppression. Those at higher risk of melanoma should be counseled on sun protection and how to perform self-examination in addition to having regular full body skin examinations.

If feasible, clinically suspicious nevi should always be removed in their entirety so that the entire lesion can be examined histopathologically. Partial biopsies can lead to false negative results.

Clinical Course and Prognosis

Around one-third of melanomas occur in pre-existing nevi. The other two-thirds of melanoma arise de novo. For this reason, it is important to counsel patients on monitoring existing nevi for changes while also watching for new pigmented lesions to develop, especially in later adulthood when development of new nevi is not typical.

Indications for Consultation

Consideration for referral for regular screening should be given to patients with risk factors for melanoma as listed above.

Depending on the surgical skills of the clinician, patients may be referred for excision of particularly large nevi or nevi in cosmetically sensitive areas.

Patient Information

DermNet NZ: https://dermnetnz.org/topics/mole/

▼ ATYPICAL/DYSPLASTIC NEVI

Introduction

Key points for atypical/dysplastic nevi

✓ The term *atypical nevus* refers to nevi with clinical atypia, including size greater than 5mm, irregular or ill-defined borders, asymmetry, or variation in pigmentation. *Dysplastic nevus* represents a histopathologic diagnosis.

✓ Atypical nevi can appear in childhood or adulthood and are not uncommon, occurring in up to 5% of White individuals and in 30% to 50% of patients with history of melanoma.

✓ Atypical/dysplastic nevi present as pink to brown to black macules or papules with variegated color, variable shape, irregular borders, and size >5mm.

✓ Because of the possibility of ambiguity on histopathology, atypical nevi with severe degree of architectural disorder or cytological atypia should be excised with a margin of normal tissue.

✓ Patients with atypical nevi should be referred for regular screening by a dermatologist.

The term atypical nevus refers to nevi with clinical atypia, including size greater than 5 mm, irregular or ill-defined borders, asymmetry, or variation in pigmentation. Dysplastic nevi represent a histopathologic diagnosis. Some experts use these terms interchangeably. Atypical nevi/dysplastic nevi are a controversial entity. The terms were first used to describe six families with increased risk of melanoma and clinically atypical nevi by dermatopathologist Clark in 1978.[1] Later, similar nevi were found to occur sporadically in individuals without increased familial melanoma risk. Initial reports suggested that dysplastic nevi were be premalignant. Most experts now agree that the risk of an individual dysplastic nevus progressing to melanoma is either similar to or just slightly higher than in common acquired melanocytic nevi, but that the presence of dysplastic nevi is an independent risk factor for development of melanoma.[9] Despite agreement on this, there still is lack of consensus by experts on definition, histopathologic criteria, and treatment of atypical/dysplastic nevi.

Atypical nevi can appear in adulthood or childhood and are not uncommon, occurring in up to 5% of White individuals. They are present in virtually every patient with familial cutaneous melanoma and in 30% to 50% of patients with sporadic primary cutaneous melanoma. Risk factors include a history of sun exposure, but atypical nevi can also occur in sun-protected skin. Unlike common acquired nevi, new atypical nevi may continue to appear throughout a patient's lifetime.

Pathogenesis

Atypical/dysplastic nevi were initially thought of as melanoma precursors, but now most experts agree that risk of malignant transformation is similar to that of other acquired melanocytic nevi. Most experts consider atypical nevi as potential markers for an increased risk for developing melanoma. The other important significance of atypical nevi is the potential histopathologic ambiguity. There are no widely accepted features for histopathologic diagnosis. There is significant inter-observer variability in diagnosis and grading of atypia. Because of this, what one pathologist calls an atypical nevus might be called an early melanoma by another pathologist.

Clinical Presentation

▶ History

Patients often have a history of multiple acquired nevi. There may be a family history of melanoma or removal of nevi.

▶ Physical Examination

Atypical/dysplastic nevi present as pink to brown to black macules or papules with variegated color, variable shape, irregular borders, and size >5 mm (Figure 22-10). Table 22-4 lists the clinical presentation of atypical nevi

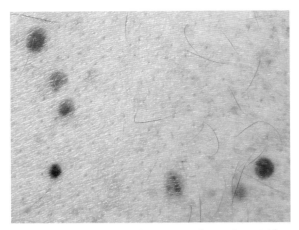

▲ **Figure 22-10.** Atypical nevi. Macules with variable colors and indistinct borders.

Table 22-4. Characteristics of typical and atypical nevi.

Features	Typical Nevi	Atypical Nevi
Color	Brown or black, uniform color	Pink to black, variegated color.
Diameter	6 mm or less	May be up to several centimeters in size.
Shape and outline	Symmetric	Variable shape or irregular borders.
Histological changes	Atypia is absent	Mild to severe architectural disorder and/or cytological atypia.

as contrasted with common typical nevi. It is difficult to evaluate a patient who does not have a "signature nevus" (a specific type of nevus pattern that most of the patient's nevi adhere to). Some patients have multiple, even hundreds of atypical nevi ranging in size from millimeters to centimeters and having a variety of colors ranging from pink to black. On dermoscopy, atypical nevi exhibit lack of uniform and symmetric pigmentation (Figure 22-11).

▷ Laboratory findings

The histopathological findings of dysplastic nevi may be similar to benign common nevi, but typically will include degrees of mild to severe architectural disorder and/or mild to severe cytological atypia.

Diagnosis

Atypical/dysplastic nevi present as pink to black macules or papules with variegated color and irregular borders. They are usually greater than 5 mm in diameter. Expertise in dermoscopy can be helpful in differentiating atypical nevi from melanoma, but often histopathology is required to rule out melanoma.

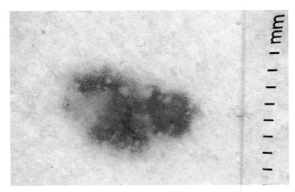

▲ **Figure 22-11.** Dermoscopy of a dysplastic nevus graded as severely atypical. Notice the lack of uniform pigmentation and symmetry in the lesion. There is loss of the reticular network near 12 o'clock. There is thickening of the reticular network near 9 o'clock. Reproduced with permission from Dr. Fiessinger.

▷ Differential diagnosis

The differential diagnosis for atypical/dysplastic nevi is listed in Table 22-4.

Management

Nevi that are changing in shape, border, size, or pigmentary features should be biopsied. The observation of these changes often originates from the patient, but ideally originates from baseline photographs, such as from total body photography or serial digital dermoscopy images.

Patients with atypical/dysplastic nevi have increased risk for melanoma and require regular skin examinations, preferably with baseline full body photography to reduce unnecessary biopsies and increase detection of early melanomas.[10]

Because of the possibility of ambiguity on histopathology, atypical nevi with severe degree of architectural disorder or cytological atypia should be excised with at least 5 mm margins. Management of atypical nevi with mild or moderate degree of architectural disorder or cytologic atypia is more controversial. While some experts still recommend re-excision of these lesions with 2–3 mm margins, newer studies have provided evidence that watching scars for repigmentation may be a reasonable alternative to re-excision of all moderately dysplastic nevi.[11]

Patients should be given color-illustrated pamphlets that depict the clinical features of atypical moles and malignant melanoma. These brochures are available through the Skin Cancer Foundation and the American Academy of Dermatology. Patients with atypical nevi should be instructed to monitor their nevi monthly with self-skin examinations. Patients should be educated on sun-protective measures, including use of a sunscreen, wearing sun-protective clothing, seeking shade, and avoiding peak sun hours. They should be instructed to avoid indoor tanning.

Clinical Course and Prognosis

Dysplastic nevi with mild or moderate architectural or cytologic atypia are considered by most to be variants of normal, but they likely are a marker for increased overall melanoma risk. Dysplastic nevi with severe architectural or cytologic atypia are less well understood biologically. Because of this and the histopathologic ambiguity of dysplastic nevi, re-excision with negative margins is recommended by most experts.[12]

Indications for Consultation

Patients with atypical nevi should be referred for regular screening by a dermatologist skilled in dermoscopic examination. In addition, if available, full body photography can be very helpful in establishing a base-line benchmark for future examinations.

Patient Information

Skin Cancer Foundation: www.skincancer.org/skin-cancer-information/dysplastic-nevi

▼ MELANOMA

Introduction

Key points for melanoma

- ✓ Melanoma is the fifth most frequently diagnosed cancer in men (lifetime risk of 3.6%) and the sixth most common in women (lifetime risk of 2.5%).
- ✓ Most melanomas begin as de novo lesions, with only about 30% arising in preexisting nevi.
- ✓ Most melanomas have the following characteristics: **A**symmetry, **B**order that is irregular, notched or blurred, **C**olor that is variable or irregularly distributed, **D**iameter >6 mm and is **E**volving.
- ✓ The first step in management of a suspected melanoma is confirmation of the diagnosis with a skin biopsy and/or referral to a dermatologist.
- ✓ Wide local excision with appropriate surgical margins prevents local recurrence and is curative for those without occult nodal or distant metastases.

Malignant melanoma is a cancer of melanocytes. Melanoma incidence is on the rise, with estimates for 2020 including 95,710 new cases of melanoma in situ and 100,350 new cases of invasive melanoma.[13] It is the fifth most frequently diagnosed cancer in men (lifetime risk of 3.6%) and the sixth most common in women (lifetime risk of 2.5%).[13] Malignant melanoma attracts a great amount of publicity, because it is one of the most common potentially lethal malignancies of young adults. When diagnosed early, melanoma is treatable, so there are national educational campaigns in most countries emphasizing the importance of self-examination of the skin. While still a very serious cancer, melanoma mortality is on the decline due to availability of new treatments for late-stage disease.[14]

Melanoma can occur at any age but is rare in childhood. Lifetime risk factors include the following:[12]

- Genotypes with specific risk enhancement (e.g., CDKN2A gene mutation)
- Family history of melanoma in first-order relatives
- Prior personal history of melanoma
- One or more atypical nevi
- Large numbers of nevi
- Advancing age
- Outdoor occupations or aviation flight occupation
- Fair skin
- History of blistering sunburn and a history of indoor tanning

Pathogenesis

Most melanomas begin as de novo lesions, with only about 30% arising in pre-existing nevi. The cancer genetics for melanoma are complex, but certain oncogenes have become important because of their frequencies and because of potential therapeutic implications for targeted therapy. Around 50% of melanoma have a mutation in BRAF, which can be targeted with BRAF-inhibitors and MEK-inhibitors which work upstream of BRAF. Other mutations in addition to BRAF (most common in superficial spreading melanoma) include KIT (most common in acral-lentiginous melanoma), NRAS, and CDKN2A (the most common specific mutation in familial melanoma).[1] Germline mutations in CDKN2A can be detected on blood test if there is concern for familial melanoma.

Clinical Presentation

▶ History

Patients often have a history of a change in size, shape, or color or pruritus in a new or existing nevus.

▶ Physical Examination

Melanoma can occur on any skin surface irrespective of sun exposure. The most common locations in men are the trunk (55%), especially the upper back, followed by the legs, arms, and face; in women, the most common location is the legs (42%), followed by the trunk, arms, and face.[15]

Melanomas typically have the clinical features as listed in Table 22-1. Figure 22-12 demonstrates many of these

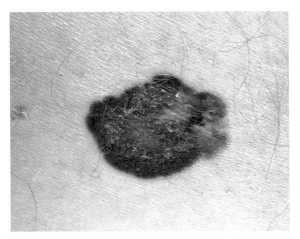

▲ **Figure 22-12.** Melanoma. Demonstrating the ABCD rule with asymmetry, irregular border, variable color, and diameter >6 mm.

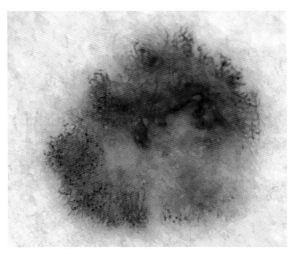

▲ **Figure 22-13.** Dermoscopy of a superficial spreading melanoma. This images shows multiple colors, including shades of pink, brown, blue, and gray. There are asymmetrically distributed dark brown to black globules on a background of a reticular network that has some normal areas, some regressed areas, and some thickened areas. There is a blue-gray smudgy area in the superior half of the image. Reproduced with permission from Dr. Fiessinger.

clinical features. There have been several dermoscopic features of melanoma described, including thickened network, blue-white veils, asymmetric pseudopods, radial streaming, scar-like depigmentation, negative networks, and polymorphous vessels. Figure 22-13 shows thickened network and asymmetrically distributed dark brown to black globules. These features will be addressed in more detail in Chapter 7.

Main Types of Melanoma

- *Superficial spreading melanoma* usually occurs on sun exposed skin as can occur in sun exposed skin, as high intensity intermittent sun exposure has been implicated in its pathogenesis. It can also occur on non sun exposed skin. It is the most common subtype of invasive melanoma, characterized by a superficial radial growth phase that occurs before an invasive vertical growth phase (Figure 22-14). These melanomas account for the majority of invasive melanomas (about 70% of melanomas) and have an excellent prognosis when detected early.

- *Nodular melanomas* are less common, accounting for 15–30% of invasive melanomas (Figure 22-15). They lack a radial growth phase. They grow rapidly over months and are often advanced at the time of diagnosis.

- *Lentigo maligna* occurs most commonly in chronically sun-damaged skin of the head and neck of elderly patients (Figure 22-16). These are very often diagnosed while still in the in situ phase and referred to as lentigo maligna versus invasive disease which is called lentigo maligna melanoma. Lentigo maligna melanoma accounts for 10–15% of invasive melanomas.

- *Acral lentiginous melanoma* occurs on the palms and soles (Figure 22-17). They account for only about 2–8% of invasive melanomas in Caucasians but are the most common subtype of melanomas in Asian and Black patients. These are often advanced at diagnosis because of the inattentiveness of patient to the sole of the foot or lack of awareness of the features of melanoma.

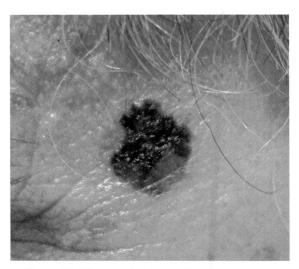

▲ **Figure 22-14.** Superficial spreading melanoma. Dark brown plaque with variable colors and irregular borders on temple.

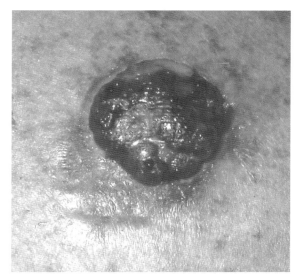

▲ **Figure 22-15.** Nodular melanoma. Black–dark grey dome shaped ulcerated papule on a pink erythematous base.

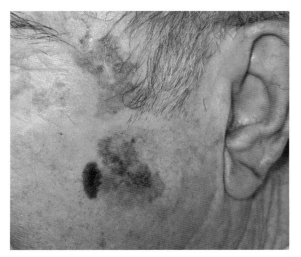

▲ **Figure 22-16.** Lentigo maligna melanoma. Four-centimeter lentigo maligna on cheek with indistinct and irregular borders and variable colors with an invasive melanoma component on medial border. A benign lentigo is above the melanoma.

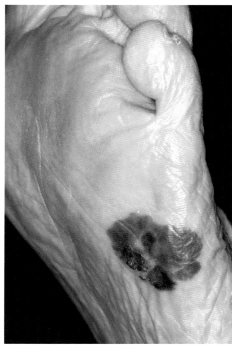

▲ **Figure 22-17.** Acral lentiginous melanoma. Dark brown patch with variable colors and irregular border with crust and superficial ulceration on the plantar and lateral aspect of the foot.

- *Metastatic melanoma from an unknown primary* occurs when melanoma is found in lymph nodes, subcutaneous tissue, or visceral organ without a primary melanoma being found on cutaneous and mucosal surface examinations. This occurs in about 3% of all melanoma diagnoses. If the metastasis is limited to skin or lymph nodes, the prognosis is actually better than patients with visceral metastases from a known primary.[16]
- *Primary mucosal melanoma of the head and neck* is a rare subtype which occurs in about 1% of melanomas. This includes both oral and nasal mucosal melanomas.
- *Vulvo/vaginal melanoma* accounts for a small number of melanomas. However, melanoma in this location is important because the detection is often delayed. Melanomas are often advanced at the time of diagnosis.
- *Subungual melanoma* accounts for up to 3% of melanomas. It most commonly presents with pigmentary changes of the nail bed (Figure 22-19). Pigment can also involve the proximal nail fold, which is referred to as Hutchinson's sign. The diagnosis is aided by dermoscopy. Early diagnosis is essential as the prognosis is otherwise poor compared to other melanoma locations.

▷ Other Presentations of Melanoma

- *Melanoma in situ* is a proliferation of malignant melanocytes confined to the epidermis. The most common subtype of melanoma in situ is lentigo maligna which occurs in sun-exposed skin (Figure 22-18).

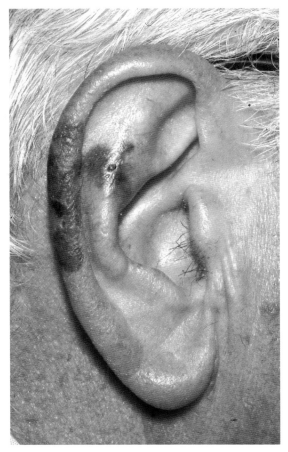

▲ **Figure 22-18.** Melanoma in situ on ear. Poorly defined borders and multiple shades of brown.

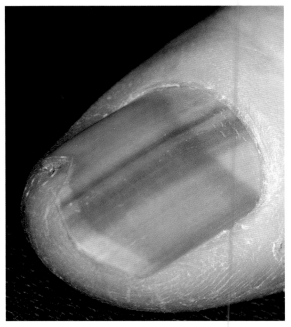

▲ **Figure 22-19.** Subungual melanoma. Acral lentiginous melanoma originating in the nail matrix of the great toe. Note the irregular bands of pigmentation in the nail bed.

- *Primary ocular melanoma* is extremely rare. Lesions may be uveal, ciliary, or choroidal and are not easily amenable to biopsy. Patients usually present with visual loss or pain. The diagnosis is based on physical findings. Despite both ocular and cutaneous melanoma arising from melanocytes, ocular melanoma has unique genetic mutations and responds differently to melanoma treatments compared to cutaneous melanoma.[17]

- *Pediatric melanoma* in pediatric patients is exceedingly rare. When it occurs, melanoma can be subclassified as congenital melanocytic nevus-associated (typically presents by 3–5 years of age), Spitz melanoma (occurs most commonly in younger adolescents), and conventional (looks and behaves similar to adult melanomas, occurs most commonly in older adolescents). The traditional clinical criteria for melanoma diagnosis (ABCDE rules, Table 22-3) may not capture pediatric melanomas, so alternative pediatric-ABCD criteria have been proposed to include **A**melanotic, **B**leeding or **B**ump, **C**olor uniformity, and **D**e novo at any **D**iameter.[18] Traditional melanoma criteria on dermoscopy are present in both childhood and adolescent melanoma.[19]

- *Amelanotic melanoma* is a variant of melanoma without visible pigment. It usually presents as a pink lesion (Figure 22-20). Clinical diagnosis can be challenging, often resulting in delay of diagnosis and later stage at diagnosis. They are often nodular and may be confused with pyogenic granulomas. Dermoscopy can be very helpful in diagnosis. Dermoscopy will sometimes show pigment not apparent on clinical examination.[20] The presence of polymorphic vessels on dermoscopy can also aid in diagnosis.[20]

- *Desmoplastic melanoma* is another rare subtype, accounting for only 1–4% of melanomas. These most commonly present as flesh-colored, scar-like, or pink papules or nodules, most commonly on chronically sun exposed areas like the head and neck.[20] Although often invasive at the time of diagnosis, the prognosis is better for pure desmoplastic melanomas than for comparably thick nodular melanomas.[21]

- *Familial melanoma:* 5% to 10% of melanomas occur in familial clusters. When a mutation is identified, it is most commonly in the CDKN2A suppressor gene. These patients also are at increased risk for pancreatic

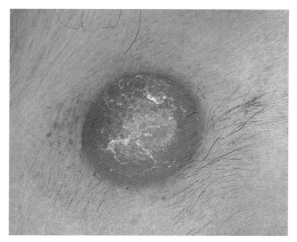

▲ **Figure 22-20.** Amelanotic melanoma. Pink dome-shaped nodule on temple. The lesion has scale on the surface and crust on the periphery.

cancer. Indications for genetic screening include individuals with three or more primary melanomas or personal history of melanoma with two first-degree family members affected by melanomas or pancreatic cancers.[22] Awareness of a gene mutation within a family can lead to earlier screening for melanoma and earlier diagnosis.

▶ Laboratory Findings

The histopathological findings of a melanoma include irregular distribution of cytologically atypical cells in nests and individually with disruption of normal nevus architecture, asymmetry, violation of boundaries, and a host response evident by an inflammatory infiltrate.

A histopathology report of melanoma should include a number of important variables. The subtype of melanoma is given if possible. The Breslow depth is a measurement of thickness of the tumor measured from the surface of the skin to the deepest level of tumor invasion. Ulceration of the epidermis is an important prognostic factor. Tumor staging is based in part on the Breslow depth and presence of ulceration which make up the T category staging.[23] Additional prognostic factors not incorporated into the current American Joint Committee on Cancer (AJCC) staging classification, which have shown prognostic significance in some studies, include mitotic figures, radial and vertical growth phases, regression, angiolymphatic invasion, angiotropism, perineural invasion, and tumor-infiltrating lymphocytes. The Clark classification, which is an older measurement of tumor invasion, is not used any more as it was considered too subjective. Atypical melanocytic hyperplasia is a term that describes lesions that are ambiguous histopathologically and may be difficult

to distinguish from melanoma. Most experts treat these lesions as melanoma in situ.

Diagnosis

Larger melanomas can present with one or more features as listed in the ABCDE rule (Table 22-1).

With appropriate training, dermoscopy can improve both sensitivity and specificity for skin cancer diagnosis compared to naked eye examination.[24] Dermoscopy can allow for diagnosis of smaller melanomas and less invasive melanomas.[24] Dermoscopy melanoma specific criteria are discussed in the dermoscopy chapter of this book.

Total body photography allows for monitoring of nevi for changes over time. This is especially useful in detecting new pigmented lesions in patients with large numbers of nevi. The combination of total body photography with serial digital dermoscopy photographs of individual nevi is increasingly being used to monitor patients at high risk of melanoma. Combination of the two modalities allows for better detection of new lesions (total body photography) and better monitoring of lesions for subtle changes (serial digital dermoscopy). The combination leads to detection of melanomas at early stages, many at the in situ stage.[25] Most interestingly, melanomas can be detected by presence of a new lesion on total body photography or subtle changes on dermoscopy in lesions that do not have any clinical or dermoscopic criteria of melanoma.[26]

Reflectance confocal microscopy can be helpful in diagnosing melanoma. Studies have shown higher sensitivity than dermoscopy for diagnosis of melanoma, especially in hypopigmented or amelanotic melanomas.[25] Reflectance confocal microscopy is particularly helpful in confirming suspicion of lentigo maligna or lentigo maligna melanoma in pigmented facial lesions where patients can be hesitant to agree to biopsy due to cosmetic concerns and dermoscopy can be equivocal.[27] Reflectance confocal microscopy is not yet widely available in the United States, but may become more available now that machine costs are decreasing and there are established current procedural terminology (CPT) codes that allow for reimbursement.

While histopathology remains the gold standard in diagnosis of melanoma, molecular techniques may offer more objective diagnosis in the future. There are a few commercially available molecular tests. Of note, none of these are currently widely used in practice, mostly due to lack of prospective studies.

The Pigmented Lesion Assay (PLA) is a noninvasive test meant to be used prior to biopsy. The assay uses tape stripping to generate lesional RNA which is tested for two genes preferentially expressed in melanoma. The Pigmented Lesion Assay has shown high negative predictive value (meaning negative test result is very unlikely to be melanoma), leading to hope that this could be a tool to reduce biopsies in the future. Because the test sensitivity is 91–95%, there is still a chance of missing a melanoma diagnosis with it.[28]

myPath®Melanoma is a genetic test done on tissue aimed at differentiating melanocytic lesions that are challenging to diagnose on histopathology. RNA is obtained from tissue blocks and examined for the presence of 23 genes that show differential expression in benign and malignant melanocytic lesions. Expression of genes leads to a numerical score of likely benign, indeterminate, or likely malignant. While an objective test for difficult to diagnosis melanoma cases sounds very appealing, more prospective studies with long-term outcomes are needed before this test will be widely used.[28]

Differential Diagnosis

Table 22-2 lists the differential diagnosis for pigmented lesions.

Management

The first step in management of a suspected melanoma is confirmation of the diagnosis with a skin biopsy. Prebiopsy photographs are helpful to aid in clinical/histopathologic correlation and to reduce the risk of wrong site surgery. The purpose of the biopsy for a suspected melanoma is to confirm the diagnosis and to provide staging and prognostic information. Ideally, a suspicious lesion should be removed in its entirety with a 1–3 mm of normal appearing skin at the margin. This can be completed with an elliptical excisional biopsy, deep shave/saucerization/scoop biopsy to the deep reticular dermis to prevent transection of the deep margin, or punch biopsy excision around the lesion with appropriate margin of normal tissue.[29] While elliptical excisional biopsy is ideal to encompass both deep and lateral margins, most dermatologists in the United States utilize deep shave/saucerization/scoop biopsies due to ease and time efficiency. Partially biopsied lesions should be avoided as they can result in false negative histopathology and inaccurate staging leading to inappropriate management. In cosmetically challenging areas like the face, removing a lesion in entirety might not be possible without leaving an unsightly scar. In these cases, multiple small scouting biopsies for the lesion or referral to a dermatologist, is appropriate.

Surgical Management

Surgery is the primary treatment of cutaneous melanoma. Wide local excision with appropriate surgical margins prevents local recurrence and is curative for those without occult nodal or distant metastases. Margins depend on the depth of the melanoma.

Melanoma in situ: This is typically treated with the surgical excision. Lentigo maligna (the most common subtype of melanoma in situ) should be excised with a wide

Table 22-5. Primary surgical management of melanoma.

Breslow depth (thickness) and ulceration status	Indications for a sentinel node biopsy	Clinical surgical margin (cm)
Melanoma in situ.	No	0.5–1
Thickness < 0.8 mm without ulceration.	No	1
Thickness < 0.8mm with ulceration. Thickness 0.8–1.0mm without ulceration.	Yes	1
1.0–2.0 mm, with or without ulceration.	Yes	1–2
>2 mm, with or without ulceration.	Yes	2

local excision with 0.5 to 1 cm margins. Use of Wood's lamp, dermoscopy, or reflectance confocal microscopy prior to excision may help to delineate margins. The depth of excision should be to the deep subcutis. Mohs micrographic surgery is often used for ill-defined or large lesions of lentigo maligna in cosmetically challenging areas like the face. The advantage of Moh's surgery is that 100% of the peripheral margin is examined following the excision. Disadvantages are unique technical problems resulting from freeze artifacts and the presence of benign melanocytic hyperplasia common to sun-damaged skin. In patients with lentigo maligna that are poor surgical candidates, topical imiquimod cream has been used off label as either monotherapy or adjuvant treatment following surgery with positive margins. Most studies have shown reduced recurrence rates. Radiotherapy can also be considered as second line in poor surgical candidates. Discussion of risks, benefits, and uncertainties of long-term prognosis of the second-line treatments with patients is important.[29]

Invasive melanoma: Surgical margins are based on tumor thickness (Table 22-5) and consideration of sentinel lymph node biopsy is based on tumor thickness and ulceration status. The depth of excision is typically down to the muscular fascia. If sentinel lymph node biopsy is needed, this should be completed prior to excision to preserve lymphatic flow.

Sentinel lymph node biopsy: The AJCC Melanoma Staging Committee recommends that patients with more advanced stages of melanoma (Table 22-5) and with clinically uninvolved regional nodes have sentinel node biopsy performed.[29] The status of the sentinel node is of clear prognostic value. Status is likely the best predictor of recurrence risk and survival. However, it is unclear if sentinel lymph node biopsy offers any survival benefit, and there is potential morbidity from the procedure. Sentinel lymph node biopsy is important in determining eligibility for adjuvant treatment or clinical trials. All patients that have melanomas eligible for sentinel lymph node biopsy should be counseled on the pros and cons and offered consultation with surgical oncology.

Completion lymph node dissection: Prior to 2017, it was standard of care to complete lymph node dissection after a positive sentinel lymph node biopsy even though it was unknown if this improved survival. In 2017, the Multicenter Selective Lymphadenectomy Trial II (MSLT-II) found that while completion lymph node dissection may offer prognostic information (worse outcomes in patients with positive nodes outside the sentinel node), it did not increase melanoma specific survival.[30] For this reason, immediate completion lymph node dissection after positive sentinel lymph node biopsy is no longer standard of care. Ultrasonography of nodal basins to monitor for disease recurrence is now often completed to follow patients with a history of a positive sentinel lymph node biopsy.

Staging

American Joint Committee on Cancer (AJCC) Eighth Edition is currently used. T (tumor– Breslows depth and ulceration status), N (positive or negative nodes), and M (presence or absence of metastatic disease) criteria are used for staging. The "Melanoma TNM8" app uses a guided approach to the AJCC 8th edition criteria to quickly and simply reach the correct staging for melanoma. This app can be downloaded from the Apple App Store.

Systemic treatments

For many years, the only treatment option for metastatic melanoma that was not surgically resectable was marginally effective traditional chemotherapy. We now have two classes of medications that can be used for unresectable Stage IV melanoma or for adjuvant treatment of Stage III and Stage IV melanoma.

The targeted therapies encompass treatments that aim to regulate the dysfunctional signaling through the Mitogen-activated protein kinase (MAPK) pathway in melanoma. Around 50% of melanomas have a mutation in this pathway at BRAF which can be targeted. Most commonly used is the combination of a BRAF-inhibitor (e.g., vemurafenib, dabrafenib, or encorafenib) with a MEK-inhibitor (e.g., trametinib, cobimetinib, binimetinib, selumetinib). Targeted therapy can only be used in melanomas with certain genetic mutations. It has the advantages of quick onset of action and high response rates. Unfortunately, over time resistance to treatment will develop in most treated with these medications.[31]

The second class of approved medication is immunotherapies. This class is made up of monoclonal antibodies that are directed against receptors that work to downregulate T cell response. By blocking this interaction, there is improved immune response against melanoma. Examples of these include ipilimumab, nivolumab, and pembrolizumab. Immunotherapy has the advantage that it can occasionally result in sustained, durable response, and long-term survival.[31]

▶ Monitoring of Patients With Asymptomatic Melanoma

Asymptomatic melanoma patients are still at risk of recurrence with either local or distant disease and risk of additional primary melanomas. Risk of recurrence is dependent on stage. Around 10% of melanoma patients in the United States go on to have a second primary melanoma. Follow-up with special attention to review of systems for symptoms concerning for distant metastases, total body skin examination including visual inspection and palpation of melanoma scar, and lymph node examination especially of potential drainage basins are important in detecting recurrence, metastases, and new primaries. Frequency of follow-up is not uniformly agreed on. Recently published guidelines in the Journal of the American Academy of Dermatology by a cutaneous melanoma working group recommended variable intervals based on staging.[29] Follow-up every 6–12 months from 1 to 2 years, and then annually was recommended for stage 0 melanoma. For stage IA-IIA, follow-up was recommended every 6–12 months from 2 to 5 years, and then annually. For stage IIB and higher, follow-up was recommended every 3–6 months for 2 years, and then every 6 months for 3 years, and then annually. In addition to in-office examinations, patients should be educated on the importance of interval self-examination of skin and lymph nodes.

Baseline imaging or laboratory studies are not recommended in stage 0-II patients in the absence of concerning symptoms. As mentioned earlier, serial ultrasonography of nodal basins in sentinel lymph node biopsy positive disease should be considered. Other surveillance imaging can be considered in later stage patients in conjunction with medical oncology.

DecisionDx-Melanoma is a commercially available test aimed at identifying patients at higher risk of melanoma recurrence or metastasis. The test is a 31-gene profile that classifies patients as "low risk" or "high risk" by gene expression. Marketing of the test has mostly been for early stage melanoma with the goal of identifying the very rare patients at higher risk of recurrence or metastatic disease for possible increased monitoring. While this test may show promise in the future, more prospective studies with long-term follow-up are needed to determine its clinical utility. The AJCC 8 guidelines do not include use of DecisionDx-Melanoma.[28]

Clinical Course and Prognosis

Melanoma survival depends on early diagnosis. Stage I melanoma has an excellent overall 5-year survival rate of 98%.[23] Stage II and Stage III melanoma have 5-year survival rates of 90% and 77%, respectively.[23] The availability of targeted therapies and immunotherapies has improved survival for both stage III and IV melanoma.

Primary Prevention and Detection

Ultraviolet radiation exposure, including radiation from commercial tanning beds, increases the risk of malignant melanoma. For this reason as well as for primary prevention of other skin cancers, patients should be counseled on the value of sun safe behavior, including use of sun protective clothing, shade, and sunscreens.

Indications for Consultation

All melanoma patients should also be referred to dermatology for a total body examination and follow-up examinations. For patients that do not need sentinel lymph node biopsy, surgical management can be completed by a primary care provider comfortable with excisions or referred to dermatology, surgical oncology, or a surgical subspecialty depending on availability in your area. Patients with melanoma who are candidates for sentinel lymph node biopsy should be referred to surgical oncology for melanoma on the body or ear, nose, and throat (ENT) for melanoma on the head/neck. Patients with positive sentinel lymph nodes or with melanomas with poor prognostic characteristics should be referred to medical oncology. Many academic centers offer multidisciplinary care teams for melanoma. Genetic counseling referral should be considered in patients with three or more melanomas, especially if diagnosed before 45 years of age, and in patients with personal history of melanoma and family history of melanoma or pancreatic cancer in three or more relatives.[22]

Patient Information

- American Academy of Dermatology: www.aad.org/skin-conditions/dermatology-a-to-z/melanoma
- Skin Cancer Foundation: www.skincancer.org/skin-cancer-information/melanoma
- Melanoma Research Foundation: www.melanoma.org
- American Society of Clinical Oncology: www.cancer.net/patient/Cancer+Types/Melanoma

REFERENCES

1. Jean L Bolognia JLJ, Julie V Schaffer, Jeffrey P Callen, Lorenzo Cerroni, Warren R Heymann, George J Hruza, Anthony J Mancini, James W Patterson, Martin Röcken, and Thomas Schwarz. *Dermatology*: Elsevier Limited; 2012.
2. MacKie RM, English J, Aitchison TC, Fitzsimons CP, Wilson P. The number and distribution of benign pigmented moles (melanocytic naevi) in a healthy British population. *Br J Dermatol*. 1985;113:167-74.
3. Vezzoni R, Conforti C, Vichi S, Giuffrida R, Retrosi C, Magaton-Rizzi G et al. Is there more than one road to nevus-associated melanoma? *Dermatol Pract Concept*. 2020;10:e2020028.
4. Alikhan A, Ibrahimi OA, Eisen DB. Congenital melanocytic nevi: where are we now? Part I. Clinical presentation,

epidemiology, pathogenesis, histology, malignant transformation, and neurocutaneous melanosis. *J Am Acad Dermatol*. 2012;67:495.e1-17; quiz 512-4.
5. Ibrahimi OA, Alikhan A, Eisen DB. Congenital melanocytic nevi: where are we now? Part II. Treatment options and approach to treatment. *J Am Acad Dermatol*. 2012;67:515.e1-13; quiz 28-30.
6. Kinsler VA, O'Hare P, Bulstrode N, Calonje JE, Chong WK, Hargrave D et al. Melanoma in congenital melanocytic naevi. *Br J Dermatol*. 2017;176:1131-43.
7. Moustafa D, Blundell AR, Hawryluk EB. Congenital melanocytic nevi. *Curr Opin Pediatr*. 2020;32:491-7.
8. Haynes D, Strunck JL, Said J, Tam I, Varedi A, Topham CA et al. Association between halo nevi and melanoma in adults: a multi-center retrospective case series. *J Am Acad Dermatol*. 2020.
9. Mesbah Ardakani N. Dysplastic/Clark naevus in the era of molecular pathology. *Australas J Dermatol*. 2019;60:186-91.
10. Rademaker M, Oakley A. Digital monitoring by whole body photography and sequential digital dermoscopy detects thinner melanomas. *J Prim Health Care* 2010;2:268-72.
11. Hiscox B, Hardin MR, Orengo IF, Rosen T, Mir M, Diwan AH. Recurrence of moderately dysplastic nevi with positive histologic margins. *J Am Acad Dermatol*. 2017;76:527-30.
12. Wall N, De'Ambrosis B, Muir J. The management of dysplastic naevi: a survey of Australian dermatologists. *Australas J Dermatol*. 2017;58:304-7.
13. Siegel RL, Miller KD, Jemal A. Cancer statistics, 2020. *CA Cancer J Clin*. 2020;70:7-30.
14. Berk-Krauss J, Stein JA, Weber J, Polsky D, Geller AC. New systemic therapies and trends in cutaneous melanoma deaths among US whites, 1986-2016. *Am J Public Health* 2020;110:731-3.
15. Tuong W, Cheng LS, Armstrong AW. Melanoma: epidemiology, diagnosis, treatment, and outcomes. *Dermatol Clin*. 2012;30:113-24, ix.
16. De Andrade JP, Wong P, O'Leary MP, Parekh V, Amini A, Schoellhammer HF et al. Multidisciplinary care for melanoma of unknown primary: experience in the era of molecular profiling. *Ann Surg Oncol*. 2020.
17. Hurst EA, Harbour JW, Cornelius LA. Ocular melanoma: a review and the relationship to cutaneous melanoma. *Arch Dermatol*. 2003;139:1067-73.
18. Cordoro KM, Gupta D, Frieden IJ, McCalmont T, Kashani-Sabet M. Pediatric melanoma: results of a large cohort study and proposal for modified ABCD detection criteria for children. *J Am Acad Dermatol*. 2013;68:913-25.
19. Carrera C, Scope A, Dusza SW, Argenziano G, Nazzaro G, Phan A et al. Clinical and dermoscopic characterization of pediatric and adolescent melanomas: Multicenter study of 52 cases. *J Am Acad Dermatol*. 2018;78:278-88.
20. Pampena R, Lai M, Lombardi M, Mirra M, Raucci M, Lallas A et al. Clinical and dermoscopic features associated with difficult-to-recognize variants of cutaneous melanoma: a systematic review. *JAMA Dermatol*. 2020;156:430-9.
21. Yang K, Mahalingam M. Differing biologic behaviors of desmoplastic melanoma subtypes: Insights based on histopathologic, immunohistochemical, and genetic analyses. *J Am Acad Dermatol*. 2020;83:523-31.
22. Leachman SA, Carucci J, Kohlmann W, Banks KC, Asgari MM, Bergman W et al. Selection criteria for genetic assessment of patients with familial melanoma. *J Am Acad Dermatol*. 2009;61:677.e1-14.

23. Gershenwald JE, Scolyer RA, Hess KR, Sondak VK, Long GV, Ross MI et al. Melanoma staging: Evidence-based changes in the American Joint Committee on Cancer eighth edition cancer staging manual. *CA Cancer J Clin.* 2017;67:472-92.

24. Yélamos O, Braun RP, Liopyris K, Wolner ZJ, Kerl K, Gerami P et al. Usefulness of dermoscopy to improve the clinical and histopathologic diagnosis of skin cancers. *J Am Acad Dermatol.* 2019;80:365-77.

25. Fried L, Tan A, Bajaj S, Liebman TN, Polsky D, Stein JA. Technological advances for the detection of melanoma: Advances in diagnostic techniques. *J Am Acad Dermatol.* 2020;83:983-92.

26. Lallas A, Apalla Z, Kyrgidis A, Papageorgiou C, Boukovinas I, Bobos M et al. Second primary melanomas in a cohort of 977 melanoma patients within the first 5 years of monitoring. *J Am Acad Dermatol.* 2020;82:398-406.

27. Schneider SL, Kohli I, Hamzavi IH, Council ML, Rossi AM, Ozog DM. Emerging imaging technologies in dermatology: Part II: Applications and limitations. *J Am Acad Dermatol.* 2019;80:1121-31.

28. Fried L, Tan A, Bajaj S, Liebman TN, Polsky D, Stein JA. Technological advances for the detection of melanoma: Advances in molecular techniques. *J Am Acad Dermatol.* 2020;83:996-1004.

29. Swetter SM, Tsao H, Bichakjian CK, Curiel-Lewandrowski C, Elder DE, Gershenwald JE et al. Guidelines of care for the management of primary cutaneous melanoma. *J Am Acad Dermatol.* 2019;80:208-50.

30. Faries MB, Thompson JF, Cochran AJ, Andtbacka RH, Mozzillo N, Zager JS et al. Completion Dissection or Observation for Sentinel-Node Metastasis in Melanoma. *N Engl J Med.* 2017;376:2211-22.

31. Volpe VO, Klufas DM, Hegde U, Grant-Kels JM. The new paradigm of systemic therapies for metastatic melanoma. *J Am Acad Dermatol.* 2017;77:356-68.

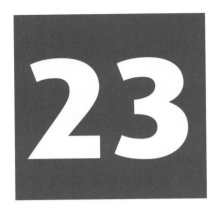

Pigmentary Disorders

Autumn L. Saizan
Nada Elbuluk

INTRODUCTION TO CHAPTER

Disorders of pigmentation, although not life-threatening, may cause significant psychosocial impairment in patients due to their visibility and associated stigma. Certain pigmentary disorders may also have associated symptoms. Management of pigmentary disorders requires accurate diagnosis and treatment in addition to careful assessment and monitoring of associated psychological conditions, such as depression and anxiety.

MELANOCYTE BIOLOGY

Melanocytes are neural crest-derived, pigment-producing cells located in the basal layer of the epidermis (stratum basale) as well as the middle layer of the eye (the uvea), the inner ear, vaginal epithelium, meninges, bones, and heart.[1] Melanocytes typically migrate to the epidermis by the eighth week of life. Each melanocyte is attached to the basal layer via hemidesmosomes; however, there are no attachments between melanocytes and neighboring keratinocytes. Instead, they are connected through dendrites extending from each melanocyte to several keratinocytes. It is estimated that each melanocyte makes contact with roughly 36 keratinocytes in the suprabasal and basal layers.[2] This contact between the two cell types is important in forming the epidermal-melanin unit,[3] which allows for the transfer of packed pigmented granules called melanosomes.[1,3]

Melanosomes are the site for synthesis, storage, and transport of melanin. Melanin is formed via a four-step process (Figure 23-1). The first step involves the enzyme tyrosinase, which is formed in the rough endoplasmic reticulum and then processed in the Golgi apparatus of the melanocyte before accumulating in vesicles. Tyrosinase converts tyrosine into 3,4-dihydroxyphenylalanine (DOPA), which is then formed into polymers to create the different types of melanin, eumelanin, and pheomelanin.[1]

Once formed, the melanosomes or melanin granules migrate to the tips of the melanocyte dendrites to be ingested by neighboring keratinocytes.[3] Once in the keratinocyte, these melanin granules migrate toward the nucleus of the keratinocyte to aid in protection of the cell's DNA from ultraviolet light damage. This is referred to as a "supranuclear cap."[1,3] As a result, keratinocytes contain more pigment than do melanocytes. Melanin pigment serves a protective function in melanocytes as well by protecting the membrane from ultraviolet A and B damage.[1]

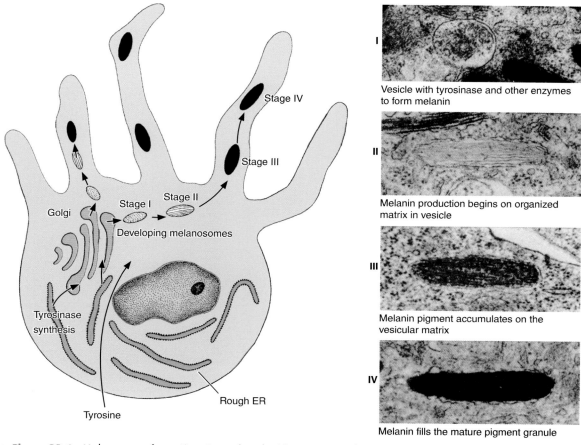

Stage IV

Stage III

Stage II

Stage I

Golgi

Developing melanosomes

Tyrosinase synthesis

Tyrosine

Rough ER

I

Vesicle with tyrosinase and other enzymes to form melanin

II

Melanin production begins on organized matrix in vesicle

III

Melanin pigment accumulates on the vesicular matrix

IV

Melanin fills the mature pigment granule

▲ **Figure 23-1.** Melanosome formation. Reproduced with permission from *Mescher AL: Junqueira's Basic Histology: Text and Atlas,* 16th ed. New York, NY: McGraw Hill; 2021.

The number of melanocytes does not determine differences in skin color. Rather, it is variation in melanosome number, size, and distribution that lead to the different skin phototypes.[1] Individuals with darker skin have a greater number of melanosomes that are typically larger and more dispersed than those with lighter skin. The type of pigment produced by melanocytes may also contribute to differences in skin and hair color. Eumelanin is a black or brown pigment, while pheomelanin is a red or yellow pigment.[1]

NORMAL SKIN VARIANTS

There are several benign and normal skin variants involving altered pigmentation that can be mistaken as a skin disorder, particularly in patients of color. It is important that physicians understand these nuances in skin pigmentation so as to avoid incorrect diagnoses, unnecessary procedures, and increased patient anxiety. The following diagnoses are common and normal skin variations that are most prevalent and noticeable in skin of color:[4] (Figure 23-2 A and B)

Pigmentary Demarcation Lines

Pigmentary demarcation lines are distinct changes in pigmentation that create a line between a lighter and darker side of skin. There are eight groups for pigmentary demarcation lines with different anatomic locations, referred to as groups A through H.[4]

- **Group A (Futcher lines)**

  Group A or Futcher lines (Figures 23-2A, 23-3) are typically located on the flexor surfaces of the upper extremity,[4] extending roughly 10 cm down the lateral edge of the biceps muscle.[5] They are also known as Voigt's lines, Futcher-Voigt lines, or Ito's lines. Futcher lines are most prevalent in adults and are very rarely seen in infants and children. They do not have a gender or skin phototype predilection, nor do they follow the anatomic distribution of a specific nerve, muscle, or blood vessel. Futcher lines are usually bilateral, although unilateral lines are possible. Forearm lines are typically seen on the medial aspect of the forearm. Very rarely these lines may

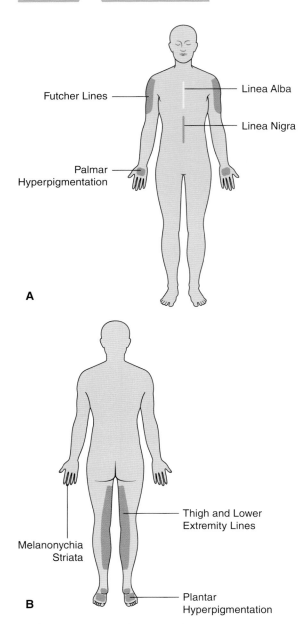

A

B

▲ **Figure 23-2.** A and B. Normal variations pigmentation in patients of color.

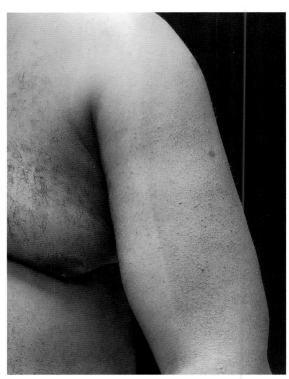

▲ **Figure 23-3.** Fuchter line on arm. Pigmentary demarcation line with darker dorsal pigmentation and lighter ventral pigmentation. Reproduced with permission from Charles E. Crutchfield III, MD.

- **Group B (thigh and lower extremity lines)**

  Group B or leg lines are typically located on the posteromedial aspect of the thigh, although they may continue down to the calf and ankle (Figure 23-2B). Leg lines, if they do not extend from the thigh, start at the popliteal fossa and extend down to the medial ankle. Such lines are commonly associated with pregnancy.[4] Leg lines may be hard to appreciate on dark skin, as this area is prone to scaling from dry skin. Moisturizing the area prior to assessment can help delineate the lines.[8]

- **Group C (linea alba and linea nigra)**

  Linea alba and linea nigra are normal skin variants located on the trunk (Figure 23-2A).[4] Linea alba is represented by vertical hypopigmentation that may begin on one side of the midline before crossing to the opposite side after reaching the umbilicus.[6] Linea nigra is a vertical linear hyperpigmentation that typically extends from the suprapubic region up to the umbilicus.[7]

- **Groups D – H**

  Group D refers to posteromedian demarcation, while group E refers to bilateral, symmetric hypopigmented macules on the chest. Groups F through H are more

be a continuation of the Futcher lines from the upper extremity.[4] When using light microscopy, no appreciable difference in melanin concentration between the two sides has been documented. Interestingly, previous cases have reported drug reactions that affected only one side of a Futcher line, suggesting the two areas may have different embryonic origin.[5]

recent classifications and refer to facial pigmentary demarcation lines. Line F is an inverted cone-shaped patch that extends from the orbital rim. Line G is similar; however, there are two inverted cones with normal pigmentation in between, uniquely forming a W-shaped patch. Finally, line H refers to linear hyperpigmentation extending bilaterally from the corners of the mouth.[4]

Palmar and Plantar Hyperpigmentation

Hyperpigmentation of the palms and soles of the feet is common in darker skinned adults (Figure 23-2 A and B).[6] Patients may present with a few to dozens of macules. Trauma and inflammation are the proposed etiologies, as there are no documented cases of children with palmar or plantar hyperpigmentation.[8] When looking at the palms and soles, it is important to rule out secondary syphilis and acral lentiginous melanoma, which is the most common form of melanoma in people of color.[9]

Areas of Localized Hyperpigmentation in Infants

With respect to infants, some may present with one or multiple areas of hyperpigmentation. Helices of the ears, lips, fingernails, the matrices of toenails, genitals, nipples, axillae, umbilicus, and anal orifice are all common areas of hyperpigmentation.[6] Most of these areas remain hyperpigmented throughout one's life, except the ears and axillae, which typically resolve one year after birth. The prevalence or location of hyperpigmentation is not dependent on the infant's skin color or gender.[8]

Circumscribed dermal melanocytosis, also known as Mongolian spots (Figure 23-4), can also occur in infants. These involve dark gray-blue macules that gradually resolve throughout childhood. The most common locations are the buttocks and hips. Patches are due to failure of the melanocytes to reach the epidermis. Instead, as the melanocytes travel from the neural crest, they stay in the dermis, leading to notable patches of pigmentation.[10]

Mucocutaneous Hyperpigmentation

Mucous membranes are another common location for hyperpigmentation. Some individuals, typically older adults, have darker lips or gums. The most common locations in decreasing order of frequency are the gingiva, buccal mucosa, lips, and palate. It is important to obtain a good medical history of adult patients to rule out more concerning causes for pigmented oral mucosa. Duration, symmetry, associated symptoms, past medical history, current medications, and more may all prove to be helpful in generating the differential diagnosis.[11] Additionally, infants may have a darker upper lip at birth. It typically disappears after a few weeks and it is hypothesized that the hyperpigmentation is the result of in-utero sucking.[8]

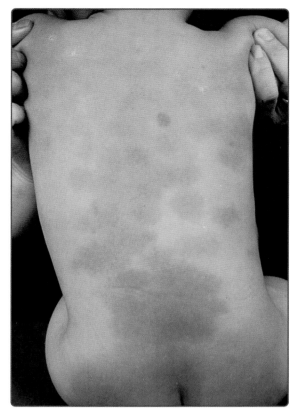

▲ **Figure 23-4.** Mongolian spots. Dark blue-gray patches of circumscribed dermal melanocytosis on back and buttock of an infant. Reproduced with permission from Kang S, Amagai M, Bruckner AL, et al: *Fitzpatrick's Dermatology, 9th ed. New York,* NY: McGraw Hill; 2019.

Melanonychia Striata

Melanonychia striata also known as longitudinal melanonychia is a vertical linear streak extending from the proximal nail fold to the distal the nail plate (Figure 23-5). Several nails may have one of these lines or a single nail can have multiple melanonychia striata. Like palmar and plantar hyperpigmentation, it is rarely seen in children and thus, proposed to be secondary to injury. Additionally, the most common locations for these streaks are the thumb and index finger, further suggesting trauma as the main etiology. When evaluating patients with these linear streaks, it is important to visualize the entire nail fold and determine if the pigment extends into the surrounding skin so as to rule out a more serious diagnosis, such as melanoma. Single nail involvement with a linear streak that is 3 mm or more is concerning. In fact, nails with multiple streaks can provide reassurance. Certain drugs can cause nail pigmentation as well. Examples include zidovudine, minocycline, antimalarials, and methotrexate.

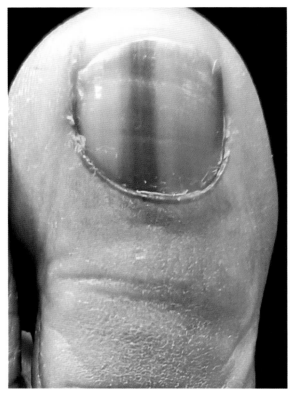

▲ **Figure 23-5.** Longitudinal melanonychia also known as melanonychia striata. Vertical linear brown streak on the left first toenail. Reproduced with permission from Charles E. Crutchfield III, MD.

Additionally, systemic diseases such as Addison's disease, hemochromatosis, vitamin B12 deficiency, and several other diseases can also potentially cause nail hyperpigmentation.[12]

▼ POSTINFLAMMATORY HYPERPIGMENTATION

Introduction

Postinflammatory hyperpigmentation is an acquired pigmentary disorder that occurs secondary to endogenous inflammation or exogenous trauma. Examples of common inciting factors include acne, folliculitis, insect bites, atopic dermatitis, medication reactions, and procedures (Figure 23-6).[13,14] Although it occurs in all skin phototypes, it is most prevalent among patients with skin of color. Postinflammatory hyperpigmentation may occur anywhere on the skin surface and does not have a predilection for any gender or age group.[13]

Pathogenesis

There are two main histopathologic types of postinflammatory hyperpigmentation, epidermal and dermal. Epidermal

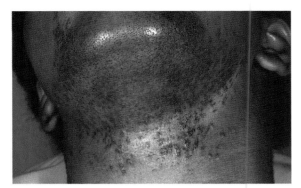

▲ **Figure 23-6.** Postinflammatory hyperpigmentation due to pseudofolliculitis barbae on chin and neck.

postinflammatory hyperpigmentation is caused by either an increase in melanin production and/or increased keratinocyte uptake of melanosomes. Outside of an increase in melanocyte size and activity, the number of melanocytes typically remains the same in postinflammatory hyperpigmentation.[15] This process is likely genetic and dependent on the individual's unique melanocyte properties, rather than their skin phototype. Additionally, inflammatory mediators, such as prostaglandins and leukotrienes, may further enhance melanin production and keratinocyte uptake.[13] In dermal postinflammatory hyperpigmentation, there is damage to the basement membrane, allowing melanosomes to travel from the epidermis to the dermis where melanosomes are engulfed by resident macrophages and ultimately become melanophages, a process also referred to as pigment incontinence.[15] Dermal melanin is traditionally slower to improve and more challenging to treat.[13]

Clinical Presentation

▷ History

Dark spots, discoloration, or an uneven skin tone are the most common chief complaints among patients with postinflammatory hyperpigmentation. Patients are typically asymptomatic, although there may be some residual irritation from previous inciting factors. It is important to obtain a detailed history to determine potential underlying causes. This includes a history of current or prior inflammatory skin conditions, medications, exposures as well as prior procedures or injuries.[13]

▷ Physical Examination

The physical examination will reveal hyperpigmented macules and patches ranging from light to dark brown or gray-blue to gray-brown in color, sometimes with poorly demarcated borders. Some patients may not have visible inflammation on physical examination. Epidermal macules tend to appear light to dark brown and dermal macules tend to be more gray-blue in color. Initially, affected areas may appear more erythematous before transitioning to a darker brown or gray color. Wood's lamp examination is helpful in distinguishing epidermal from dermal postinflammatory hyperpigmentation since epidermal hyperpigmentation will typically enhance. Patients with darker skin may have more ambiguous results with the Wood's lamp due to their high concentrations of melanin in the dermis or having a mixed epidermal and dermal component.[13]

Laboratory Findings

No laboratory findings are associated with postinflammatory hyperpigmentation. Occasionally, a biopsy will help with diagnosis, especially in those with no visible evidence of inflammation or history of prior skin condition or trauma. Histopathology may reveal increased epidermal melanin and/or dermal melanophages.

Diagnosis

The key diagnostic features of postinflammatory hyperpigmentation are light to dark brown or gray-blue hyperpigmented macules with indistinct margins that occur as a sequela of inflammation or injury.

Differential Diagnosis

✓ Drug-induced hyperpigmentation: Common culprits include anti-malarials, chemotherapy, amiodarone, minocycline, and heavy metals. Patch testing may help distinguish between an allergy or a medication toxicity as the primary cause.

✓ Melasma: Refer to "Melasma" section.

✓ Café au lait spots: Present with well-defined borders and are not preceded by inflammation or trauma.

✓ Acanthosis nigricans: Refer to "Acanthosis Nigricans" section.

✓ Pityriasis versicolor: Refer to "Pityriasis Versicolor" section.

✓ Cutaneous hyperpigmentation related to Addison's disease: Generalized and diffuse pigmentation in patients who also have signs and symptoms of hypocortisolism.

✓ Lichen planus pigmentosus: A variant of lichen planus characterized by violaceous, gray to dark brown macules, most commonly located on sun-exposed areas such as the face and upper extremities.

✓ Erythema dyschromicum perstans: A rare pigmentary disorder also known as ashy dermatosis. Patients present with gray-to-brown macules and patches sometimes with an erythematous border, typically in sun-protected sites.

✓ Riehl melanosis: A type of pigmented contact dermatitis, most commonly seen in young to middle-aged women with skin of color. Patients may present after repeated exposure to an allergen, causing diffuse, brown-to-gray hyperpigmentation, most commonly on the face and neck.

✓ Hyperpigmented mycosis fungoides (Cutaneous T-cell lymphoma): A rare variant of cutaneous T-cell lymphoma in which patients present with hyperpigmented macules and patches. It is most common in dark-skinned individuals.

Management

The first step in management is to treat any potential underlying causes to prevent the continued development of postinflammatory hyperpigmentation. Sun protection and daily sunscreen application with a minimum sun protection factor of 30 are important to prevent worsening pigmentation from light exposure.[16] With these measures, postinflammatory hyperpigmentation may improve over time and can be combined with medical treatment. Some patients may also benefit from use of mineral sunscreens to provide expanded ultraviolet and visible light protection. Mineral sunscreens can be more opaque on application which may be less appealing to patients, particularly those with darker skin.[16,17] However, newer formulations have improved this issue. The importance of sun protection should be further emphasized in patients with skin of color, as there is a common misconception among this population that use of sunscreen on a regular basis is not necessary.[18]

Topical treatments can help improve epidermal pigmentation[19] through several different processes, including inhibition of melanin production and melanosome transfer, decreasing keratinocyte proliferation, and reducing the effects of anti-inflammatory mediators. Commonly used topical agents include hydroquinones, retinoids, and combination products.[17]

Topical hydroquinone a tyrosinase inhibitor, can be used as monotherapy and is considered one of the gold standard treatments for skin lightening.[16] Hydroquinone 2% is available over-the-counter and higher concentrations may be given as a prescription. Side effects may include contact dermatitis or lightening of normal skin around areas of pigmentation. A more serious side effect is ochronosis, which is a paradoxical darkening of the skin. There is also an associated risk of cancer with hydroquinone in animals, although there have been no documented cases in humans.[17] Mequinol, a hydroquinone derivative and a substrate for tyrosinase, may be used as an alternative. Mequinol acts as a competitive inhibitor in melanin synthesis without causing toxicity to melanocytes. Additionally, glycosylated hydroquinones, arbutin and its synthetic form, deoxyarbutin, are over the counter products that work by inhibiting tyrosinase activity and melanosome maturation.[17]

Topical retinoids are also commonly used for treating postinflammatory hyperpigmentation. Topical retinoids are proposed to increase keratinocyte turnover, decrease melanosome transfer, and increase the efficacy of depigmenting agents. These agents can be used as monotherapy or in combination with other agents.[17] Topical retinoids are encouraged in patients with acne-related postinflammatory hyperpigmentation due to their ability to prevent acne and improve skin pigmentation and texture.[14] Treatment should be stopped if irritation occurs, as some people may develop "retinoid dermatitis" characterized by erythema, irritation, and desquamation as well as subsequent dyspigmentation in darker skin patients.[17] Combination products may contain hydroquinone, tretinoin, and/or a low potency steroid and have shown greater efficacy compared to monotherapy in treatment of certain pigmentary disorders.

Other therapeutic options for postinflammatory hyperpigmentation include azelaic acid, kojic acid, L-ascorbic acid, and alpha- and beta-hydroxy acid as well as licorice extracts, niacinamide, soy, and N-acetyl glucosamine. Azelaic acid, a natural derivative of Pityrosporum ovale, inhibits tyrosinase and thus, decreases melanin production. Other tyrosinase inhibitors include kojic acid, a product of fungi, and licorice extracts from Glycyrrhiza glabra, which also increase melanin dispersion. Ascorbic acid, or vitamin C, reduces the conversion of L-dopa to L-dopaquinone, decreasing melanogenesis; niacinamide inhibits melanosome transfer; soy products prevent keratinocyte phagocytosis of melanosomes and inhibit ultraviolet B

pigmentation; and N-acetyl glucosamine inhibits glycosylation of tyrosinase. Although not as effective as hydroquinone, these alternatives are acceptable options when hydroquinone is not well-tolerated or when a therapeutic break from hydroquinone is needed (Table 23-1).[16,17]

Procedural treatments can also be used alone or as adjunctive treatment to medical therapy in treating postinflammatory hyperpigmentation. Caution should be used with procedural therapies particularly in darker skin as they can also cause skin trauma and lead to further dyspigmentation.[16] Procedural treatments for postinflammatory hyperpigmentation include chemical peels, dermabrasion, microneedling, and light and laser therapies.[17]

Chemical peels can help to increase absorption of skin-lightening agents while also increasing epidermal turnover and decreasing epidermal pigment. Superficial peeling agents include glycolic acid, salicylic acid, 10–20% trichloroacetic acid, modified jessners, and retinols. The depth of these superficial peels is limited to the stratum corneum. However, medium and deeper peels affect the papillary and reticular dermis, respectively and are typically avoided in darker skin patients.[20] In cases of acne-induced postinflammatory hyperpigmentation, salicylic acid peels can help in treating both the acne and postinflammatory hyperpigmentation. Peels in combination with topical therapy are often more effective than topical treatments alone.[17]

Laser and light techniques for hyperpigmentation include the Q-switched and picosecond lasers as well as

Table 23-1. Common topical products for treating hyperpigmentation

Topical Products	Mechanism of action	Notes
Sunscreen	Helps prevents worsening of hyperpigmentation.	Apply broad spectrum sunscreen SPF 30 or greater daily. Needs to be reapplied every 2 hours if outside for prolonged periods.
Hydroquinone	Tyrosinase inhibitor.	Available in 2% over the counter and 4% and above in prescription form.
Mequinol	Tyrosinase inhibitor. Decreased melanosome transfer Increased epidermal turnover.	Does not cause toxicity to melanocytes.
Azelaic acid	Tyrosinase inhibitor.	Available in foam, cream, and gel in prescription strengths. Also available over the counter in cosmeceuticals at lower strengths.
Kojic acid	Tyrosinase inhibitor.	Available over the counter in concentrations ranging from 1% to 4%.
Licorice extract	Tyrosinase inhibitor.	Available in numerous cosmeceutical products.
Retinoids	Increased keratinocyte turnover. Decreases melanosome transfer.	Vitamin A derivative, particularly useful in patients with acne and hyperpigmentation.
L-ascorbic acid	Reduces conversion of L-dopa to L-dopaquinone, thus decreasing melanogenesis.	Ascorbic acid is Vitamin C.
Soy products	Decreased melanosome transfer.	
N-acetyl glucosamine	Inhibits glycosylation of tyrosinase.	

intense pulsed light therapy, ablative and nonablative lasers, including fractionated lasers.[17] Lasers are typically considered a second- or third-line therapy for refractory postinflammatory hyperpigmentation.

Of note, cosmetic camouflage is another option which can improve quality of life for patients dealing with postinflammatory hyperpigmentation whether or not they choose to pursue treatment.

Clinical Course and Prognosis

The duration and response to treatment is highly dependent on the type of postinflammatory hyperpigmentation, the etiology, as well as the individual's skin phototype. Unlike epidermal hyperpigmentation which may resolve or fade naturally after 6–12 months, dermal hypermelanosis is more likely to persist for months to years or become permanent due to the presence of melanophages. Additionally, those with skin of color tend to have more persistent pigmentation. Chronic inflammation, recurring injuries and ultraviolet exposure can exacerbate and prolong the hyperpigmentation.[13] Topical and procedural treatments have been used successfully to treat and improve postinflammatory hyperpigmentation but treatment typically requires months of consistent compliance.

Indications for Consultation

Consultation can be helpful in cases where pigmentation has not improved on its own or seems to be worsening. In addition to a wood's lamp, there are several other noninvasive assessment techniques, such as dermoscopy and reflectance confocal microscopy that can be used to help assess and monitor postinflammatory hyperpigmentation. However, these are not needed for the diagnosis and management of postinflammatory hyperpigmentation.

- **Wood's Lamp**: A tool that uses ultraviolet light to detect fluorescence, which may be associated with abnormal pigmentation or a cutaneous fungal or bacterial infection.
- **Dermoscopy**: A helpful diagnostic method that uses a dermatoscope with LED lighting to magnify various structures in the epidermis and dermis, including melanin and blood vessels.
- **Reflectance Confocal Microscopy**: This method is highly correlated with histology. It produces a high-resolution image from near-infrared light that is reflected from the various cellular structures. The images can be reconstructed to form a 3-D image.[13]

Patient Information

- Skinsight: https://www.skinsight.com/skin-conditions/adult/post-inflammatory-hyperpigmentation
- Skin of Color Society: https://skinofcolorsociety.org/dermatology-education/post-inflammatory-hyperpigmentation-postinflammatory hyperpigmentation/

Introduction

Melasma, also known as the "mask of pregnancy" and chloasma is an acquired hypermelanosis characterized by symmetric hyperpigmented patches with irregular borders, occurring most commonly on sun-exposed regions of the face.[21,22] It is the most common cause for hyperpigmentation in the world and is most prevalent in young- to middle-aged women of color. In some populations, it affects nearly 30% of child-bearing women.[19] Prevalence is variable and highly dependent on the population studied. Women of Latino, African, Native American, and Asian descent are the most likely to present with melasma. Common inciting and exacerbating factors are sun exposure, hormone exposure, including oral contraceptives and pregnancy, as well as genetics.[16]

Pathogenesis

The pathogenesis of melasma is complicated and not fully elucidated. It is suspected that ultraviolet and visible light exposure along with hyperestrogenic states, such as pregnancy, oral contraceptives, and hormone replacement therapy can contribute to a potential increase in cytokines leading to an increase in melanin production.[21] Nevertheless, recent studies have revealed that less than 20% of pregnant women get melasma and that almost 10% get melasma after menopause. Additionally, there is minimal improvement of melasma after oral contraceptive pill discontinuation suggesting female hormones may play a minimal role in pathogenesis.[19]

Over the last decade, studies have suggested that melasma may also be considered a photoaging skin disorder that also involves an increase in fibroblasts, mast cells, sebocytes, and endothelial cells.[20] Photoaging skin is further characterized by solar elastosis, a disrupted basal membrane, and increased vascularization.[19,21] Additionally, while the cheeks, forehead, and upper lips are sun-exposed areas, they are also areas rich in sebaceous glands, which produce cytokines and growth factors that further increase vascularization, melanocyte activity, and the hyperpigmentation seen in melasma. Studies suggest that promelanogenic growth factors and vascularization may contribute to hyperpigmentation in melasma. Additionally, patients tend to have a positive family history, suggesting a genetic component as well. It is possible that all of these mechanisms act synergistically to cause melasma in genetically susceptible individuals.[19]

Clinical Presentation

▶ History

Patients, most commonly women of color, will report dark spots on the face or uneven skin tone as their chief complaint. Melasma may also occur less commonly off the face and this has been called extrafacial melasma. A previous study conducted in Brazil suggests extrafacial melasma, although rare, is most prevalent in menopausal women and tends to have an earlier age of onset among those with a family history of melasma.[23] Melasma tends to get worse in the summer and improves in the winter months.[19] Determining the patient's line of work and hobbies can help determine their level of sun exposure, especially since some patients may not appreciate their daily light exposure. Medication history should also be obtained. Anticonvulsants, such as phenytoin, and other phototoxic drugs may aggravate melasma.[16]

▶ Physical Examination

Patients will typically present with symmetric bilateral light to dark brown irregularly shaped macules coalescing into reticulated patches (Figure 23-7). The symmetric involvement is helpful in distinguishing melasma from other causes of hyperpigmentation. There are three classic patterns of melasma: centrofacial, malar, and mandibular.

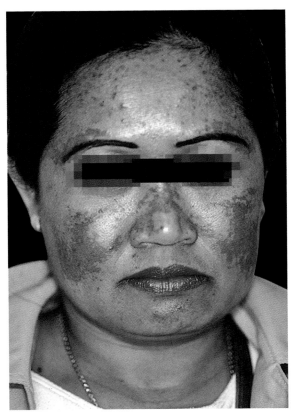

▲ **Figure 23-7.** Melasma. Dark brown reticulated macules and patches on the face. Reproduced with permission from Charles E. Crutchfield III, MD.

Centrofacial is the most common and it involves the cheeks, forehead, nose, upper lip, and chin, while sparing the nasolabial folds and philtrum. Malar melasma, the second most common, affects the cheeks and nose, while mandibular affects only the jawline. Mandibular melasma is thought to be more prevalent in older individuals.[22] Many patients present with more than one pattern and classification does not influence management. Patients with extrafacial melasma may present with it on their forearms or trunk.[23] Wood's lamp may be helpful in distinguishing epidermal from dermal melasma, as epidermal hyperpigmentation will typically enhance. However, recent studies have proposed that Wood's lamp may not correlate with histologic findings and many patients have mixed melasma with epidermal and dermal involvement.[19]

▶ Laboratory Findings

No laboratory findings are associated with melasma. Occasionally, a biopsy can help with diagnosis if the presentation is atypical. Based on histology, there are three different types of melasma: epidermal, dermal, or mixed. Epidermal melasma presents as enlarged melanocytes with numerous dendrites as well as melanin located in the basal and suprabasal layers of the skin. Dermal melasma is associated with melanophages and melanosomes in the dermis and a limited amount of melanin in the epidermis. Solar elastosis and increased blood vessels may also be noted in dermal melasma. Mixed melasma combines histologic features of both epidermal and dermal melasma.[22]

Diagnosis

Symmetric light- to dark-brown macules and patches involving sun-exposed regions, especially the centrofacial areas of women.[22]

▶ Differential Diagnosis

- ✓ Postinflammatory hyperpigmentation: Refer to "Postinflammatory hyperpigmentation" section.
- ✓ Ephelides/Freckles: 1–3 mm light-brown macules in sun exposed areas that typically present before puberty.
- ✓ Solar lentigines: Light- to dark-brown macules associated with sun exposure that can increase in number with age.
- ✓ Facial acanthosis nigricans: Refer to "Acanthosis Nigricans" section.
- ✓ Drug-induced hyperpigmentation: Refer to "Postinflammatory Hyperpigmentation" differential diagnosis section.
- ✓ Bilateral acquired nevus of Ota: Blue-gray and brown macules that typically occur symmetrically on the face without involvement of the mucosa. Most prevalent in Asian women.

Management

Melasma and postinflammatory hypopigmentation have similar management and treatment options, although no definitive cure for melasma exists. Like postinflammatory hypopigmentation, management involves preventive measures, disruption of melanin production via tyrosinase inhibitors and melanin uptake by keratinocytes, as well as treatments for melanin removal. Topical skin-lightening agents are used as first-line therapies along with proper sun protection and cosmetic camouflage when necessary. Procedural treatments such as chemical peels often serve as adjunctive and second-line therapies while lasers and light-based therapies serve as third-line options.

Traditional skin-lightening agents include hydroquinone, topical tretinoin, and combination therapies. Triple combination therapy containing hydroquinone, tretinoin, and a low-potency steroid is commonly used in the treatment of melasma. Side effects with chronic cutaneous steroid use include atrophy, acne, striae, and lightening of the skin.[22]

Non-hydroquinone alternatives overlap with those used in postinflammatory hypopigmentation, including azelaic acid, kojic acid, vitamin C, arbutin, cysteamine, and methimazole. These alternative therapies may be helpful in those who have experienced adverse side effects with hydroquinone or combination therapy. Additionally, certain skin-lightening agents should be avoided in pregnant and breast-feeding women, including hydroquinone and retinoids.[16]

Chemical peels including glycolic acid, trichloroacetic acid, salicylic acid, or retinols may be used as adjunctive treatments. Light-based therapies and lasers may be used in recalcitrant cases although they carry a risk of worsening hyperpigmentation by causing rebound melasma, especially in those with darker skin. Irritation and hypopigmentation are also potential complications of these treatment modalities. Treatments should be tailored to the patient's Fitzpatrick skin type and their unique medical history. It is important to consider prior dermatologic history including inflammatory skin conditions, history of cosmetic procedures, and history of infections, such as herpes simplex virus which can reactivate with procedural treatments.[19]

Systemic agents have also been studied in the treatment of melasma. Tranexamic acid, commonly used to treat hemophilia and menorrhagia, has been more recently studied orally and topically in the treatment of melasma. It is thought to inhibit ultraviolet light-induced plasminogen to plasmin conversion in keratinocytes. Plasmin is responsible for breaking down clots in the body, hence it is used for disorders of abnormal fibrinolysis.[17] More recently, plasmin has been found to contribute to pigmentation by increasing inflammatory mediators, such as prostaglandins and arachidonic acid, which trigger melanogenesis. Therefore, a decrease in plasmin reduces the level of circulating inflammatory mediators, subsequently decreasing

melanocyte tyrosinase activity and melanin production.[16] Tranexamic acid may also treat the vascular component of melasma by decreasing angiogenesis.[19] Hypercoagulability and thromboembolic events are concerning side effects of oral tranexamic acid. Clinicians should screen for potential contraindications to tranexamic acid therapy, including a previous history of thromboembolic events, such as pulmonary embolism and deep venous thrombosis, smoking, familial clotting disorders, such as protein S deficiency, hormonal therapy, certain medications, cancer, recent surgery, and prolonged immobility.[16] Other side effects include abdominal bloating, headaches, and tinnitus.[22]

Clinical Course and Prognosis

Melasma is an asymptomatic skin condition and can have a good prognosis. However, lack of uniform treatment, inconsistent results, and constant relapses make it a frustrating disorder for both patients and physicians.[19] It may persist for months after pregnancy or years after discontinuation of oral contraceptives. In women with lighter skin, melasma tends to fade more quickly after pregnancy. However, for some individuals, melasma may be permanent without treatment. Patients who receive topical treatment for epidermal hyperpigmentation will require months of treatment in order to see improvement. Patients who receive chemical peels or laser therapy should be counseled on the temporary results and the risk of relapse despite the high economic burden these treatments may impose.[16]

Indications for Consultation

Consultation with a dermatologist is helpful in creating a tailored treatment plan that may include topical, procedural, and/or oral treatments. Due to the chronicity of the condition and potential side effects from treatments, it may be helpful to transfer care to a dermatologist for long-term treatment of melasma. The same non-invasive techniques used to assess and monitor postinflammatory hyperpigmentation including wood's lamp, dermoscopy, and reflectance confocal microscopy, may be used for melasma.

Patient Information

- Skinsight: https://www.skinsight.com/skin-conditions/adult/melasma
- Skin of Color Society: https://skinofcolorsociety.org/dermatology-education/1406-2/
- American Academy of Dermatology: https://www.aad.org/public/diseases/a-z/melasma-overview

ACANTHOSIS NIGRICANS

Introduction

Acanthosis nigricans is a common cutaneous manifestation of insulin resistance, usually secondary to diabetes and/or obesity. However, acanthosis nigricans can be classified into eight different types based on the underlying etiology. These include benign, obesity-associated, syndromic, malignant, acral, unilateral, drug-induced, and mixed acanthosis nigricans. Obesity and insulin resistance remain the most common causes for acanthosis nigricans, although rarely acanthosis nigricans may be one of the first signs of malignancy. The most common cancer associated with acanthosis nigricans is gastric adenocarcinoma.[24] Other less common causes of insulin resistance include Cushing syndrome, Addison disease, acromegaly, polycystic ovarian syndrome, Prader-Willi Syndrome, and Down Syndrome.[25] The prevalence of acanthosis nigricans is unclear and appears to vary widely with age, gender, and skin phototype.[24] Those of Native American, African, and Hispanic descent tend to represent the most high-risk populations in the United States.[25]

Pathogenesis

It is proposed that increased levels of circulating insulin bind to insulin-like growth factor 1 receptors on fibroblasts and keratinocytes, leading to their proliferation and the cutaneous manifestation of hyperpigmented plaques. Additionally, high levels of insulin in those with metabolic syndrome may increase the amount of free insulin-like growth factor-1, leading to even more keratinocyte proliferation and growth. Individuals with familial syndromes may have defects in their fibroblast growth factor receptor genes. For example, those with familial acanthosis nigricans have a mutation in fibroblast growth factor receptor 3. For those with malignant acanthosis nigricans, the exact mechanism is unclear. However, it is suspected that these individuals have high levels of transforming growth factor-alpha that act on epidermal growth factor receptors causing cell proliferation and growth. Transforming growth factor-alpha is increased in individuals with gastric adenocarcinoma and tends to normalize after surgical removal of the tumor.[25]

Clinical Presentation

History

A detailed history including the time of onset, progression, patient age, family history, and medication list are all important for determining the underlying cause of acanthosis nigricans.[24] For example, unilateral acanthosis nigricans, although rare, is typically inherited in an autosomal dominant fashion. Drug-induced acanthosis nigricans is associated with several medications, such as testosterone, insulin, oral contraceptives, systemic glucocorticoids, and protease inhibitors.[25]

A detailed review of systems should be done to assess for diabetes or malignancy. Overall, the majority of patients who present will be obese and have a family history positive for diabetes or polycystic ovarian syndrome.[26]

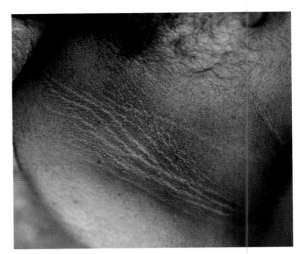

▲ **Figure 23-8.** Acanthosis nigricans. Dark brown velvety plaques on the posterior neck.

Individuals with malignancy-associated acanthosis nigricans may report rapid onset[25] mucosal and palmar involvement, and numerous skin tags and seborrheic keratoses, all of which are atypical for obesity-related acanthosis nigricans.[26] Individuals may have cutaneous manifestations before any signs of cancer and can have associated pruritus.[25] Endocrinopathies causing acanthosis nigricans will typically have a more gradual onset that is less extensive.

Physical Examination

Clinical examination will reveal thick velvety brown to black plaques, most commonly located on the neck, axillae, and groin (Figure 23-8). Some patients may also present with hyperpigmentation of the lips, umbilicus, areolae, elbows, and hands. Acral acanthosis nigricans, more common in skin of color, is limited to the elbows, knees, knuckles, and dorsal surfaces of the feet. More extensive involvement may even involve the mucosa.[25] Some patients may develop tripe palms (acanthosis palmaris) which may be a sign of malignancy. In severe cases, tripe palms have a rugose appearance, characterized by thick, velvety palms and exaggerated dermatoglyphics secondary to epidermal hyperkeratosis. Tripe palms with acanthosis nigricans can be a sign of gastric cancer, while tripe palms alone may be associated with lung cancer.[27]

Laboratory Findings

Laboratory results should be reviewed to help detect possible metabolic syndrome, dyslipidemia, or an endocrine disorder. If an insulin-resistant state is suspected, fasting glucose, hemoglobin A1C, liver function tests, and a lipoprotein profile should all be completed in addition to body weight and blood pressure. Additional laboratory work may be done if an endocrinopathy is suspected. If there is concern for malignancy, further steps in management may include imaging, such as x-ray, computerized tomography, or magnetic resonance imaging.[26]

Biopsy may be helpful if the diagnosis is unclear. Histopathology typically reveals hyperkeratosis with increased pigmentation of the basal layers and papillomatosis. The hyperpigmentation in acanthosis nigricans is likely secondary to hyperkeratosis and thickening rather than by increased melanin. In malignancy-associated acanthosis nigricans, hyperkeratosis is the dominant feature rather than hyperpigmentation.[25]

Diagnosis

Symmetrical, velvety, light- to dark-brown plaques most commonly located in intertriginous areas, such as the neck, axillae, and elbows.

▷ Differential Diagnosis

✓ Seborrheic dermatitis: Erythematous to hyperpigmented or hypopigmented scaly patches commonly presenting on scalp, eyebrows, and nasolabial folds.

✓ Tinea versicolor: Refer to : "Pityriasis Versicolor" section.

✓ Erythrasma: A superficial bacterial skin infection caused by the overgrowth of *Corynebacterium minutissimum* in the stratum corneum. Commonly occurs in moist, intertriginous areas of the body such as the groin and axillae. Patients present with pink to red patches with distinct borders and fine scale.

✓ Pellagra: Patients will usually have a history of poor nutrition and are deficient in vitamin B_3. Patients typically present with dermatitis, diarrhea, and dementia. The dermatitis typically consists of scaly erythematous patches and plaques which become hyperpigmented and hyperkeratotic.

✓ Linear epidermal nevus: Skin-colored or hyperpigmented papules coalescing to form a linear plaque that commonly presents at birth or develops during childhood.

✓ Granular parakeratosis: Erythematous, scaly macules that occur in the intertriginous regions of the body, especially the axillae.

Management

Treatment of acanthosis nigricans is multifactorial and also relies on addressing the underlying cause of the cutaneous manifestations. Patients should be reminded that acanthosis nigricans is not a primary skin disorder.

For those with insulin resistance and obesity, tight glycemic control and weight loss are key to management of acanthosis nigricans. Metformin and dietary modification may be helpful in reducing insulin resistance. Some patients may benefit from addition of another oral agent such as thiazolidines, dipeptidyl peptidase 4 inhibitors, and oral contraceptives. Pharmacotherapy for weight loss management may also be considered. Clinicians should be careful not to undermine the difficulty patients may have with weight loss and dietary modification.[26]

For those with malignancy-associated acanthosis nigricans, treatment requires locating and removing the underlying cancer.[25] Those with an endocrinopathies must treat the underlying cause and those with drug-induced acanthosis nigricans require discontinuation of their medication.[26]

Concurrent dermatologic treatment of acanthosis nigricans may also be helpful and includes topical retinoids, vitamin D analogs, alpha-hydroxy acids, oral retinoids, and combination therapies.[26]

Histologically, these medications lead to improvement through reduction of the hyperkeratosis.[26,28] Topical alpha-hydroxy acids are similar to retinoids and help decrease the papillomatosis associated with acanthosis nigricans.[28] Oral retinoids have been considered in management of both benign and syndromic acanthosis nigricans. However, large dose requirements, lengthy treatment courses, and risk of relapse make it a less preferred option.[26] Finally, several reports have documented improvement with calcitriol, which is proposed to increase keratinocyte proliferation.[26,28]

Alternative therapies that have been documented in case reports are podophyllin, fish oil, and combination therapy with urea, salicylic acid, and triple-combination depigmenting cream.[26,28] There are also studies highlighting the success of combination therapies with tretinoin and ammonium lactate or the common triple-combination cream of hydroquinone, tretinoin, and a low potency steroid.[28]

Chemical peels may improve pigmentation, skin texture and overall appearance. Additionally, chemical peels are considered to be safe, and easily accessible, making these a favorable option for cosmetic treatment.[26,28] Laser therapy is another treatment option, although it is not the most cost-effective.

Clinical Course and Prognosis

Patients with benign acanthosis nigricans have a good prognosis and a high likelihood of resolution with treatment. Acanthosis nigricans responds well to therapies treating the primary etiology. Duration and risk of relapse is dependent on adequate management of underlying chronic diseases that are causing the hyperkeratosis. Additionally, there is variable improvement and risk of relapse with dermatologic therapies, as they do not address the underlying cause. Patients with malignant acanthosis nigricans may have a worse prognosis if the cancer has metastasized.

Indications for Consultation

Dermatology referral may prove beneficial when the diagnosis is unclear, patient has not had sufficient improvement or for dermatologic treatment to occur concurrently with the treatment of the underlying cause. Referral to an endocrinologist should also be considered for difficulty managing diabetes or other metabolic disorders.

Patient Information

- Skinsight: https://www.skinsight.com/skin-conditions/child/acanthosis-nigricans
- American Academy of Dermatology: https://www.aad.org/public/diseases/a-z/acanthosis-nigricans-overview

▼ POSTINFLAMMATORY HYPOPIGMENTATION

Introduction

Postinflammatory hypopigmentation, similar to postinflammatory hyperpigmentation, is a common sequelae of cutaneous inflammation or injury. It affects both genders and all ages equally and is more common and more apparent in darker skin types.[29]

Pathogenesis

Melanocytes respond to inflammation and trauma in postinflammatory hypopigmentation through a decrease in melanogenesis. This means that there may be a decrease in melanin synthesis, transport, and/or keratinocyte uptake.[29] As in postinflammatory hyperpigmentation, it is proposed that the melanocyte response to inflammation and trauma is genetic, with some individuals responding with increased melanocyte activity and subsequent hyperpigmentation and some with decreased activity and hypopigmentation.[29]

Clinical Presentation

▶ History

Patients will typically have a history of cutaneous inflammation or injury that preceded the hypopigmentation. Review of medical history, medication history, and procedural history can be helpful, especially when inflammation is not visible at the time of presentation. A thorough history may also reveal or help exclude underlying disorders that can present similarly, such as sarcoidosis, leprosy, and mycosis fungoides.[30]

▶ Physical Examination

The physical examination will reveal hypopigmented macules and/or patches with indistinct borders in areas

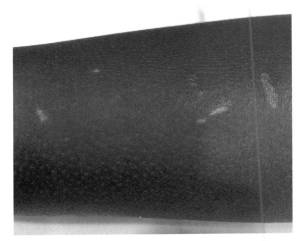

▲ **Figure 23-9.** Postinflammatory hypopigmentation. Linear hypopigmented macules on the leg of a young child secondary to trauma.

of previous inflammation or injury (Figure 23-9).[30] The Wood's lamp can help distinguish postinflammatory hypopigmentation from other depigmenting disorders, such as vitiligo. Postinflammatory hypopigmentation may become more visible under Wood's lamp examination but will not accentuate as brightly as vitiligo.

▶ Laboratory Findings

No laboratory findings are associated with postinflammatory hypopigmentation. Occasionally, a biopsy will help with diagnosis. Histopathology is nonspecific and will show decreased melanin in the epidermis, melanophages in the upper dermis, and lymphohistiocytic infiltrate superficially.

Diagnosis

The characteristic features of postinflammatory hypopigmentation are poorly defined, light tan to white-appearing macules and patches located in areas of previous inflammation or trauma.

▶ Differential Diagnosis

- ✓ Vitiligo: Refer to "Vitiligo" section.
- ✓ Tinea Versicolor: Refer to "Pityriasis Versicolor" section.
- ✓ Pityriasis alba: Refer to "Pityriasis Alba" section.
- ✓ Idiopathic guttate hypomelanosis: Refer to "Idiopathic Guttate Hypomelanosis" section.

✓ Nevus depigmentosus and hypomelanosis of Ito: Long standing-fixed, hypopigmented patches present at birth.

✓ Leprosy: Chronic bacterial infection caused by *Mycobacterium leprae* that can present with an array of cutaneous and systemic manifestations including hypopigmentation and loss of sensation.

✓ Sarcoidosis: A granulomatous skin disease with various cutaneous presentations, including a hypopigmented variant. May present with macules, papules, patches, plaques, or nodules.

✓ Hypopigmented Mycosis Fungoides: A variant of cutaneous T-cell lymphoma presenting with hypopigmented patches more common in skin of color.

✓ Drug-induced hypopigmentation: Common culprits are topical and intralesional steroids.

Management

Accurate diagnosis and treatment of the underlying cause will help resolve and prevent postinflammatory hypopigmentation. Most areas of hypopigmentation will improve in a few weeks to months without treatment and some patients may benefit from cosmetic camouflage in the meantime. Repigmentation may occur from sun exposure or ultraviolet radiation leading to melanocyte stimulation. Nevertheless, there are several treatment options that have been examined in small studies. These include topical, photo-based, procedural, and combination therapies. Topical therapies include topical immunomodulators, such as pimecrolimus prostaglandin analogs, including topical bimatoprost and psoralen plus ultraviolet A photochemotherapy. Procedural treatments may involve lasers, microneedling, and phototherapy.[29] Procedural therapies often require referral to a specialist. Combination therapies have also been utilized with varying degrees of success. Any treatments causing irritation should be discontinued due to risk of worsening or new postinflammatory hypopigmentation.

Clinical Course and Prognosis

This condition may resolve spontaneously over the course of a few weeks to months. Severe cases of hypopigmentation or complete depigmentation can persist for years or may be permanent. Response to therapy and risk of relapse is dependent on the underlying cause, which should be addressed first. If the underlying condition is treated, patients typically have a good prognosis with little risk of recurrence.

Indications for Consultation

Consultation with a dermatologist is usually unnecessary, unless the diagnosis is unclear, the patient is not improving with time, or the patient is interested in more specialized treatments that may accelerate resolution of the condition.

Patient Information

- Skinsight: https://www.skinsight.com/skin-conditions/adult/post-inflammatory-hypopigmentation
- Australian College of Dermatologist: https://www.dermcoll.edu.au/atoz/post-inflammatory-hypopigmentation/

▼ PITYRIASIS ALBA

Introduction

Pityriasis alba is a common skin disorder causing hypopigmentation most commonly on the face, neck, and trunk and typically affects children and adolescents, particularly those with Fitzpatrick skin types IV to VI. Both genders are affected equally. It is common in patients with a history of atopy and is often considered a form of atopic dermatitis.[31]

Pathogenesis

The pathogenesis for pityriasis alba is unknown; however, it is thought to be a manifestation of atopic dermatitis with subsequent postinflammatory hypopigmentation. Resulting hypopigmentation may be secondary to impaired melanosome transfer between melanocytes and keratinocytes. Dry skin from frequent bathing as well as nutritional and vitamin deficiencies, particularly copper deficiency, have been associated with pityriasis alba as well.[31]

Clinical Presentation

▶ History

Most patients with this skin disorder are children or adolescents, with a majority of cases occurring in children less than 12 years of age. Patients are typically asymptomatic. Although, some patents have associated pruritus. Family history may help narrow the diagnosis, as atopic dermatitis, allergic rhinitis, and asthma are all common in patients with pityriasis alba.[30] Most patients present for cosmetic reasons, especially during the summer months when the hypopigmented patches become more apparent.

▶ Physical Examination

Visual assessment may reveal erythematous macules or patches with indistinct borders. However, these areas usually fade after a few weeks and become scaly, round, or ovoid-shaped hypopigmented macules or patches (Figure 23-10). The erythematous phase may go unnoticed, as most

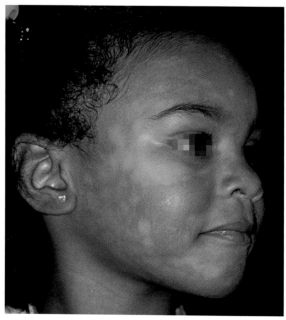

▲ **Figure 23-10.** Pityriasis alba. Scattered ill-defined hypopigmented macules and patches on face of young girl. Reproduced with permission from Charles E. Crutchfield III, MD.

patients present once hypopigmentation has occurred. It is most commonly located on the face. Multiple affected macules and patches ranging from 0.5 cm to 5 cm can also be present on the neck, upper arms, and trunk. Clinicians may also note signs of atopic dermatitis as well.[31]

▶ Laboratory Findings

There are no associated laboratory findings with pityriasis alba. If biopsy is performed, histology will usually reveal a decreased number of active melanocytes, smaller and fewer melanosomes, and less melanin in the basal layer. It may also reveal evidence of spongiosis, perivascular infiltrates, hyperkeratosis, parakeratosis, and acanthosis, all of which are consistent with a nonspecific dermatitis.[32]

Diagnosis

Erythematous, well-defined macules and patches that persist for several weeks before becoming hypopigmented with overlying scale.[31]

If the diagnosis is uncertain, Wood's lamp may be used. Unlike vitiligo, pityriasis alba does not fluoresce under Wood's lamp. Additionally, skin scrapings and potassium hydroxide preparation will help rule out fungal etiologies, such as tinea versicolor or tinea corporis.

▶ Differential Diagnosis

✓ Postinflammatory hypopigmentation: Refer to "Postinflammatory hypopigmentation" section.

✓ Tinea versicolor: Refer to "Pityriasis Versicolor" section.

✓ Vitiligo: Refer to "Vitiligo" section.

✓ Nevus depigmentosus, Nevus anemicus, Hypomelanosis of Ito: Long standing-fixed, hypopigmented lesions present at birth or soon after birth.

✓ Seborrheic dermatitis: Refer to differential diagnosis in 'Acanthosis Nigricans' section.

✓ Ash-leaf macules of tuberous sclerosis: Hypopigmented, white macules typically present at birth, suggesting tuberous sclerosis. May be accompanied by perilingual fibromas, angiofibromas, and connective tissue nevi.

✓ Hypopigmented Mycosis fungoides: A cutaneous T-cell lymphoma that may present with hypopigmented macules and patches.

✓ Drug-induced hypopigmentation: Topical and intralesional steroids are common culprits.

Management

Pityriasis alba will typically resolve on its own. However, adequate sun protection, and proper moisturization with emollients and lubricants is encouraged.[32] Some patients may also benefit from bathing less often, as frequent baths and exfoliation may remove the protective factors of the skin. Those with hypopigmentation limited to the face may benefit from low potency topical steroids. Higher potency steroids are typically reserved for affected areas on the body. Topical steroids should be used with caution as to avoid side effects associated with chronic cutaneous use. Safer alternatives include calcineurin inhibitors, but in some cases this may be cost prohibitive. Calcitriol, a topical Vitamin D analog, has also shown some efficacy. Patients with extensive disease who have been unsuccessful with topical therapy may benefit from phototherapy, specifically psoralen plus ultraviolet A or ultraviolet B light alone.[31]

Clinical Course and Prognosis

It is suspected that pityriasis alba will spontaneously resolve with time, usually after one year. Complete repigmentation will occur in most individuals. Treatment may shorten the duration of hypopigmentation.[32]

Indications for Consultation

Consultation with a dermatologist is typically not needed, unless the patient is interested in more specialized therapies for cosmetic purposes.

Patient Information

- Skinsight: https://www.skinsight.com/skin-conditions/teen/pityriasis-alba
- DermNet NZ: https://www.dermnetnz.org/cme/dermatitis/pityriasis-alba-cme/

PITYRIASIS VERSICOLOR (TINEA VERSICOLOR)

Introduction

Tinea versicolor is a cutaneous manifestation of fungal colonization causing hypopigmentation. The most common involved species are *Malassezia globosa* and *Malassezi furfur*. Malassezia yeasts are a part of the normal skin microbiota. Colonization occurs at birth and increases with age.[33] Incidence increases during the summer months and tinea versicolor is most common in tropical climates. It is most prevalent in young adults and likely does not have a predilection for gender, although increased sebaceous activity in males may make them more susceptible.[34]

Pathogenesis

Tinea versicolor occurs when the *Malassezia* yeast transforms from the saprophytic, round-celled, yeast phase to the mycelial phase. It is proposed that *Malassezia* produces azelaic acid and lipoxygenase which inhibit melanin synthesis and leads to hypopigmentation. Melanosomes in tinea versicolor are small and poorly pigmented. There is also decreased melanosome transfer to keratinocytes.[34]

Tropical climates increase the transformation of Malassezia to the mycelial phase, thus explaining the increased disease prevalence in hotter and more humid climates.[32] Immunodeficiency, inadequate nutrition, increased sweating, pregnancy, oral contraceptives, and corticosteroids may also contribute.[33] A genetic component is also likely. Further, *Malassezia* genus is lipophilic, meaning frequent use of oils or other products with high lipid concentrations may increase overgrowth. These products may also clog the skin leading to altered pH and microflora and increased carbon dioxide thus enhancing fungal colonization. Sebum production is also a likely contributor and may explain the lower disease prevalence in pre-pubescent and elderly individuals.[34]

Clinical Presentation

History

Most patients will present with concern for asymptomatic white spots; however, some may have associated pruritus.

Physical Examination

Because *Malassezia* is lipophilic and requires certain lipids to grow, it affects sebum rich areas of the skin. Clinical

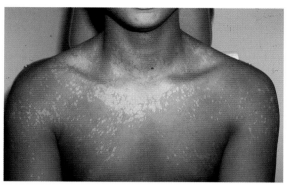

▲ **Figure 23-11.** Pityriasis versicolor (Tinea versicolor). Hypopigmented scaly macules coalescing centrally into patches on the upper chest, neck, and bilateral upper extremities.

examination will reveal numerous scaly, round, or ovoid hypopigmented macules that coalesce into patches, typically on the trunk and upper extremities (Figure 23-11).[32] For some individuals the patches may also have erythema. With the exception of children and immunocompromised patients, involvement of the face or lower extremities is rare. Tinea versicolor can be diagnosed clinically and is best confirmed with a potassium hydroxide preparation.[32]

Laboratory Findings

There are no associated laboratory findings with tinea versicolor. A potassium hydroxide preparation can be helpful with diagnosis and will reveal short, thick pseudohyphae and spores on microscopy. "Spaghetti and meatballs" is a common term used to describe the strands of mycelium and spores. If a biopsy is done, staining can be done to confirm hyphae and spores[32] within a thick basket-weave stratum corneum.[34] For patients who have atrophic lesions, effacement of the rete ridges, subepidermal fibroplasia, pigment incontinence, and elastolysis is seen in addition to epidermal colonization.[35]

Diagnosis

The key diagnostic features are hypopigmented to skin colored macules and patches on the trunk with associated pruritus that can worsen during summer months.

Differential Diagnosis

- ✓ Seborrheic dermatitis: Refer to differential diagnosis in "Acanthosis Nigricans" section.
- ✓ Pityriasis rosea: Faint erythematous macules to patches often in a "Christmas tree-like" distribution on the trunk. Patients can have history of a larger

herald patch preceding the diffuse eruption of macules.

✓ Pityriasis alba: Refer to "Pityriasis Alba" section.

Management

Several topical agents have been shown to treat tinea versicolor. Imidazoles, triazoles, selenium sulfide, sulfur preparations, ciclopirox olamine, and zinc pyrithione have all shown efficacy.[32] Selenium sulfide lotion is the most cost-effective option. Selenium sulfide shampoo is recommended for those with overgrowth on the scalp and trunk. Another cost-effective treatment is zinc pyrithione soap. The most effective topical azole is ketoconazole. Many topicals are initially used daily for several weeks. Shampoos can also be used long-term for maintenance treatment as well.[34]

Patients with extensive disease may benefit from oral medications such as itraconazole or fluconazole for treatment or prophylaxis.[32] Oral terbinafine is typically ineffective, although topical terbinafine has proven to be effective.[36]

Clinical Course and Prognosis

Without treatment, tinea versicolor can be a chronic disease. It may take several weeks to months for areas of hypopigmentation to resolve, even after completing treatment. Without occasional prophylactic therapy, recurrence is likely. After initial treatment, patients may occasionally use the following as prophylaxis: selenium sulfide, topical ketoconazole, econazole, and bifonazole shampoo, zinc pyrithione wash, or oral therapy.[34]

Indications for Consultation

Consultation with a dermatologist is typically not needed, unless the diagnosis is unclear and further work-up is needed or the patient is not improving.

Patient Information

- Skinsight: https://www.skinsight.com/skin-conditions/child/tinea-versicolor
- Skin of Color Society: https://skinofcolorsociety.org/dermatology-education/tinea-versicolor/
- American Academy of Dermatology: https://www.aad.org/public/diseases/a-z/tinea-versicolor-overview

IDIOPATHIC GUTTATE HYPOMELANOSIS

Introduction

Idiopathic guttate hypomelanosis is an acquired pigmentary disorder causing areas of hypopigmentation, most commonly on sun-exposed areas of the upper and lower extremities. Although more noticeable in patients with skin of color, idiopathic guttate hypomelanosis occurs in all skin phototypes and has equal gender prevalence.[30] Prevalence increases with age and idiopathic guttate hypomelanosis is most common in the elderly population, particularly those 70 years and older with a prolonged history of sun exposure.[32]

Pathogenesis

The pathogenesis of idiopathic guttate hypomelanosis is unknown. Genetics, aging, trauma, and sun exposure have been suggested as possible etiologies.[30] Idiopathic guttate hypomelanosis is characterized as a melanopenic as well as melanocytopenic process. This means that there is both a decrease in melanin production due to reduced tyrosinase activity as well as a decrease in the transfer of melanin from melanocytes to keratinocytes.[2]

Clinical Presentation

▶ History

The patient will report several scattered light brown to white spots that have likely increased in number over time and with no associated symptoms.

▶ Physical Examination

Visual assessment will reveal smooth, flat, and symmetric hypopigmented to depigmented macules that are typically 2–5 mm in diameter with irregular or jagged borders. Occasionally, patients may present with patches reaching up to 10 mm in size.[2] Hair within the macules maintains its pigmentation (Figure 23-12).

▶ Laboratory Findings

There are no associated laboratory findings with idiopathic guttate hypomelanosis. However, biopsy may be done if the diagnosis is unclear. Histology will typically reveal epidermal atrophy with flattening of the dermal–epidermal junction. Decreased melanin granules in the basal and suprabasal layers and 3,4-dihydroxyphenylalanine negative melanocytes are also present.[37]

Diagnosis

The characteristic features of idiopathic guttate hypomelanosis include multiple, small, porcelain-white macules, most commonly on the upper and lower extremities.

▶ Differential Diagnosis

✓ Tinea versicolor: Refer to "Pityriasis Versicolor" section.

✓ Vitiligo: Refer to "Vitiligo" section.

✓ Pityriasis alba: Refer to "Pityriasis Alba" section.

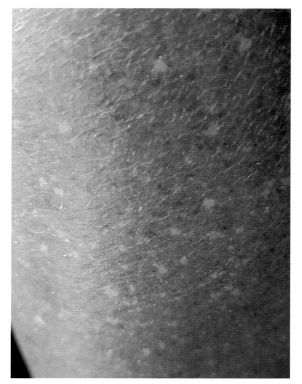

▲ Figure 23-12. Idiopathic guttate hypomelanosis. Small 2–5 mm hypopigmented macules with scalloped borders on lower extremity. Reproduced with permission from Charles E. Crutchfield III, MD.

✓ Postinflammatory hypopigmentation: Refer to "Postinflammatory Hyperpigmentation" section.

✓ Chemical leukoderma: Occupational exposure causing melanocyte destruction and depigmentation. Patients have a history of toxin exposure, specifically aromatic derivatives of catechols and phenols. Presents in a "confetti-like" distribution with associated pruritus.

Management

Medical treatment is not necessary, although some patients may be interested in cosmetic therapies. There are no gold standard treatments for this condition though several topical and procedural treatments have been tried, many with minimal success. These include topical corticosteroids as well as cryotherapy, dermabrasion, surgical mini-grafting, fractional lasers and microneedling with transdermal delivery of 5-fluorouracil.[30] Camouflage may also be used. Patients are also encouraged to be diligent with sun protection since this may play a role in the pathogenesis of this condition.

Clinical Course and Prognosis

Idiopathic guttate hypomelanosis is a benign and permanent condition. There is currently no treatment that reliably results in significant improvement. The hypopigmented macules typically remain the same size and do not coalesce.[32]

Indications for Consultation

Consultation with a dermatologist is typically not needed, unless the patient is interested in more specialized cosmetic procedural treatments.

Patient Information

- DermNet NZ: https://dermnetnz.org/topics/idiopathic-guttate-hypomelanosis/
- Dermatology Advisor: https://www.dermatologyadvisor.com/home/decision-support-in-medicine/dermatology/idiopathic-guttate-hypomelanosis-leukopathia-symmetrica-progressiva/

▼ VITILIGO

Introduction

Vitiligo is a pigmentary disorder of depigmentation of the skin and hair. Disease prevalence is around 0.5–1% in most countries, although this varies by region with 0.38% prevalence in Denmark and nearly 8% prevalence in certain regions of India. Vitiligo does not have a predilection for any particular gender, race, age, or geographic location. Peak onset typically occurs between ages 10 and 30 with nearly 50% of individuals presenting before age 20.[38]

Pathogenesis

The exact pathogenesis of vitiligo is unknown. Possible etiologies include genetic, autoimmune, neural, biochemical, and cytotoxic mechanisms. With respect to genetics, there is increased disease frequency and presence of autoimmune disorders among relatives. In a study conducted by Alkhateeb et al., the risk of a patient's sibling developing vitiligo was 6%, while the risk for an identical twin was 23%, thus highlighting the heritability of vitiligo.[39] Genome-wide association studies have identified 50 genetic loci that contribute to the risk of vitiligo and associated autoimmune disorders in European and Chinese patients. Many of these genes are involved in immune regulation, cellular apoptosis, and melanocyte function,[40,41] further highlighting autoimmune dysfunction as part of the pathogenesis. Additionally, many individuals with vitiligo have other autoimmune disorders such as hypothyroidism or pernicious anemia, and many have elevated circulating antibodies against melanocytes and other organs in which melanocytes may be present, such as the eye and the heart.[38] The immune pathway of vitiligo is complex and may serve as a protective factor to the development of melanoma.[41]

There are studies suggesting oxidative stress may also play a role in the pathogenesis of vitiligo, in which melanocytes with intrinsic defects are unable to manage cellular stress. Environmental triggers, such as ultraviolet radiation, may increase production of reactive oxygen species, causing DNA damage and worsening cellular stress in already vulnerable melanocytes.[39]

The loss of pigmentation is also caused by destruction of melanocytes via cytotoxic CD8[+] T cells. Recent studies have demonstrated a correlation between the circulating level of cytokines and disease activity. Levels of CXCL9 and 10 have been found to be lower among healthy controls as well as those with vitiligo who have been successfully treated, suggesting these cytokines may be used to assess disease activity and treatment response.[39]

Biochemical etiologies may include dysfunction of the melanocortic system, such as low alpha–melanocyte stimulating hormone or decreased pro-opiomelanocortin (POMC) mRNA expression in affected skin.[39,40]

Clinical Presentation

▶ History

Patients commonly report a slow progression of white, well-circumscribed spots usually without associated symptoms. However, pruritus is occasionally reported among vitiligo patients, even in the absence of irritation and prior to the presence of depigmented patches.[42,43] One study noted pruritus in 20.2% of patients with vitiligo.[43] Rarely, patients may have an inflammatory variant of vitiligo characterized by redness, scaling, and itching.[40] The initial onset of disease can be rapid. A thorough family history may help narrow the diagnosis, considering nearly 25–50% of vitiligo patients have an affected relative.[32] Additionally, a personal or family history of autoimmune disease is common, particularly autoimmune thyroid disease. Patients may also more rarely have a history of ocular or auditory dysfunction, as melanocytes exist in these tissues as well.[38] Clinicians should address potential occupational exposures if there is concern for chemical leukoderma.[40] Some patients may present with the halo phenomenon, in which there is an initial loss of pigmentation surrounding a nevus.[43] Many patients seek medical care after sun exposure due to increased visibility of the vitiligo.

▶ Physical Examination

Visual assessment reveals several depigmented macules and patches of varying size and shape with smooth, distinct borders (Figures 23-13 and 23-14). Areas of depigmentation

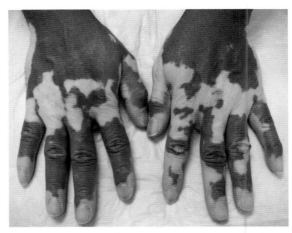

▲ **Figure 23-13.** Vitiligo. Symmetric depigmented patches on the bilateral dorsum of the hands.

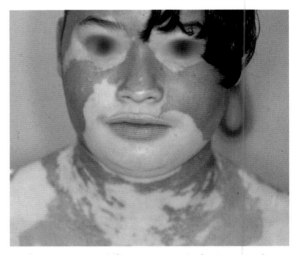

▲ **Figure 23-14.** Vitiligo. Symmetric depigmented patches on the face. Reproduced with permission from Charles E. Crutchfield III, MD.

typically range from a few millimeters to several centimeters.[32] Rarely, patients may present with erythematous, inflamed margins. Wood's lamp examination accentuates areas of nonscaly depigmentation. There are six possible patterns for patients with vitiligo including:

1. Focal: Limited to one specific anatomic location and can be asymmetric or non-dermatomal.
2. Segmental: Typically, present early in life and often in a unilateral blaschkoid pattern that correlates with the pathway of epidermal migration occurring during fetal development. It is the least common subtype and usually the most difficult to treat.

3. Generalized: Typically, symmetric and have a predilection for the face, upper chest, axillae, dorsal surfaces of the hands, groin, areas of trauma such as the elbows and knees and skin around orifices such as the eyes, nose, and mouth.

4. Universal: Complete depigmentation of 50% or more of the body.

5. Acrofacial: Affects the distal fingers and facial orifices.

6. Mucosal: Limited to mucosal sites including lips and genitalia.

The most common pattern is generalized vitiligo. Some patients may present with trichrome vitiligo, especially early on in the disease course.[40] This is characterized by three skin color variations including normal pigmentation, hypopigmentation, and complete depigmentation. Patients may also have loss of hair pigment in vitiliginous areas.[32]

▶ Laboratory Findings

There are no specific laboratory findings associated with vitiligo. However, many patients have associated autoimmune disorders that they should be screened for, the most common being autoimmune thyroid disease.[38] At the time of diagnosis, baseline laboratories can be obtained including a complete blood count, comprehensive metabolic panel, and thyroid function tests. Additional laboratory screening should be based on their review of systems if the patient presents with other signs and symptoms. Other common autoimmune diseases to be aware of include Addison disease, systemic lupus erythematosus pernicious anemia, and inflammatory bowel disease.[44] Biopsies are only necessary if the diagnosis is unclear. Histopathology will reveal an absence of melanocytes in the affected regions.[32]

Diagnosis

The diagnosis is typically a clinical one. Vitiligo is characterized by its well-defined completely depigmented white patches and its asymptomatic, progressive disease course.

▶ Differential Diagnosis

✓ Tinea versicolor: Refer to "Pityriasis Versicolor" section.

✓ Pityriasis alba: Refer to "Pityriasis Alba" section.

✓ Postinflammatory hypopigmentation: Refer to "Postinflammatory Hypopigmentation" section.

✓ Idiopathic guttate hypomelanosis: Refer to "Idiopathic Guttate Hypomelanosis" section.

✓ Chemical leukoderma: Refer to differential diagnoses in "Idiopathic Guttate Hypomelanosis" section.

✓ Ash leaf spots of tuberous sclerosis: Hypopigmented, white macules typically present at birth, suggesting tuberous sclerosis. May be accompanied by perilingual fibromas, angiofibromas, and connective tissue nevi.

✓ Piebaldism: Genetic condition involving loss of melanocytes and depigmentation that is present at birth.

✓ Nevus depigmentosus, Nevus anemicus, and Hypomelanosis of Ito: Congenital and typically do not change over one's life course.

✓ Other: Under the appropriate clinical context, mycosis fungoides, Hansen's disease, and sarcoidosis may also be considered, as they too can present as hypopigmented macules and patches.

Management

Treatment is not required but is chosen by many patients due to the profound psychosocial effects of the disease. Optimization of treatments is dependent on multiple factors including disease subtype, extent and distribution, and activity as well as patient age and effect on quality of life. With respect to disease severity, categorizing the patient to one of the four categories of body surface area involvement may help in determining the best treatment options.

- Limited: < 10% involvement
- Moderate: 10–25% involvement
- Moderately severe: 26–50% involvement
- Severe: >50% involvement

For patients interested in treatment, there are medical and procedural options available including topical corticosteroids, topical calcineurin inhibitors, phototherapy, laser therapy, nutritional supplements, and surgery.[45] Certain treatments may help to stop progression of the disease, lead to regimentation, or both. It is also common to combine different treatment modalities to increase efficacy. For all patients, regardless of their choice of management, sun protection is the key to prevent sunburns, exacerbation of existing lesions, or increased risk of skin cancer.

Topical treatments are appropriate for those with less than 20% body surface area involvement. Topical steroids are often used cyclically to treat the disease and avoid side effects of chronic topical steroid use. Duration of steroid use should never exceed 4–6 months and patients should receive "days off" from the medication.[45] The potency of the steroid is dependent on the location of depigmentation. Higher potency steroids may be used for the trunk and extremities, while lower potency steroids are preferred for the face and intertriginous sites. Topical calcineurin inhibitors are also commonly used. These immunomodulators allow for prolonged use given their lack of side effects and are often considered first-line treatment. Nevertheless, high costs may prevent their use. These calcineurin inhibitors may be used concurrently with topical steroids or on "off days" from topical steroids for patients interested in continuous treatment.[45] Additionally, the vitamin D analog, calcipotriol is well-tolerated and proposed to increase melanocyte and keratinocyte growth and differentiation. Additionally, a short course of systemic steroids may be prescribed to stabilize rapidly progressive disease.[40]

Procedural treatments for vitiligo include phototherapy, laser therapy, and surgery. Phototherapy is currently the mainstay of treatment and current options include sunlight, ultraviolet A, psoralen plus ultraviolet A, broadband ultraviolet B, narrow-band ultraviolet B, and excimer. Narrowband ultraviolet B, however, is the most effective and is considered first-line for individuals with moderate to severe vitiligo. Compared to the previous gold standard, psoralen plus ultraviolet A, narrowband ultraviolet B has minimal side effects.[40] Many patients receive treatment 2–3 times per week and many can achieve more than 75% repigmentation of the face and extremities.[45] Combination of topical treatments with phototherapy often leads to enhanced repigmentation rates.[40,45] The excimer laser, which uses gases to produce a 308 nm ultraviolet wavelength that lies within the ultraviolet B spectrum, can be used to treat more localized areas.[40] Combination with a topical corticosteroid may enhance efficacy. The hardest areas to treat are usually the elbows, knees, wrists, and dorsal surfaces of the hands and feet. Surgery is a good alternative for patients who have failed treatment with previous methods and have more focal stable depigmentation with less than 2–3% body surface area involvement. Individuals with segmental and stable vitiligo are good candidates. Surgical methods include minigrafting, transplantation of autologous epidermal cell suspension, and ultrathin epidermal grafts. Ultraviolet phototherapy is often used adjunctively after surgery.

Depigmentation therapy with topical monobenzyl ether of hydroquinone can be considered for individuals with greater than 80% body surface area involvement. Psychological consultation is recommended before proceeding with depigmentation. Given the irreversible nature of the treatment, it is best done under the care of an experienced dermatologist.[45]

Studies on more targeted therapies that address melanocyte stress, autoimmune response, and melanocyte regeneration are emerging. Supplements with antioxidant properties may prove beneficial by reducing production of reactive oxidative species. Immunomodulator therapies that target specific signaling pathways, such as interferon-gamma and janus kinase inhibitors, are also being studied topically and orally.[39,45] Prostaglandins, like bimatoprost, may help with melanocyte stimulation and immunomodulatory effects. All of these therapies, however, require further investigation.[39] Lastly, for patients who desire cosmetic camouflage, several options exist including makeups, tattooing, and self-tanning creams containing dihydroxyacetone, which can last for several days.

Clinical Course and Prognosis

Vitiligo is a chronic disease currently without a cure. Areas of depigmentation may remain stable or they may progress over time. Very rarely, in less than 25% of cases, spontaneous regimentation occurs. Response to treatment is highly dependent on the duration and stability of disease and the extent and distribution. The earlier in the disease course treatment is started, the more likely the patient is to see significant improvement.[32]

Vitiligo located in areas with a large number of hair follicles is more likely to achieve regimentation, specifically when the hair in these areas, are still pigmented. The response to treatment is slow, with many patients not seeing results until after several months. Segmental vitiligo is considered to be the least treatment responsive pattern to traditional topical and oral treatments for vitiligo, but does appear to have good results with surgical treatment.[45]

The duration of treatment and the risk of relapse is dependent on the form of treatment. For example, those receiving phototherapy may not see significant improvement until they have received at least 3 months of therapy.[32] For those receiving surgical treatment, relapse is uncommon.[45]

Indications for Consultation

For patients who do not respond to topical therapy, consultation with a dermatologist may be necessary for more specialized procedures including phototherapy, surgery, and combination therapy. Additionally, clinicians should know when to consult an esthetician to help patients who are interested in cosmetic camouflage or a psychiatrist for patients experiencing significant psychosocial impairment. Consultation with an endocrinologist or rheumatologist may also be needed for those with associated autoimmune diseases.

Patient Information

- Global Vitiligo Foundation: https://globalvitiligofoundation.org/
- Skin of Color Society: https://skinofcolorsociety.org/dermatology-education/vitiligo/
- American Academy of Dermatology: https://www.aad.org/public/diseases/a-z/vitiligo-overview

⏷ QUALITY OF LIFE ISSUES

Pigmentary disorders can be mistaken as merely "cosmetic disorders." However, not only do many pigmentary disorders have a medical etiology, but many also carry with them significant psychosocial burden and mental health issues. Uneven skin tone can lead to many patients experiencing both a lack of societal and self-acceptance. This can lead to life-long struggles with shame, fear of rejection, and social isolation. One study, highlighting the prevalence of stigmatization among patients with vitiligo, reported that 90% of participants had been approached by a stranger regarding their appearance.[46] The impact of pigmentary disorders on quality of life (QoL) has been assessed with several validated tools including the Dermatology Quality of Life Index (DQLI), the Vitiligo Life Quality Index, and the Melasma Quality of Life Scale (MelasQoL).

Several studies report high DLQI scores, correlating with lower QoL, among patients with vitiligo. In one study, 96.43% of males and 97.73% of females with vitiligo experienced a reduced QoL based on their scores. Fify-two percent of these patients also suffered from depression, with a higher prevalence in women, and 48% avoided certain activities due to fear of stigmatization.[47] In a study on hyperpigmentation and QoL, melisma, and postinflammatory hyperpigmentation had the highest DLQI scores and lowest QoL scores compared to other disorders of hyperpigmentation, such as lentigo and seborrheic keratosis.[48] Studies on patients with acne-related postinflammatory hyperpigmentation have found that these individuals have significantly greater psychosocial impairment compared to those with acne alone. These individuals report higher levels of anxiety, decreased socialization, feelings of self-consciousness, and difficulties finding a partner.[49,50] There is also an increased psychosocial burden among obese adolescent girls with acanthosis nigricans and high levels of testosterone. One study revealed that hyperandrogenism in addition to acanthosis nigricans results in even higher reports of anxiety, depression, and low self-esteem than acanthosis nigricans alone.[51]

Pigmentary disorders can be challenging to treat and in order to ensure holistic treatment of patients, the emotional and psychological effects of these conditions must be taken into consideration. Physicians should assess how their patients are coping and in addition to medical treatment of their condition, can suggest cosmetic camouflage and mental health support when appropriate. An international observational study assessing the impact of corrective cosmetics on quality of life revealed that 81.6% of participants who applied corrective cosmetics once daily for four weeks had a significant improvement in their well-being.[52]

INSURANCE COVERAGE

Treatments for pigmentary disorders can be costly to patients, particularly when insurances deny coverage for treatment and dismiss pigmentary disorders as being cosmetic conditions. In addition to a lack of insurance coverage, high co-pays, long commutes, and lost wages from missed work days all contribute to the economic burden that may accompany medical treatment for chronic conditions such as vitiligo.[53,54] Because chronic pigmentary disorders may require years of treatment, a good outcome-to-cost ratio is important for reducing the financial burden and increasing patient adherence.[55] Several studies have demonstrated greater cost-effectiveness with home phototherapy compared to office-based therapy; however, few insurance companies offer coverage for home phototherapy.[54] Additionally, many topical treatments including lightening agents used for melasma and postinflammatory hyperpigmentation are often denied coverage and can be quite costly as an out-of-pocket expense for patients.[53] Working with insurance companies to obtain increased insurance coverage is an important and ongoing challenge facing physicians today.

REFERENCES

1. Lin JY, Fisher DE. Melanocyte biology and skin pigmentation. *Nature*. 2007;445(7130):843-850.
2. Rani S, Kumar R, Kumarasinghe P, et al. Melanocyte abnormalities and senescence in the pathogenesis of idiopathic guttate hypomelanosis. *Int J Dermatol*. 2018;57(5):559-565.
3. Yaar M, Gilchrest BA. Melanocyte biology: before, during, and after the fitzpatrick era. *J Invest Dermatol*. 2004;122(2):27-29.
4. Zieleniewski Ł, Schwartz RA, Goldberg DJ, Handler MZ. Voigt-Futcher pigmentary demarcation lines. *J Cosmet Dermatol*. 2019;18(3):700-702.
5. Shelley ED, Shelley WB, Pansky B. The drug line: The clinical expression of the pigmentary Voigt-Futcher line in turn derived from the embryonic ventral axial line. *J Am Acad Dermatol*. 1999;40(5):736-740.
6. George AO, Shittu OB, Enwerem E, Wachtel M, Kuti O. The incidence of lower mid-trunk hyperpigmentation (linea nigra) is affected by sex hormone levels. *J Natl Med Assoc*. 2005;97(5):685-688.
7. Bieber AK, Martires KJ, Stein JA, Grant-Kels JM, Driscoll MS, Pomeranz MK. Pigmentation and pregnancy: knowing what is normal. *Obstet Gynecol*. 2017;129(1):168-173.
8. Kelly AP, Heidelberg KA. Nuances in skin of color. In: Kelly AP, Taylor SC, Lim HW, Serrano AMA, eds. *Taylor and Kelly's Dermatology for Skin of Color*. 2nd ed. McGraw-Hill Education; 2016. Accessed August 17, 2020. accessmedicine.mhmedical.com/content.aspx?aid=1161545089
9. Gately LE, Krementz AB, Reed RJ, Krementz ET. Nevi, Lentigines, and Melanomas in Blacks. *Arch Dermatol*. 116:4.
10. Gupta D, Thappa D. Mongolian spots. *Indian J Dermatol Venereol Leprol*. 2013;79(4):469-478.
11. Rosebush MS, Briody AN, Cordell KG. Black and brown: nonneoplastic pigmentation of the oral mucosa. *Head Neck Pathol*. 2019;13(1):47-55.
12. Leung AKC, Lam JM, Leong KF, Sergi CM. Melanonychia striata: clarifying behind the Black Curtain. A review on clinical evaluation and management of the 21st century. *Int J Dermatol*. Published online 2019:7.
13. Silpa-archa N, Kohli I, Chaowattanapanit S, Lim HW, Hamzavi I. Postinflammatory hyperpigmentation: A comprehensive overview. *J Am Acad Dermatol*. 2017;77(4):591-605.
14. Shenoy A, Madan R. Post-Inflammatory Hyperpigmentation: A Review of Treatment Strategies. 2020;19(8):6.
15. Park JY, Park JH, Kim SJ, et al. Two histopathological patterns of postinflammatory hyperpigmentation: epidermal and dermal. *J Cutan Pathol*. 2017;44(2):118-124.
16. Huerth KA, Hassan S, Callender VD. Therapeutic insights in melasma and hyperpigmentation management. *J Drugs Dermatol*. 2019;18(8):718-729.
17. Chaowattanapanit S, Silpa-archa N, Kohli I, Lim HW, Hamzavi I. Postinflammatory hyperpigmentation: A comprehensive overview. *J Am Acad Dermatol*. 2017;77(4):607-621.
18. Fatima S, Braunberger T, Mohammad TF, Kohli I, Hamzavi IH. The role of sunscreen in melasma and postinflammatory hyperpigmentation. *Indian J Dermatol*. 2020;65(1):5-10.

19. Passeron T, Picardo M. Melasma, a photoaging disorder. *Pigment Cell Melanoma Res.* 2018;31(4):461-465.

20. Shokeen D. Postinflammatory hyperpigmentation in patients with skin of color. *Cutis.* 2015;97:E9-E11.

21. Rajanala S. Melasma pathogenesis: a review of the latest research, pathological findings, and investigational therapies. *Dermatol Online J.* 25(10):7.

22. Ogbechie-Godec OA, Elbuluk N. Melasma: an up-to-date comprehensive review. *Dermatol Ther (Heidelb).* 2017;7(3):305-318.

23. Hexsel D, Lacerda DA, Cavalcante AS, et al. Epidemiology of melasma in Brazilian patients: A multicenter study. *Int J Dermatol.* 2014;53(4):440-444.

24. González-Saldivar G, Rodríguez-Gutiérrez R, Ocampo-Candiani J, González-González JG, Gómez-Flores M. Skin manifestations of insulin resistance: From a biochemical stance to a clinical diagnosis and management. *Dermatol Ther (Heidelb).* 2017;7(1):37-51.

25. Popa M-L, Popa AC, Tanase C, Gheorghisan-Galateanu A-A. Acanthosis nigricans: To be or not to be afraid. *Oncol Lett.* 2019;17(5):4133-4138.

26. Patel NU, Roach C, Alinia H, Huang WW, Feldman SR. Current treatment options for acanthosis nigricans. *Clin Cosmet Investig Dermatol.* 2018;11:407-413.

27. Barman B, Devi LP, Thakur BK, Raphael V. Tripe palms and acanthosis nigricans: a clue for diagnosis of advanced pancreatic adenocarcinoma. *Indian Dermatol Online J.* 2019;10(4):453-455.

28. Phiske MM. An approach to acanthosis nigricans. *Indian Dermatol Online J.* 2014;5(3):239-249.

29. Madu PN, Syder N, Elbuluk N. Postinflammatory hypopigmentation: a comprehensive review of treatments. *J Dermatolog Treat.* Published online July 20, 2020:1-5.

30. Saleem MD, Oussedik E, Picardo M, Schoch JJ. Acquired disorders with hypopigmentation: A clinical approach to diagnosis and treatment. *J Am Acad Dermatol.* 2019;80(5):1233-1250.e10.

31. Miazek N, Michalek I, Pawlowska-Kisiel M, Olszewska M, Rudnicka L. Pityriasis Alba—common disease, enigmatic entity: Up-to-date review of the literature. *Pediatr Dermato.* 2015;32(6):786-791.

32. Brown AE, Qiu CC, Drozd B, Sklover LR, Vickers CM, Hsu S. The color of skin: white diseases of the skin, nails, and mucosa. *Clin Dermatol.* 2019;37(5):561-579.

33. Prohic A, Sadikovic TJ, Krupalija-Fazlic M, Kuskunovic-Vlahovljak S. Malassezia species in healthy skin and in dermatological conditions. *Int J Dermatol.* 2016;55(5):494-504.

34. Kallini JR, Riaz F, Khachemoune A. Tinea versicolor in dark-skinned individuals. *Int J Dermatol.* 2014;53(2):137-141.

35. Moon SY, Lee WJ, Lee S-J, Kim DW, Jang YH. Pityriasis versicolor atrophicans: Is it true atrophy or pseudoatrophy?: Letter to the Editor. *J Cutan Pathol.* 2016;43(2):187-189.

36. Gupta A, Foley K. Antifungal treatment for pityriasis versicolor. *J Fungi.* 2015;1(1):13-29.

37. Kim SK, Kim EH, Kang HY, Lee E-S, Sohn S, Kim YC. Comprehensive understanding of idiopathic guttate hypomelanosis: clinical and histopathological correlation. *Int J Dermatol.* 2010;49(2):162-166.

38. Baldini E, Odorisio T, Sorrenti S, et al. Vitiligo and autoimmune thyroid disorders. *Front Endocrinol (Lausanne).* 2017;8.

39. Rashighi M, Harris JE. Vitiligo pathogenesis and emerging treatments. *Dermatol Clin.* 2017;35(2):257-265.

40. Bishnoi A, Parsad D. Clinical and molecular aspects of vitiligo treatments. *Int J Mol Sci.* 2018;19(5).

41. Spritz R, Andersen G. Genetics of vitiligo. *Dermatol Clin.* 2017;35(2):245-255.

42. Levai M. The relationship of pruritus and local skin conditions to the development of vitiligo. *Arch Dermatol.* 1958;78(3):372.

43. Vachiramon V, Onprasert W, Harnchoowong S, Chanprapaph K. Prevalence and clinical characteristics of itch in vitiligo and its clinical significance. *Biomed Res Int.* 2017;2017.

44. Alkhateeb A, Fain PR, Thody A, Bennett DC, Spritz RA. Epidemiology of vitiligo and associated autoimmune diseases in caucasian probands and their families. *Pigment Cell Res.* 2003;16(3):208-214.

45. Rodrigues M, Ezzedine K, Hamzavi I, Pandya AG, Harris JE. Current and emerging treatments for vitiligo. *J Am Acad Dermatol.* 2017;77(1):17-29.

46. Krüger C, Schallreuter K. Stigmatisation, avoidance behaviour and difficulties in coping are common among adult patients with vitiligo. *Acta Derm Venerol.* 2015;95(5):553-558. 1

47. Sawant NS, Vanjari NA, Khopkar U. Gender differences in depression, coping, stigma, and quality of life in patients of vitiligo. *Dermatol Res Pract.* 2019;2019:1-10.

48. Maymone MBC, Neamah HH, Wirya SA, et al. The impact of skin hyperpigmentation and hyperchromia on quality of life: A cross-sectional study. *J Am Acad Dermatol.* 2017;77(4):775-778.

49. Akinboro A, Ezejiofor OI, Olanrewaju FO, et al. The impact of acne and facial post-inflammatory hyperpigmentation on quality of life and self-esteem of newly admitted Nigerian undergraduates. *Clin Cosmet Investig Dermatol.* 2018;Volume 11:245-252.

50. Darji K, Varade R, West D, Armbrecht ES. Psychosocial impact of postinflammatory hyperpigmentation in patients with acne vulgaris. *J Clin Aesthet Dermatol.* 2017;10.

51. Pirgon Ö, Sandal G, Gökçen C, Bilgin H, Dündar B. Social anxiety, depression and self-esteem in obese adolescent girls with acanthosis nigricans. *J Clin Res Pediatr E.* 2015;7(1):63-68.

52. Andra C, Suwalska A, Dumitrescu AM, et al. A corrective cosmetic improves the quality of life and skin quality of subjects with facial blemishes caused by skin disorders. *Clin Cosmet Investig Dermatol.* 2020;Volume 13:253-257.

53. Chen T, Grau C, Suprun M, Silverberg NB. Vitiligo patients experience barriers in accessing care. *Cutis.* 2016;98:385-388.

54. Smith MP, Ly K, Thibodeaux Q, Bhutani T, Nakamura M. Home phototherapy for patients with vitiligo: challenges and solutions. *Clin Cosmet Investig Dermatol.* 2019;12:451-459.

55. Ezzedine K, Sheth V, Rodrigues M, et al. Vitiligo is not a cosmetic disease. *J Am Acad Dermatol.* 2015;73(5):883-885.

The Differential Diagnosis of Purpura

24

Nikifor K. Konstantinov
Ryan M. Wells

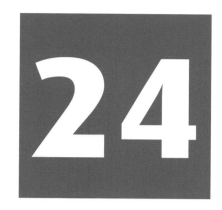

▼ INTRODUCTION TO CHAPTER

Purpura Key Points

- ✓ Purpura is caused by extravasation of red blood cells into the skin or mucous membranes due to disorders of blood vessels or some component or disorder of the hemopoietic system.
- ✓ Purpura can present as petechiae, ecchymosis, palpable lesions or retiform lesions.
- ✓ Purpura may be associated with serious diseases of several organ systems.
- ✓ A skin biopsy of a new lesion less than 2 days old and laboratory studies are usually needed to confirm the diagnosis of purpura and its underlying cause.

Purpura is extravasation of red blood cells into the skin or mucous membranes. For this reason, purpuric lesions do not blanch on diascopy (pressing on the lesion with a glass slide or finger). The differential diagnosis for purpura is broad, but it can be quickly narrowed by classifying the lesions based on their morphology, as well as other clinical and laboratory findings. A flowchart for the differential diagnosis of purpura is in Figure 24-1.

The clinical descriptive terms for purpura are listed below, and their respective tables describing the differential diagnosis are referenced.

- Petechiae: Flat lesions, macules ≤ 4 mm (Figure 24-2). Typically, initially bright red and then fade to a rust color (Tables 24-1 and 24-2).
- Ecchymosis: Flat lesions, macules and/or patches, >5 mm (Figure 24-3). Typically, initially red or purple, but may fade to yellow, brown, or green (Table 24-3).
- Palpable purpura: Elevated, round or oval, red or purple papules and/or plaques (Figure 24-4), sometimes barely palpable (Table 24-4).
- Retiform purpura: Stellate or branching lesions, with angular or geometric borders (Figure 24-5). These are often palpable plaques but can present as non-palpable patches as well (Tables 24-5 and Table 24- 6).

▼ EVALUATION

- A careful history and review of underlying medical conditions, medications, and a complete physical examination can be crucial to the diagnosis.
- Laboratory studies listed in the tables may assist with narrowing the differential.
- A skin biopsy is often necessary for further evaluation, at which time referral to a dermatologist is recommended. An optimal biopsy involves appropriate selection of the biopsy type, site, timing, and interpretation of results. At times, an additional biopsy needs to be done for direct immunofluorescence (DIF).
  - Indications for skin biopsy: Palpable and retiform purpura should prompt a skin biopsy. Other

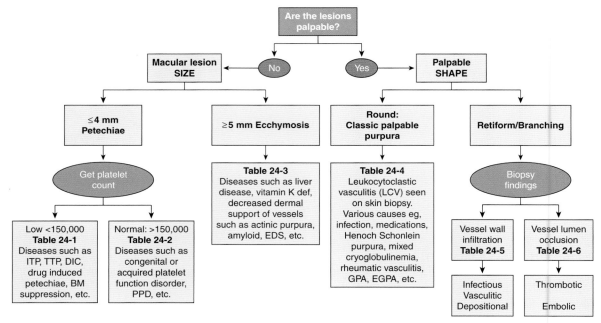

Figure 24-1. Flowchart for the differential diagnosis of purpura. BM, bone marrow; DIC disseminated intravascular coagulation; EDS, Ehlers-Danlos syndrome; EGPA, eosinophilic granulomatosis with polyangiitis; GPA, granulomaatosis with polyangiitis; ITP, immune thrombocytopenic purpura; PPD, pigmented purpuric dermatitis; TTP, Thrombotic thrombocytopenic purpura.

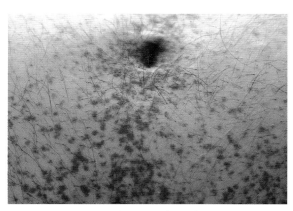

Figure 24-2. Petechiae. Bright red macules < 4 mm on abdomen.

indications include purpura whose cause cannot be determined by history, physical examination, and laboratory testing.

- Timing of biopsy: A new lesion less than 2 days old is ideal for biopsy. It is important to make note of the age of the lesion, as a disease process can appear different on histopathologic examination at various stages. For example, late stage leukocytoclastic vasculitis (LCV) and early micro-occlusive purpura can have similar histopathologic findings. It is important to let the pathologist reading the biopsy know how long the process has been present. Distinguishing between vasculitis and microocclusive disease is important because the two disorders require different treatments.

  - Biopsy for direct immunofluorescence (DIF): In addition to the standard 4 mm punch biopsy, an additional biopsy should be sent for DIF in Michel's medium if cutaneous small vessel vasculitis (CSVV) is in the differential. This is particularly useful early in the process of CSVV and can assist in the diagnosis of IgA-mediated diseases.

- Findings on biopsy: Vasculitis is characterized by inflammation within vessel walls, often leading to extravasation of red blood cells and fibrin deposition in vessel walls. Vasculitis that manifests on the skin is limited to involvement of vessels found in the dermis and/or subcutis. The size of the affected vessels may give clues to the diagnosis.

  - Small (e.g., Henoch-Schonlein purpura, acute hemorrhagic edema of infancy, urticarial vasculitis, mixed cryoglobulinemic vasculitis)
  - Small-medium (e.g., ANCA-associated vasculitides)
  - Medium (e.g., polyarteritis nodosa).

DIF findings can give additional information relating to the type of antibody visualized. For example, HSP demonstrates perivascular IgA deposition.

Table 24-1. Causes of petechiae (primary lesion is a macule ≤ 4mm) with platelets <150,000 μL

Disease/Disorder	Clinical Features and Associations	Initial Diagnostic Evaluation
Thrombocytopenia (<150,000/μL; though petechiae not usually observed until platelet count <50000/μL)	Mucocutaneous bleeding (e.g., epistaxis, increased bleeding with menses or minor cuts). Splenomegaly and lymphadenopathy may be present.	CBC with differential and peripheral smear; If anemic, check reticulocyte count, LDH, haptoglobin, bilirubin. If hemolysis is present, check PTT, PT/INR, fibrinogen, D-dimer, Coombs, ANA. If inconclusive, consider bone marrow biopsy.
Immune Thrombocytopenic Purpura (ITP)[10]	F>M. Primary: Insidious onset Secondary: Associated with underlying disease, for example, viral infections (HIV, HCV, CMV, VZV, Zika virus, *H. pylori*), or disorders of immune alteration (SLE, antiphospholipid syndrome, or lymphoproliferative disorders).	Platelets <100,000. Diagnosis of exclusion. Primary: Isolated decreased platelets. Secondary: May relate to viral process (can obtain serology for HIV, HCV, HBV, EBV or PCR for parvovirus and CMV), *H. pylori*, ANA, pregnancy, APLA, or TSH.
Thrombotic Thrombocytopenic Purpura (TTP)[1]	Pentad: thrombocytopenia, hemolytic anemia, changes in mental status, fever, renal dysfunction. Do not need all five for diagnosis. It may be idiopathic, familial, drug-induced, from pregnancy, HIV, autoimmune disease, or hematopoietic stem cell transplant. HUS: Thrombocytopenia, MAHA, and renal dysfunction; usually in children with prodrome of bloody diarrhea	Labs that can be observed: ↓Platelets and MAHA, schistocytes on peripheral smear, ↑reticulocyte count, positive hemolysis labs (↑LDH, ↑indirect bilirubin, ↓haptoglobin), normal PTT & INR, ↑creatinine, ↓ADAMSTS13 (in idiopathic TTP).
Disseminated Intravascular Coagulation (DIC)[14]	Spectrum in hematologic abnormalities can have bleeding and/or thrombosis. May also have soft-tissue bleeding in muscles and joints. May be related to trauma, shock, infection, malignancy, obstetric complication.	↑PT/INR, ↑PTT, ↓fibrinogen, Positive fibrin degradation product/D-dimer and hemolysis labs.
Drug-induced[1]	Petechiae, purpura due to drugs such as quinine, trimethoprim-sulfamethoxazole	Generally isolated thrombocytopenia.
Bone marrow suppression[1]	Associated with aplastic anemia, MDS, drugs (e.g., thiazides and antibiotics), alcohol, cirrhosis, myelofibrosis, granulomas from infections, hematologic, or solid malignancies.	Peripheral smear may show pancytopenia, blasts, hypersegmented neutrophils, leukoerythroblastic changes (teardrop cells, nucleated RBCs, immature WBCs).

CBC, complete blood count; LDH, lactate dehydrogenase; PTT, partial thromboplastin time; PT/INR, prothrombin time/international normalized ratio; ANA, antinuclear antibody; bx, biopsy; F, female; M, male; HIV, human immunodeficiency virus; HCV, hepatitis C virus; HBV, hepatitis B virus; EBV, Epstein-Barr virus ; PCR, polymerase chain reaction; CMV, cytomegalovirus; H. pylori, Helicobacter pylori; APLA, anti-phospholipid antibody; dx, diagnosis; MAHA, microangiopathic hemolytic anemia; TSH, thyroid stimulating hormone; ADAMTS13, a disintegrin and metalloproteinase with a thrombospondin type 1 motif, member 13; HUS, hemolytic uremic syndrome; MDS, myelodysplastic syndrome; RBC, red blood cells; WBC, white blood cells

Table 24-2. Causes of Petechiae (primary lesion is a macule ≤4 mm), with normal to high platelets (>150,000/μL)

Disease/Disorder	Clinical Features and Associations	Initial Diagnostic Evaluation
Platelet Function Disorder[15, 16]	Mucocutaneous bleeding	Look for splenomegaly and LAD. Labs: CBC with differential, peripheral smear, BUN, creatinine, LFTs and platelet aggregation tests. If suspect vWD or dysproteinemia, obtain vWF studies or SPEP/UPEP, respectively.
Congenital or Inherited[15]	vWD: Usually AD	vWD: ↓vW factor, ↓vWF activity (measured by ristocetin co-factor assay) ↓factor VIII, confirm with vWF multimer analysis.

(continued)

Table 24-2. Causes of Petechiae (primary lesion is a macule ≤4 mm), with normal to high platelets (>150,000/μL) (Continued)

Disease/Disorder	Clinical Features and Associations	Initial Diagnostic Evaluation
Acquired (e.g., drug-induced, liver disease, uremia, dysproteinemia, acquired vWD)[15]	Associated medications include: ASA, NSAIDS, clopidogrel, ticlopidine. Acquired vWD may be associated with malignancy, autoimmune disease, hypothyroidism, or drugs	Liver disease may show abnormal LFTs or ↑PT/INR, ↑PTT. Uremia will show ↑BUN. Dysproteinemias will show abnormalities on SPEP/UPEP.
Thrombocytosis secondary to myelofibrosis[16]	Myelofibrosis may be primary or secondary to other malignancy. Massive splenomegaly, +/- fatigue, weight loss, fever.	Peripheral smear shows leukoerythroblastic changes and bone marrow biopsy shows a "dry tap" with severe fibrosis.
No Platelet Abnormality		
Pigmented purpuric eruptions, capillaritis	Clustered petechial hemorrhage, often with a background of yellow brown discoloration often on lower extremities. Most common in middle aged to older men, for example, Schamberg's disease, 'cayenne pepper' appearance (Figure 24-6).	No systemic findings. A biopsy may be needed to differentiate lesions from vasculitis.
Hypergamma globulinemic purpura of Waldenstrom	Often in women, with recurrent crops of petechiae/purpura on lower extremities that burn/sting. Primary or secondary to autoimmune disease (e.g., Sjogren's or SLE), RA, less likely hematologic malignancy.	Hypergammaglobulinemia on SPEP. ↑titer of IgG or IgA RF (standard RF tests only detect IgM RF). ↑ESR. +/- positive ANA, Anti Ro, Anti La.
Intravascular, local pressure, or trauma	Can be caused by valsalva (e.g., from vomiting or constipation) or blood pressure cuff.	Can occur without an underlying lab abnormality.

LAD, lymphadenopathy; CBC, complete blood count; BUN, blood urea nitrogen; LFT's, liver function tests ; vWD, Von Willebrand disease; vWF, Von Willebrand factor; SPEP/UPEP, serum protein electrophoresis/urine protein electrophoresis; AD, autosomal dominant; ASA, aspirin; NSAIDs non-steroidal anti-inflammatory drugs; PT/INR, prothrombin time/international normalized ratio ; SLE, systemic lupus erythematosus; RA, rheumatoid arthritis; RF, rheumatoid factor; ANA, anti-nuclear antibody; ESR, erythrocyte sedimentation rate

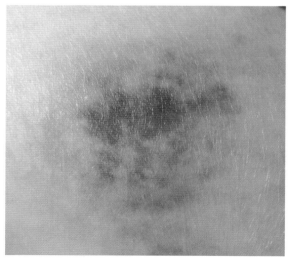

▲ **Figure 24-3.** Ecchymosis. Resolving purpura leaving red, purple, blue, and yellow patch.

The presence of granulomas also narrows the differential. Microgranulomas with an eosinophilic infiltrate are found in eosinophilic granulomatosis with polyangiitis (EGPA; previously called Churg-Strauss disease), necrotizing granulomatous inflammation of the vessel in granulomatosis with polyangiitis (GPA; formally called Wegener's disease), and necrotizing pauci-immune inflammation in microscopic polyangiitis (MPA).

In chilblains, lymphocytic vasculitis with edema and thickening of dermal vessel wall is seen.

Retiform purpura without inflammation generally reveals bland thrombi with no inflammation of vessel wall. Other retiform purpuras can have specific features, for example, cryoglobulinemia shows periodic acid-Schiff (PAS) stain positive hyaline intramural deposits, cholesterol emboli show needle-shaped clefts, and oxalate crystal emboli show yellow-gray birefringent crystals in the subcutis and vessel walls.[2] A skin biopsy for calciphylaxis shows calcification of small and medium vessels.

Below, we describe a more in-depth approach to two important categories of purpura—palpable purpura and retiform purpura; both of which may be signs of important underlying disease processes.

Table 24-3. Causes of Ecchymosis (primary lesion is a macule ≥ 5 mm)

Disease/Disorder	Clinical Features and Associations	Initial Diagnostic Evaluation
Procoagulant Defects[1]	Susceptible to having deeper bleeding into soft tissue.	↑PT/INR, +/- ↑PTT.
Anticoagulant	E.g., warfarin.	↑PT/INR.
Liver disease	History of alcohol abuse, hepatitis, primary liver disease.	↑PT/INR, ↑PTT, abnormal LFTs
Vitamin K deficiency	State of malnutrition (e.g., alcoholic), malabsorption (e.g., from antibiotics), liver disease.	↑PT/INR.
DIC	See Table 24-1	
Platelet Disorders	See Table 24-1	
Decreased Dermal Support of Vessels and Minor Trauma[1]		
Solar or senile purpura	Older age and sun damaged skin usually on forearms.	None
Corticosteroid therapy (systemic and topical)	Cushing's syndrome stigmata (e.g., central obesity, dorsocervical fat pad, moon facies). Skin may reveal atrophy and telangiectasia.	None
Scurvy (vitamin C deficiency)	Diet lacking in vitamin C. Perifollicular hemorrhage, cork-screw hairs, gingival bleeding, and tooth loss.	↓Serum ascorbic acid deficiency and possibly other vitamins (e.g., B12 and folate).
Systemic Amyloidosis	All have hepatosplenomegaly, GI involvement (diarrhea, protein loss) and macroglossia. May also have cardiac, renal, and liver involvement. Periorbital waxy ecchymotic papules, purpura with minor trauma, 'pinch-purpura'.	SPEP/UPEP and free light chain, +/- bone marrow bx. CBC with differential, LFTs, BUN, creatinine, urinalysis, and EKG. Biopsy of abdominal subcutis fat pad reveals apple-green birefringence on Congo red stain. Consider genetic testing for hereditary form.
Genetic Disease with collagen or elastin defects	Ehlers-Danlos Syndrome: stretchable skin and flexible joints, usually AD inheritance. Pseudoxanthoma elasticum: appearance of 'plucked chicken skin' on neck.	Genetic testing for specific mutations depending on the suspected condition.

SPEP/UPEP, serum protein electrophoresis/urine protein electrophoresis ; PT/INR, prothrombin time/international normalized ratio; PTT, partial thromboplastin time; GI, gastrointestinal; bx, biopsy; CBC, complete blood count; LFTs liver function tests; BUN, blood urea nitrogen; EKG, electrocardiogram; AD, autosomal dominant

APPROACH TO PALPABLE PURPURA

Palpable purpura presents with round to ovoid, red or purple papules and or plaques that may sometimes be only subtly palpable to the astute clinician. There is a broad differential for palpable purpura with some etiologies being relatively benign and others representing more serious systemic illness that require additional workup and systemic therapies. Etiology of palpable purpura can be divided into conditions that primarily affect cutaneous small vessels and those that can affect a mix of small- and medium-sized vessels. Those conditions that affect both small and medium vessels can have a spectrum of presentation that ranges from palpable purpura to retiform or stellate purpura.

Cutaneous small vessel vasculitis (CSVV) is characterized histologically by leukocytoclastic vasculitis (LCV) that primarily affects small postcapillary venules in the dermis. LCV is defined by neutrophilic inflammation of the blood vessels with large amounts of nuclear breakdown with associated debris (leukocytoclasis). Cutaneous small vessel vasculitis most often presents clinically as palpable purpura, however, there are subclasses of CSVV that tend to present with other features besides palpable purpura which will not be discussed in this section. For example, urticarial vasculitis presents with urticarial plaques, acute hemorrhagic edema of infancy presents abruptly with large red patches or urticarial plaques that may evolve, and erythema elevatum diutinum presents as violaceous, red-brown or yellowish papules, plaques and nodules on extensor surfaces.

Cutaneous small vessel vasculitis that primarily presents as palpable purpura can be grouped into either primary CSVV or secondary CSVV. Approximately 50% of all cases of secondary CSVV are idiopathic and an underlying cause is never identified. Infection (15–20%), autoimmune connective tissue diseases (AI-CTD) (15–20%), drugs (10–15%), and underlying neoplasm (5%) are the most common known causes of secondary CSVV. Treatment of

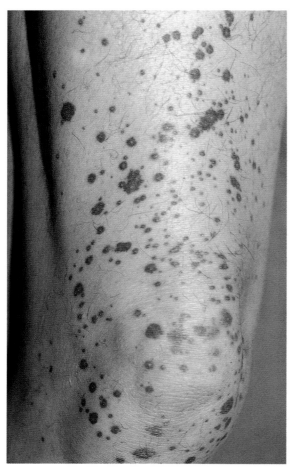

Figure 24-4. Palpable purpura. Multiple red papules on leg of patient with Henoch-Schönlein Purpura.

above consists of supportive measures, discontinuation of the offending agent in the case of drug associated CSVV, and treatment of the underlying AI-CTD, infection, or neoplasm.[1–4]

Primary causes of cutaneous small vessel vasculitis that typically present as palpable purpura include Henoch-Schönlein Purpura (HSP), also known as IgA vasculitis, and type II and III cryoglobulinemia (also called mixed cryoglobulinemic vasculitis). HSP is the most common form of vasculitis in children less than 10 years of age and has a reported incidence of 30–270 per million children per year.[5–7] It has a bimodal distribution related to age and can also affect older adults, although at approximately half the incidence seen in children. There is seasonal fluctuation in the number of cases with peaks occurring in the fall and winter which is likely due to its association with the preceding infection. Upper respiratory tract infections are the most common preceding infection associated with HSP

and typically occur 1–2 weeks prior to onset of palpable purpura. HSP results from IgA-containing immune complexes that deposit in tissue leading to a robust inflammatory response. HSP affects the skin, musculoskeletal system with arthritis/arthralgias, gastrointestinal system with abdominal pain and rarely intussusception, and renal system with acute renal failure. In boys, HSP can cause orchitis and scrotal edema. In adults, palpable purpura tend to progress to necrotic lesions in 60% of patients, whereas this only occurs in < 5% of children.[6] Adults are much more susceptible to developing chronic renal failure and it is unclear if this is related to their baseline lower kidney function in older adults or if it is an inherent difference of the HSP disease process in adults.[6]

Cryoglobulinemia II and III (mixed cryoglobulins) are due to monoclonal and polyclonal cold-precipitable immunoglobulins that can result in vasculitis that typically affects the skin, peripheral nervous system, and kidneys. Cryoglobulinemia varies due to geography and there is a higher prevalence in Southern Europe than compared with Northern Europe and North America. There is an association with cryoglobulinemia II and III with the viral hepatitides, with HCV having the highest association (70–90% of cases of cryoglobulinemia).[8]

Mixed small- and medium-sized vessel vasculitides (including the ANCA-associated vasculitides microscopic polyangiitis, granulomatosis with polyangiitis, and eosinophilic granulomatosis with polyangiitis) can also result in palpable purpura. As mentioned earlier, these etiologies can result in a clinical spectrum of presentations from palpable purpura to retiform purpura.

APPROACH TO RETIFORM PURPURA

Retiform purpura is characterized by non-blanching purpuric patches that are arranged in a branching or reticular pattern.[9] These lesions may also ulcerate or develop necrosis. The ability to recognize retiform purpura and diagnose the underlying disease process is of utmost importance, as this skin pattern is often a sign of serious illness that may warrant rapid treatment.

Retiform purpura may be confused with livedo reticularis and livedo racemosa. Although all three patterns result from disorders of vascular etiology and have a reticulate pattern, there are notable differences. Livedo reticularis is characterized by patches arranged in complete rings that result from partial or intermittent reduction of blood flow.[10] Livedo racemosa may look similar; however, the patches are more irregular, broken, and do not form complete rings. This is due to more significant reduction of blood flow. These morphologies do not usually become necrotic or ulcerate, as in retiform purpura.[11]

Retiform purpura results from disorders that either 1) cause vessel wall damage, or 2) cause vessel lumen occlusion. Retiform purpura due to vessel wall damage occurs from depositional disease (e.g., calciphylaxis), severe

Table 25-4. Causes of palpable purpura, inflammatory

Disease/Disorder	Clinical Features and Associations	Initial Diagnostic Evaluation
Cutaneous Small Vessel Vasculitis[2-4]	**Purpuric papules or plaques typically on distal legs or dependent areas.**	Skin biopsy for routine histology and another for DIF.
Idiopathic (IgG, IgM, or IgA), secondary to drugs or infection	May appear targetoid.	In addition to skin biopsies, careful review of medications and recent/current infections.
Henoch-Schönlein Purpura (Figure 24-4)	M>F. Usually age <20 years. Tetrad: Purpura (universal), arthritis (82%), nephritis (40%), abdominal pain (63%) or gastrointestinal hemorrhage (33%). May appear targetoid, on extensor areas and buttock. Extension to trunk/upper extremities can indicate renal involvement.	Two skin biopsies should be done, one for routine histology and one for DIF.
Urticarial vasculitis	Persistence of hive-like lesions>24 hours, often burn> itch. Can have concomitant systemic symptoms (e.g., LAD, arthralgia, angioedema, fever). Can be caused by drug (e.g., ACE inhibitors, penicillin, and sulfonamides), autoimmune disease, hematologic or other malignancies, and infections.	In addition to skin biopsies, the following lab findings may be helpful: ↓Complement (e.g., CH50, C4, C3, Clq) may relate to a variety of systemic processes, e.g., SLE, malignancy, infection. Creatinine and UA. For suspected infection screen for HBV, HCV, and heterophile serology. For suspected autoimmune condition screen with autoantibody test.
Mixed cryoglobulinemic vasculitis[8] (Type II and III)	Usually acral distribution. Weakness, livedo reticularis, leg ulcers, HSM, Raynaud's phenomenon. Can also have glomerulonephritis and peripheral neuropathy.	In addition to skin biopsies, the following labs may be helpful: Cryoglobulins (proteins that precipitate from serum or plasma when cooled). Type II: Sjogren's, SLE evaluation. Type III: Hepatitis C RNA, ESR, C4, RF.
Rheumatic Vasculitis (e.g., RA, SLE, Sjogren's syndrome)	Digital ischemia, livedo reticularis, pericarditis, bowel ischemia, peripheral neuropathy.	In addition to skin biopsies, the following lab findings may be helpful: +ANA and ↓complement (SLE) +RF, Anti-CCP (RA) +ANA, RF, Anti-Ro or La (Sjogren's).
Anti-Neutrophil Cytoplasmic Antibody (ANCA) Associated		
Granulomatosis with polyangiitis (Wegener's granulomatosis)	Usually young and middle-aged adults. Can have a nasal or oral (e.g., sinusitis, saddle-nose deformity), pulmonary (e.g., infiltrate, diffuse alveolar hemorrhage, nodule, cavity), or renal involvement (hematuria, RBC casts).	In addition to skin biopsies, +ANCA (90%), c-ANCA (anti-PR3).
Eosinophilic granulomatosis with polyangiitis (Churg-Strauss syndrome)	Usually age 30–40 years, with HLA-DRB4. Can also involve lungs (e.g., asthma), peripheral nerves, heart, and kidneys.	In addition to skin biopsies, CBC with differential, showing eosinophilia. +ANCA (50%), p-ANCA (anti-MPO) or c-ANCA (anti-PR3).
Microscopic polyangiitis	Can involve the kidney and lungs.	In addition to skin biopsies, +ANCA (70%), p-ANCA (anti-MPO).

DIF, direct immunofluorescence; LAD, lymphadenopathy; SLE, systemic lupus erythematosus; CH50, total hemolytic complement; C, complement; Cr, creatinine; UA, urinalysis; HBV, hepatitis B virus; HCV,hepatitis C virus; HSM, hepatosplenomegaly; RNA, ribonucleic acid; ESR, erythrocyte sedimentation rate; RF, rheumatoid factor; PAS, Periodic acid-Schiff stain; RA, rheumatoid arthritis; ANA, antinuclear antibody; anti-CCP, anti-citrullinated protein; c/p ANCA, cytoplasmic/peri-nuclear anti-neutrophil cytoplasmic antibodies; CBC, complete blood count; RBC, red blood cells; PR 3, proteinase 3; MPO, myeloperoxidase

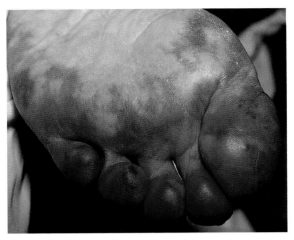

▲ **Figure 24-5.** Retiform purpura. Purpura on toes with retiform pattern on foot in patient with cholesterol emboli.

infections (e.g., angioinvasive fungal infections), or certain vasculitides (e.g., polyarteritis nodosa). Embolic disorders (e.g., septic emboli) or thrombotic disorders (e.g., due to hypercoagulable states) fall within the spectrum of vessel lumen occlusion (Tables 24-5 and 24-6, adapted and modified from Georgesen et al.).[11]

When approaching a patient in whom retiform purpura is suspected, knowledge of the chronicity of the lesions is paramount. Patients that develop retiform purpura require rapid diagnosis and often empiric treatment for the severe underlying conditions mentioned earlier, particularly if any concern for infection. A punch biopsy for hematoxylin and eosin stain (H&E) should be performed at the border of the purpuric rim. The clinician should have a low threshold to obtain a second punch biopsy (usually from the center of the lesion) for tissue culture of bacteria, acid-fast bacteria, and fungal organisms. Laboratory workup and imaging should be tailored based on the suspected underlying etiology, but in the severely ill patients, diagnostic workup is appropriate.

Table 24-5. Causes of retiform purpura due to vessel wall damage[11]

Disease/Disorder	Clinical Features and Associations	Initial Diagnostic Evaluation
Infections		
Angioinvasive Fungal Infections[17] (e.g., *Aspergillus, Fusarium,* and Zygomycetes)	Acute, rapidly evolving, often fatal infections, due to vasculotropic invasive mycoses. Primary inoculation can occur in children and immunocompetent adults. Disseminated disease is usually seen in the immunosuppressed. Besides retiform purpura morphology, a targetoid, or "bull's eye" dusky purpuric patch may occur.	Biopsy for H&E and tissue culture (can consider touch prep for more rapid preliminary diagnosis). Blood cultures and biologic markers such as galactomannan *Aspergillus* antigen and (1-3)-beta-D-glucan (fungal wall component). CT imaging of chest, sinus and brain should be considered.
Ecthyma Gangrenosum[18]	Classically occurs secondary to *Pseudomonas aeruginosa* sepsis in immunocompromised patients, but can occur due to fungal infections (*Aspergillus* and *Candida*) or gram-positive organisms (Staphylococcus aureus); usually with bacteremia or fungemia.	CBC with differential. Blood and urine cultures. Skin biopsy from ulcer edge and tissue culture (from more central portion). Imaging may be indicated if concern for deeper soft tissue infection.
Meningococcemia[19]	*Neisseria meningitidis* is a gram-negative bacterium which causes meningitis and rapidly progressive sepsis, high mortality without prompt treatment. Patients with asplenia, immunodeficiency or C5-C9 complement deficiency are at increased risk.	CBC with differential. Coagulation studies for DIC (platelets, PT/INR, aPTT, fibrinogen, D-dimer). Lumbar puncture with gram stain and culture; PCR testing of plasma or CSF when available. Blood cultures.
Strongyloides[20]	Caused by *S. stercoralis* (endemic to Africa, Asia, SE Asia, Central and South America). Variable clinical presentation. Purpuric form characterized by retiform purpura typically involving trunk and proximal extremities with classic "thumbprint" appearance.	CBC w/ differential (peripheral eosinophilia may be seen). Stool O&P, Strongyloides IgM and IgG, HIV.

(continued)

Table 24-5. Causes of retiform purpura due to vessel wall damage[11] (Continued)

Disease/Disorder	Clinical Features and Associations	Initial Diagnostic Evaluation
Vasculitis		
Small or small/medium vessel vasculitis (i.e., IgA vasculitis, ANCA vasculitis, cryoglobulinemia (type II, III), cocaine-levamisole vasculopathy/ vasculitis, leukemic vasculitis, rheumatic vasculitis)	See Table 24-4.	Punch biopsy for H&E and DIF (if palpable purpura in morphology). Labs: should be tailored to suspect cause.
Medium vessel vasculitis[1, 21,22] (e.g., Polyarteritis Nodosa)	Males more affected than females in classic PAN, but cutaneous PAN may be more common in female. Age ~50 years. Can have palpable subcutis nodules (Figure 24-7). Often multisystemic (e.g., constitutional, renal, abdominal pain, livedo reticularis, peripheral neuropathies). Associated with HBV.	Rule out other systemic vasculitis (CBC, creatinine, UA, ANA, ANCA, RF, complement levels, cryoglobulins). Hepatitis B/C serologies, HIV, and ASO titers/throat culture in children (to rule out strep infection). Punch biopsy (larger sample preferred to have adequate subcutaneous tissue). Additional workup may include angiography, CXR, EMG.
Depositional		
Calciphylaxis[23, 24]	Frequently fatal disorder of progressive vascular calcification that results in skin and soft tissue necrosis. Commonly occurs in patients with ESRD, but a nonuremic variant also exists. Lesions are painful that may lead to necrotic ulceration. Occurs in areas with increased adiposity.	Deep and large skin biopsy to get adequate sample. Lab workup: CMP, PTH (hypercoagulable workup and vasculitis workup may be indicated to exclude alternative causes).
Oxalosis[25]	Acral distribution, can cause nephrolithiasis, nephrocalcinosis, AKI, CKD, and ESRD.	Skin biopsy. Serum/urine oxalates.

H&E, Hematoxylin and eosin; CT, computed tomography; CBC, complete blood count; DIC, disseminated intravascular coagulation; PT/INR, prothrombin/international normalized ratio; aPTT, activated partial thromboplastin time; PCR, polymerase chain reaction; CSF, cerebrospinal fluid; O&P, ova and parasites; PAN, polyarteritis nodosa; HBV, hepatitis B virus; DIF, direct immunofluorescence; UA, urinalysis; ANA, anti-nuclear antibody; ANCA, anti-neutrophil cytoplasmic antibodies; RF, rheumatoid factor; ASO, anti-streptolysin O; CXR, chest-x-ray; EMG, electromyography; CMP, comprehensive metabolic panel; PTH, parathyroid hormone; AKI, acute kidney injury; CKD, chronic kidney disease; ESRD, end-stage renal disease

Table 24-6. Causes of retiform purpura due to vessel lumen occlusion[11]

Disease/Disorder	Clinical Features and Associations	Initial Diagnostic Evaluation
Thrombosis from Platelet Occlusion[1, 14, 16, 26]		In addition to a skin biopsy, the following lab findings may be helpful.
Heparin necrosis (from heparin or low molecular weight heparin), Heparin-induced thrombocytopenia (HIT), type II[26]	Often on the abdomen>extremities. Lesions may be distant sites or sites of heparin infusion or injection. New venous or arterial thrombus (venous>arterial). Onset 4-10 days after treatment or <24 hours if drug used within 100 days. Post-op highest risk. Type I is with platelets >100,000/µL and benign course.	CBC (Platelets <100,000/µL or >50% drop from original with a + HIT antibody).
Thrombocytosis, from myeloproliferative disorder[16]	See Table 24- 2.	
Paroxysmal nocturnal hemoglobinuria (PNH)	Complement-mediated hemolytic anemia, hypercoagulability state, smooth muscle dystonia, cytopenia, aplastic anemia, MDS, evolution to AML, Budd-Chiari syndrome.	CBC with differential and flow cytometry, showing ↓CD55 and CD59. Urine hemosiderosis.

(continued)

Table 24-6. Causes of retiform purpura due to vessel lumen occlusion[11] (Continued)

Disease/Disorder	Clinical Features and Associations	Initial Diagnostic Evaluation
TTP	See Table 24-1	
Cold-related gelling or agglutination[1] (e.g., cryoglobulinemia, cold agglutinins)	See Table 24 4. In addition, cryoglobulinemia Type I (monoclonal) is associated with multiple myeloma and Waldenstrom's macroglobulinemia. Cold agglutinins in adults is associated with lymphoproliferative disease and in children infections (e.g., *Mycoplasma* pneumonia, mononucleosis, and HIV).	
Thrombosis from systemic coagulopathies[1, 9, 21, 27]		
Inherited hypercoagulable states	Venous or arterial thrombi, miscarriages in women.	↑PT/INR, PTT. Protein C and S, antithrombin III, prothrombin 20210A, factor V Leiden mutation.
Warfarin necrosis[1]	Onset 1–10 days after exposure. Large irregular bullae with eventual necrosis on breasts, buttocks, thighs and penile skin. More common in obese women or those with underlying hypercoagulopathy (e.g., protein C or S or ATIII deficiency). May be post-infectious. May have purpura fulminans.	Non-specific.
Purpura fulminans[1, 28]	Dermatologic emergency characterized by acute onset retiform purpura (Figure 24-8). Predilection for buttocks and lower extremities. 3 types: 1. Neonatal purpura fulminans (due to hereditary deficiency in protein C or S). 2. Acquired purpura fulminans- most commonly 1–2 weeks after Group A Streptococcal or varicella infection. 3. Acute infectious purpura fulminans- associated with bacteremia and DIC (refer to Table 24-1).	↑PT/INR, PTT, D-dimer, fibrin degradation products ↓fibrinogen, platelets. Bacteria cultures may be positive. Peripheral smear shows schistocytes.
Antiphospholipid Antibody Syndrome[1, 21, 29] (APLS)	Characterized by venous and/or arterial thrombosis (Figure 24-9). Usually presents in women <40. May have history of spontaneous abortions. APLS may be primary or secondary. Secondary APLS associated with SLE (40–50% of SLE patients) malignancy, infection, or drugs.	+Anti-cardiolipin or β2-glycoprotein antibodies. +Lupus anti-coagulant (↑PTT). Can check dRVVT.
Thrombosis from Reticulocytes		
Sickle Cell Disease	Can have symptoms of anemia from chronic hemolysis, infections with encapsulated organism from infracting spleen, osteomyelitis from infracting bone, and pain crisis.	CBC shows anemia. Sickle shaped RBCs or Howell-Jolly bodies on peripheral smear. Hemoglobin electrophoresis.
Occlusion from Emboli[1]		
Cholesterol	Males > females. Acral distribution. Arterial or cardiac catheter, prolonged anticoagulation, acute thrombolytic therapy, atherosclerosis, hypertension, tobacco use are risk factors. Can be multi-systemic.	In addition to characteristic skin biopsy findings, CBC with differential, showing eosinophilia. Other lab abnormalities will depend on affected organ.
Endocarditis/septic emboli	Associated with IV drug use and prosthetic valves. Stigmata include Osler's nodes, Janeway lesions, and splinter hemorrhages.	Blood cultures, EKG. Transthoracic and/ or transesophageal echocardiogram.

HIT, heparin-induced thrombocytopenia; CBC, complete blood count; MDS, myelodysplastic syndrome; PT/INR, prothrombin time/international normalized ratio; PTT, partial thromboplastin time; DIC, disseminated intravascular coagulation; APLS, anti-phospholipid syndrome; SLE, systemic lupus erythematosus; RBCs red blood cells; dRVVT, dilute Russell's viper venom time

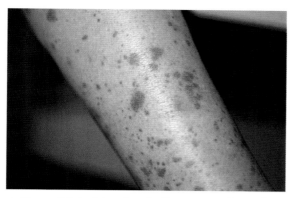

▲ **Figure 24-6.** Schamberg's disease. Macules and patches of petechial hemorrhage on lower leg.

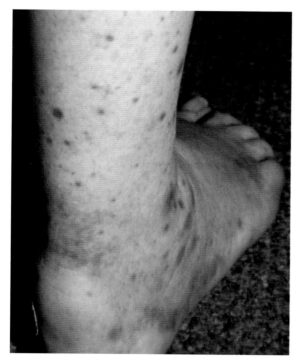

▲ **Figure 24-7.** Polyarteritis nodosa. Painful palpable purpura on legs with depressed areas at sites of healing "punched- out" ulcers.

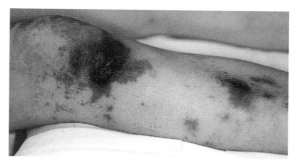

▲ **Figure 24-8.** Purpura fulminans. Retiform purpura on knee and shin with areas of early necrosis.

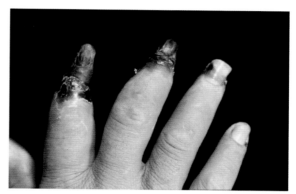

▲ **Figure 24-9.** Purpura in antiphospholipid antibody syndrome. Purpura with necrosis of the fingertips in woman with systemic lupus erythematosus.

PURPURIC MANIFESTATIONS OF COVID-19

Toward the end of 2019, the novel Severe Acute Respiratory Syndrome Coronavirus-2 (SARS-CoV-2) was first reported and subsequently spread worldwide, resulting in the Coronavirus Disease (COVID)-19 pandemic. The cutaneous manifestations of COVID-19 are diverse and include variably distributed erythema, chilblain-like lesions, urticaria, a vesicular eruption, petechiae, livedo reticularis, retiform purpura, and necrosis.[12] Although the pathogenesis is not completely understood, severely ill patients with this virus present with coagulopathy and disseminated intravascular coagulation (DIC)-like intravascular clot formation, so it is hypothesized that an occlusive phenomenon may result in at least some of the purpuric skin findings.[13] Recognizing the skin manifestations of COVID-19 may play a pivotal role in diagnosis, particularly for otherwise asymptomatic patients and may provide further insights on the pathogenesis of this deadly virus.

REFERENCES

1. Piette WW. The differential diagnosis of purpura from a morphologic perspective. *Adv Dermatol.* 1994;9:3-23; discussion 24.
2. Sunderkötter C, Sindrilaru A. Clinical classification of vasculitis. *Eur J Dermatol.* 2006 Mar-Apr 2006;16(2):114-24.
3. Carlson JA, Chen KR. Cutaneous vasculitis update: small vessel neutrophilic vasculitis syndromes. *Am J Dermatopathol.* Dec 2006;28(6):486-506.

4. Gonzalez-Gay MA, Garcia-Porrua C, Salvarani C, Lo Scocco G, Pujol RM. Cutaneous vasculitis: a diagnostic approach. *Clin Exp Rheumatol.* 2003 Nov-Dec 2003;21(6 Suppl 32): S85-8.

5. Penny K, Fleming M, Kazmierczak D, Thomas A. An epidemiological study of Henoch-Schönlein purpura. *Paediatr Nurs.* Dec 2010;22(10):30-5.

6. Watts RA, Scott DG. Epidemiology of the vasculitides. *Semin Respir Crit Care Med.* Oct 2004;25(5):455-64.

7. Gardner-Medwin JM, Dolezalova P, Cummins C, Southwood TR. Incidence of Henoch-Schönlein purpura, Kawasaki disease, and rare vasculitides in children of different ethnic origins. *Lancet.* Oct 2002;360(9341):1197-202.

8. Cacoub P, Comarmond C, Domont F, Savey L, Saadoun D. Cryoglobulinemia Vasculitis. *Am J Med.* Sep 2015;128(9):950-5.

9. Weinstein S, Piette W. Cutaneous manifestations of antiphospholipid antibody syndrome. *Hematol Oncol Clin North Am.* Feb 2008;22(1):67-77.

10. McCrae K. Immune thrombocytopenia: no longer 'idiopathic'. *Cleve Clin J Med.* Jun 2011;78(6):358-73.

11. Georgesen C, Fox LP, Harp J. Retiform purpura: A diagnostic approach. *J Am Acad Dermatol.* Apr 2020;82(4):783-796.

12. Zhao Q, Fang X, Pang Z, Zhang B, Liu H, Zhang F. COVID-19 and cutaneous manifestations: A systematic review. *J Eur Acad Dermatol Venereol.* Jun 2020.

13. Iba T, Levy JH, Levi M, Thachil J. Coagulopathy in COVID-19. *J Thromb Haemost.* Jun 2020;

14. Kitchens CS. Thrombocytopenia and thrombosis in disseminated intravascular coagulation (DIC). *Hematology Am Soc Hematol Educ Program.* 2009:240-6.

15. Nichols WL, Hultin MB, James AH, et al. von Willebrand disease (VWD): evidence-based diagnosis and management guidelines, the National Heart, Lung, and Blood Institute (NHLBI) Expert Panel report (USA). *Haemophilia.* Mar 2008;14(2):171-232.

16. Tefferi A. Polycythemia vera and essential thrombocythemia: 2012 update on diagnosis, risk stratification, and management. *Am J Hematol.* Mar 2012;87(3):285-93

17. Stephen S. Angioinvasive Fungal Infections. In: Rosenbach M, Wanat KA, Micheletti RG, Taylor LA, eds. *Inpatient Dermatology.* 1st ed. Springer International Publishing AG; 2018:193-197:chap Angioinvasive Fungal Infections.

18. Stewart CL. Ecthyma Gangrenosum. In: Rosenbach M, Wanat KA, Micheletti RG, Taylor LA, eds. *Inpatient Dermatology.* 1st ed. Springer International Publishing AG; 2018:119-121:chap Echthyma Gangrenosum.

19. Stewart CL. Meningococcal Infection. In: Rosenbach M, Wanat KA, Micheletti RG, Taylor LA, eds. *Inpatient Dermatology.* 1st ed. Springer International Publishing AG; 2018:127-129:chap Meningococcal Infection.

20. Suh K, Keystone J. Helminthic Infections. In: Kang S, Amagai M, Bruckner A, et al, eds. *Fitzpatrick's Dermatology 9th Edition.* McGraw Hill Education; 2019:3271-3272:chap Helminthic Infections.

21. Khenifer S, Thomas L, Balme B, Dalle S. Livedoid vasculopathy: thrombotic or inflammatory disease? *Clin Exp Dermatol.* Oct 2010;35(7):693-8.

22. Noe MH. Polyarteritis Nodosa. In: Rosenbach M, Wanat KA, Micheletti RG, Taylor LA, eds. *Inpatient Dermatology.* Springer International Publishing AG; 2018:251-255:chap Polyarteritis Nodosa.

23. Mathur RV, Shortland JR, el-Nahas AM. Calciphylaxis. *Postgrad Med J.* Sep 2001;77(911):557-61.

24. Wanat KA. Calciphylaxis. In: Rosenbach M, Wanat KA, Micheletti RG, Taylor LA, eds. *Inpatient Dermatology.* 1st ed. Springer International Publishing AG; 2018:281-283:chap Calciphylaxis.

25. Glew RH, Sun Y, Horowitz BL, et al. Nephropathy in dietary hyperoxaluria: A potentially preventable acute or chronic kidney disease. *World J Nephrol.* Nov 2014;3(4):122-42.

26. Ortel TL. Heparin-induced thrombocytopenia: when a low platelet count is a mandate for anticoagulation. *Hematology Am Soc Hematol Educ Program.* 2009:225-32.

27. Wysong A, Venkatesan P. An approach to the patient with retiform purpura. *Dermatol Ther.* 2011 Mar-Apr 2011;24(2):151-72.

28. Wanat KA. Purpura Fulminans. In: Rosenbach M, Wanat KA, Micheletti RG, Taylor LA, eds. *Inpatient Dermatology.* 1st ed. Springer International Publishing AG; 2018:123-126.

29. Moye M. Antiphospholipid Antibody Syndrome. In: Rosenbach M, Wanat KA, Micheletti RG, Taylor LA, eds. *Inpatient Dermatology.* 1st ed. Springer International Publishing AG; 2018:277-280:chap Antiphospholipid Antibody Syndrome.

Pruritus in Patients with No Underlying Skin Disease

Rehana Ahmed

INTRODUCTION TO CHAPTER

Pruritus (itch) is the unpleasant sensation of the skin that results in an urge to scratch. It is a major symptom of many cutaneous and systemic diseases. Pruritus can range from mild to severe and may be intermittent or chronic (lasting longer than 6 weeks). Pruritus can have a significant impact on health-related quality of life (HRQOL), and has been associated with depression, decreased sleep quality, and a negative impact on most quality of life categories.[1] The authors of a case-control study of patients with chronic pruritus observed that the impact of chronic pruritus on HRQOL may be similar to that of chronic pain.[2] Pruritus has multiple etiologies in patients with and without underlying skin disease. The International Forum for the Study of Itch recently published a clinical classification of pruritus[3] in which they proposed six categories for pruritus based on the underlying origin:

1. Dermatological: Pruritus associated with diseases of the skin, including diseases which feature prominent pruritus such as atopic dermatitis, allergic contact dermatitis, xerotic dermatitis, lichen simplex chronicus, lichen planus, scabies, and urticaria. These diseases typically have characteristic skin findings.
2. Systemic: Pruritus associated with diseases in organs other than the skin, such as the liver, kidneys, hematopoietic system, malignancy, nutrient deficiency,

medications, or illicit substances with pruritus as a side-effect.
3. Neurological: Pruritus associated with damage to nerve fibers from diseases or disorders of the central nervous system (e.g., brain and spinal cord injury, brain tumors) or peripheral nervous system (e.g., damage from diabetes mellitus or herpes zoster, narrowing of bony foramina from osteoarthritis).
4. Psychogenic/Psychosomatic: Pruritus associated with psychiatric disorders and defined as itch not related to dermatologic or systemic causes.
5. Mixed: Pruritus from combinations of categories 1–4.
6. Other: Pruritus of undetermined origin.

Typically, the pruritus in categories 2–6 is associated with no primary skin lesions. However, secondary lesions from scratching or rubbing, such as excoriations (Figure 25-1), prurigo nodularis (Figure 25-2), or lichenification (Figure 25-3) can be seen. Additionally, a patient's pruritus may span multiple categories. For example, pruritus in the elderly may occur due to decreased function of the stratum corneum, including reduced lipid production, compounded by polypharmacy, low iron levels, or neuropathy from diabetes mellitus. It is important to determine the etiology of chronic pruritus, because it can be an early symptom of the diseases in categories 2–4. Table 25-1 contains information about selected diseases that are associated with chronic pruritus starting with the most likely diseases.

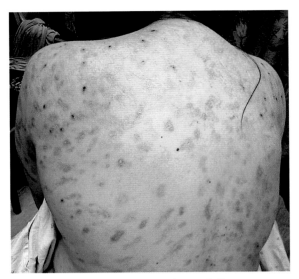

▲ **Figure 25-1.** Excoriations with post inflammatory hyperpigmentation on back of patient with no underlying skin disease.

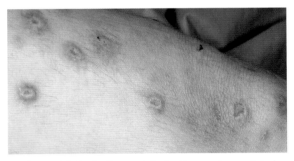

▲ **Figure 25-2.** Purigo nodularis. Grouped excoriated papules secondary to scratching.

APPROACH TO DIAGNOSIS

The approach to the diagnosis of pruritus with no underlying skin disease relies on a careful history and physical examination. A thorough review of the patient's medical history, medications, and substance abuse is essential. Additional evaluation with a skin biopsy, laboratory

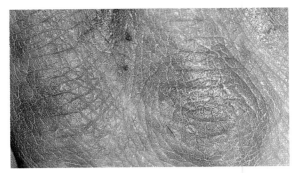

▲ **Figure 25-3.** Lichenification of skin due to chronic scratching.

testing, or imaging may be required to further determine whether or not there is an underlying medical condition contributing to the patient's pruritus (Table 25-2).

For psychogenic pruritus, building a relationship with the patient helps, as patients may find it difficult to accept that a psychiatric component may be part of their condition;[13,17] ultimately a psychiatric screen may aid in diagnosis and management when other workup is negative. It is also important to rule out skin disorders which may be very pruritic, but may have subtle skin lesions, such as dry skin, scabies (Figure 25-5), pediculosis, and dermatitis herpetiformis (Figure 25-6).

MANAGEMENT

The neurophysiology of pruritus is quite complex and comprises an active area of research[10] and a better understanding of pruritus will lead to more targeted treatment strategies. Correction of underlying conditions may improve pruritus (such as for pruritus related to iron-deficiency).[10] While a complete review of all treatment options for pruritus is beyond the scope of this chapter, Table 25-3 lists topical antipruritic medications that may be helpful in the management of patients with pruritus. Treatments may include emollients, zinc oxide, menthol, topical capsaicin, topical vitamin D modulators, topical doxepin, lidocaine, calcineurin inhibitors or corticosteroids, antihistamines (sedating and non-sedating), and light therapy (narrow or broad-band UVB). Other systemic treatments are guided by the underlying cause of pruritus (including anticholestatics, antidepressants, anticonvulsants, thalidomide, and opioid inhibitors).[10] Recent review articles outline in detail options for the treatment of chronic pruritus.[18,19]

Table 25-1. Pruritus: Etiology and presentation in patients with no underlying skin disease.[a]

Disease	Epidemiology/Etiology	History and Clinical Presentation of Pruritus
Endocrine and metabolic disorders		
Renal failure	Occurs in 15–48% of patients with end-stage renal failure, up to 90% on hemodialysis.[4] Etiology poorly understood.	Generalized pruritus is more common than localized. Peaks at night. Often resolves with transplantation.[5]
Hepatic disorders	Common in up to 80% of patients with primary biliary cirrhosis. Seen more in intrahepatic than extrahepatic obstruction: primary biliary cirrhosis, primary sclerosing cholangitis, obstructive choledocholithiasis, carcinoma of the bile duct, cholestasis, hepatitis. Pruritus of pregnancy (pruritus gravidarum) occurs in 1–8% of pregnancies.	Generalized, migratory. Worse on the hands, feet, and areas constricted by clothing. Worse at night. May precede other manifestations of liver disease such as chronic cholestasis.[6] Pruritus of pregnancy presents with pruritus of the hands and feet, may generalize. Usually presents in the 3rd trimester and resolves with delivery.[7]
Thyroid disease	More common with hyperthyroidism. Pruritus with hypothyroidism, hypoparathyroidism, and pseudohypoparathyroidism may be due to xerosis.[7]	Usually more severe and generalized with hyperthyroidism. Generalized or localized with hypothyroidism.[8]
Diabetes mellitus	Approximately 7% of diabetics are affected. Reported with poor glycemic control, mechanism unknown.[8]	May be localized, especially in genital and perianal areas (may be due to neuropathy or infection).
Infections and Infestations		
Human immunodeficiency virus (HIV)/ Acquired immunodeficiency syndrome (AIDS)	May be presenting symptom of HIV infection. HIV infected patients develop several pruritic dermatoses but may develop pruritus without other cutaneous findings.[9]	Local or generalized. Intractable pruritus may correlate with HIV viral loads. Elevated serum IgE, peripheral hypereosinophilia and altered TH1/TH2 profile are associated with poor prognosis.[9]
Hepatitis C	Present in approximately 15% of patients with chronic hepatitis C.[10]	Generalized or localized (See cholestasis, above).
Parasites	Several, including ancylostoma tungiasis, schistosomiasis myiasis, helminthosis, toxicosis, trypanosomiasis.[10]	Local or generalized. Often with other skin findings.
Hematologic disorders		
Iron deficiency	May be a sign of malignancy.[10]	Generalized or localized. Perianal or vulvar regions may be involved.
Myelodysplasia	Prevalence unknown.	Generalized or localized. May present as aquagenic pruritus.
Polycythemia vera (PCV)	30–50% of patients with PCV experience pruritus.	Generalized. Usually occurs within 5 minutes of contact with water.[11] Aquagenic pruritus may precede development of PCV by years.
Hodgkin's Disease	30% have pruritus. Severe persistent pruritus associated with poor prognosis. May predict recurrence. Less prevalent in non-Hodgkin's lymphoma and leukemia.[12]	Persistent, generalized. Mild to intractable.

(continued)

Table 25-1. Pruritus: Etiology and presentation in patients with no underlying skin disease.[a] (Continued)

Disease	Epidemiology/Etiology	History and Clinical Presentation of Pruritus
Tumors		
Solid organ tumors	May precede a cancer diagnosis. Occurs in 5–27% of patients in palliative care. Unknown whether or not rates of malignancy are increased in patients with unexplained pruritus.	Often generalized. Mild to intractable. Intensity or extent of pruritus not correlated with extent of tumor involvement.[12]
Carcinoid	Flushing and gyrate (wave-like) erythema common. May experience pruritus during flushing episode.	Upper half of body more commonly affected. Other symptoms are often present.
Drug induced: virtually any drug may be associated with pruritus		
	Common: antihypertensives, antiarrhythmics, anticoagulants, antidiabetic drugs, hypolipidemics, antimicrobials and chemotherapy agents, psychotropics, antiepileptics, cytostatic agents, cytokines, growth factors, and monoclonal antibodies, plasma volume expanders, nonsteroidal anti-inflammatory drugs (NSAIDs).[10]	Generalized pruritus is more common. Mechanisms include cholestasis, hepatotoxicity, reduction in sebum production, xerosis, phototoxicity, neurologic, histamine release, deposition, idiopathic.
Neurologic (Neurogenic/Neuropathic)		
	Diverse etiology: brachioradial pruritus, multiple sclerosis, spinal or cerebral neoplasms, abscess, or infarcts; phantom itch, post-herpetic neuralgia, notalgia (Figure 25-4) or meralgia paresthetica, conditions associated with nerve damage, compression (e.g., from osteoarthritis), or irritation (including diabetes mellitus or vitamin B12 deficiency).[10]	Usually localized. Occurs due to dysfunction of signaling, synthesis or sensation at any level of afferent pathway from skin to brain.
Psychogenic/Psychosomatic		
	Delusions of parasitosis, psychogenic excoriations, somatoform pruritus. Associated with psychiatric disorders.[13]	Generalized or localized. Important to rule out other causes.
Mixed		
	Combination, such as uremic itch with xerosis, or neurologic and dermatologic itch in HIV/AIDS.	
Other (of Unknown Origin)		
Pruritus of the elderly	Many causes: chronic disease, polypharmacy, xerosis, institutionalized care, age-related alterations of skin including atrophy, decreased cutaneous vascular supply, altered lipid composition, altered peripheral nerve innervation, and compromised moisture retention.[14]	Generalized or localized.
Aquagenic Pruritus	Generally secondary to systemic disease or other skin disorders. There are strict criteria for true idiopathic aquagenic pruritus.	Prickling, stinging, burning, tingling sensation occurs within 30 minutes of water exposure and lasts up to 2 hours. Begins on lower extremities and generalizes. Spares head, palms, soles, and mucosa.[15]
Pruritus in anorexia nervosa	Etiology unknown. Not related to other behaviors or internal abnormalities. Resolves with weight restoration.[16]	Intermittent or constant. May also experience burning or tingling. Often localized: neck, thighs, forearms, buttocks, ankles and upper arm.

[a] Based on the International Forum for the Study of Itch (IFSI) clinical classification.

Table 25-2. Evaluation of pruritus.

Initial Laboratory and Imaging Studies for Selected Diseases
- Complete blood count with differential (leukemia, myeloma, iron-deficiency anemia, B12 deficiency, polycythemia, infection, HIV)
- Chemistry profile with liver function tests including aspartate aminotransferase (AST), alanine aminotransferase (ALT), alkaline phosphatase (ALP), and total bilirubin (cholestasis, hepatitis)
- Creatinine and blood urea nitrogen (uremia)
- Thyroid function with thyroid stimulating hormone and reflex free T4 (thyroid disease)
- Chest X-ray (lymphoma, lung cancer)

Additional testing may be guided by the patient's history and physical findings including:
- Sedimentation rate
- Glucose (diabetes) Hemoglobin A1C
- Iron studies: transferrin, percent saturation, ferritin, total iron (anemia)
- Serum protein electrophoresis (myeloma)
- Other: urine drug screen, HIV antibody test, hepatitis serology, antinuclear antibody, anti-mitochondrial antibody, anti-gliadin antibody, anti-transglutaminase antibody, parathyroid hormone, calcium, phosphate, specific immunoglobulin (Ig)E, serum tryptase, serotonin and its metabolites, stool for ova and parasites, stool for occult blood, and age and gender appropriate malignancy workup

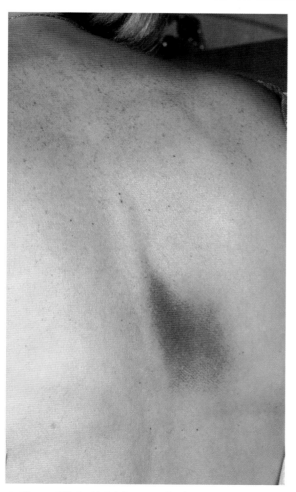

▲ **Figure 25-4.** Notalgia paresthetica. Hyperpigmented, slightly lichenified plaque on back caused by chronic rubbing and scratching.

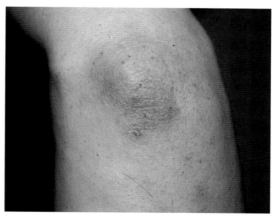

▲ **Figure 25-5.** Bites from scabies mite on elbow. Subtle excoriated papules.

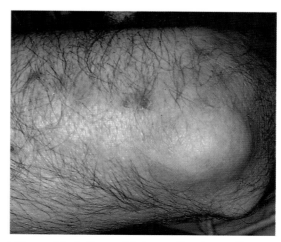

▲ **Figure 25-6.** Dermatitis herpetiformis on elbow. Subtle excoriated vesicles.

Table 25-3. Examples of topical over the counter product for pruritus.

Product Examples	Active ingredients
Aspercreme with Lidocaine	Lidocaine 4%
Aveeno Anti-Itch Lotion	Calamine 3%, Pramoxine 1%
Aveeno Soothing Oatmeal Bath Treatment	Colloidal Oatmeal 100%
Benadryl Extra Strength Itch Stopping Gel	Diphenhydramine 2%
Calamine lotion	Calamine 8%, Pramoxine 1%
Capzasin-HP Cream	Capsaicin 0.1%
CeraVe Itch Relief Cream	Pramoxine 1%
Eucerin Skin Calming Itch Relief	Menthol 0.1%
Gold Bond Anti-Itch Cream	Menthol 1%, Pramoxine 1%
Sarna Lotion Original	Camphor 0.5%, Menthol 0.5%
Sarna Lotion Sensitive	Pramoxine 1%
Vanicream Anti-Itch Cream	Hydrocortisone 1%

▼ REFERENCES

1. Tessari G, Dalle Vedove C, Loschiavo C, et al. The impact of pruritus on the quality of life of patients undergoing dialysis: a single centre cohort study. *J Nephrol.* 2009; 22(2):241-8.
2. Kini SP, Delong LK, Veledar E, McKenzie-Brown AM, Schaufele M, Chen SC. The impact of pruritus on quality of life: the skin equivalent of pain. *Arch Dermatol.* 2011; 147(10):1153-6.
3. Ständer S, Weisshaar E, Mettang T, et al. Clinical classification of itch: a position paper for the International Forum for the Study of Itch. *Acta Derm Venerol.* 2007; 87(4):291-294.
4. Narita I, Iguchi S, Omori K, Gejyo F. Uremic pruritus in chronic hemodialysis patients. *J Nephrol.* 2008; 21(2):161-5.
5. Verduzco HA, Shirazian S. CKD-Associated Pruritus: New Insights into Diagnosis, Pathogenesis, and Management. *Kidney Int Rep.* 2020;5(9):1387-1402.
6. Kremer AE, Beuers U, Oude-Elferink RP, Pusl T. Pathogenesis and treatment of pruritus in cholestasis. *Drugs.* 2008; 68(15):2163-82.
7. Weisshaar E, Diepgen TL, Luger TA, Seeliger S, Witteler R, Ständer S. Pruritus in pregnancy and childhood--do we really consider all relevant differential diagnoses? *Eur J Dermatol.* 2005; 15(5):320-31.
8. Welz-Kubiak K, Reszke R, Szepietowski JC. Pruritus as a sign of systemic disease. *Clinics in Dermatology.* 2019;37(6): 644-656.
9. Singh F, Rudikoff D. HIV-associated pruritus. Etiology and management. *Am J Clin Dermatol.* 2003;4(3):177-88.
10. Cassano N, Tessari G, Vena GA, Girolomoni G. Chronic pruritus in the absence of specific skin disease. An update on pathophysiology, diagnosis and therapy. *Am J Clin Dermatol.* 2010; 11(6):399-411.
11. Lelonek E, Matusiak Ł, Wróbel T, Szepietowski J. Aquagenic Pruritus in Polycythemia Vera: Clinical Characteristics. *Acta Derm Venereol.* 2018;98(5):496-500.
12. Yosipovitch G. Chronic pruritus: a paraneoplastic sign. *Dermatol Ther.* 2010; 23(6):590-6.
13. Buteau A, Reichenberg J. Psychogenic pruritus and its management. *Dermatol Clin.* 2018; 36: 309-314.
14. Clerc C-J, Misery L. A literature review of senile pruritus: from diagnosis to treatment. *Acta Derm Venereol.* 2017;97(4):433-440.
15. Wang F, Zhao Y-K, Luo Z-Y, et al. Aquagenic cutaneous disorders. *JDDG: Journal der Deutschen Dermatologischen Gesellschaft.* 2017;15(6):602-608.
16. Morgan JF, Lacey JH. Scratching and fasting: a study of pruritus and anorexia nervosa. *Br J Dermatol.* 1999;140(3):453-6.
17. Rattanakaemakorn P, Suchonwanit P. Scalp pruritus: review of the pathogenesis, diagnosis and management. *Biomed Res Int.* 2019; e-collection.
18. Pereira MP, Ständer S. Chronic Pruritus: Current and Emerging Treatment Options. *Drugs.* 2017;77(9):999-1007.
19. Weisshaar E, Szepietowski JC, Dalgard F et. al. European S2K guideline on chronic pruritus. *Acta Derm Venereol.* 2019; 99: 469-506.

Fever and Rash

Kristen Hook

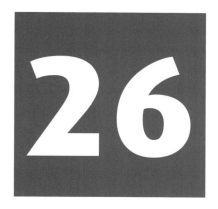

INTRODUCTION TO CHAPTER

Bacterial and viral infections are frequently associated with fever and rash in children. Many of these rashes have known etiologies and characteristic features. Recognizing the clinical features of the rash and identifying key points in the history can help with diagnosis. In the Table 26-1, key points in a number of pediatric exanthems are summarized, as well as other rashes associated with fever. Most exanthems are self-limited and require only symptomatic treatment. Hypersensitivity reactions, such as those due to viruses or medications, can also present with fever and maculopapular rash. Vaccinations have significantly decreased the incidence of measles, rubella, varicella, and their congenital complications. However, isolated outbreaks of imported measles still occur, especially in unvaccinated populations.[1,2] COVID-19 has emerged as a novel cause of fever and rash in children and adults.[3] With travel to endemic areas, infections such as Zika and West Nile virus should be considered. Tick-borne infections such as Rocky Mountain spotted fever and Ehrlichiosis require identification and treatment.

APPROACH TO DIAGNOSIS

- Prodrome: Many exanthems are preceded by a prodromal period with fever, sore throat among others.
- Enanthem: Oral findings may precede the development of skin signs or occur in conjunction.
- Morphology: Morphology is commonly described as erythematous and papular or maculopapular. The color

of the rash, characteristic primary lesion, presence of desquamation, and swelling can all aid in diagnosis. Associated key features such as "sandpaper" texture or "dew drop on a rose petal" may be helpful for diagnosis. Rarely a skin biopsy is needed to confirm the diagnosis. Serologic evaluation can help in some cases to identify a specific viral etiology, but is not necessary for diagnosis or treatment in most cases.

- Distribution: The distribution and chronology of the clinical presentation are important defining characteristics. Cephalocaudad spread and resolution is characteristic of many exanthems such as measles and rubella. Additionally, some rashes may be unilateral, or present only in dependent areas, such as unilateral laterothoracic exanthem and Henoch-Schonlein purpura, respectively.
- Associated signs and factors: Frequently included in the clinical differential diagnosis are drug rash, heat rash (miliaria rubra), urticaria among a host of possible viral etiologies. Consideration of exposures, travel, severe illness, and other clinical signs will narrow the differential.

EVALUATION

- Most rashes can be diagnosed clinically based on the patient's history and physical findings. Ask questions such as: Did you notice any clinical signs before the rash started or associated with the rash? Were any new medications started recently? Is anyone else sick at home? Any recent travel? Description of the rash: where did it start and how has it changed over time?

- Most viral exanthems will be associated with elevated white count and lymphocytosis. Bacterial infections will demonstrate neutrophilia.
- If the diagnosis is not clear, serologic blood studies as listed in the table may be helpful. PCR is widely available for many viruses listed.
- If varicella (chickenpox) is suspected, polymerase chain reaction (PCR), direct fluorescent antibody test (DFA), and viral cultures can be done. A Tzanck smear or a skin biopsy can be done but does not distinguish between herpes simplex and varicella zoster infections.
- A skin biopsy is rarely helpful in establishing the diagnosis of most viral exanthems. A skin biopsy can be diagnostic for erythema multiforme and Henoch-Schonlein purpura. Varicella and cytomegalovirus infections may show specific changes on biopsy. A biopsy can be helpful in staphylococcal scalded skin syndrome, especially if toxic epidermal necrolysis is considered, but is not necessary for diagnosis.

- Kawasaki disease should be considered in any child with prolonged fever of unknown origin.
- Vaccine preventable diseases should be considered in unvaccinated populations and the immunocompromised.
- Meningococcemia can result in tissue necrosis and autoamputation.
- Rocky Mountain spotted fever can be associated with low platelets and severe illness.
- Appropriate services should be consulted and inpatient hospitalization considered for patients with meningococcemia, toxic-shock syndrome, staphylococcal scalded skin syndrome, Kawasaki's disease, tick and travel borne diseases.
- https://www.cdc.gov/ is useful for available testing and reporting requirements.

Table 26-1. Diseases associated with fever and rash.

Disease/Etiology	History	Clinical signs	Laboratory evaluation
Viral			
Measles [2,4,5,6] (Rubeola; 1st disease) Paramyxovirus ssDNA	Incubation: 8-14 days. Prodrome: Fever, cough, coryza, conjunctivitis. Rash lasts 4-7 days.	Erythematous macules and papules appear on scalp along hairline and behind ears. Spreads in cephalocaudad distribution (Figure 26-1) and by 5th day, clears in same direction. Koplik spots (red macules with a white blue center) may be seen on the buccal mucosa. Complications: Otitis, pneumonitis, encephalitis, myocarditis.	Fourfold increase in acute and convalescent titers confirm diagnosis. PCR and ELISA are also available.
Varicella [5,6] (Chicken pox) Varicella zoster virus dsDNA	Incubation: 10-21 days Prodrome: Malaise and low grade fever. Late fall, winter, spring.	Tear drop vesicles, "dew on a rose petal" (Figures 26-2 A and B). Multiple lesional stages present at once. Immunocompromised patients at increased risk of disseminated disease, pneumonia, and secondary infection. Reye syndrome associated with aspirin use. Congenital varicella is associated with hypoplastic limbs.	Clinical diagnosis usually sufficient. PCR, DFA are available for rapid diagnosis, viral cultures take several days. Acute and convalescent IgM and IgG antibody titers confirmatory.
Cytomegalovirus [7] (CMV) dsDNA	Post-natal infection in immune competent usually asymptomatic, but mononucleosis like syndrome may occur.	Erythematous macules and papules in diffuse distribution. Skin or mucosal ulcerations are possible. Complications include congenital CMV: 'Blueberry muffin' baby resulting in hearing loss, seizures, intracranial calcifications.	Urine virus isolation, serologic evaluation, antigen (blood), PCR analysis (blood). Skin biopsy may show intracytoplasmic, intranuclear viral inclusions in endothelial cells.
Mononucleosis [8] Epstein-Barr virus, Human Herpesvirus 4 (HHV-4) dsDNA	Incubation: 30-50 days. Prodrome: Fever, pharyngitis, lymphadenopathy, malaise, anorexia. Rash following use of amoxicillin/ampicillin.	Morbilliform rash spreads over entire body (Figure 26-3A). Periorbital edema. Petechiae on palate (Figure 26-3B). Painful mucosal ulcerations (especially vaginal/perineal).	Leukocytosis with 50% lymphocytosis. Elevated LFT's. Monospot test for IgM heterophile antibodies, usually positive by second week of infection. Not reliable in children <4 years of age.
Rubella [9] (German measles; 3rd disease) Togavirus ssRNA	Incubation: 16-18 days. Prodrome: Fever, headache and upper respiratory symptoms. Late winter, early spring.	Rose-pink macules (1-4 mm) in cephalocaudad spread and clear in 2-3 days in same manner. May have soft palate petechiae, (Forscheimer's spots), posterior auricular/occipital lymphadenopathy. Self-limited. Complications: Teratogenic (congenital rubella syndrome characterized by deafness, cataracts, congenital heart disease and CNS signs), hepatitis, myocarditis, pericarditis, hemolytic anemia, thrombocytopenic purpura. Arthritis in adults.	IgM anti-rubella antibody presence, and/or 4-fold increase in IgG antirubella antibody are most diagnostic. Despite vaccination, 10% of US citizens remain susceptible to infection. Risk higher in unvaccinated or those who reject vaccination.
Roseola [5,6] (Exanthema subitum 6th disease) HHV6 and 7 dsDNA	Incubation: 5-15 days Prodrome: High fever for 2-3 days, followed by rash on trunk, which then spreads to extremities and face, for 1-2 days. Usually in children <3 years old.	Erythematous, blanchable, macules and papules. Periorbital edema is a common association. Rash appearing after fever defervescence is key finding. Complications: seizures secondary to fever.	Serologic confirmation available with ELISA or PCR.

(continued)

Table 26-1. Diseases associated with fever and rash. (Continued)

Disease/Etiology	History	Clinical signs	Laboratory evaluation
Parvovirus B19[5,10] (Erythema infectiosum, 5th disease) Parvovirus B19 ssDNA	Incubation: 4-14 days. Prodrome: Headache and fever	Slapped cheeks (red plaques) at 1-4 days (Figure 26-4), then lacy reticular rash in 4-9 days, which can wax and wane for several weeks. Arthritis alone can be seen in adults as presenting sign. Associated papular-purpuric, gloves and sock syndrome in adolescents. Complications include: hydrops fetalis, aplastic crises in sickle cell patients.	Clinical diagnosis is usually sufficient. Serologic studies available for detection of anti-B19 IgM and IgG antibodies. PCR studies also available. In a pregnant female who has been exposed to B19, serologic testing for IgM and IgG antibodies should be performed.
Hand, Foot, Mouth Disease[6] Coxsackie A16 (most common serotype) Picornavirus ssRNA	Incubation: 3-6 days. Prodrome: Fever, malaise.	Macules progress to vesicles on red base on the hands and feet (especially on palms and soles) and oral mucosa (Figures 26-5 A and B). Oral lesions are painful and quickly erode.	Testing usually not indicated, but PCR is available.
Herpangina[5] Coxsackie groups A and B most common, Other echoviruses ssRNA	Incubation: 4-14 days Prodrome: Fever. Most common in children 3-10 years old.	Oral erosions and ulceration in posterior pharynx and buccal mucosa. Exanthem usually absent.	Testing usually not indicated, but PCR is available.
Gianotti-Crosti syndrome[5,11] (Acrodermatitis of childhood) Most commonly Hepatitis B in developing countries, EBV in USA. Other causes include numerous viruses, bacteria and vaccinations.	Most common in spring/early summer. Most common in 2 year olds with range 6 months to 14 years old, average age 2 years, May have associated low grade fever and lymphadenopathy. Hepatosplenomegaly less often.	Symmetric papular eruption of face, buttocks and extremities (Figure 26-6). Papules are pink, to erythematous, "juicy" and have acral predilection.	Evaluate for specific viral etiology, only if indicated.
Unilateral Laterothoracic Exanthem[4] AKA (Asymmetric periflexural exanthem of childhood (APEC)) No confirmed etiology, but considered a viral exanthem.	Most common in 2-year olds with range 6 months to 10 years. Preceded by URI or GI symptoms. Associated with low grade fever, lymphadenopathy, diarrhea or rhinitis and pruritus.	Rash usually starts in unilateral axilla and spreads in centrifugal fashion to contralateral side as the disease progresses (Figure 26-7). Erythematous papules, plaques with associated scale, with unilateral predominance. May appear urticarial.	Laboratory tests not indicated.
Pityriasis Rosea[5] **(PR)** HHV-6/7 dsDNA	Usually asymptomatic.	Guttate erythematous papules and plaques with characteristic 'trailing scale' centrally and occur in characteristic 'Christmas tree' distribution on the back most notably (Figure 26-8).	No confirmatory test necessary in most cases. Skin biopsy can help distinguish between PR and guttate psoriasis if needed. PCR is available for HHV-6/7
COVID-19[3] SARS-CoV-2 Coronavirus ssRNA	Incubation: 7-14 days. Prodrome: Fever, cough, fatigue, anosmia.	No known signature rash: morbilliform, pernio-like (Figure 26-9) urticarial, macular erythema, vesicular, papulosquamous, retiform purpura all reported. Enanthem: petechial macules on upper palate seen rarely. Late effects: possible telogen effluvium.	PCR (nasal swab, throat swabs, oral rinse). Antigen tests available but less sensitive. Antibody testing following seroconversion.

Non-specific viral exanthem[5] Non-polio enteroviruses (most common cause in summer) and respiratory viruses (most common cause in winter).	Prodrome: Fever, myalgia, malaise or gastrointestinal symptoms. Most are self-limited, resolve in one week.	Blanchable erythematous papules and macules in diffuse distribution involving trunk (Figure 27-10), and extremities, and less often the face.	Laboratory tests not required. Enterovirus culture can be obtained from throat or stool.
Bacterial			
Scarlet Fever[12] (2nd disease) Group A beta hemolytic streptococcus (GABHS): pyrogenic exotoxin -A, B or C)	Incubation: 1-4 days. Prodrome: Fever, chills, sore throat, headache. Signs of strep pharyngitis likely. Rash lasts 4-5 days. Primarily a disease of children 1-10 years old.	Clinical signs of streptococcal pharyngitis likely. Enanthem appears as white coating on the tongue, which sloughs in 4-5 days leaving the classic "strawberry tongue" (Figure 26-11). Fine, erythematous papules and macules (sandpaper-like rash), accentuated in flexures with petechial component (Pastia's lines). Circumoral pallor characteristic. Rash resolves over 4-5 days and commonly heals with significant desquamation.	Gold standard is throat culture with growth of GABHS. Rapid strep test has a high sensitivity and specificity. Anti-streptococcal serologic studies are also available and may be useful.
Staphylococcal Scalded Skin Syndrome[13] (Ritter's disease) Staphylococcus aureus, phage group II, exfoliative toxin (ETA, ETB)	Fever, malaise, lethargy, irritability, and poor feeding with rapid onset of generalized tender erythema. Cutaneous or systemic staphylococcal infection may be present.	Tender erythema with flexural, perioral accentuation which progresses to large, superficial fragile blisters that rupture easily, leaving behind denuded, desquamating, erythematous, and tender (Figure 26-12). The Nikolsky sign (progression of the blister cleavage plane induced by gentle pressure on the edge of the bulla) is positive.	Culture of causative lesion (if present). Blood cultures positive rarely. Skin culture of rash will not yield organisms. The organism is most easily recovered from pyogenic (not exfoliative) foci on the skin, conjunctivae, nares, or nasopharynx.
Toxic shock syndrome (TSS)[14] Staphylococcus aureus, TSS toxin-1 or streptococcal (GABHS)	Menstrual and non-menstrual forms; the latter more common. Caused by toxin-producing strains of S. aureus. Prodrome of malaise, myalgias, chills precedes rash. Fever, lethargy, diarrhea, altered mental status ultimately develop.	Diffuse, scarlatiniform rash that later desquamates palms and soles involved (Figure 26-13). Accentuation in skin folds may be seen, and in rare cases, inguinal folds or perineal area may be only area of involvement. Hypotensive symptoms, shock, hyperemia of the mucous membranes and pharyngitis, "strawberry tongue." Skin or muscle tenderness may be associated. Edema of hands/feet. Streptococcal disease: Usually characterized by a focal tissue or blood infection with GABHS. Necrotizing fasciitis, myonecrosis may be associated. Extremely painful. Shock develops rapidly with renal impairment, DIC and respiratory distress syndrome.	Evidence of multiorgan involvement required. To meet criteria, 3 of 7 organ systems must be involved. Clinical diagnosis usually acceptable, but if positive culture or toxin production can be demonstrated, this is supportive. Biopsy not helpful usually. Leukocytosis, anemia, thrombocytopenia, elevated creatinine and CK, hypocalcemia, abnormal liver function studies and evidence of disseminated coagulopathy may be present. Cultures may be obtained from blood, throat, CSF, peritoneal fluid. Tissue biopsy for culture if streptococcus is suspected.

(continued)

Table 26-1. Diseases associated with fever and rash. (Continued)

Disease/Etiology	History	Clinical signs	Laboratory evaluation
Meningococcemia[15] *Neisseria meningitidis* Serogroups A,B,C	Incubation: 2–10 days, average is 4 days. Presentation varies from fever to fulminant disease. Upper respiratory prodrome, followed by high fever and headache. Meningitis associated with stiff neck, nausea, vomiting, and coma. Leading cause of bacterial meningitis in children.	Petechial rash of skin and mucous membranes. Other morphologies may be seen including macular (Figure 26-14 A), morbilliform, urticaria and gray-colored acrocyanosis. Trunk and lower extremities are commonly involved. Palms, soles and head tend to be spared. Extensive hemorrhagic lesions seen in fulminant disease Figure 26-14B). Progression to purpura fulminans (purpuric patches with sharply marginated borders, progressing to necrosis and eschar formation) when associated with consumptive coagulopathy (Autoamputation is a potential complication.	Culture blood and CSF. Meningococci isolation from nasopharynx is not diagnostic. Petechial lesions may be cultured for organisms. Serology detecting *N. meningitidis* capsular polysaccharide antigen in CSF, urine, serum, and other bodily fluids is available. PCR available and useful if antibiotics already used.
Multiple Etiologies			
Urticaria multiforme[16] Multiple etiologies	Upper respiratory infections, viral infections, fever can occur as prodrome. Abrupt presentation of rash. Fever commonly associated.	Abrupt presentation of annular erythematous wheals that may have associated central clearing (Figure 27-15). Generally widespread. Hand/foot edema common. May have associated lip swelling.	Skin biopsy may be helpful if other entities are considered including erythema multiforme.
Serum-sickness like reaction[17] Cefaclor most common cause. Amoxicillin, griseofulvin also described, among others.	Develops 1–3 weeks after initiation of inciting drug with mild fever, rash, joint pain.	Targetoid or annular to polycyclic erythematous plaques. Violaceous center of plaques very characteristic.	None.
Erythema multiforme[18] HSV, mycoplasma, medications most common cause.	Herpes simplex infection may precede rash.	Targetoid erythematous plaques, that are persistent and non-migratory for days (Figure 26-16). Palm/sole involvement common.	HSV titers, cold agglutinins for mycoplasma. Skin biopsy diagnostic.
Viral-induced rash with mucositis[19] Mycoplasma pneumoniae, chlamydia pneumoniae, influenza B, likely others	Prodrome: fever, mild URI symptoms.	Hemorrhagic desquamation of the lips with possible associated involvement of palate, buccal mucosa, tongue, conjunctiva, cornea, urethra, and vagina. Skin manifestations may include erythematous targetoid lesions with bullae.	PCR/culture/titers for causative pathogens.
Henoch-Schonlein purpura (HSP)[20] Etiology unclear, but linked to GABHS, viral infections, drugs, immunizations.	Small vessel vasculitis that occurs in children. Most common 2–11 years old. Antecedent upper respiratory infection suggests hypersensitivity phenomenon.	Initial lesions appear urticarial, but quickly progress to purpuric (non-blanchable) papules with primary distribution on lower extremities (Figure 26-17) and buttocks. Scrotal involvement common. Edema of hands, face, feet commonly seen, especially in younger patients. Individual lesions resolve in 4–5 days. Associated with abdominal pain, arthritis, and glomerulonephritis.	IgA immune complexes in affected organs. Direct immunofluorescence of skin specimens may document IgA, but absence should not exclude diagnosis. 1/3 of patients will have elevated serum IgA.

No Confirmed Etiology/Other		
Kawasaki's Disease[21] (acute febrile mucocutaneous lymph node syndrome) Unknown etiology, but probably due to infection.	Winter or spring most common. Most common in children <5 years old, peak incidence <2 years old.	Need 4 of 5 criteria: (1) fever >5 days (2) palmoplantar erythema/desquamation (3) conjunctivitis (4) strawberry tongue/red fissured, crusted lips (5) cervical lymphadenopathy. A polymorphous rash on the trunk and extremities usually occurs presenting as a maculopapular rash or targetoid rash or a scarlet fever-like rash with accentuation in body fold areas. "Atypical" cases more commonly diagnosed. Complications: Coronary artery aneurysms, myocarditis and other cardiovascular disease.	No reliable diagnostic test. The histopathologic features of a skin biopsy are nonspecific. Clinical diagnosis required.
Exanthematous eruption Drug or hypersensitivity	4–21 days after new drug initiation. High risk drugs include: carbamazepine, phenytoin, lamotrigine, penicillin, cephalosporins, sulfonamides.	Diffuse, symmetric, erythematous maculopapular rash; often with low-grade fever. May have truncal predominance.	Skin biopsy may be helpful if more severe drug reactions are considered.

TICK-BORNE ILLNESS			
Rocky Mountain Spotted Fever[5] *Rickettsia Rickettsii* Gram negative bacteria Highest incidence in men >40 years. North Carolina, Oklahoma, Arkansas, Missouri, Tennessee. Winter peak.	Transmitted by tick bites with *Dermacentor variabilis* (American Dog Tick) most commonly, and also *Dermacentor andersoni* (Rocky Mountain wood tick), *Amblyomma americanum* (lone star tick) and *Rhipecephalus sanguineus* (brown dog tick).	Incubation 3–12 days. Presentation with fever, headache, nausea, vomiting. 2–4 days later, rash develops. Small pink macules on wrists (Figure 26-18) and ankles and spread to trunk. Palms and soles involved. Development of petechiae 5–6 days after illness onset indicative of severe disease. Other signs noted in children: altered mental status, periorbital edema, and dorsum of hands. Untreated complications include seizures, encephalitis, shock, respiratory and renal failure.	Sera may be negative 7-10 days after infection and cannot be relied on for diagnosis. Treatment: doxycycline first line for all patients including children <8 years. *tetracyclines usually avoided in children < 8 years old due to risk of permanent tooth staining.
Ehrlichiosis[5] *Ehrlichia chaffeensis Ehrlichia ewingii, Ehrlichia muris-like.* Gram-negative bacteria South central/southeast US Summer peak	*Amblyomma Americanum (Lone star tick).* Transmission requires tick carrying bacteria to feed for 24 hours. Lone star tick can also transmit Lyme, babesiosis and anaplasmosis, so consider multiple infections.	Incubation 7–14 days. Fever, headache, myalgia, malaise. GI upset, cough, dyspnea rare. Rash appears 5 days after symptom onset. Widespread erythema, petechiae, maculopapular. Palms and soles may be involved. Rash more common in children.	Serology available. Antibody levels may not rise during infection. Wright or Giemsa stained peripheral blood smear may reveal morulae within monocytes (*E. chaffeensis*) or granulocytes (*E. ewingii*)

(continued)

Table 26-1. Diseases associated with fever and rash. (Continued)

Disease/Etiology	History	Clinical signs	Laboratory evaluation
TRAVEL-BORNE ILLNESS			
Dengue[5] Dengue virus *Flaviviridae* Flavivirus ssRNA Caribbean, Central and South America, Pacific Islands, Southeast Asia.	Travel to endemic area. Transmitted by Aedes genus mosquitos from infected animal or human.	Incubation 3–14 days. 50% may be asymptomatic. 3 phases: (1) Febrile: 2–7 days: high fever, nausea, vomiting, headache, joint pain "break-bone fever" "bone crusher disease." Facial flushing followed by maculopapular rash of trunk and extremities with islands of clear skin. Petechiae may be associated. Mucosal findings: vesicles, crusting, gingival bleeding, epistaxis. (2) critical or leakage (24–48 hours) (3) convalescence (2–9 days). 95% of patients enter convalescence following febrile stage, 5% enter critical stage with pulmonary edema, ascites and shock.	PCR serologic testing. Leukopenia in mild cases, thrombocytopenia, increased LFT's and signs of organ failure in severe cases.
Zika[4] Zika virus *Flaviviridae* ssRNA Africa, South east Asia, Pacific Islands, Caribbean, South and Central America.	Travel to endemic area. Transmitted by *Aedes* genus, *Calicudae* family mosquitoes from infected animal or human.	Most infections asymptomatic or mild. 14-day incubation. Conjunctival injection, cervical lymphadenitis, maculopapular or scarlatiniform exanthem that starts on the trunk and spreads to involve lower extremities. Gingival bleeding, petechiae. Strong link between maternal infection and birth defects established.	Nucleic acid amplification test (NAAT) available. False positives possible. Antibody testing available. Antibodies may form as early as 1 week after infection.
Chikungunya[4] *Togaviridae* Alphavirus ssRNA Africa, southeast Asia, Indian subcontinent, Pacific Islands. Probably sub-tropical Americas.	Transmitted by bites from *Aedes aegypti* and *Aedes albopictus* infected mosquitos Blood borne transmission possible.	Fever, polyarthralgia (bilateral and symmetric), cutaneous. Most patients asymptomatic. Incubation 1–12 days. Morbilliform or generalized macular erythema with areas of sparing. 50% children present with hyperpigmentation shortly after rash, or in absence of rash. Face and extremities most common. vesiculobullous possible in infants. Symptoms resolve in 1–3 weeks, arthralgias may persist for months to years.	ELISA available Detection of virus, virus nucleic acid, viral specific IgM antibodies and neutralizing antibodies No specific treatment. Symptomatic relief with NSAIDS and fluids. Lymphopenia, thrombocytopenia, elevated creatinine, elevated transaminases.

CK, Creatine kinase; CNS, central nervous system; CSF, cerebrospinal fluid; DFA, direct fluorescent antibody; DIC, disseminated intravascular coagulation; ds, double stranded; EBV, Epstein-Barr virus; ELISA, enzyme-linked immunosorbent assay; GI, gastrointestinal; LFTs, liver function tests; PCR, polymerase chain reaction; ss, single stranded; URI, upper respiratory infection; USA, United States of America.

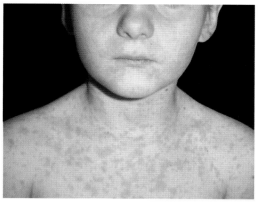

⚴ **Figure 26-1.** Measles. Erythematous macules and papules with symmetrical, diffuse distribution.

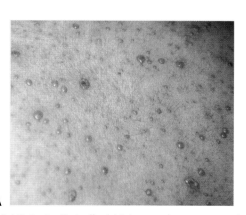

A

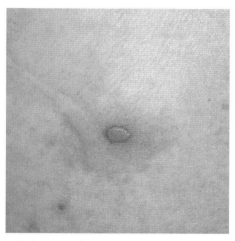

B

⚴ **Figure 26-2 A, B.** Varicella (chicken pox). A. Scattered diffusely distributed vesicles on an erythematous base on chest. B. Vesicle on pink base "dew on a rose petal."

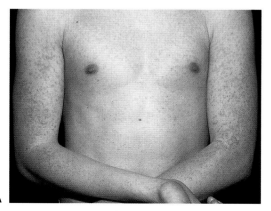

A

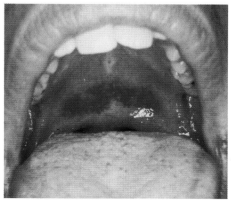

B

⚴ **Figure 26-3A, B.** Mononucleosis. A. Diffuse erythematous morbilliform rash on trunk and arms. B. Petechiae on palate.

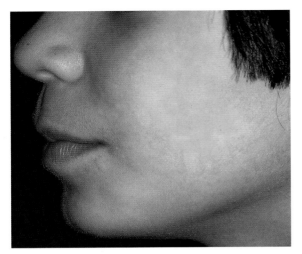

▲ **Figure 26-4.** Parvovirus B19 infection (fifth's disease). Red patch on cheek.

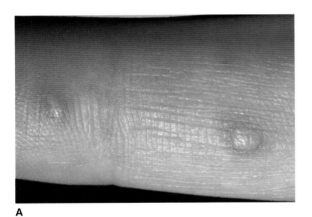

A

B

▲ **Figure 26-5 A, B.** Hand, foot, mouth disease exanthem and enanthem. A. Vesicles on an erythematous base on finger B. Vesicles on hard palate.

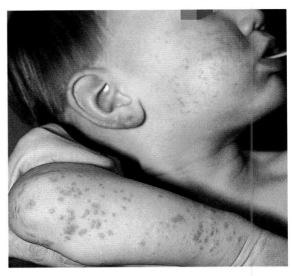

▲ **Figure 26-6.** Gianotti-Crosti syndrome. Pink papules on cheek and acral arm.

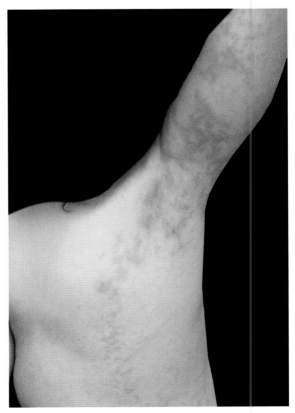

▲ **Figure 26-7.** Unilateral laterothoracic exanthema. Erythematous papules along the lateral chest and flexural arm.

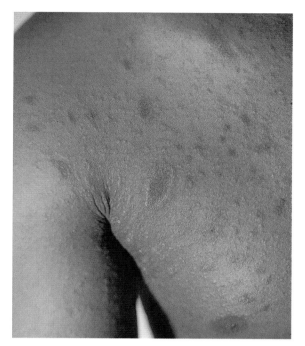

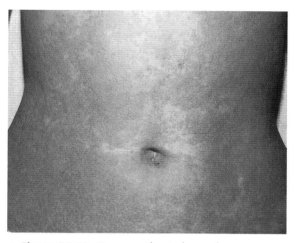

△ **Figure 26-10.** Non-specific viral exanthem. Erythematous macules in diffuse distribution on trunk in patient with upper respiratory symptoms.

△ **Figure 26-8.** Pityriasis rosea. Oval thin plaques with trailing scale on arm and chest.

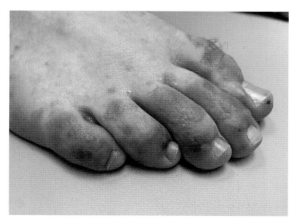

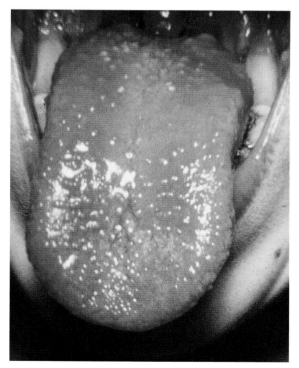

△ **Figure 26-9.** COVID-19 toes. Tender, pernio-like changes with purple color and vesicles.

△ **Figure 26-11.** Scarlet fever. "Strawberry tongue" enathem with bright red tongue with enlarged papillae and white patches.

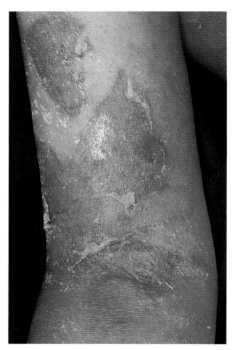

▲ Figure 26-12. Staphylococcal scalded skin syndrome. Diffuse erythema and sloughing of the epidermis leaving areas of denuded skin on the arm.

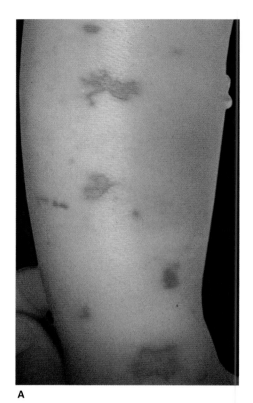

A

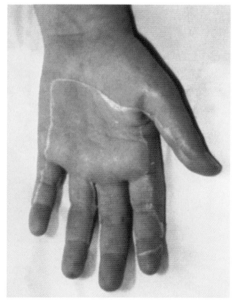

▲ Figure 26-13. Toxic shock syndrome. Diffuse erythema with desquamation of skin on palm. Reproduced with permission from Centers for Disease Control and Prevention. PHIL Collection ID# 5113.

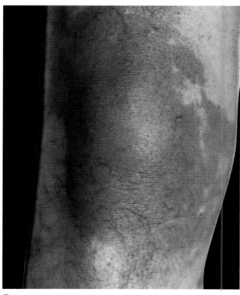

B

▲ Figure 26-14. A, B. Meningococcemia. A. Erythematous irregularly shaped plaques with a grey center on a child's leg. B. Purpuric plaque on knee.

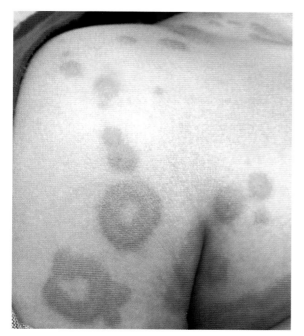

▲ **Figure 26-15.** Urticaria multiforme. Annular erythematous wheals on child's trunk and thighs.

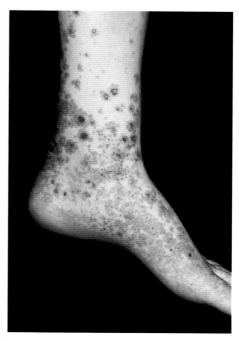

▲ **Figure 26-17.** Henoch-Schoenlein purpura. Confluent, non-blanchable purpuric papules on lower leg.

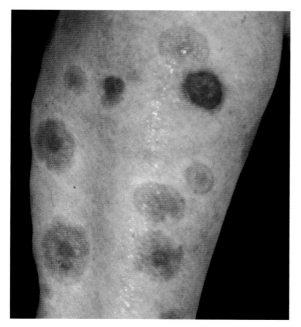

▲ **Figure 26-16.** Erythema multiforme. Targetoid erythematous plaques on leg.

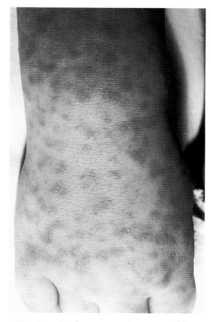

▲ **Figure 26-18.** Rocky Mountain spotted fever. Pink macules and petechiae on arms and dorsal hand. Reproduced with permission from Centers for Disease Control and Prevention. PHIL Collection ID# 1962.

REFERENCES

1. Pickering L K, Baker C J, Freed G L,et al: Immunization programs for infants, children, adolescents, and adults: clinical practice guidelines by the Infectious Diseases Society of America. *Clini Infect Dis.* 2009;49(6):817-840.
2. Centers for Disease Control and Prevention. Measles – United States, 2011. *MMWR Morb Mortal Wily Rep.* 2019; 68(40):893-896.
3. Freeman EE,et.al. The spectrum of COVID-19 associated dermatologic manifestations: An international registry of 716 patients from 31 countries. *J Am Acad Dermatol.* 2020;83(4):1118-1129.
4. Knöpfel N, Noguera-Morel L, Latour I, Torrelo A. Viral exanthems in children: A great imitator. *Clin Dermatol.* 2019;37(3):213-226.
5. Drago F, Ciccarese G, Gasparini G, et al. Contemporary infectious exanthems: an update. *Future Microbiol.* 2017;12: 171-193.
6. Muzumdar S, Rothe MJ, Grant-Kels JM. The rash with maculopapules and fever in adults. *Clin Dermatol.* 2019 Mar-Apr;37(2):109-118.
7. Kabani N, Ross SA. Congenital cytomegalovirus infection. *J. Infect. Dis.* 2020;221: S9-S14.
8. Womack J, Jimenez, M. Common questions about infectious mononucleosis. *Am Fam Phys.* 2015;91(6):372-376.
9. Lambert N. Strebel P, Orenstein W, Icengole J, Poland G. Rubella. *Lancet.* 2015; 385:2297-307.
10. Sim JY, Chang L-Y, Chen J-M, Lee P-I, Huang L-M, Lu C-Y. Human parvovirus B19 infection in patients with or without underlying diseases. *J Microbiol Immunol Infect.* 2019;52(4):534-541.
11. Leung AKC, Sergi CM, Lam JM, Leong KF. Gianotti–Crosti syndrome (papular acrodermatitis of childhood) in the era of a viral recrudescence and vaccine opposition. *World J Pediatr.* 2019;15(6):521-527.
12. Pardo S, Perera TB. Scarlet Fever. In: *StatPearls.* StatPearls Publishing; 2021. Accessed February 28, 2021. http://www.ncbi.nlm.nih.gov/books/NBK507889/
13. Leung AKC, Barankin B, Leong KF. Staphylococcal-scalded skin syndrome: evaluation, diagnosis, and management. *World J Pediatr.* 2018;14(2):116-120.
14. Wilkins AL, Steer AC, Smeesters PR, Curtis N. Toxic shock syndrome - the seven Rs of management and treatment. *J Infect.* 2017;74:S147-S152.
15. Siddiqui JA, Ameer MA, Gulick PG. Meningococcemia. In: *StatPearls.* StatPearls Publishing; 2021. Accessed February 28, 2021.
16. Gavin M, Sharp L, Stetson CL. Urticaria multiforme in a 2-year-old girl. *Proc (Bayl Univ Med Cent).* 2019;32(3):427-428.
17. Rixe N, Tavarez MM. Serum Sickness. In: *StatPearls.* StatPearls Publishing; 2021. Accessed February 28, 2021. http://www.ncbi.nlm.nih.gov/books/NBK538312/
18. Trayes KP, Love G, Studdiford JS. Erythema multiforme: recognition and management. *Am Fam Physician.* 2019;100(2):82-88.
19. Canavan TN, Mathes EF, Frieden I, Shinkai K. Mycoplasma pneumoniae-induced rash and mucositis as a syndrome distinct from Stevens-Johnson syndrome and erythema multiforme: a systematic review. *J Am Acad Dermatol.* 2015;72(2):239-245.
20. Hetland LE, Susrud KS, Lindahl KH, Bygum A. Henoch-Schönlein Purpura: A Literature Review. *Acta Derm Venereol.* 2017;97(10):1160-1166.
21. Rife E, Gedalia A. Kawasaki Disease: an Update. *Curr Rheumatol Rep.* 2020;22(10):75.

Hospital Acquired Rashes

Barbara D. Wilson

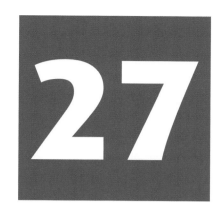

INTRODUCTION TO CHAPTER

Hospitalized patients frequently have cutaneous problems that the attending physician will need to assess. Skin disorders occur in as many as one third of all inpatients.[1,2] These problems range from those unrelated to the hospitalization and inconsequential at that time, to those that could indicate life threatening disorders of the skin or serious underlying systemic disease. The challenges to correctly diagnosing and treating a skin problem in a hospitalized patient is influenced by both access to timely dermatological consultation and the lack of adequate dermatologic training received by many non-dermatologist physicians or advanced care providers.[3] It is well known that referring physicians' dermatologic diagnoses and those of dermatologic consultants concur in less than half of inpatient episodes.[4–8] Implicit in this observation is the risk that many patients could receive improper, costly or even harmful treatments or no treatment at all. Improper or delayed diagnoses and treatment can lead to prolonged hospitalizations and higher readmission rates.[8,9] Some papers now address ways for inpatient dermatology to be more available by including the utilization of teledermatology.[10–12]

For the non-dermatologist attending, it is important to be familiar with both common and serious dermatoses seen in the hospital setting and how the hospital setting might contribute to these.

The type and scope of problems seen in a hospital setting are often dependent on the nature of the hospital itself (pediatric, academic, tertiary, community) and the population that it serves as well as the specialty origin of the consultation (i.e., internal medicine vs. neurology). Certain problems are seen frequently, including dermatitis (atopic, seborrheic, contact), psoriasis, infectious problems (bacterial, fungal and viral, and especially candidiasis and cellulitis), and drug reactions.[1,5,7,12,13]

The hospital setting can predispose a patient to many dermatological problems. It has been estimated in one study that approximately 36% of dermatological problems in hospitalized patients occurred after the admission.[6] The hospitalized patient is especially vulnerable to infections for many reasons including exposure to prevalent and sometimes resistant hospital organisms, lowered or altered immunity due to underlying disease or treatment (e.g., chemotherapy),[14] and the loss of skin integrity caused by trauma, surgeries, and intravenous lines creating portals of entry. Searching for and discerning a portal of entry in the skin is especially important in diagnosing skin infections. In addition, some infections are caused by overgrowth, not contagion, resulting from ecologic changes (e.g., candida after antibiotics), moist environments (e.g., tinea in groin in bedridden patients) or by autoactivation (e.g., herpes simplex virus (HSV) in immunosuppressed individuals).

In addition to exposure to potentially infectious agents, the hospital setting also provides a challenge for regular and careful cleansing/bathing of the skin which can exacerbate many skin problems. Also, many potential products that can cause allergic or irritant contact dermatitis are also found in the hospital setting including soaps, cleansers, disinfectants, topical therapies, bed clothes, adhesives, and bandages. Other factors that might contribute to hospital-acquired skin problems include the immobility of seriously ill patients resulting in pressure on the skin and nutritional impairment.

It is very important to remember that drug reactions are common in the hospital setting, with the number of medications that hospitalized patients receive contributing directly to this trend. Adverse drug reactions in the skin of hospitalized patients can be the result of many mechanisms not all of which are clearly "allergic." Some dermatologic reactions might be expected after exposure to a certain drug (e.g., mucositis after chemotherapy) while other reactions might represent toxicity, overdose, or hypersensitivity. Hypersensitivity can be seen with many patterns. The most common pattern by far is a morbilliform exanthem[1] occurring in up to 2% of inpatients. Fortunately, about 95% of these are uncomplicated.[1] Careful assessment is still needed in discerning the likely culprit drug, assessing the need for discontinuation, and diagnosing those reactions that are more serious and complicated. In general, drug reactions that are serious tend to be those with fever, systemic signs and symptoms, and severe skin involvement. Viral exanthems can be difficult to clinically discern from drug exanthems, but are expected to be less frequent in the hospital in adult patients than drug exanthems overall. Viral exanthems are more frequently seen in the hospital setting in those with compromised immune systems and in pediatric patients. Graft versus host disease, which can occur in the setting of bone marrow and stem cell transplantation may be particularly difficult to differentiate from viral exanthems and drug hypersensitivities and could require special expertise.

Finally, hospitalized inpatients are often chronically or acutely immunosuppressed. Immunosuppression can take many forms. Examples are myriad but include immunosuppression can be due to the following:

- Solid organ transplant medications
- Cancer and cancer chemotherapy
- Serious rheumatologic and inflammatory conditions and the treatment of these diseases with immunosuppressive drugs
- Bone marrow transplantation and graft versus host disease treatment
- Administration of high dose steroids for a prolonged period
- Poorly controlled diabetes
- Human immunodeficiency virus (HIV) infection
- Prolonged neutropenia, lymphopenia, or other hematologic abnormalities especially related to underlying leukemias and lymphomas

The type and duration of immunosuppression are important in determining the risk of a skin complication. Immunosuppressed patients characteristically have atypical or severe morphologies and their skin diseases can also disseminate and evolve very rapidly with dire consequences if a diagnosis is delayed. As a result, these patients require a great deal of surveillance and a very high index of suspicion for timely diagnosis, often with the aid of a consulting dermatologist.

APPROACH TO DIAGNOSIS

Important factors to consider in evaluating the patient's skin problem in the hospital setting include the previous known dermatologic history, underlying systemic diagnoses, systemic medications taken over the past 3 weeks including over the counter medications, as well as the topical products the patient has used recently. It is important to have a total body skin baseline skin examination with findings recorded at admission. It is also important to know immediately if the patient is experiencing rapid changes in their skin condition or has evidence of acute skin failure. Skin pain, intense pruritus, fever, skin blisters, mucosal lesions, purpura, necrosis, target lesions, or other specific signs of toxicity may indicate a serious condition and an immediate response.

A dermatologic problem seen in the hospital setting can also be that of a pre-existing skin disease exacerbated by the current illness or treatment for which the hospitalization is occurring. Studies have shown that common rashes in hospitals include pre-existing atopic dermatitis, seborrheic dermatitis, psoriasis, and stasis dermatitis. It is therefore important to inquire about pre-existing diagnoses of skin disease and to be familiar with reasons that these diseases might flare. Examples might include a flare of atopic dermatitis due to secondary bacterial infection, a flare of seborrheic dermatitis due to inability to bathe, a flare of bullous pemphigoid due to the withdrawal of systemic steroids, or a flare of stasis dermatitis due to immobility and the resultant increased edema of the lower extremities. In the most extreme settings, the pre-existing underlying dermatitis could even evolve into erythroderma, defined as involvement of >90% of the body surface area.

Contact dermatitis is common in hospital settings but is rarely the initial cause of the hospitalization. Most contact dermatitis in the hospital is probably irritant and not allergic contact caused by exposure to strong cleansers for skin, disinfectants and adhesives. One very important opportunity for misdiagnosis due to "hidden" contact dermatitis is the "red leg."

The "red leg," often erroneously assumed to be cellulitis, can be easily misdiagnosed. In one study, one-third of those suspected of having cellulitis had alternative diagnoses.[1,15–17] The red leg due to presumed cellulitis can be the result of allergic contact dermatitis due to application of topical products. The clinician needs to be aware of what products the patient was using in the hospital setting to avoid the possibility of inappropriate antibiotic use for presumed cellulitis. When diagnosing a "red leg," the physician must also look for history and clinical evidence of stasis dermatitis, lipodermatosclerosis, or even acute venous thrombosis as well as previously mentioned allergic contact dermatitis. As admission and readmission for cellulitis is common and costly,[15] and limiting inappropriate antibiotics is important, it is essential that every attending physician early in the admission process is aware of the possibilities for misdiagnosis of the "red leg" especially when the patient is not responding to therapy.

The careful approach to the immunosuppressed patient requires diligence. The attending physician should understand the context, duration, and type of immunosuppression as this will help to understand the patient's risks for infections and other problems. Travel, occupation, hobbies, pets, behaviors, and preceding trauma are essential parts of the history. A complete examination of the entire skin, including mucous membranes is required, including a search for any potential portals for infection (trauma, surgery, intravenous (IV) lines). The physician should be aware that infections in immunosuppressed patients occur with unusual and "opportunistic" organisms including bacteria, acid fast organisms, yeast and fungi and even parasites and "contaminants" should not be dismissed.[18] To make things more challenging, neutropenic patients may not demonstrate erythema and purulence and infections might instead show minimal lesions or atypical necrosis. Synchronous multiple infections can occur as well as "auto-activated" infections. As a rule, infectious processes can move quickly in this population. The attending physician should therefore request an appropriate consultation as soon as possible as skin biopsies for pathology, read by an experienced pathologist who is aware of the setting may be required to make a diagnosis. In addition, tissue biopsies should be done for culture of organisms including bacterial, fungal, and acid-fast bacilli (AFB).

Common dermatologic disorders seen in the hospital as well as several high-risk problems seen less commonly are listed in the table format.

- Table 27-1 lists common inflammatory cutaneous diseases.
- Table 27-2 lists common infections.
- Table 27-3 lists some uncommon cutaneous diseases with moderate to high morbidity.
- Table 27-4 has guidelines in approaching an immunosuppressed patient. This table is not intended to be exhaustive and the reader is directed to seek consultation if needed.

Table 27-1. Common inflammatory dermatoses in the hospital.

Disease and Pertinent chapter	Epidemiology	History	Physical Examination	Laboratory
Drug Rash (See chapter 17)	All ages and races. Relative risk factors: female, older age, multiple medications, immunosuppression (HIV), some concurrent viral infections. Especially common with sulfonamides, penicillins, cephalosporins, aromatic anticonvulsants, and allopurinol. Drug eruptions are overall about 10% of all hospital consults; morbilliform eruptions are most common form.	Onset 4–14 days after drug initiation most common. Variable pruritus. More serious reactions such as DRESS and SJS/TEN may present with high fever, skin tenderness, severe edema, extensive purpura, targets, and mucosal lesions.	Morbilliform (like measles): pink, red or dull red macules and papules with confluence especially on trunk> extremities. Dependant areas often more affected. May have polymorphous features, some areas may appear urticarial.	Skin biopsy generally not helpful. CBC can help differentiate viral syndrome. More serious reactions may have abnormal chemistry profile and liver function tests.
Urticaria (See Chapter 16)	All ages, races, and both genders. Underlying causes include URI, drug ingestions, foods, and systemic diseases including infectious, hematologic, vasculitic, and immunologic diseases. In hospital setting, drugs are the most common cause, but systemic diseases need to be considered.	Abrupt appearance of transient pruritic edematous wheals. May have associated oral mucosal swelling (angioedema).	Edematous pink or red wheals of all sizes and shapes anywhere on body and transient over 24 h May have associated angioedema (soft tissue swelling of the face). Fever, target lesions, persistence of wheals, bruising, purpura, toxicity indicate need to look for causes of complex urticaria.	Mild eosinophilia. Urticaria due to serious systemic disease may have cytopenias, profound eosinophilia, hypocomplementemia, evidence of renal or liver problems.

(Continued)

Table 27-1. Common inflammatory dermatoses in the hospital. (Continued)

Disease and Pertinent chapter	Epidemiology	History	Physical Examination	Laboratory
Contact dermatitis (CD) (See Chapter 8)	All ages, races and both genders. Allergic CD (e.g., metals, adhesives, fragrances, preservatives, formaldehyde, topical antibiotics) probably less common in hospital setting than irritant CD (e.g., strong soaps, disinfectants, surgical preps, bedclothes, paper products).	Irritant CD is immediate if contact irritant is strong and can have burning or pain. Cumulative irritancy with weaker irritants more commonly subacute. Allergic CD is classically delayed 1–2 days after exposure to allergen and pruritic.	Well demarcated erythematous dermatitis in areas of exposure. Irritant CD can be eczematous and scaling when subacute and sometimes erosive when acute. Allergic CD can have vesicles or bullae if severe.	Skin biopsy generally not indicated. Patch tests of specific allergens can later elucidate cause if allergy is suspected.
Seborrheic dermatitis (See Chapter 9)	All ages, races, both genders; common in infants and postpubertal adults; especially common in some neurological diseases, in those on chronic steroids and patients with HIV.	Acute exacerbations of chronic dermatitis with variable pruritus. Often worse when bathing is diminished.	Greasy, loose scale overlying pink dermatitis in seborrheic distribution on scalp, face, ears, intertriginous areas, chest, and upper back.	None helpful.
Atopic dermatitis (See Chapter 8)	All ages, races, both genders atopic diathesis, family history of atopy.	Chronic pruritic eczematous dermatitis with exacerbations.	Infantile-extensor and face. Child and adult-flexural and possibly widespread. Poorly marginated, pink eczematous plaques often with lichenification and excoriations.	Possible elevated serum IgE and eosinophilia.

CBC, complete blood count; DRESS, drug rash with eosinophilia and systemic symptoms; HIV, human immunodeficiency virus; IgE, immunoglobulin E; URI, upper respiratory infection; SJ/TEN, Stevens Johnson/toxic epidermolysis

Table 27-2. Common cutaneous infections in the hospital.

Disease and Pertinent chapter	Epidemiology	History	Physical Examination	Laboratory
Viral Exanthem (See Chapter 26)	All ages, both genders. More common in children and immunosuppressed. Less common than drug exanthems in hospital setting. Exposure in community and autoactivation are important factors.	Abrupt onset with gradual worsening. Variable pruritus. Dependent on underlying virus but typically associated fever, cough, sore throat, myalgias, headache, lymphadenopathy, conjunctivitis, nausea, vomiting, and diarrhea.	Maculopapular, morbilliform, urticarial and vesicular lesions. Often mucosal lesions. Consider: HIV, EBV, CMV, HHV-6, HHV-7, rubella, rubeola, enteroviruses, adenoviruses, parvovirus B-19, varicella. Varies depending on specific causative virus.	CBC with atypical lymphocytes, lymphopenia or lymphocytosis; LFTs, viral specific antibody tests; nasopharyngeal, throat, stool washings, and swabs.
Herpes simplex(HSV) Herpes Zoster(VZV) (See Chapter 13)	All ages, races, both genders. Worldwide. VZV more common >age 50. Severe, recurrent HSV and VZV in immunosuppressed patients.	Tingling, pain, burning sensation may precede rash. VZV is dermatomal with possible dissemination. Rare cutaneous dissemination of HSV in atopic individuals.	Grouped vesicles and crusting on red base. HSV usually recurrent in same place. VZV is dermatomal. Severe, widespread, ulcerating disease in immunosuppressed.	Tzanck smear of lesion. DFA, PCR, or NAAT. Viral culture required for drug sensitivities.

(Continued)

Table 27-2. Common cutaneous infections in the hospital. (Continued)

Disease and Pertinent chapter	Epidemiology	History	Physical Examination	Laboratory
Cellulitis (See Chapter 11)	All ages, races, both genders. More common with trauma, portals, broken skin.	Abrupt onset of tenderness and pain with variable chills, malaise, and fever.	Sudden appearance of tender, red, warm, edematous ill-defined or sharply demarcated advancing erythema, generally unilateral.	CBC with leukocytosis and left shift. Cultures from definite portal may be helpful. Biopsy for tissue cultures if unresponsive to treatment or immunosuppressed.
Pyoderma (Abscess) (See Chapter 11)	All ages, races, both genders. More common with trauma, portals, broken skin	Acute or subacute onset of variably tender or pruritic areas of skin	Pyoderma with weeping, eroded, crusted, purulent lesions with surrounding erythema Abscesses with tender fluctuant red nodules with or without surrounding erythema.	Skin culture after incision for abscess.
Candidiasis (See Chapter 12)	All ages, races, both genders. Risk factors: broad spectrum antibiotics, diabetes, hyperhidrosis, occlusion, corticosteroid use.	Acute or sub-acute. Pruritus, tenderness, burning.	Bright red moist or erosive dermatitis, poorly marginated with satellite and lesional pustules in intertriginous areas, genitals, scrotum and areas of occlusion. Mucous membranes with white removable exudates on red patches.	KOH with budding yeast and pseudohyphae. Cultures recommended if unresponsive to treatment.
Fungal Infection (See Chapter 12)	All races, both genders. T. capitis prepubertal, all other forms commonly post-pubertal. M>F for T. cruris, T. pedis. Severity and extent can be worse in immunosuppressed. Relative risk factors: Obesity, hyperhidrosis, age, occlusion. Tinea is an important cause of broken skin and portals for bacterial infection (cellulitis).	Generally subacute or chronic with exacerbations. Tinea pedis can be portal for bacterial infections.	Generally dry, scaling on body on and groin with annular configuration and central clearing /active border. Spares scrotum. On feet, moccasin or interdigital distribution. Rarer inflammatory with vesicopustules. Nails with powdery scale and subungual debris.	KOH with branching hyphal structures. PAS stain of nail or skin will demonstrate same. Fungal culture to identify species.

CBC, complete blood count; CMV, cytomegalovirus; DFA, direct fluorescent antibody; F, female; HHV, human herpes virus; HIV, human immunodeficiency virus ; KOH, potassium hydroxide; LFTs, liver function tests; M, male; NAAT, Nucleic acid amplification test; PAS, periodic acid-Schiff; PCR, polymerase chain reaction; T., tinea.

Table 27-3. Uncommon dermatoses in the hospital.

Disease and Pertinent Chapter	Epidemiology	History	Physical Examination	Laboratory
Vasculitis (See Chapter 24)	All ages, races, both genders. More common in adults with associated underlying diseases (rheumatologic, hematologic, infectious) and also after use of certain drugs.	Generally painful or burning lesions on the skin with accompanying symptoms of underlying disease.	Range from non-blanching palpable purpura on the lower extremities and dependant areas as to purpuric nodules and ulcers corresponding in size to that of the involved underlying vessel.	Directed at diagnosing underlying disease and defining which organ systems may be involved. Biopsy of appropriate site can show pathologic evidence of the type of vessel involved and type of inflammation present.

(Continued)

Table 27-3. Uncommon dermatoses in the hospital. (Continued)

Disease and Pertinent Chapter	Epidemiology	History	Physical Examination	Laboratory
Erythroderma (See Chapter 18)	All ages, races, both genders. Most common in adults. Idiopathic type most common in adult males. Other causes: underlying severe dermatitis, Sezary syndrome, drug reaction, pityriasis rubra pilaris.	Usually acute or subacute over days or weeks. Often with pre-existing milder underlying dermatologic disease (atopic, psoriatic, seborrheic). Medications added in past weeks.	Extensive pink inflamed plaques or dull erythema with and without scale covering 90% of body surface area. May have appearance of underlying skin disease.	Biopsy may be diagnostic, but often not in evolving disease. If chronic erythroderma, concern for hypoalbuminemia, anemia, electrolyte disturbances. CBC and flow cytometry for cutaneous T cell lymphoma/leukemia.
DRESS Syndrome (Drug Reaction with Eosinophilia and Systemic Symptoms) (See Chapter 17)	All ages, genders. Women>men. More common in adults. More common in immunosuppressed patients and also after the use of certain drugs including sulfonamides, penicillins, aromatic anticonvulsants, allopurinol.	Onset of variable exanthem along with fever and other organ dysfunction. Significant mortality especially if not recognized.	Exanthem is variable. Can be morbilliform and minimal, but purpura, targets, blisters can occur. Often extensive edema of face and extremities and lymphadenopathy.	Eosinophilia and dysfunction of other organs including kidney, liver, lung, GI tract, or other. Imperative screening for organ dysfunction if suspected. Most important management is to stop offending drug.
Erythema Multiforme EM (See Chapter 18)	More common in children and young adults. Respiratory viral or bacterial infection or herpes simplex may precede rash.	URI-like symptoms may precede rash. Sudden onset of red target lesions.	Target lesions often with multiple rings on trunk, extremities, and palms. Lips may have ulcerations and crusts, but oral cavity usually has limited disease.	Biopsy findings variable depending on stage of disease.
Stevens-Johnson Syndrome/Toxic Epidermal Necrolysis SJ/TEN (See Chapter 18)	Can occur at any age, but more common and severe after age 65. More common in women. Majority of cases are caused by medications or less likely infections. Causes significant morbidity and mortality.	Sudden onset of painful dusky patches often following URI- or flu-like symptoms. Patients require hospitalization often in burn units.	Rapid development of areas of erythematous dusky red patches and atypical target like lesions. Within hours the lesions form flaccid blisters and leave large areas of necrotic, sloughing skin. Mucosal areas, especially oral, ocular, and genital areas are affected. Nikolsky sign is positive.	Skin biopsy shows epidermal necrolysis. May develop electrolyte imbalance, decreased serum albumin and protein. Sepsis is a risk from impaired skin integrity.
Pyoderma Gangrenosum (See Chapter 28)	All ages, races, both genders. More common in adults and those with underlying predisposing disease (inflammatory bowel disease, hematologic and rheumatologic diseases). Recent surgery or trauma to site.	Rapid evolution of painful necrotic or purulent ulcer that grows quickly. Initial lesion often very painful pustule. Variable fever.	Purulent, necrotic deep ulcer with undermined dusky border. Most common on lower legs, but also abdomen, peristomal, site of surgery.	Biopsy is confirmatory but not diagnostic. Need to consider infection, vasculitis and trauma. Tissue culture may be needed to rule out infection. Avoid debridement due to pathergy.

CBC, complete blood count; HIV, human immunodeficiency virus; GI, gastrointestinal.

Table 27-4. Dermatoses in the immunosuppressed hospitalized patient.

Disease and Pertinent Chapter	Epidemiology	History	Physical Examination	Laboratory
GVHD (Graft vs. Host Disease) (See Chapter 15)	Transplant of (mismatched or altered) immunologically active graft with allogeneic or autologous bone marrow transplant, stem cell transplant, transfusion or rarely, solid organ transplant.	Variable onset: Acute< 100 days or with change in immunosuppression Chronic > 100 days. GVHD often associated diarrhea, liver changes, rarely lung.	Generally (lacy reticular) exanthem often involving face, hands and trunk in acute GVHD. Occasional severe necrosis of skin. Exanthem or lichenoid cutaneous and mucosal involvement in chronic GVHD.	Biopsy with characteristic changes and keratinocyte apoptosis. Associated elevated bilirubin, diarrhea volumes.
Sweets syndrome (Acute febrile neutrophilic disorder) (See Chapter 15)	Occurs accompanying some acute infections and rheumatologic conditions. Especially common in myeloproliferative disease, acute leukemias.	Sudden onset of pink edematous tender plaques with fever.	Tender edematous pink to red plaques on the face, trunk > extremities. Occasionally bullous, purpuric or atypical.	CBC with neutrophilia in normal host. Associated CBC abnormalities in leukemia. Pathology demonstrates dermal edema with infiltrate of numerous neutrophils without prominent vasculitis or leukemic cells.
Chemotherapy-related rashes (See Chapter 17)	Common in those receiving cytotoxic, targeted chemotherapy, and immunotherapy.	Generally, within days of cytotoxic agents although some effects are cumulative. Targeted chemotherapies with variable onset. Immunotherapy with variable onset.	Dependent on the nature of the chemotherapy. Be familiar with certain patterns: • Hand foot syndrome • Mucositis • Toxic erythema of chemotherapy • Acneiform eruptions • Immunologic reactions • Numerous isolated skin, hair and nail changes	Pathology dependent on type of reaction.
Drug reactions in immunosuppressed patients (See Chapter 17)	Morbilliform exanthems and complicated hypersensitivity like DRESS reactions more common in patients with immunosuppression including HIV.	Dependent on type of reaction-some hypersensitivity reactions require longer exposures to drug (3 weeks + for DRESS).	Dependent on nature of reaction. If systemic hypersensitivity, could cause GI problems, transaminitis, other liver problems, pneumonitis, and fever.	Look for and track systemic symptoms and signs.
Herpes and VZV (See Chapter 13)	Occurs in those with and without immunosuppression, all forms.	Often acute onset in normal host but can be recurrent or chronic infection in immunosuppression.	Typical isolated grouped vesicles for HSV in normal but disseminated or chronic painful ulcers periorificial or perianal/groin in immunosuppressed patients. May not have vesicles in this setting. Typical dermatomal vesicles in VZV in normal but ulcerated or disseminated in immunosuppressed patients.	PCR, NAAT, and biopsy. Culture required if sensitivity to antivirals is required.

(Continued)

Table 27-4. Dermatoses in the immunosuppressed hospitalized patient. (Continued)

Disease and Pertinent Chapter	Epidemiology	History	Physical Examination	Laboratory
Subcutaneous and deep mycoses (See Chapter 12)	Can occur in normal host but especially common in immunosuppressed patients including solid organ transplant.	Often history of trauma, travel for exposure but also disseminated from lung, sinus, or another portal.	Extremely variable: can mimic bacterial cellulitis, subcutaneous nodules, ulcerating necrotic lesions, molluscum-like lesions, bullae, pustules, or other.	Early pathology with special stains and tissue cultures for all possible organisms.
Atypical mycobacteria (See Chapter 12)	Can occur in normal host but especially common in immunosuppressed patients including solid organ transplant.	Often history of trauma or exposure to organism (fish tank, etc.).	Extremely variable: can mimic bacterial cellulitis, but also subcutaneous nodules, ulcers, necrotic lesions, or other.	Early pathology with special stains and tissue cultures for all possible organisms.
Scabies (See Chapter 14)	Can occur in normal or immunosuppressed host with contact to infested person.	Contact with person with scabies. Variable or even absent pruritus in immunosuppressed patients, unlike in normal. Extremely large number of mites-isolation required.	Variable but can cause large areas of gray hyperkeratotic debris, crusts overlying erythema with thousands of burrows. Does not resemble typical scabies in webs, etc.	Scraping, dermoscopy, rarely biopsy. Follow up exams required as relapse is common.
Gram-positive bacteria (See Chapter 11)	Can occur in normal or immunosuppressed persons where infection is more likely severe, atypical, or resistant to treatment. Very common in patients with prolonged neutropenia.	Often portal is traumatic, surgical, IV line or other, including dissemination or sepsis.	Extremely variable and dependent on host and organism but includes cellulitis, pustules, nodules, necrosis, abscesses, other.	Culture of blood and culture of tissue biopsy of skin for organism and sensitivities. Pathology and special stains of skin biopsy for diagnosis.
Gram negative bacteria (See Chapter 11)	Can occur in normal or when in immunosuppressed persons, infection is more likely to be severe, atypical, or resistant to treatment. Very common in patients with prolonged neutropenia.	Often portal is traumatic, surgical, IV line or other, including dissemination or sepsis.	Extremely variable and dependent on host and organism, but includes cellulitis, pustules, nodules, necrosis, abscesses, other.	Culture of blood and culture of tissue biopsy of skin for organism and sensitivities. Pathology and special stains of skin biopsy for diagnosis.

CBC, complete blood count; DRESS, drug rash with eosinophilia and systemic symptoms; IV, intravenous; PCR, polymerase chain reaction; NAAT, nucleic acid amplification test; VZV, varicella zoster virus.

REFERENCES

1. Biesbroeck L, Shinohara,M: Inpatient Consultative Dermatology. *Med Clin N Am.* 2015; 99(6): 1349-1364.
2. Arnold J, Yoon S, Kirkorian Y: The national burden of inpatient dermatology in adults. *J Am Acad Dermatol.*2019; 80: 425-32.
3. Ahmad K, Ramsay B: Analysis of inpatient dermatologic referrals: insight into the educational needs of trainee doctors. *Ir J Med Sci.* 2009; 178(1):69-71.
4. Hughey LC: Why perform inpatient consultations? (editorial). *Dermatol Ther.* 2011; 24(2):149-150.
5. Falanga V, Schachner LA, Rae V, et al: Dermatologic consultations in the hospital setting. *Arch Dermatol.* 1994; 130(8): 1022-1025.
6. Mancusi S, Festo Neto C: Inpatient dermatologic consultations at a university hospital. *Clinics.* 2010; 65(9): 851-855.
7. Davila M, Christenson LJ, Sontheimer RD: Epidemiology and outcomes of dermatology inpatient consultations in a Midwestern U.S. university hospital. *Dermatol Online J.* 2010; 16(2):12.

8. Hu L, Haynes H, Ferrazza D, Kupper T, Qureshi A: Impact of Specialist Consultations on Inpatient Admissions for Dermatology-Specific and Related DRGs. *J Gen Intern Med*.2013; 28(11): 1477-82.

9. Galimberti F, Guren L, Fernandez A, Sood A: Dermatology consultations significantly contribute quality to care of hospitalized patients: a prospective study of dermatology inpatient consults at a tertiary care center. *Int J of Dermatology*. 2013;55: 547-551.

10. Strowd L: Inpatient dermatology: a paradigm shift in the management of skin disease in the hospital (editorial). Br J Derm.2019;180: 966-67.

11. Fox L, Madigan L: Where are we now with inpatient consultative dermatology? Assessing the value and evolution of this subspecialty over the past decade. *J Am Acad Dermatol*. 2019;80:1804-8.

12. Barbieri JS, Nelson CA, James WD, et al: The reliability of teledermatology to triage inpatient dermatology consultations. *JAMA Dermatol*.2014; 150:419-424.

13. Phillips G, Lacouture ME et al: Inflammatory Dermatoses, infections and drug eruptions are the most common skin conditions in hospitalized cancer patients. *J Am Acad Dermatol*. 2018; 78(6):1102-1109.

14. Tracey E, Forrestel A, Rosenbach M, Micheletti R: Inpatient dermatology consultation in patients with hematologic malignancies.. *J Am Acad Dermatol*. 2016;75(4):835-836

15. Fisher J, Feng J, Tan S, Mostaghimi A: Analysis of Readmissions Following Hospitalization for Cellulitis in the United States. *JAMA Dermatol*. 2019;155(6):720-723.

16. Ko L, Kroshinsky D, et al: Effect of Dermatology Consultation on Outcomes for Patients with Presumed Cellulitis. A Randomized Controlled Trial. *JAMA Dermatol*. 2018;154(5): 529-536.

17. Hirschmann J, Raugi G: Lower Limb Cellulitis and its Mimics: Part I and II. *J Am Acad Dermatol*. 2012;67(2): 163.e1-163.e12 and 177.e1- 177.e9.

18. Grossman ME, Fox LP, Kovarik C, Rosenbach M. Cutaneous Manifestations of Infection in the Immunocompromised Host. Second Edition. New York, NY: Springer; 2011.

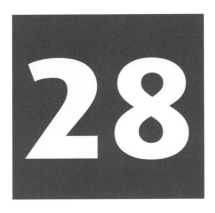

Leg Ulcers

Neal Foman

▼ INTRODUCTION TO CHAPTER

An understanding of the pathophysiology, diagnosis, and management of leg ulcers is very important to healthcare providers as these occur in a significant number of patients. Approximately 1–3% of the population, or up to 10 million people in the United States are affected.[1] The annual cost of leg ulcers is proposed to be $8–10 billion per year, with an estimated loss of 2 million workdays per year.[2] The majority of leg ulcers are seen in middle-aged to elderly patients, and there is a female:male predilection of 2:1. The three most common types of leg ulcers are venous, arterial, and neuropathic, although leg ulcers can also be multifactorial in origin. Defining the underlying etiology is of the utmost importance to designing a successful treatment plan.

▼ VENOUS ULCERS

Introduction

Key Points for Venous Ulcers

✓ Venous ulcers are caused by venous insufficiency and account for 70–80% of all leg ulcers.

✓ They present as well-marginated ulcers with sloped borders on the lower leg usually over or proximal to the medial malleolus. Stasis dermatitis and varicosities are often seen in conjunction with these ulcers.

✓ Pedal pulses are usually present.

✓ The use of inelastic or elastic compression products is the gold standard for the treatment of venous leg ulcers.

Ulcers caused by venous insufficiency, are the most common type of leg ulcerations, accounting for 70–80%. They are often called stasis ulcers. 10–20% of leg ulcerations have a mixed venous and arterial etiology. Leg ulcers caused by chronic venous insufficiency lead to significant morbidity and can have a long-term negative impact on an individual's quality of life. The ability of affected patients to work, be active, and function well in society can be greatly compromised. Diagnosis can be challenging, and management is often expensive and labor-intensive for both the patient and the healthcare provider.

Pathogenesis

Venous ulcers most commonly arise secondary to varicose veins or postphlebitic syndrome. They may also be seen in patients with a history of a deep vein thrombosis (DVT), obesity, or previous leg injury or surgery. When a patient with normal venous return stands or walks, the calf muscle acts in concert with veins and associated valves to empty the venous system and reduce its pressure.[3] When the valves become incompetent secondary to some form of injury, blood pools in the lower extremities and venous hypertension develops. This leads to tissue hypoxia and ultimately to skin destruction and breakdown. In addition, wound healing processes are compromised, and autolytic processes take action. The result is loss of the epidermis and dermis and the formation of an ulcer.

Clinical Presentation

▶ History

Patients with venous insufficiency usually complain of a heavy or swollen feeling in the affected leg(s). Pain ranges from mild with a superficial ulceration to severe with a deep ulceration. Patients may describe limitation of movement of the affected extremity, depending on the location of the ulcer. There may be a small, moderate, or significant amount of drainage from the ulcer itself or even from other areas of the affected extremity. In addition, patients with venous stasis and dermatitis may have pruritus and inflammation of the skin surrounding an ulcer.

▶ Physical Examination

Most patients with venous ulceration have some degree of non-pitting or pitting edema. Varicosities may be visible and there is often hyperpigmentation from hemosiderin deposition over the shin (Figure 28-1). Typically, venous ulcers occur over or proximal to the medial malleolus, but they may occur anywhere below the knee. They can be

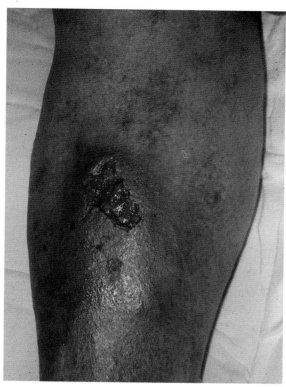

▲ **Figure 28-2.** Venous ulcer. Sharply marginated ulcer with irregular border in area of stasis dermatitis.

single or multiple, small or large, shallow or deep. They are usually well-marginated with sloped borders but can present with irregular shapes (Figure 28-2). Often, there is fibrinoid material and/or granulation tissue at the base. The surrounding skin may have an inflamed and eczematous appearance. These ulcers can sometimes have copious drainage. Pedal pulses are usually present. Clinical findings of venous insufficiency can sometimes be confused with cellulitis, leading to unnecessary and costly hospitalizations and treatments. Early consultation by dermatologists for patients with presumed cellulitis can reduce inappropriate antibiotic use and hospitalizations.[4]

▶ Laboratory Findings

There are no specific laboratory findings that point toward a diagnosis of venous ulceration. However, a complete blood count (CBC), erythrocyte sedimentation rate (ESR), and blood glucose can help to diagnose an underlying hematologic, inflammatory, or diabetic condition. A culture will likely yield mixed flora and may not be relevant unless the wound appears clinically infected. Consider culturing a wound when it becomes painful, more inflamed,

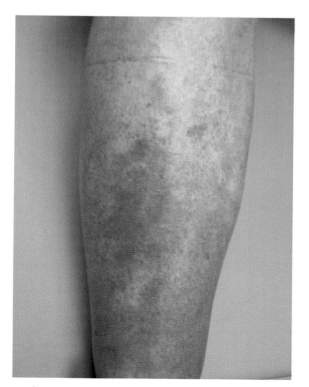

▲ **Figure 28-1.** Venous Insufficiency with stasis dermatitis, varicosities, and edema.

Table 28-1. Differential diagnosis of leg ulcers.

Type of Ulcer	Risk Factors	History and Physical	Notes
Venous	Deep venous thrombosis (DVT), varicose veins, previous lower extremity surgery or injury, obesity.	Lower extremity edema, varicosities, hyperpigmentation, and dermatitis; ulcer over shin, or medial malleolus.	Compression is the key to treatment. Pulses usually palpable.
Arterial	Peripheral arterial disease, smoking, hyperlipidemia, hypertension, diabetes.	Intermittent claudication, painful ulcer, shiny skin, eschar may be present at base of ulcer, ulcer over distal lower extremities.	Low threshold for referral to vascular surgery. Pulses usually not palpable. Do **not** use compression.
Neuropathic	Diabetes, spinal cord injury or disease, alcohol abuse, leprosy.	Ulcer over pressure points of plantar foot, surrounded by callus, foot deformities, insensate lower extremities, deep.	Prevention is critical as a significant number of these ulcers can lead to amputation.
Inflammatory	Vasculitis, systemic lupus erythematosus.	May have signs and symptoms of systemic inflammatory disease.	Systemic workup is appropriate.
Infectious	Diabetes, obesity.	Significant exudate, foul odor, pain and warmth of surrounding skin	Culture prior to starting treatment with antibiotics.
Pyoderma Gangrenosum	Inflammatory bowel disease, arthritis, myeloproliferative disorder.	Irregularly shaped ulcer with undermined edges (Figure 28-3).	Diagnosis of exclusion.
Malignancy	History of ionizing radiation.	Non-healing ulcer (Figure 28-4).	Must be considered if standard therapy fails.

has increased exudate, or becomes malodorous. A venous Doppler ultrasound can help to locate venous occlusion or incompetent perforating veins.

Diagnosis and Differential Diagnosis

The key diagnostic findings of venous ulcers are well-circumscribed ulcerations usually located over the shins or medial malleolus, on a backdrop of hyperpigmentation, varicosities, and lower extremity edema. Pedal pulses are usually present. Fibrinoid material or granulation tissue is often observed at the base of the ulcer. The most likely differential diagnosis is an arterial ulcer, or an ulcer caused by mixed arterial and venous insufficiency.

See Table 28-1 for the differential diagnosis of leg ulcers.

Management

One must always know the cause of an ulcer before designing a treatment plan. Once a diagnosis of a venous ulcer has been definitively made, the primary goal is to reverse venous hypertension so that there is an environment amenable to wound healing.[5] The most effective way to accomplish this is with compression, the gold standard for the treatment of venous leg ulcers. Compression reverses venous hypertension, has positive effects on microcirculation, reduces deep venous reflux, reduces lower leg edema, and allows for improved oxygenation of the skin. To treat venous insufficiency, there should be a goal to provide at least 20–30 mm Hg compression for several hours a day. The more severe edema there is, the more compression

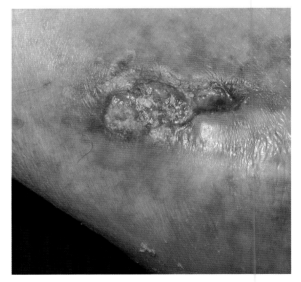

▲ **Figure 28-3.** Pyoderma gangrenosum. Deep ulcer with violaceous border and undermined edges.

should be applied. There are two categories of compression products available.

- Inelastic compression products which are used for reduction of edema and healing of ulcers.
- Elastic compression products which are used for maintenance to prevent ulcer recurrence.

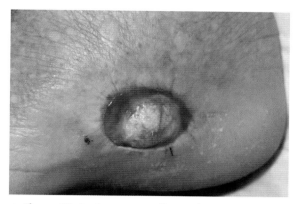

Figure 28-4. Squamous cell carcinoma on foot presenting as a leg ulcer.

The most widely used inelastic products are Unna boots (single layer) or Profore boots (multiple layer). These are occlusive wraps that are applied as an ace wrap would be applied in the office and removed 1 week later. They may also be applied at the patient's residence by a trained home health professional. An important companion to the use of these leg wraps is frequent elevation of the legs.

Elastic compression is achieved with products such as TEDS or Jobst stockings which can be worn on a regular basis for maintenance, once a venous ulcer has healed. Another option is a mechanical pneumatic compression device which can be ordered for a patient.

Compression should always be a component of treating a venous ulcer, but **one must rule out the possibility of arterial insufficiency** prior to applying a compressive dressing to a patient.

In addition to compression, the treatment of the wound itself is very important. The ulcer bed must be prepared so as to allow for optimum healing.[6] Tissue removal or debridement may be necessary, as the fibrinoid material present in some wounds interferes with healing. This may be accomplished surgically or mechanically with scissors, a curette, or a scalpel, and may require local anesthesia. Enzymatic or proteolytic agents (e.g., Santyl, Panafil, or Accuzyme) can also be used to more slowly debride a wound when necessary. One can also apply a hydrocolloid dressing (e.g., Duoderm or Restore) every 2–3 days, and this will serve to slowly debride a wound as well.

The moisture balance in an ulcer can have a significant effect on healing. In particular, most wounds heal more quickly in a moist environment. This is accomplished by using dressings that absorb excess fluid in a very exudative wound, or that retain fluid in an otherwise dry wound.[7]

- When there is significant exudate, some appropriate absorptive dressing choices are Kerlix, Mepilex, gauze sponges, abdominal combine pads (ABD), hydrophilic foam dressings (e.g., COPA), or hydrocellular polyurethane dressings (e.g., Allevyn).

- When a wound is dry, some appropriate dressing choices are Telfa, Vaseline petroleum gauze, or a non-adhering oil emulsion dressing (e.g., Curity).

An ulcer often needs help with reepithelialization. There are several products that aid in providing contact between the wound edges so that they are stimulated to grow back together. Hydrocolloid dressings (e.g., Duoderm or Restore) provide this function. They should be replaced over a wound every 2–3 days. Extracellular matrix dressings (e.g., Oasis, or Matristem) create a scaffold over which growth factors and keratinocytes can migrate, thus helping to bring a wound together. Biologic agents (e.g., Apligraf or Dermagraft) provide live building blocks for new skin to regenerate. Newer advanced therapies such as human placental membrane allografts (e.g., Biovance) are also available and easy to apply in the office.

One last item to be addressed in the treatment of a venous ulcer is the possibility of infection. Most ulcers are colonized with bacteria, but this is not often to the level of frank infection. In these cases, the bacteria are coexisting with the host, and these ulcers do not require antibiotic treatment. Certainly, if there are clinical signs of infection such as thick odorous exudate, surrounding erythema, or increasing warmth or pain, one should consider the use of an oral antibiotic after a culture has been taken. The daily use of a diluted bleach or vinegar soak can be important in preventing bacterial infection of a wound. If a patient has stasis dermatitis adjacent to an ulcer, this should be treated with a mid-potency topical steroid, such as triamcinolone 0.1% ointment. The latter will help to maintain the integrity of the skin, thus decreasing the risk of cellulitis.

Although leg ulcers due to venous insufficiency can often be successfully treated with medical interventions, a recent study has shown that early treatment with endovenous ablation can accelerate the healing of venous ulcers and reduce the overall incidence of ulcer recurrence.[8]

Clinical Course and Prognosis

Ongoing treatment may be necessary for many months before a venous ulcer will heal. Control of the patient's comorbidities plays an important role in the success of treatment. Recurrence is common, seen in 54–78% of all venous ulcers.[9] Compared with standard care, some advanced wound care therapies may improve the proportion of ulcers healed and reduce time to healing.[10]

Indications for Consultation

If the underlying etiology of a leg ulcer can't be determined, a specialist such as a vascular surgeon or a dermatologist should be consulted. If an ulcer is not healing despite appropriate treatment, referral to a wound care clinic should be considered. Also consider referral if the necessary management products are not available at the patient's primary clinic.

ARTERIAL ULCERS

Introduction

Key Points for Arterial Ulcers

✓ The major risk factors for arterial ulcers are peripheral arterial disease, cigarette smoking, and diabetes.

✓ They are caused by compromised arterial blood flow which leads to tissue ischemia and necrosis. Pedal pulses are often absent.

✓ Arterial ulcers present as painful, round, punched-out ulcers with sharp edges usually on the feet, often over bony prominences.

✓ Compression should not be used in patients with arterial ulcers.

It is important to note that 6–10% of leg ulcers are found in the setting of peripheral arterial disease and are usually referred to as arterial or ischemic ulcers, and 10–20% of leg ulcers have a mixed venous-arterial component. It is very important to determine the underlying etiology so that the appropriate management plan can be followed. Diagnosis can be challenging, and often a multidisciplinary approach is necessary for diagnosis and treatment.

Pathogenesis

The major risk factors for arterial ulcers are peripheral arterial disease, cigarette smoking, and diabetes. Other factors which contribute to the risk are hyperlipidemia and hypertension. In contrast to venous ulcers, arterial ulcers are seen more commonly in men. The underlying etiology in most cases is a decrease in or complete obstruction to arterial blood flow in the lower extremities. This is often the result of narrowing of the vessel lumen by an atherosclerotic plaque. The compromised blood flow leads to tissue ischemia and necrosis, and ultimately a skin ulceration forms.

Clinical Presentation

▶ History

The most common complaint of a patient with an arterial ulcer is intermittent claudication. The patient experiences pain around the calf muscles during exercise early in the disease and at rest in late disease. The pain tends to be relieved when the patient places the leg in a dependent position.[11] In general, arterial leg ulcers are significantly more painful than venous ulcers. The patient may report that their feet are usually cold, and they may notice that their feet and legs become pale with elevation.

▶ Physical Examination

Arterial ulcers present in distal locations, often over bony prominences such as the toes. They tend to have a round,

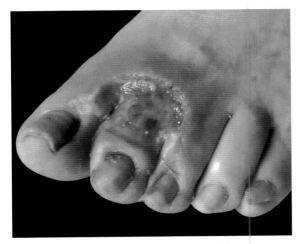

Figure 28-5. Arterial ulcer with round sharply defined edges.

punched-out appearance with sharp edges (Figure 28-5). The base of the ulcer is often dry and may be covered with necrotic debris, presenting as an eschar. These ulcers are sometimes so deep that bone or tendon might be exposed. Perhaps the most important clinical feature in making a diagnosis of an arterial ulcer is the absence of pedal pulses. The skin on the lower legs of these patients is often shiny and atrophic appearing with little or no hair. The feet of a patient with arterial insufficiency may be cold to palpation.

▶ Laboratory Findings

It is very important to measure the ankle-brachial index (ABI) in a patient who is suspected of having arterial insufficiency. This is the ratio of the ankle systolic pressure of the affected limb to the higher of the brachial systolic pressures measured in each arm. An ABI <0.8 indicates occlusive arterial disease.[12] An ABI test can be conducted in the office or in a vascular laboratory. Of note, those with diabetes or advanced age may have falsely elevated ABI results, because their vessels are highly calcified or noncompressible. A Duplex ultrasound can also be helpful to identify arterial occlusion or atherosclerotic disease. Inaudible pedal pulses would be highly suspect for arterial insufficiency. As with venous ulcers, a CBC, ESR, and blood glucose can help to diagnose an underlying hematologic, inflammatory, or diabetic condition. A culture will likely yield mixed flora and may not be relevant unless the wound appears clinically infected.

Diagnosis and Differential Diagnosis

The key diagnostic findings of arterial ulcers are punched-out appearing, well-circumscribed, and sometimes quite deep ulcerations, usually present in distal locations over bony prominences such as the toes. Pedal pulses tend to be absent. The base of the ulcer tends to be dry and might appear necrotic. The surrounding skin is often shiny and hairless. This is all likely to be found in the setting of intermittent claudication. The most likely differential diagnosis is a venous ulcer, a mixed venous-arterial ulcer, or a neuropathic ulcer.

See Table 28-1 for the differential diagnosis of leg ulcers.

Management

If an arterial etiology is suspected, **compression should not be part of the treatment plan** as this can lead to ischemia and necrosis of tissue.

Therapy of arterial ulcers should be targeted at locating an occlusion, and then reestablishing adequate arterial blood supply. One should have a low threshold for referring the patient to vascular surgery for evaluation and/ or treatment. Surgical interventions may include angioplasty, stent placement, atherectomy, endarterectomy, or bypass. In addition, the patient should be encouraged to stop smoking, eat a low-fat diet, and gain better control of their blood pressure and blood sugar. Antiplatelet medications such as aspirin and Plavix can be helpful in preventing ischemic events. An exercise program where a patient exercises on a regular basis to the threshold of tolerable pain is an important part of the patient's recovery; this should be discussed with the patient's primary care provider.

Pain control is another important element of the care of patients with arterial ulcers. This may include systemic medication in addition to good local wound care. If an arterial ulcer is exudative or there is surrounding erythema, one should consider a systemic antibiotic after culture. Again, it is important to pay attention to the level of moisture in a wound, to the level of bacteria in the wound, and to the surrounding skin.

Clinical Course and Prognosis

Patients with an identifiable vessel obstruction who undergo surgical intervention will often have rapid healing of their ulcer. About 10% of patients with peripheral arterial disease and associated ulcers will have severe enough ischemia to lead to amputation of a digit or a limb. The likelihood of amputation is greater in diabetics and smokers. A small percentage of patients will spontaneously develop collateral blood flow that leads to improvement of their symptoms. The 5-year mortality for patients with intermittent claudication is 30%, with death largely attributed to cardiovascular causes.[13]

Indications for Consultation

Most patients with arterial ulcers should be evaluated by and co-managed with vascular surgery as surgical intervention might be a necessary part of their treatment.

▼ NEUROPATHIC ULCERS

Introduction

Key Points for Neuropathic Ulcers

✓ Neuropathic ulcers are caused by peripheral neuropathy usually due to diabetes.

✓ They present as painless, deep, punched-out ulcers over the pressure points of the plantar surface of the foot.

✓ Prevention and early detection of these ulcers is important.

Ulcerations secondary to peripheral neuropathy account for up to 10% of all leg ulcers. Some patients have both an ischemic and a neuropathic component to their ulcers. The most common cause of neuropathic foot ulcers in the United States is diabetes. Approximately 20% of those with diabetes (3 million people) will develop a foot ulcer in their lifetime.[14] Unfortunately, up to 25% of these patients will require an amputation.

Pathogenesis

The vast majority of diabetic patients have peripheral neuropathy which predisposes them to the development of an ulcer. The neuropathy interferes with the patient's ability to perceive pain thus leading to repeated trauma to pressure points on the feet. In addition, neuropathy can lead to the development of foot deformity resulting in further trauma to susceptible areas.[15] Hyperglycemia can impede wound healing by leading to impaired function of neutrophils, macrophages, and fibroblasts. Lastly, autonomic dysfunction contributes to hypohidrosis which causes skin to become fissured and callused. The result is the formation of a neuropathic ulcer. Less common causes of neuropathic ulcers are spinal cord disease or injury, alcohol abuse, and leprosy.

Clinical Presentation

▶ History

The neuropathic ulcer is usually painless. It may not be apparent to the patient until it is advanced because it is asymptomatic and not easily visible on the bottom of the foot. The patient will often complain of burning, numbness, or other paresthesias of the feet and lower legs.

▶ Physical Examination

The typical location of a neuropathic ulcer is over a pressure point of the plantar foot, such as the great toe, metatarsal head, or heel (Figure 28-6). A callus often surrounds and hides the full extent of the wound (Figure 28-7). The patient may have claw toes, flat feet, or Charcot joints. These ulcers tend to be deep and bone or tendon might be visible.

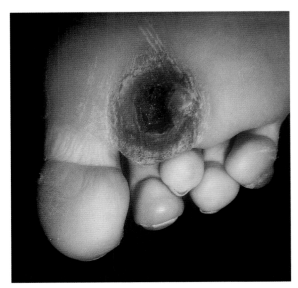

Figure 28-6. Neuropathic ulcer. Ulcer with callous over metatarsal head in diabetic patient.

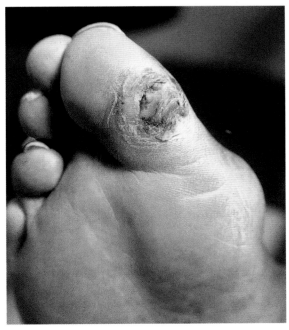

Figure 28-7. Neuropathic ulcer with overlying callus.

▶ Laboratory Findings

As with venous and arterial ulcers, a CBC, ESR, and blood glucose can help to diagnose an underlying hematologic, inflammatory, or diabetic condition. If infection is suspected, one should not only culture the wound, but also consider an x-ray or MRI to rule out osteomyelitis. Tissue and/or bone cultures should be taken prior to the initiation of antibiotic therapy.

Diagnosis and Differential Diagnosis

The key diagnostic findings of neuropathic ulcers are deep, punched-out appearing ulcerations mainly over pressure points of the plantar foot. There may be symmetric distribution of ulcers over both feet. These ulcers are often surrounded by callus and the foot might exhibit some deformity. The most likely differential diagnosis would be an arterial ulcer or a mixed neuropathic-arterial ulcer.

See Table 28-1 for the differential diagnosis of leg ulcers.

Management

Of paramount importance in the care of a diabetic patient is the prevention and early detection of lower extremity ulcers. The largest cause of amputation other than traumatic injury is a non-healing diabetic foot ulcer.[16]

Proper care of the ulcer itself is very important, with a goal of keeping the ulcer environment moist and clean. Once a wound is prepared properly, an engineered product such as a collagen matrix product, a biologic skin product, or a human placental membrane allograft can be quite useful in helping an ulcer to reepithelialize.

Identification and early management of infection in a neuropathic ulcer will significantly decrease morbidity and even mortality. If osteomyelitis is suspected or confirmed, appropriate parenteral antibiotic therapy should be instituted promptly.

Aggressive debridement of the surrounding callus and non-viable tissue should be performed either surgically (with a scalpel), mechanically (with wet-to-dry dressings), or enzymatically (with a collagenase-containing product).[17]

Another important component of treatment of a neuropathic ulcer is off-loading of pressure.[18] Repeated trauma to high pressure areas of an insensate foot is the underlying cause of many neuropathic ulcers. There are a number of different devices used to reduce foot pressure and one should consider consultation with a podiatrist to aid in the selection of the appropriate device for a patient. Most commonly, orthotic devices with cushioning are chosen for this purpose.

Clinical Course and Prognosis

Because diabetes is a chronic disease and the most common underlying cause of a neuropathic ulcer, management can be challenging. Those ulcerations that are discovered early and when they are shallow and small have the best prognosis in terms of complete healing. Deeper and larger ulcerations will take longer to heal, may require more advanced wound care tools, and are more likely to be complicated by a secondary soft tissue or bone infection which then also has to be treated. In addition, even in cases where healing is achieved, the same patients seem to return repeatedly with ulcers at the same or different sites.[19]

Indications for Consultation

It is often useful to co-manage a patient with a neuropathic ulcer with a podiatrist who has expertise in orthotics and procedures involving the foot. If there is also an arterial component, consultation with a vascular surgeon might be appropriate as well.

Patient Information

- American Diabetes Association: www.diabetes.org/living-with-diabetes/complications/foot-complications/
- Overview of Guidelines for the Prevention and Treatment of Leg Ulcers: https://www.ncbi.nlm.nih.gov/pmc/articles/PMC3930479

REFERENCES

1. Valencia IC, Falabella A, Kirsner RS, Eaglstein WH. Chronic venous insufficiency and venous leg ulceration. *J Am Acad Dermatol* 2001; 44:401-421.
2. Philips T, Stanton B, Provan A, Lew R. A study of the impact of leg ulcers on quality of life: financial, social, and psychological implications. *J Am Acad Dermatol.* 1994; 31:49-53.
3. Sackheim K, DeAraujo TS, Kirsner RS. Compression modalities and dressings: their use in venous ulcers. *Dermatol Ther.* 2006; 19:338-347
4. Li, DG, Xia, FD, Khosravi, H, et. al. Outcomes of early dermatology consultation for inpatients diagnosed with cellulitis. *JAMA Dermatol.* 2018; 154(5):537-543.
5. Lund J, Miech D. Leg ulcers. In: Schwarzenberger K, Werchniak AE, Ko CJ, eds. *General Dermatology.* 1st ed. Philadelphia, PA: Elsevier; 2009:346.
6. Schultz GS, Sibbald RG, Falanga V, et. al. Wound bed preparation: systematic approach to wound management. *Wound Repair Regen* 2003;11:1-28.
7. Palfreyman SJ, Nelson EA, Lochiel R, Michaels JA. Dressing for healing venous leg ulcers. *Cochrane Database Syst Rev* 2006 Jul 19;3:CD001103.
8. Gohel, MS, Mora, J, Szigeti, M, et. al. Long-term clinical and cost-effectiveness of early endovenous ablation in venous ulceration. *JAMA Surg.* 2020, Sept. doi:10.1001/jamasurg.20203845.
9. Abbade LP, Lastoria S. Venous ulcer: epidemiology, diagnosis and treatment. *Int J Dermatol.* 2005;44(6):449-56.
10. Greer, N, Foman NA, MacDonald, R, et. al. Advanced wound care therapies for nonhealing diabetic, venous, and arterial ulcers. *Ann Int Medi.* 2013, Oct.
11. Hiatt WR. Medical treatment of peripheral arterial disease and claudication. *N Engl J Med.* 2001;344:1608-21.
12. Vowden K, Vowden P. Doppler and the ABPI; how good is our understanding? *J Wound Care.* 2001; 10:197-202.
13. Newman, SA. Cutaneous Changes in Arterial, Venous, and Lymphatic Dysfunction. In: *Fitzpatrick's Dermatology*, 9th Edition. New York, NY: McGraw-Hill.
14. Pham HT, Rich J, Veves A. Wound healing in diabetic foot ulceration: a review and commentary. *Wounds.* 2000; 12: 79-81.
15. Caputo GM, Cavanagh PR, Ulbrecht JS, et. al. Assessment and management of foot disease in patients with diabetes. *N Engl J Med.* 1994; 331:854-60.
16. Browne AC, Sibbald RG. The diabetic neuropathic ulcer: an overview. *Ostomy Wound Manage.* 1999;45(1A suppl.):65-205.
17. Dinh TL, Veves A. Treatment of diabetic ulcers. *Dermatologic Therapy.* 2006; 19:348-355.
18. Armstrong DG, Nguyen HC, Lavery LA, et. al. Offloading the diabetic foot wound: a randomized clinical trial. *Diabetes Care.* 2001; 24:1019-1022.
19. Cavanagh, P, Owings, T. Nonsurgical strategies for healing and preventing recurrence of diabetic foot ulcers. *Foot Ankle Clin N AM.* 11(2006) 735-743.

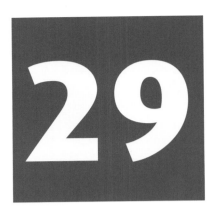

Cutaneous Signs of Psychiatric Disorders

David R. Pearson
Maria K. Hordinsky

INTRODUCTION TO CHAPTER

Psychiatric diseases are commonly associated with cutaneous pathology. *Psychophysiologic skin disorders* result from precipitation or exacerbation of skin disease by psychosocial stress.[1] These are particularly common in acne, lupus erythematosus, psoriasis, telogen effluvium, and many other dermatologic diseases are well-known examples.[1–3] This chapter will focus on primary psychiatric skin disorders, including *delusional infestation, dermatitis artefacta,* and *obsessive compulsive disorders* affecting the skin, where an underlying psychiatric disease results in self-induced cutaneous findings. In contrast, secondary psychiatric skin disorders describe primary skin diseases that result in stress, anxiety, or depression.

DELUSIONAL INFESTATION

Introduction

Delusional infestation describes the fixed, false belief of mucocutaneous infestation with parasites, particles, fibers, or other living or non-living material.[4] Patients do not have other delusions, although comorbid psychiatric disease, such as anxiety, depression, or substance use, is common.[5] The prevalence is approximately 80 per million in the outpatient setting.[5] *Delusions of parasitosis* (delusional parasitosis) refers specifically to delusional infestation of living

parasites, often arthropods or worms. *Morgellons disease* is a variant of delusional infestation attributed to inanimate fibers or particles.

Clinical Presentation

▶ History and Physical Examination

Patients frequently note the sensation of crawling, biting, or stinging on the skin. Reported visualization of parasites, particles, or fibers is common, and many patients bring previously collected samples to their visit for clinical evaluation (specimen sign) (Figure 29-1). By definition, patients lack insight and are unable to accept alternative explanations for their symptoms. Excoriations from extraction attempts may result in erosions, ulcers, (Figure 29-2) prurigo nodularis, lichenification, hair loss, and secondary infection.

Self-isolation and fear of contamination of family members or friends are common, but 8–12% present with folie à deux, shared delusions in a close contact.[5] Many patients describe repeated courses of topical and systemic antiparasitic agents from past providers, repeated use of home exterminators, or frequent moves to attempt to escape recurrent infestation.

▶ Laboratory Findings

No laboratory abnormalities are commonly observed.

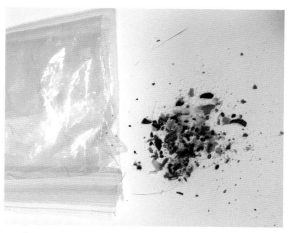

▲ **Figure 29- 1.** Delusional parasitosis. Collection of cloth fibers, food particles, black seeds, dust and skin debris that patients interpret as being "bugs" (specimen sign).

Diagnosis

Diagnosis is based on characteristic clinical presentation and exclusion of other causes of symptoms. It is particularly important to rule out true infestation, as well as other potential underlying medical, metabolic, neurologic, substance abuse, or psychiatric disorders that may cause similar symptoms. Examination of the patient's entire body and clothing should be performed (body lice may not be present on the skin, but may be present on clothing). Initial laboratory workup is warranted, including complete blood count (CBC), comprehensive metabolic panel (CMP), thyroid studies, vitamin B12, folate, iron studies, and urine or serum toxicology. A skin scraping should be obtained and examined microscopically to rule out scabies infestation. Skin biopsies and cultures may be appropriate to aid in correct diagnosis.

▶ Differential Diagnosis

Evidence of true infestation (see Chapter 14 Infestations and Bites) is absent in delusional infestation. Underlying cutaneous dysesthesia disorders associated with unwanted, uncomfortable, or inappropriate sensations such as itching, burning, tingling, prickling, pins-and-needles, electrical jolts, or pain should be ruled out. Examples of such syndromes include notalgia paresthetica, brachioradial pruritus, and erythromelalgia.[6] Patients with formication or neuropathy may have similar cutaneous dysesthesia, but usually do not lack insight or believe they are infested. Substance use and underlying psychotic disorders usually do not demonstrate fixed, encapsulated delusions and demonstrate more widespread symptoms.

Management

It is critical to create a strong, non-judgmental therapeutic relationship, and to neither challenge nor affirm the delusion.[4,7] Confrontation with the patient over the nature of their delusions may rapidly erode the therapeutic relationship and in some cases, exacerbate symptoms. In contrast, providing repeated courses of antiparasitic agents despite evidence that an infestation is absent violates the ethical principles of patient autonomy and non-maleficence. After an appropriate workup has been completed, there should be an open-ended discussion with the patient that validates their symptoms without endorsing them. Data that supports a lack of infestation should be presented clearly. Because they lack insight, patients may not be convinced by the available data and are typically resistant to psychiatric referral or initiation of antipsychotic agents. The process of building rapport may take several visits over weeks to months.

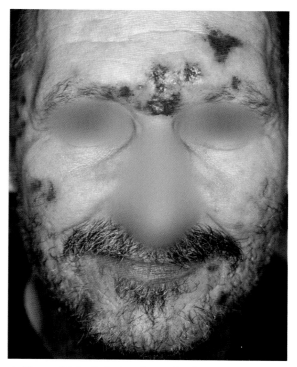

▲ **Figure 29-2.** Delusional parasitosis. Numerous excoriations from extraction attempts are apparent, resulting in erosions and shallow ulcers.

After trust has been established, patients are more likely to become receptive to initiation of antipsychotic agents. Pimozide, a typical antipsychotic, is traditionally used; however, the newer atypical antipsychotics such as risperidone, olanzapine, quetiapine, or aripiprazole may have fewer extrapyramidal side effects. Patients may respond to lower doses than those used for other psychotic disorders.[5]

Psychotherapy is typically unsuccessful.

Clinical Course and Prognosis

Successful treatment of delusional infestation is particularly challenging. Patients frequently transition care to another clinician if they perceive their infestation is not taken seriously or if they do not receive requested treatments (typically antiparasitic agents). Even with appropriate treatment with antipsychotics, delusions may remain, thus the primary goal of treatment is reducing their intrusiveness and improve function.[7]

Indications for Consultation

Patients will frequently request referral to a dermatologist or infectious disease specialist. They are often resistant to psychiatric referral, but a psychiatrist may be able to assist with pharmacotherapy.

Patient Information

- Minnesota Department of Health: https://www.health.state.mn.us/diseases/pests/dp.html
- Harvard Mental Health Letter: https://www.health.harvard.edu/newsletter_article/delusions-of-infestation
- Psychology Today: https://www.psychologytoday.com/us/conditions/delusional-disorder

▼ DERMATITIS ARTEFACTA

Introduction

Dermatitis artefacta is a factitial disorder whereby patients knowingly create skin lesions in order to assume the sick role; it is distinct from *malingering*, where the motivation is overtly due to secondary gain (tangible physical, social, or emotional advantage due to illness). Patients with dermatitis artefacta deny the self-inflicted nature of their injuries and the history of acquisition may be obscure or intentionally vague (hollow history). By definition, patients have an underlying psychiatric disease, and personality disorders are common.

Clinical Presentation

The clinical presentation may include geometric, superficial erosions that do not follow any clear disease pattern (Figures 29-3 and 29-4). These changes may be caused by chemical or thermal injuries, or injection of exogenous

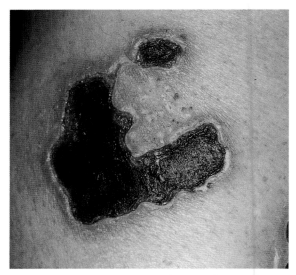

▲ **Figure 29-3.** Dermatitis artefacta. A chemical burn from acid intentionally applied to the skin, resulting in ulceration with eschar formation. Reproduced with permission from Charles E. Crutchfield III, MD.

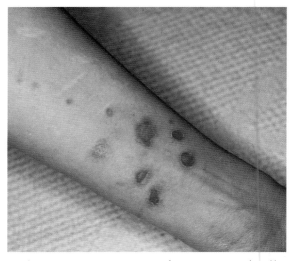

▲ **Figure 29-4.** Dermatitis artefacta. Intentional, self-administered cigarette burns on the ventral forearm.

substances into the skin or subcutaneous tissue. Secondary infection may occur; in some cases, this may be severe or life-threatening. *Other diagnoses, including delusional infestation and skin-picking disorder, must be excluded.*

Management

Treatment must target the resultant skin injury as well as aggressive psychotherapy and concomitant pharmacotherapy. A multidisciplinary approach led by a psychologist and psychiatrist is usually necessary.

Patient Information

- DermNet NZ https://dermnetnz.org/topics/dermatitis-artefacta/
- Stat Pearls https://www.statpearls.com/ArticleLibrary/viewarticle/20376

OBSESSIVE-COMPULSIVE DISORDERS

Introduction

Skin diseases associated with obsessive-compulsive disorder (OCD) and obsessive-compulsive tendencies are characterized by intrusive, unwanted thoughts or urges (obsessions) that compel the patient to perform repetitive behaviors to alleviate the associated intolerable anxiety (compulsions). In the following section, *skin-picking disorder*, *hair-pulling disorder*, and *body dysmorphic disorder* will be reviewed.

Skin-Picking Disorder

▷ Introduction and Pathogenesis

Skin-picking disorder (neurotic excoriations, psychogenic excoriations, dermatillomania) results from repetitive picking of the skin that result in tissue damage, distress, or functional impairment.[5,8] Prevalence is estimated between 1% and 5% of the population and is more common in females; onset usually occurs in adolescence or young adulthood, although in may appear later in life.[5,7] Concomitant psychiatric illness, including anxiety, depression, post-traumatic stress disorder, and body dysmorphic disorder (see below) are common.

▷ History and Physical Examination

In skin-picking disorder, patients often demonstrate numerous angulated, superficial ulcerations on the face, extremities, and upper back (Figure 29-5). Regions on the mid-back that are difficult to reach tend to be spared. Lesions may originate from a primary skin condition such as acne (resulting in *acne excoriée*), arthropod bites, or keratosis pilaris. Repetitive picking may lead to the development of lichen simplex chronicus (Figure 29-6) or prurigo nodularis. Lesions may be complicated by secondary infection or bleeding. While patients may initially deny knowledge of how lesions develop, they generally have some insight but may be unable to control the compulsion to excoriate, or experience significant associated shame.[9]

▷ Laboratory Findings

Unless complicated by infection, no laboratory abnormalities are observed.

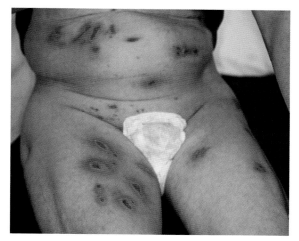

▲ **Figure 29-5.** Skin-picking disorder. Angulated and linear superficial ulcerations on the torso and thighs in easily accessible areas

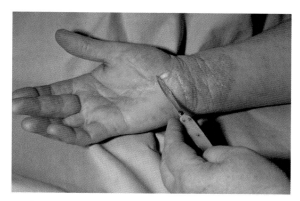

▲ **Figure 29-6.** Lichen simplex chronicus on the right ventral wrist from repetitive rubbing and scratching with a pocket knife.

▷ Diagnosis

Diagnosis is based on typical clinical appearance and exclusion of alternative diagnoses. Laboratory workup may include CBC, CMP, iron studies, thyroid studies, vitamin B12, skin scrapings to rule out parasitic infestation, and skin culture, depending on the clinical presentation. Skin biopsy may be warranted.

▷ Differential Diagnosis

- ✓ Organic causes of pruritus such as renal disease, thyroid disease, xerosis, atopic dermatitis, cutaneous dysesthesia.
- ✓ Primary psychiatric skin disorders including delusional infestation and dermatitis artefacta.

Management

Behavioral modification including patient-directed intentional cessation of picking is often of limited use. Practical approaches such as covering involved areas may offer some benefit and allow wound healing. General principles of adequate wound care should also be followed. More organized psychotherapy, including cognitive-behavioral therapy (CBT) may be more beneficial, particularly when techniques of habit reversal therapy are employed.

N-acetylcysteine, an over-the-counter nutraceutical that modulates the glutamatergic and neuroinflammatory systems, has demonstrated improvement in controlled studies.[5,8] Selective serotonin reuptake inhibitors (SSRIs) may be of benefit, particularly if there is underlying anxiety, depression, or OCD. Other agents, including gabapentin, naltrexone, and antipsychotics, may be considered but rigorous evidence is limited.

In cases where an underlying skin disorder precipitates picking, such as acne excoriée, treatment of that condition is warranted.

Clinical Course and Prognosis

Patients often follow a chronic course, and relapses are common. Successful treatment of underlying organic and psychiatric conditions may improve outcome.

Indications for Consultation

A dermatologist may be useful to confirm the diagnosis. A team-based approach with a clinical psychologist and psychiatrist is usually helpful.

Patient Information

- Mental Health America: https://www.mhanational.org/conditions/excoriation-disorder-skin-picking-or-dermatillomania
- Harvard Health blog: https://www.health.harvard.edu/blog/picking-your-skin-learn-four-tips-to-break-the-habit-2018112815447

Hair-Pulling Disorder

Introduction and Pathogenesis

Hair-pulling disorder (trichotillomania, trichotillosis) is due to repetitive pulling of hair that results in hair loss. Like skin-picking disorder, prevalence is estimated between 1% and 4% of the population and is more common in females.[5] Hair-pulling disorder usually begins in early adolescence.[9] Like skin-picking disorder, coexistent psychiatric diseases such as anxiety, depression, and post-traumatic stress disorder are common. In children, acute psychosocial stressors (e.g., parental divorce) may trigger onset of symptoms.

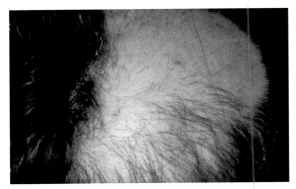

▲ **Figure 29-7.** Hair-pulling disorder (trichotillomania). Sharply demarcated, geometric areas of hair loss with broken hairs of variable lengths.

History and Physical Examination

The scalp is the most common site of involvement, followed by the eyebrows and eyelashes; however, any site may be affected. Hair loss may be significant, and sharply demarcated, geometric configurations are typical with broken hairs of variable lengths (Figure 29-7). Asymmetry favoring the patient's dominant hand side is frequently observed. Patients, particularly children, may not readily admit to hair pulling. This may be due in part to shame, but at least some hair pulling occurs unconsciously.

Laboratory Findings

No laboratory abnormalities are observed. Skin biopsy of the scalp demonstrates trichomalacia, pigment casts, increased catagen hairs, and trauma to the hair bulbs.

Diagnosis

Diagnosis is based on typical clinical appearance and exclusion of alternative diagnoses. In the appropriate clinical scenario, skin biopsy may be warranted.

Differential Diagnosis

Alternative causes of hair loss, especially those that are common in pediatric populations such as alopecia areata and tinea capitis, should be considered.

Management

There is good evidence that habit reversal therapy is effective in hair-pulling disorder. Other forms of CBT may be useful. SSRIs and other antidepressants and *N*-acetylcysteine have been used with variable success.[10] Combining psychotherapy and pharmacotherapy may lead to the best outcomes.

Clinical Course and Prognosis

Most patients achieve remission, but patients with onset later in childhood or in adulthood tend to have a more chronic course. Management of comorbid psychiatric disease is important.

Indications for Consultation

Like skin-picking disorder, a dermatologist may be useful to confirm the diagnosis, and a psychologist and psychiatrist are helpful in further management.

Patient Information

- The American Hair Research Society- North, South, and Central: https://www.americanhairresearchsociety. org/trichotillomania/
- Mayo Clinic: https://www.mayoclinic.org/diseases-conditions/trichotillomania/symptoms-causes/syc-20355188

Body Dysmorphic Disorder

Introduction

Body dysmorphic disorder is an intrusive preoccupation with perceived defects in physical appearance that are minor or not readily apparent to others. It is characterized by repetitive mirror checking, grooming, or picking behaviors that cause significant distress and may interfere with functioning with up to 40% of patients spending 3 to 8 hours a day engaged in these activities.[5] Underlying major depressive disorder and social anxiety disorder are particularly common, and suicidal ideation is endorsed by the majority of patients.[5,11] Cognitive behavioral therapy with adjunctive SSRI pharmacotherapy is the treatment of choice.[11]

Patient Information

- Mental Health America: https://www.mhanational.org/ conditions/body-dysmorphic-disorder-bdd
- Mayo Clinic: https://www.mayoclinic.org/diseases-conditions/body-dysmorphic-disorder/symptoms-causes/ syc-20353938

REFERENCES

1. Koo JYM, Lee CS. General approach to evaluating psychodermatological disorders. In: Koo JYM, Lee CS, eds. Psychocutaneous Medicine. New York, NY: Marcel Dekker, Inc. 2003: 1-29.
2. Roussou E, Iacovou C, Weerakoon A, Ahmed K. Stress as a trigger of disease flares in SLE. Rheumatol Int. 2013; 33:1367-70.
3. Chien Yin GO, Siong-See JL, Wang ECE. Telogen Effluvium - a review of the science and current obstacles. J Dermatol Sci. 2021; 101:156-163.
4. Campbell EH, Elston DM, Hawthorne JD, Beckert DR. Diagnosis and management of delusional parasitosis. J Am Acad Dermatol. 2019; 80:1428-1434.
5. Kuhn H, Mennella C, Magid M, Stamu-O'Brien C, Kroumpouzos G. Psychocutaneous disease: Clinical perspectives. J Am Acad Dermatol. 2017; 76:779-791.
6. Hylwa S, Davis M, Pittelkow M. Dysesthetic syndromes. Practical Psychodermatol. 2014; 164-172.
7. Jafferany M, Ferreira BR, Abdelmaksoud A, Mkhoyan R. Management of psychocutaneous disorders: A practical approach for dermatologists. Dermatol Ther. 2020:e13969.
8. Lochner C, Roos A, Stein DJ. Excoriation (skin-picking) disorder: a systematic review of treatment options. Neuropsychiatr Dis Treat. 2017; 13:1867-1872.
9. Jones G, Keuthen N, Greenberg E. Assessment and treatment of trichotillomania (hair pulling disorder) and excoriation (skin picking) disorder. Clin Dermatol. 2018; 36:728-736.
10. Sani G, Gualtieri I, Paolini M, et al. Drug treatment of trichotillomania (hair-pulling disorder), excoriation (skin-picking) disorder, and nail-biting (onychophagia). Curr Neuropharmacol. 2019; 17:775-786.
11. Krebs G, Fernández de la Cruz L, Mataix-Cols D. Recent advances in understanding and managing body dysmorphic disorder. Evid Based Ment Health. 2017; 20:71-75.

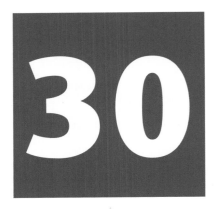

Hair Disorders

Maria K. Hordinsky

INTRODUCTION TO CHAPTER

The hair follicle is a complex structure which produces a hair fiber consisting of a cortex, medulla and cuticle (Figures 30-1, 30-2). Hair follicles demonstrate the unusual ability to completely regenerate themselves. Hair grows, falls out, and then regrows. In the normal human scalp, up to 90% of hair follicles are in the growth phase called anagen, 1% in the transition phase catagen and up to 10% in telogen or the loss phase. The anagen phase lasts approximately 3 years, catagen 2–3 weeks and telogen 3 months.[1]

Hair disorders are broadly grouped into the following categories:

- The nonscarring alopecias associated with hair cycle abnormalities.
- The scarring or cicatricial alopecias associated with inflammation and injury to the stem cell region of the hair follicle.

Hair loss is common and can occur with a variety of medical conditions. The workup of this chief complaint starts with a thorough history and physical examination as outlined in Tables 30-1 and 30-2, respectively.

The *nonscarring* hair disorders associated with abnormalities in the hair cycle include three very common hair disorders:

- Androgenetic alopecia (with or without androgen excess)
- Alopecia areata
- Telogen effluvium

These nonscarring hair diseases are associated with changes to the anagen, or growing stage of the hair cycle.

The scarring alopecias are characterized by lymphocytic, neutrophilic, or mixed inflammatory infiltrates which involve the bulge or stem cell region of the hair follicle, leading to fibrosis and permanent hair loss (Figure 30-1). The scarring alopecias may be primary or secondary as in the case of a burn or radiation injury, but in either case permanent loss of hair follicles occurs.

Hair loss may also occur with inherited or acquired structural hair abnormalities. When present, hair fibers break easily resulting in the chief complaint of "hair loss."

EXAMINATION OF THE PATIENT WITH A HAIR DISORDER

Examination of the patient presenting with the chief complaint of "hair loss" should focus on assessing the presence or absence of the following and if applicable, the use of trichoscopy.[2,3]

- Vellus, indeterminate, and terminal fibers ideally using scoring systems such as the Ludwig or Hamilton

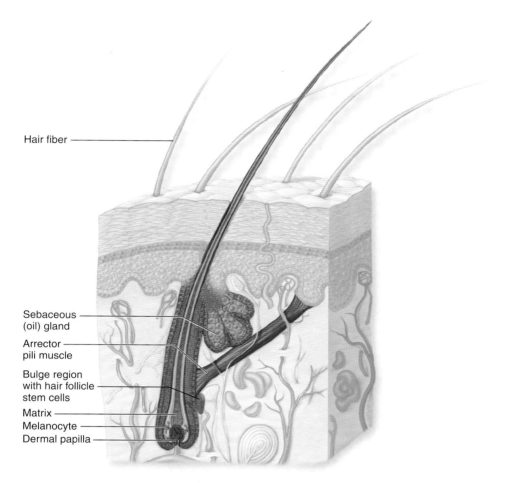

- Hair fiber
- Sebaceous (oil) gland
- Arrector pili muscle
- Bulge region with hair follicle stem cells
- Matrix
- Melanocyte
- Dermal papilla

▲ **Figure 30-1.** Pilosebaceous unit. Reproduced with permission from McKinley M, O'Loughlin VD, Pennefather-O'Brien EE: Human Anatomy, 6th ed. New York, NY: McGraw Hill; 2021.

Norwood classification systems, or the Severity of Alopecia ScoringTool (SALT score).[2–4] Vellus fibers are short, fine, light-colored, and barely noticeable. Terminal fibers are long, have a wider diameter and are pigmented. Indeterminate fibers clinically are somewhere in between vellus and terminal fibers.

- Scale, erythema, folliculitis, scarring or atrophy in the affected area.
- Eyebrow, eyelash, or body hair loss.
- Nail abnormalities which if present can be a clue to an underlying medical problem associated with the chief complaint of hair loss.
- Findings of androgen excess.

Trichoscopy or dermoscopy of the scalp can complement the clinical examination and is usually performed with a handheld dermatoscope (10× magnification) or in some centers, with a videodermoscope (up to 1000× magnification). The instrument is directly applied to the scalp to assess findings such as perifollicular and erythema, diffuse scale hyperkeratosis, or scarring.

ANDROGENETIC ALOPECIA – MALE AND FEMALE PATTERN ALOPECIA

Introduction

Androgenetic alopecia (AGA) in males is commonly called male pattern baldness and is the most common type of hair loss in men, affecting approximately 50% of men by age 50.[4] Androgenetic alopecia is characterized by the progressive miniaturization of terminal hairs or shortening of the anagen phase and transition to "baby" vellus fibers on the scalp in a characteristic distribution frequently classified using the

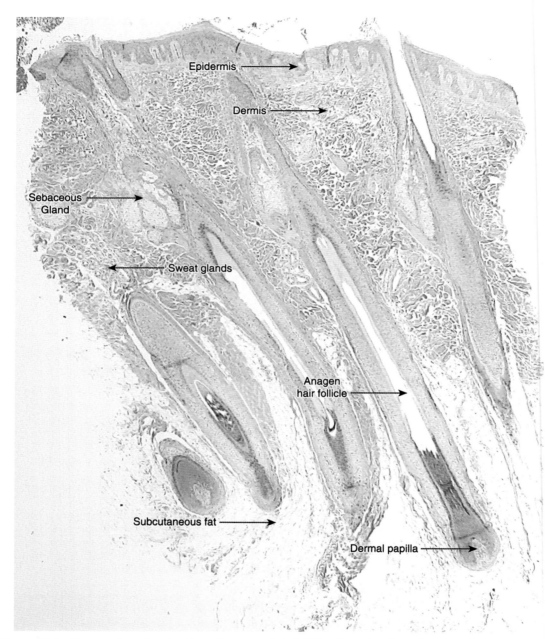

▲ **Figure 30-2.** Cross section of scalp skin with anagen hair follicles. Hematoxylin and eosin stain.

Hamilton-Norwood scale. (Figure 30-3A). Androgenetic alopecia is considered an androgen-dependent trait and the mode of inheritance polygenic with variable penetrance. Balding usually starts in the late teens or early twenties. However, approximately 10% of males will be bald in a pattern that resembles female androgenetic alopecia.

Androgenetic alopecia in females is also commonly called female pattern baldness and can be classified using the Ludwig classification scale. [5] (Figure. 30-3B). Classic androgenetic alopecia in women is also polygenic and androgen dependent with full expression usually by the mid-twenties. This pattern of alopecia may also occur in

Table 30-1. Questions for the patient presenting with the chief complaint of "hair loss."
Ask about the following:

- The chief complaint – is it "loss" or "thinning"?
- Hair care habits.
- Prescription and nonprescription medications.
- Symptoms – pain, itch, burning, whether there is a hair care product relationship.
- Body hair – is there too much or too little?
- Nail abnormalities.
- Use of supplements, herbals/botanicals.
- Family history of hair diseases.
- Signs of androgen excess.
- History of autoimmune/endocrine diseases.
- Recent or chronic illnesses.
- Recent surgical procedures.
- For females, query about the menstrual cycle/pregnancies.

Table 30-2. Physical examination of the patient with the chief complaint of "hair loss."

- Closely examine the scalp.
- Document:
  - Erythema
  - Scale
  - Folliculitis
  - Evidence of scarring
- Look for new hair growth (fibers with tapered ends) or hair breakage.
- Pull test.
- Note body hair density and distribution.
- Document any nail abnormalities.
- Use scales – Ludwig, Hamilton/Norwood, SALT or Ferriman Gallwey.

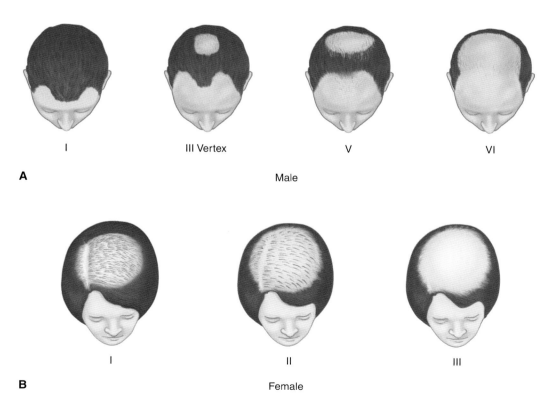

A Male

I   III Vertex   V   VI

B Female

I   II   III

▲ **Figure 30-3.** Androgenetic alopecia in males and females. A. Hamilton-Norwood scale. Types I, III, V and VII progressive patterns of male androgenetic alopecia. B. Ludwig Classification Scale for Females. Reproduced with permission from Wolff K, Johnson R, Saavedra AP, et al: Fitzpatrick's Color Atlas and Synopsis of Clinical Dermatology, 8th ed. New York, NY: McGraw Hill; 2017.

the perimenopausal and menopausal periods and may be a presenting feature of ovarian or adrenal gland abnormalities. A clinically useful classification system for women with pattern thinning is as follows: [6]

- Early Onset
  - With androgen excess
  - Without androgen excess
- Late Onset
  - With androgen excess
  - Without androgen excess

Pathogenesis

Androgenetic alopecia occurs in genetically susceptible individuals in response to the conversion of testosterone to dihydrotestosterone (DHT) by 5-alpha reductase at the level of the hair follicle resulting in miniaturization and a shortened anagen phase of the hair cycle. Androgenetic alopecia may be associated with hirsutism in women who have excess androgen production from the adrenal gland or ovaries or only in the end organ, the hair follicle.

Clinical Presentation

▶ History

Patients usually report hair shedding and a noticeable decrease in hair density following one of the patterns described previously.

▶ Physical Examination

Males may present with balding initially in the bitemporal regions, followed by thinning in the vertex region and when extensive, the two areas are no longer separated as demonstrated in Type VII Hamilton balding (Figure 30-4A). Males may also bald with the thinning process occurring from the anterior scalp to the vertex. Females present with thinning in the frontal scalp region accompanied by an increase in the part width and retention of the frontal hairline. Some patients will also exhibit a "Christmas tree" pattern in the anterior scalp region (Figure 30-4B).

The Hamilton Norwood or Ludwig classification systems can be used to classify male and female pattern alopecia, respectively (Figure 30-4 A and B). The physical examination should also take into consideration the areas noted in Table 30-2.

▶ Laboratory Findings

Usually no laboratory studies are required in the evaluation and management of male androgenetic alopecia. Women who present with pattern alopecia should be evaluated for medical conditions or nutritional deficiencies. A summary of recommended laboratory tests is presented in Table 30-3.

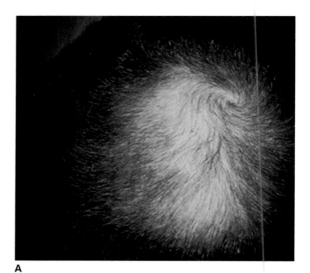

A

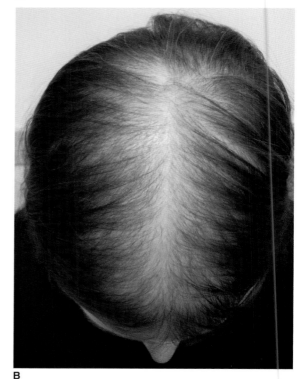

B

△ **Figure 30-4. A.** Male androgenetic alopecia. Patient demonstrates Hamilton Type IV balding with prominent thinning in the vertex region. **B.** Female androgenetic alopecia. Patient demonstrates retention of the frontal scalp hair line and pattern thinning centrally.

Table 30-3. Basic laboratory evaluation of the patient with the chief complaint of "hair loss."

- Thyroid stimulating hormone.
- Heme, ferritin, and iron studies.
- If indicated by history and physical examination: i.e., presence of hirsutism.
  - Non-cycle dependent hormones such as DHEA-S and total/free testosterone.
  - Antinuclear antibodies (ANA), other autoantibodies.
  - Other: Zinc, vitamin D, vitamin A, vitamin E, total protein, other hormones.

Diagnosis and Differential Diagnosis

The diagnosis of male androgenetic alopecia is usually straightforward. The diagnosis of female androgenetic alopecia may be slightly more complicated as thinning hair is common in women with metabolic or nutritional disorders.

The differential diagnosis includes diffuse alopecia areata and telogen effluvium both of which will be discussed next. A scalp biopsy may be needed if there is difficulty making a diagnosis.

Management

Medical, surgical, cosmetic, and device treatments can be used to treat androgenetic alopecia. Currently, minoxidil, and finasteride are Food and Drug Administration (FDA)-approved, and the HairMax LaserComb, which is FDA-cleared, are the major treatments recognized by the FDA as treatments of androgenetic alopecia. In a systematic review of randomized controlled trials, a meta-analysis was conducted separately for 5 groups of studies that tested the following hair loss treatments: low-level laser light therapy in men, 5% minoxidil in men, 2% minoxidil in men, 1 mg finasteride (Propecia) in men, and 2% minoxidil in women. All treatments were superior to placebo ($P < .00001$) in the 5 meta-analyses.[7] Rogaine 5% is available both as a solution and a foam. Finasteride is an oral inhibitor of DHT production. Clinical response can vary with some men attaining significant hair regrowth while others experience primarily a reduction in hair loss. Treatment needs to be continued to maintain the result. The HairMax LaserComb is an example of photobiomodulation (PBM) for the treatment of hair loss.

Two % topical minoxidil, 1 mL twice a day and 5% topical minoxidil once daily application are approved by the FDA in the United States for women. In a double-blind controlled study using finasteride, 1 mg daily, no efficacy was demonstrated in post-menopausal women.[8] For women with early or late onset pattern thinning and evidence of androgen excess, the use of anti-androgens or androgen receptor blocking agents may be beneficial. An example is the use of spironolactone, 100–200 mg daily.[9,10] More recently, combination therapy of spironolactone with low dose oral minoxidil has been reported to be effective in women with androgenetic alopecia.[11]

Photobiomodulation to treat androgenetic alopecia has rapidly expanded and the FDA has cleared many devices for this purpose.[12] A search by Dodd et al of the FDA 510(k) Premarket Notification database using product code "OAP" to identify all home-use devices that are FDA-cleared to treat androgenetic alopecia revealed 13 commercially available devices which varied in shape, wavelength, light sources, technical features, price, and level of clinical evidence. However, despite this rapid expansion there are still no head-to-head studies comparing the efficacy of these devices.

Regardless of which treatment or treatments are selected, a minimum of 6 months therapy is recommended to assess efficacy. The success of a therapeutic response is linked to a healthy scalp and any dermatitis or folliculitis should be managed concurrently.

Hair transplantation is also an option for patients with stable disease. Use of a scalp prosthesis or camouflaging agents such as hair fibers, powder cakes, scalp lotions or scalp sprays may also be recommended.

Clinical Course and Prognosis

Male and female androgenetic alopecia are androgen dependent genetic traits. If left untreated, there is potential for progression to extensive scalp involvement. Treatments may stabilize the thinning process as well as regrow hair. Multiple treatments are available and if prescribed, need to be used for at least 6 months. Patients need to be counseled that hair shedding may occur before improvement is seen as the hair follicles resume a normal anagen growth phase.

Indications for Consultation

Male and female patients who have not responded to a prescribed treatment such as topical minoxidil, photobiomodulation, or an oral medication should be referred to dermatology to explore other treatment options.

Patient Information

- The American Hair Research Society- North, South, and Central: https://www.americanhairresearchsociety.org/female-pattern-hair-loss/

  https://www.americanhairresearchsociety.org/male-pattern-hair-loss/

- American Academy of Dermatology: https://www.aad.org/public/diseases/hair-loss/types/female-pattern

ALOPECIA AREATA

Introduction

Alopecia areata (AA) is considered to be a complex genetic, immune-mediated disease that targets anagen hair follicles.[13] It is estimated alopecia areata affects between 4 and 5 million individuals in the United States. In alopecia areata, the hair follicle is not destroyed and maintains its potential to re-grow hair. The presence of severe nail abnormalities, atopy (asthma, allergic rhinitis, and atopic dermatitis), onset of extensive disease in children less than 5 years of age as well as alopecia totalis or universalis lasting more than 2 years, were all implicated as negative prognostic indicators until recently. The introduction of janus kinase JAK inhibitors in clinical trials and enrollment of patients with extensive disease of greater than 10 years duration who showed clinical improvement is changing the dogma about disease duration.

Both males and females of all ages can be affected and there is no known race or ethnic preponderance. Alopecia areata reportedly affects 1–2.1% of the population and has a reported lifetime risk of 1.7%. Up to 80% of cases are considered to be sporadic. Alopecia areata has been reported to occur in all age groups, males and females, and all races.

Pathogenesis

Alopecia areata is an immune-mediated disease that targets the bulb region of anagen hair follicles resulting in a shortened anagen cycle.

Clinical Presentation

▶ History

Patients typically complain of asymptomatic patchy hair loss from any hair bearing area. However, some patients may report a tingling or pruritic sensation with hair loss or hair regrowth.

▶ Physical Examination

The key diagnostic features are round or oval patches of hair loss, loss of all scalp hair (alopecia totalis), loss of all body hair (alopecia universalis), or ophiasis pattern hair loss (Figures 30-5A-D). Alopecia areata may target any hair bearing area as well as the nail matrix resulting in benign (i.e., pitting) to severe nail disease (i.e., onychodystrophy). Some patients may also present with a diffuse decrease in scalp hair density. Patches may resolve spontaneously, persist, or recur. Episodes may last for days to months to years.

The Severity of Alopecia Scoring Tool (SALT) can be used to provide an assessment of scalp hair loss and can be used as a tool to monitor therapy.[14] Disease activity can be assessed by doing light hair pull tests (Figure 30-6). Describing the types of fibers (vellus, indeterminate, terminal) present on the scalp may be helpful with setting treatment expectations. A complete examination as outlined in Table 30-2 should be done and any scalp inflammation present should be treated.

▶ Laboratory Findings

Alopecia areata may occur with other immune-mediated diseases so in addition to the laboratory studies noted in Table 30-3, additional autoantibody and immune studies may be indicated based on the history and physical examination.

Diagnosis and Differential Diagnosis

Alopecia areata is usually quite easy to diagnose. Hair diseases in the differential diagnosis for patchy disease include tinea capitis and trichotillomania, a hair disorder characterized by hair pulling in unique shapes. The differential diagnosis for extensive alopecia areata includes papular atrichia as well as an ectodermal dysplasia. For patients with the diffuse variant of alopecia areata, the clinical picture may be confused with telogen effluvium or in some cases, pattern alopecia. If the diagnosis is not straightforward, examination of a 4-mm scalp biopsy specimen may be beneficial and will demonstrate peribulbar lymphocytes around affected anagen follicles.

Management

No drug is currently approved by the U.S. Food and Drug Administration (FDA) for the treatment of alopecia areata. Many therapies are available and current treatment choices are frequently based on the disease extent, duration, and age of the patient. In some situations, patients may choose "no treatment."[15] Spontaneous remissions can occur as is seen with other autoimmune diseases. Commonly used treatments for patchy disease include application of topical class I steroids or intralesional triamcinolone acetonide (Kenalog) up to 10 mg/cc, 4 cc per session every 6 weeks. Topical minoxidil is commonly added if there are vellus or indeterminate fibers present. Anthralin and induction of allergic contact dermatitis are options. Steroid side effects need to be monitored and irritation from anthralin and contact sensitization may prevent their use. For active disease characterized by positive hair pull tests and progressive hair loss, oral corticosteroids may be prescribed in a tapering course over several weeks in an attempt to halt disease activity and in some cases; therapy may also be associated with hair growth. A challenge with oral corticosteroid therapy is that treatment may be associated with sustained hair regrowth in only about one-third of the treated patients. Other patients may be steroid non-responders or require on-going treatment to maintain hair growth.

Extensive alopecia areata (alopecia totalis and alopecia universalis) in both children and adults can be very challenging to treat and many treatments are available. These include not only oral prednisone but also other immunosuppressive drugs, such as cyclosporine, pulse methylprednisolone, narrow band ultraviolet B-light, and combination therapy.

Assessing the efficacy of treatments for patchy and extensive alopecia areata is complicated by the fact that there are few published randomized controlled trials. There are many published uncontrolled trials and reports with non-ideal criteria to evaluate treatment. Long-term follow-up is unfortunately not included in most of the published works. More clinical and translational research is

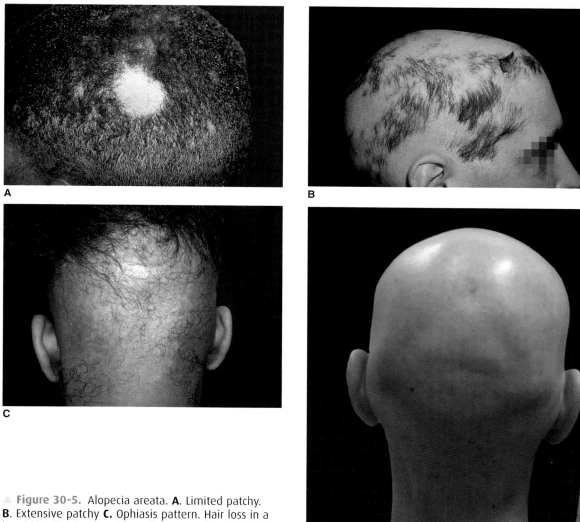

▲ **Figure 30-5.** Alopecia areata. **A**. Limited patchy. **B**. Extensive patchy **C**. Ophiasis pattern. Hair loss in a band like distribution above the ears and lower posterior scalp. **D**. Extensive. Alopecia totalis.

forthcoming particularly with the administration of janus kinase (JAK) inhibitors, several of which are currently in clinical trials.

JAK inhibitors are emerging as a novel treatment option for many immune mediated and inflammatory diseases in dermatology. Oral JAK inhibitors including tofacitinib, (a pan JAK inhibitor), and ruxolitinib (a JAK1/2 inhibitor) have proven efficacious for treatment of alopecia areata in case reports, case series, pilot studies, open-label trials, and meta-analysis. However, treatment with topical JAK inhibitors has yielded mixed results with patients in some studies experiencing significant regrowth while in other trials; outcomes have reported to be similar or inferior to clobetasol 0.05% ointment.[16–19]

Clinical Course and Prognosis

Patients with limited disease usually respond well to traditional therapies such as application of class I topical steroids or use of intralesional corticosteroids. Patients with extensive disease such as alopecia totalis or alopecia universalis may be more recalcitrant to treatment and require oral therapy with immunosuppressive medications. Such patients should also be given the opportunity to participate in clinical trials examining new evolving therapies as with the janus kinase inhibitors. As alopecia areata is an autoimmune disease, spontaneous remission may occur but is seen more commonly in patients with limited patchy disease.

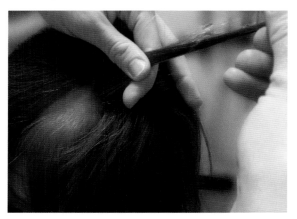

▲ **Figure 30-6.** Light hair pull test. Several fibers are grasped and pulled lightly. Presence of six or more fibers on a light hair pull test is considered to be positive.

Indications for Consultation

Patients whose disease is not responding to standard therapies or who are experiencing progressive disease should be referred to the dermatologist.

Patient Information

- National Alopecia Areata Foundation - supports research and patients and families dealing with alopecia areata: https://www.naaf.org/alopecia-areata
- The American Hair Research Society- North, South, and Central:

  https://www.americanhairresearchsociety.org/alopecia-areata/

- American Academy of Dermatology: https://www.aad.org/public/diseases/hair-loss/types/alopecia

▼ TELOGEN EFFLUVIUM

Introduction

Telogen effluvium (TE) is a very common hair loss condition that can be seen in all races and ethnic groups. The chief complaint is increased hair shedding which is the result of a shortened anagen phase and premature conversion to telogen (Figure 30-7 A). Telogen effluvium has been categorized into different subsets which may be helpful in explaining the process to patients.[20] Some examples are as follows:

- Immediate anagen release occurs after a high fever or illness.
- Delayed anagen release occurs in the postpartum period.
- Short anagen is seen in patients who report not having to cut their hair frequently or that their hair does not grow.

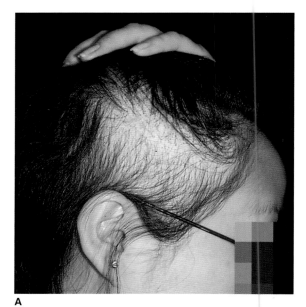

A

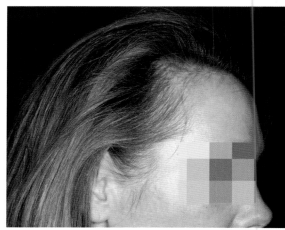

B

▲ **Figure 30-7.** Telogen effluvium. A. Female patient with diffuse hair thinning secondary to a severe telogen effluvium. Hair regrowth is expected with removal of the inciting trigger. B. Female patient with chronic telogen effluvium. Clinical clue is the significant thinning in the temporal regions.

- Immediate telogen release is typically seen after beginning topical minoxidil.
- Chronic telogen effluvium is commonly reported in middle-aged women in their fourth to sixth decades and is characterized by decreased hair density in the bitemporal regions. (Figure 30-7 B).[21]

Pathogenesis

Telogen effluvium results when more follicles than usual transition to the telogen or loss phase of the hair cycle in response to a trigger.

▶ History

The chief complaint is increased scalp hair shedding related to a trigger. Telogen effluvium can be associated with the onset of androgenetic alopecia, the postpartum period, some medications, weight loss, endocrine disorders, physiological and metabolic stress, nutritional deficiencies, acute and chronic illness, after surgeries, and with scalp inflammation. When the inciting trigger can be identified and be removed or treated, hair shedding may diminish and regrowth occur.[21,22]

▶ Physical Examination

The assessment of telogen hair loss may be made using several methods, two common methods include:

- Hair pluck. Approximately 50 hairs are plucked using a rubber-tipped hemostat and the anagen–telogen ratio is assessed by examination of the hair bulbs.
- Collection of fibers shed daily for at least 1–2 weeks. The scalp should be shampooed daily and fibers collected daily after shampooing and put into dated labeled envelopes. Anagen and telogen fibers are then qualitatively assessed. If shampooing is less frequent, it is to be expected there will be a greater number of shed telogen fibers in the sample collected on a shampoo day as hair cycling occurs and telogen fibers "rest" in follicles and are then released with the shampoo process.

▶ Laboratory Findings

If a patient is taking several supplements, additional laboratory studies to those outlined in Table 30-3 may need to be ordered. For example, high levels of Vitamin A or E may be associated with scalp hair shedding.

Diagnosis and Differential Diagnosis

The diagnosis of telogen effluvium can be established with the hair pluck test or sample collection as described previously. A scalp biopsy may also be done to confirm the shift to telogen.

The differential diagnosis includes diffuse alopecia areata, androgenetic alopecia, and possibly an inflammatory alopecia such as central centrifugal alopecia or lichen planopilaris especially when the hair loss is primarily in the central scalp region.

Management

Successful treatment depends on controlling transitions between stages of the hair cycle and moving follicles from telogen to anagen. Topical minoxidil does induce anagen differentiation and may be tried. Currently, there are no good tools to easily and safely control hair cycle transitions.

Clinical Course and Prognosis

In most cases such as after the delivery of a baby or correction of low iron stores, the telogen effluvium process will resolve. However, for those who develop chronic telogen effluvium, the ongoing hair shedding can often be psychologically distressing.

Indications for Consultation

Referral to a dermatologist is recommended if the telogen effluvium process does not resolve or is complicated by the presence of other hair diseases or underlying medical issues.

Patient Information

- The American Hair Research Society- North, South, and Central: https://www.americanhairresearchsociety.org/telogen-effluvium/
- American Academy of Dermatology: https://www.aad.org/public/diseases/hair-loss/insider/new-moms

▼ CICATRICIAL (SCARRING) ALOPECIAS

Introduction

The cicatricial or scarring alopecias are a group of diverse disorders with a common end result – permanent injury to the hair follicle.[23] Destruction may be primary as discussed in this section or secondary as the result of an injury such as a burn. The *early stages* of the cicatricial alopecias may be distinguished clinically but the *end stages* are indistinguishable and are all characterized by scarring. Treatments may arrest signs and symptoms but do not normally influence the underlying disease process and when discontinued, clinical activity frequently recurs.

Pathogenesis

The pathogenesis of the cicatricial or scarring alopecias is not well understood, but the results are the same and are related to irreversible damage to the stem cells located in the bulge region of the hair follicle. Though unique clinically, the cicatricial alopecias are broadly characterized histologically by their inflammatory infiltrate, either lymphocytic, neutrophilic, or mixed.

There are several hypotheses as to why cicatricial alopecias occur. These include the loss of follicular immune privilege, changes in the local pilosebaceous unit microbiome, abnormal lipid metabolism, and a potential role for mast cells, particularly in the lymphocytic cicatricial alopecias. Allergic contact dermatitis to chemicals as in hair care products have also been associated with a lymphocytic cicatricial alopecia.[24–26]

Clinical Presentation

History

Affected patients will frequently complain not only of hair loss but also of severe pain or burning. Some patients may describe their scalp "being on fire" while others will be almost asymptomatic.

Physical Examination

The presence or absence of follicular ostia within affected areas should be noted. The absence of follicular ostia or openings will be suggestive of a cicatricial alopecia. Pustules are most likely to be seen in neutrophilic or mixed cicatricial alopecias.

Some of the more common lymphocytic cicatricial alopecias include:

- Lichen planopilaris (Figure 30-8)
- Frontal fibrosing alopecia (Figure 30- 9)
- Discoid lupus erythematosus (Figure 30-10)
- Central centrifugal scarring alopecia (Figure 30-11)

Common neutrophilic cicatricial alopecias include:

- Folliculitis decalvans (Figure 30-12)
- Dissecting cellulitis (Figure 30-13)

Examples of mixed cicatricial alopecias include:

- Acne keloidalis (Figure 30-14)
- Acne necrotica

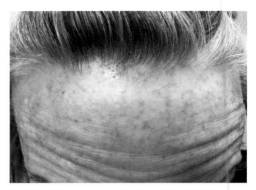

▲ **Figure 30-9.** Frontal fibrosing alopecia. There is regression of the hair line secondary to the scar process and perifollicular inflammation is present at the active margin.

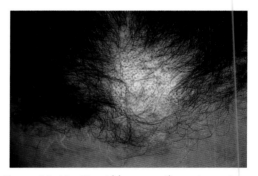

▲ **Figure 30-10.** Discoid lupus erythematosus. In contrast to lichen planopilaris, inflammation is present within the affected area rather than the periphery. Hyperkeratosis and accentuation of the hair follicle orifices is noted.

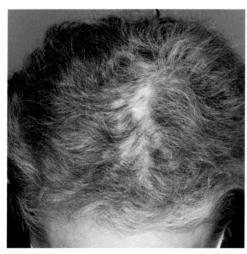

▲ **Figure 30-8.** Lichen planopilaris. Scarring with erythema and perifollicular scale.

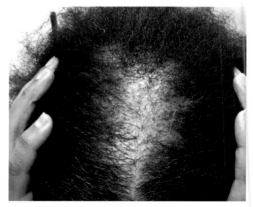

▲ **Figure 30-11.** Central centrifugal scarring alopecia. Central scalp scarring with extension to the temporal region and peripheral inflammation.

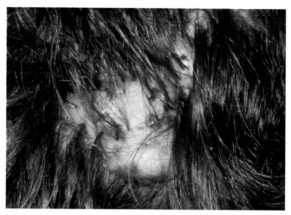

▲ **Figure 30-12.** Folliculitis decalvans. Follicular papules, patchy scarring alopecia, some crusting from draining pustules.

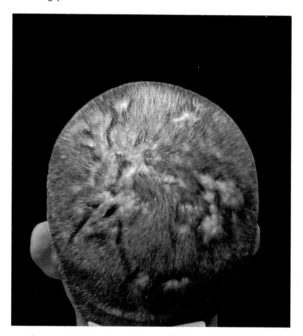

▲ **Figure 30-13.** Dissecting cellulitis. Nodules, patchy scarring alopecia, and boggy plaques with sinus tract formation.

- Erosive pustular dermatoses, an idiopathic, chronic, relapsing pustular dermatosis of the scalp which is frequently preceded by a history of trauma.

Laboratory Findings

There are no blood tests required for patients with cicatricial alopecias. Bacterial cultures may be beneficial if the pustular component does not respond to standard

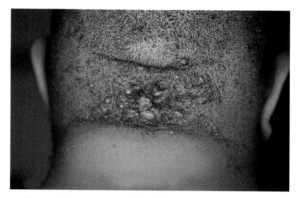

▲ **Figure 30-14.** Acne keloidalis. Discrete and grouped papules with hypertrophic scars.

treatment. In some cases, a scalp biopsy for tissue culture will be needed to isolate the organism contributing to the ongoing inflammatory process. *Staphylococcus aureus* is commonly found on tissue culture examination.

Diagnosis and Differential Diagnosis

The diagnosis of a cicatricial alopecia can be made clinically but when in doubt a scalp biopsy from an active area for histologic examination may be done to confirm the diagnosis as well as to assess the degree and extent of inflammation and follicle injury. If the question is whether there are any hair follicles left in the clinically scarred area that can respond to medical therapy, a biopsy may be helpful to confirm the presence or absence of any hair follicles.

Management

The choice of treatment for the lymphocytic cicatricial alopecias is usually based on the clinical activity, severity of symptoms, and disease activity. Treatments can be grouped into the following three tiers:

- Tier 1 treatments for patients with limited active disease include topical high potency corticosteroids or intralesional steroids or topical non-steroid anti-inflammatory creams such as tacrolimus or pimecrolimus.
- Tier 2 treatments for patients with moderate disease include hydroxychloroquine, low dose oral antibiotics for their anti-inflammatory effect or specific antimicrobial effect, or acitretin.
- Tier 3 treatments include immunosuppressive medications such as cyclosporine, prednisone, or mycophenolate mofetil.

For patients experiencing a neutrophilic cicatricial alopecia, pustules should be cultured and antibiotic sensitivities determined. Treatment may be needed for months. The addition of oral prednisone may improve efficacy and the use of retinoids may or may not be helpful. Oral L-tyrosine administration, laser hair removal, and intranasal eradication of *S. aureus* have all also been advocated.

Scientific breakthroughs related to lipid metabolism abnormalities involving peroxisomes and peroxisome proliferator-activated receptor gamma (PPAR-γ) have been made in the cicatricial alopecias, in particular lichen planopilaris. This has opened the opportunity to consider the use of drugs such as pioglitazone hydrochloride in affected individuals.[24]

For patients experiencing a mixed type of cicatricial alopecia, treatments can be any combination of those recommended for the lymphocytic or neutrophilic cicatricial alopecias.

Clinical Course and Prognosis

The goal is to make the correct diagnosis and focus on bringing the inflammatory destructive process under control. If caught early and prior to permanent destruction, hair growth promoting agents such as topical minoxidil or photobiomodulation can be tried. Patients experiencing frontal fibrosing alopecia may respond to medications like finasteride.[26]

Indications for Consultation

The cicatricial alopecias are considered by some to be a "trichologic emergency." Therefore, all patients with suspected or diagnosed cicatricial alopecias that are not responsive to tier 1 medications should be referred to dermatology as soon as possible.

Patient Information

- Cicatricial Alopecia Research Foundation supports research and provides excellent information for patients with any cicatricial or scarring alopecia: https://www.carfintl.org
- The American Hair Research Society- North, South, and Central: https://www.americanhairresearchsociety.org/cicatricial-alopeca/

HIRSUTISM

Introduction

Hirsutism is defined as the presence of terminal hair growth following a similar pattern to that developing in androgen-dependent sites in men after puberty (Figure 30-15). [28] About 2–8% of the American population are considered to have hirsutism depending on the chosen cutoff for the Ferriman-Gallwey score, a scoring system in which nine androgen sensitive sites (upper lip, chin, chest, upper and lower abdomen, arms, thighs, upper back, and lower back)

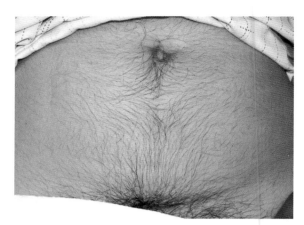

▲ **Figure 30-15.** Hirsutism. Excess terminal hair growth in the linea alba. Reproduced with permission from Hoffman BL, Schorge JO, Halvorson LM, et al: Williams Gynecology, 4th ed. New York, NY: McGraw Hill; 2020.

are assessed, with a maximum grade of 4 points for each area.[29] The degree of hair growth in each area is graded from 1 (minimal terminal hair growth) to 4 (frank virilization). The scores are then summed with a total score of 8 or more indicating hirsutism.

Hirsutism may be inherited. It is well known that East Asian, North Asian, and Southeast Asian populations have less hair, as well as hirsutism than do White individuals, or those of West Asian or Middle Eastern descent. Hirsutism may also be drug induced or associated with aging.

Hypertrichosis is defined as elongation of hair in non-androgen dependent areas and is commonly seen in patients treated with topical or oral minoxidil or who are taking cyclosporine.

Pathogenesis

Hirsutism can also be caused by any one of the following:

- An increase in the actual amount of androgens produced by any of the three major sources of androgens – the ovaries, adrenal glands, or skin.
- Increase in androgen receptor sensitivity at the level of the hair follicle.
- Enhanced activity of 5-alpha-reductase.

Two ovarian causes of hirsutism include polycystic ovarian syndrome and ovarian tumors. Two adrenal gland causes include congenital adrenal hyperplasia with 21-hydroxylase deficiency being most common and adrenal gland tumors. Other less common causes of congenital adrenal hyperplasia include 11*B*-hydroxylase deficiency and 3*B*-ol-dehydrogenase deficiency.

Clinical Presentation

History

Women with hirsutism will present with concerns about increased dark hair growth on any or all of the following areas: upper lip, chin, chest, upper and lower abdomen, arms, thighs, upper back, and lower back.

Physical Examination

The examination should be directed towards describing (1) the location and amount of excess terminal hair growth using the Ferriman-Gallwey scale and (2) identifying other signs of androgen excess including the following:

- Alopecia
- Acne
- Deepening of the voice
- Clitoral enlargement
- Signs of Cushing's syndrome
  - Central obesity
  - Acanthosis nigricans
  - Striae
  - Buffalo hump

Laboratory Findings

In addition to checking a testosterone level and when indicated, dihydrotestosterone and dehydroepiandrosterone sulfate levels, the following may be useful in ruling out a secondary cause of hirsutism:

- Androstenedione
- Dexamethasone suppression test
- Follicle stimulating hormone
- Luteinizing hormone
- Serum prolactin
- Thyroid studies
- 17-hydroxyprogesterone level

Diagnosis and Differential Diagnosis

Hirsutism can be end organ specific (hair follicle androgen excess only), inherited, or associated with ovarian or adrenal gland disease. Hirsutism may also be associated with hyperprolactinemia, acromegaly, postmenopausal androgen therapy, thyroid dysfunction, and use of anabolic steroids.

Management

13.9% Eflornithine (Vaniqua) cream is FDA-approved for the management of hirsutism and is applied topically twice a day. Several other medications can also be used off-label to treat hirsutism. The risk/benefit ratio of each of these drugs needs to be carefully considered when prescribing any of the following for the medical management of hirsutism.

Medications prescribed for hirsutism include spironolactone, finasteride, flutamide, cyproterone acetate as well as leuprolide acetate, bromocriptine, and metformin. Adrenal gland suppression of androgen production can be treated with dexamethasone or prednisone. Any combination of oral contraceptives can be used but those with non-androgenic progestins are considered to be the best.

Mechanical treatments are also available for managing hirsutism. These include epilation with tweezing, waxing, sugaring or threading, chemical depilation, bleaching, electrolysis, light treatment with Intense Pulse Light (IPL), the diode or Nd:YAG laser. The latter can be safely and effectively used to treat individuals with light and darker-skin pigmentation.

Clinical Course and Prognosis

Hirsutism is a treatable condition. The presence of hirsutism requires a thorough clinical evaluation and in most cases, a laboratory evaluation to rule out adrenal or ovarian disease.

Indications for Consultation

A consultation to dermatology should be requested when the hair disease is difficult to diagnose or if the hair loss or excessive hair growth are progressing despite appropriate therapy. If anxiety about hair loss and change in body image are the main problems, consider referral to psychology or psychiatry. If androgen excess with associated scalp hair thinning and hirsutism persists despite appropriate therapy, a referral to endocrinology is recommended.

Patient Information

- Mayo Clinic: https://www.mayoclinic.org/diseases-conditions/hirsutism/symptoms-causes/syc-20354935
- The American Hair Research Society- North, South, and Central: https://www.americanhairresearchsociety.org/#

REFERENCES

1. Paus R, Cotsarelis G. The biology of hair follicles. *N Engl J Med.* 1999. Aug 12;341(7):491-7.
2. Mubki T, Rudnicka L, Olszewska M, Shapiro J. Evaluation and diagnosis of the hair loss patient:part I. History and clinical examination. *J Am Acad Dermatol.* 2014;71(3):415.e1-415.e15.
3. Mubki T, Rudnicka L, Olszewska M, Shapiro J. Evaluation and diagnosis of the hair loss patient: part II. Trichoscopic and laboratory evaluations. *J Am Acad Dermatol.* 2014;71(3):431.e1-431.e11.
4. Hamilton JB. Patterned loss of hair in man: types and incidence. *Ann NY Acad Sci.* 1951;53(3):708-728.

5. Ludwig E. Classification of the types of androgenetic alopecia (common baldness) occurring in the female sex. *Br J Dermatol.* 1977;97(3):247-254.

6. Olsen E, Messenger AG, Shapiro J, et al. Evaluation and treatment of male and female pattern hair loss. *J Am Acad Dermatol.* 2005;52 (2) :301-311.

7. Adil A, Godwin M. The effectiveness of treatments for androgenetic alopecia: A systematic review and meta-analysis. *J Am Acad Dermatol.* 2017 Jul;77(1):136-141.e5.

8. Price VH, Roberts JL, Hordinsky M, et al. Lack of efficacy of finasteride in postmenopausal women with androgenetic alopecia. *J Am Acad Dermatol.* 2000;43(5 Pt 1):768-776.

9. Burns LJ, De Souza B, Flynn E, Hagigeorges D, Senna MM. Spironolactone for treatment of female pattern hair loss. *J Am Acad Dermatol.* 2020 Jul;83(1):276-278.

10. Burns LJ, De Souza B, Flynn E, et al. Spironolactone for treatment of female pattern hair loss. *J Am Acad Dermatol.* 2020;83(1):276-278.

11. Sinclair RD. Female pattern hair loss: a pilot study investigating combination therapy with low-dose oral minoxidil and spironolactone. *Int J Dermatol.* 2018; 57(1):104-109.

12. Dodd EM, Winter MA, Hordinsky MK, Sadick NS, Farah RS. Photobiomodulation therapy for androgenetic alopecia: A clinician's guide to home-use devices cleared by the Federal Drug Administration. *J Cosmet Laser Ther.* 2018 Jun;20(3): 159-167.

13. Gilhar A, Etzioni A, Paus R. Alopecia areata. *N Engl J Med.* 2012;366(16):1515-1525. .

14. Olson EA, Hordinsky, M, Price VH, et al. Alopecia areata investigational guidelines –Part II. *J Am Acad Dermatol.* 2004;51(3):440-447.

15. Hordinsky MK. Alopecia Areata: The clinical situation. *J Investig Dermatol Symp Proc.* 2018 Jan;19(1):S9-S11. .

16. Kennedy Crispin M, Ko JM, Craiglow BG, et al. Safety and efficacy of the JAK inhibitor tofacitinib citrate in patients with alopecia areata. *JCI Insight.* 2016; 22(15):e89776.

17. Guo L, Feng S, Sun B, Jiang X, Liu Y. Benefit and risk profile of tofacitinib for the treatment of alopecia areata: a systematic review and meta-analysis. *J Eur Acad Dermatol Venereol.* 2020;34(1):192-201.

18. Liu LY, Craiglow BG, King BA. Tofacitinib 2% ointment, a topical Janus kinase inhibitor, for the treatment of alopecia areata: A pilot study of 10 patients. *J Am Acad Dermatol.* 2018;78(2):403-404.e401.

19. Meah N, Wall D, York K, et al. The Alopecia Areata Consensus of Experts (ACE) study: Results of an international expert opinion on treatments for alopecia areata. *J Am Acad Dermatol.* 2020;83(1):123-130.

20. Headington JT. Telogen effluvium. New concepts and review. *Arch Dermatol.* 1993; 129(3):356-363.

21. Whiting DA. Chronic telogen effluvium. *Dermatol Clin.* 1996;14(4):723-731.

22. St. Pierre SA, Vercellotti GM, Donovan JC, Hordinsky MK. Iron deficiency and diffuse alopecia in women: more pieces to the puzzle. *J Am Acad Dermatol,* 2010;63(6):1070-1076.

23. Ross EK, Tan E, Shapiro J. Update on primary cicatricial alopecias. *J Am Acad Dermatol.* 2005; 53(3):1-37.

24. Karnik P, Tekeste Z, McCormick TS, et al. Hair follicle stem cell-specific PPAR gamma deletion causes scarring alopecia. *J Invest Dermatol.* 2009; 129(5): 1243-57.

25. Prasad S, Marks DH, Burns LJ, et al. Patch testing and contact allergen avoidance in patients with lichen planopilaris and/or frontal fibrosing alopecia: A cohort study. *J Am Acad Dermatol.* 2020; 83(2):659-661.

26. Sundberg JP, Hordinsky M, Bergfeld W, et al. Cicatricial alopecia research foundation meeting. May 2016: Progress toward the diagnosis, treatment and care of primary cicatricial alopecias. *Exp Dermatol.* 2018 Mar;27(3):302-310.

27. Ho A, Shapiro J. Medical therapy for frontal fibrosing alopecia: A review and clinical approach. *J Am Acad Dermatol.* 2019 Aug;81(2):568-580.

28. Rosenfield RL. Hirsutism. *N Engl J Med.* 2005;353(24): 2578-2588.

29. Ferriman D, Gallwey JD. Clinical assessment of body hair growth in women. *J Clin Endocrinol Metab.* 1961; 21: 1440-1447.

Nail Diseases

Andrea Bershow

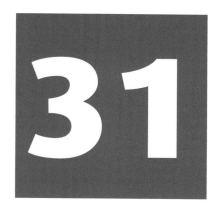

INTRODUCTION TO CHAPTER

The nails have several important functions. The nail plate acts as a protective shield for the fingertips; it assists in grasping and manipulating small objects. Nails are also used for scratching, grooming, and cosmetic adornment.

NAIL ANATOMY

The nail unit is composed of the nail plate, nail matrix, nail folds, nail bed, and hyponychium (Figure 31-1 A and B).[1]

- Nail matrix: Forms the nail plate.
- Nail plate: Hard, translucent, keratin-containing structure covering the dorsal surface of the distal digits on the hands and feet. Formed by the nail matrix, the nail plate grows out from under the proximal nail fold. The nail usually appears pink, which is due to the underlying vasculature of the nail bed. The small, white, semicircular structure at the proximal portion of the nail is the lunula, which is the visible portion of the nail matrix.
- Nail bed: Structure underlying the nail plate, which contributes to the nail plate's ability to attach to the finger.

- Hyponychium/Onychodermal band: Under the distal free edge of the nail. The hyponychium is the transition point between the nail and the normal skin of the digits. The onychodermal band is the point of strongest attachment between the nail and the underlying digit.
- Nail folds: Proximal and lateral. These are epithelial structures. The cuticle protects the matrix by sealing off the potential space between the nail plate and the proximal nail fold.

DIFFERENTIAL DIAGNOSIS

Nail disorders can be difficult to differentiate from one another. To determine the correct diagnosis takes practice and often laboratory studies such as fungal cultures. To add to the confusion, many nail disorders can have secondary fungal or bacterial infections.

The following are the common categories of nail disorders and examples of some specific diseases.

- Infectious: Dermatophyte, candida, mold, and bacteria.
- Papulosquamous: Psoriasis and lichen planus.
- Systemic: Yellow nail syndrome, clubbing, and Beau's lines.

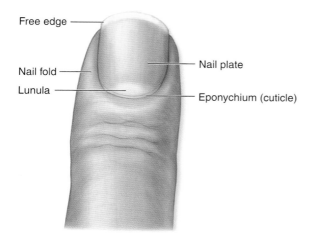

A

B

▲ **Figure 31-1.** **A** and **B**. Anatomy of the nail. Reproduced with permission from McKinley M, O'Loughlin VD, Pennefather-O'Brien EE: Human Anatomy, 6th ed. New York, NY: McGraw Hill; 2021.

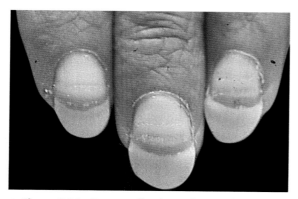

▲ **Figure 31-2.** Terrys Nails. The nails are white proximally, with a narrow pink distal band.

- Traumatic: Habit tic, some cases of onychodystrophy or onycholysis
- Tumors: Squamous cell carcinoma, melanoma, and benign tumors.
- Aging-related changes: physiologic changes in nail plate thickness, texture, and color.

Tumors involving the nail unit are an important category of nail disorders. These are covered in other sections of this textbook (see chapters 21 and 22).

A differential diagnosis of nail disorders and clinical findings that distinguish them from one another are presented in Table 31-1.

INFECTIONS

Fungal Infections

Dermatophyte, mold, and candida infections of the nails are common causes of nail disorders. They closely resemble other nail disorders such as psoriasis.

Onychomycosis is a very common nail disorder and accounts for about 50% of nail disease. The prevalence of onychomycosis in North Americans and Europeans is reportedly between 2% and 14% with the prevalence increasing with age. [2,3] Onychomycosis is rare in prepubertal children. In contrast, 60% of patients older than 70 years are affected. [1] Non-dermatophyte molds are responsible for 30–40% of cases of onychomycosis. [2]

Onychomycosis is more common in patients who are male, immunosuppressed, diabetic, infected with human immunodeficiency virus (HIV), or who have poor circulation. Trauma or nail dystrophy also predisposes patients to fungal infection. [1]

The initial most common findings in a dermatophyte nail infection are white/yellow or orange/ brown streaks or macules under the nail plate. As the infection progresses, subungual hyperkeratosis, onycholysis (separation of the nail plate from the nail bed), and a thickened nail plate may develop (Figure 31-3). White superficial onychomycosis is a less common presentation in which the nail plate appears white and chalky (Figure 31-4). It is more likely to occur in immunosuppressed individuals.

In candida species infection, mild cases may produce nothing more than diffuse leukonychia (white spot(s) under the nail plate). Severe cases may present with a yellow-brown discoloration, with a thick nail bed and lateral and proximal nail fold swelling (Figure 31-5). Onycholysis is common and subungual hyperkeratosis can occur.

It is important to confirm the diagnosis of fungus prior to initiating treatment. Fungal cultures are not always necessary but can sometimes be helpful in distinguishing between dermatophytes, mold, and yeasts. A fungal culture is the least sensitive, but most specific, method for confirming a fungal infection. The most sensitive method to detect fungus is to clip the distal portion of the nail plate, place it

Table 31-1. Differential diagnosis of nail disorders

Nail Disease	Clinical Findings
Infectious	
Onychomycosis	Brown, yellow, orange, or white discoloration, thickened nail plate, subungual hyperkeratosis, onycholysis.
Pseudomonas Infection	Green or black discoloration of nail plate. Onycholysis is usually present. Paronychia is common.
Papulosquamous	
Psoriasis	Nail matrix involvement: Pitting is broader and more irregular than pitting due to alopecia areata, leukonychia, erythema of lunula, crumbling of nail plate. Nail bed involvement: Discoloration (oil drop-yellow or salmon patch-red), splinter hemorrhage, subungual hyperkeratosis, or onycholysis.
Lichen Planus	Thinning of nail plate with longitudinal ridging and fissuring. Dorsal pterygium is almost pathognomonic for nail lichen planus. The matrix is scarred, and the nail plate is divided into two distinct sections.
Associated with Systemic Diseases	
Beau's Lines	Horizontal, depressed, white, non-blanching bands of the nail plate. Can be caused by systemic insults, drugs, or trauma.
Clubbing	Over-curvature of the nail. Can be idiopathic or related to cardiovascular, pulmonary, or gastrointestinal disorders.
Koilonychia	Also called spoon nails. The center of the nail is depressed relative to the edges. Can be caused by iron deficiency, hypothyroidism, trauma, or be congenital.
Half and Half Nails	Also called Lindsay's nails. The proximal half of the nail is normal or white and the distal half is darker. Can be caused by renal disease.
Mee's Lines	Single or multiple transverse white lines, usually present on all nail plates. Classically caused by arsenic poisoning but can be the result of many other systemic insults.
Splinter Hemorrhage	Small, longitudinal lines of dark discoloration. Should grow out with the nail plate. Usually caused by trauma, but can be related to systemic illnesses, or drugs. If the lesions occur distally on a single nail, it is less likely to be related to a systemic cause.
Terry's Nails	The nails are white proximally, with a narrow pink or brown distal band. Can be related to liver disease or aging (Figure 31-2).
Yellow Nail Syndrome	Diffuse yellow, thickened nail plates. Most commonly seen with lung disease and chronic lymphedema.
Other	
Alopecia Areata	Superficial, regular, geometric pitting most common. The pitting is much more regular than pitting due to psoriasis.
20-Nail dystrophy (trachyonychia)	Nails have a roughened surface, longitudinal ridging, and thinning. Nail plates have a sandpaper appearance. Look for skin or hair abnormalities suggestive of lichen planus, psoriasis or alopecia areata to help distinguish the underlying cause.
Habit tic deformity	Roughly parallel, horizontal depressions most often over the median nail plate.
Onycholysis	Nail plate appears white due to air between the nail plate and nail bed.

in formalin, and send it for histopathologic examination. Fungal elements stain positive with periodic acid Schiff (PAS) stain.

Oral antifungals are the gold standard of treatment for onychomycosis, but for many patients non-treatment is a viable option. Although oral antifungals are generally well-tolerated, patients may prefer not to risk the potential side effects of oral antifungal medications. Oral terbinafine has the highest cure rate of any onychomycosis therapy, with

no significant difference in rate of adverse effects when compared to azoles, and a lower rate of adverse effects compared to griseofulvin.[2,4]

Bacterial Infections

Bacteria can also infect the nail unit. Pseudomonas is a common colonizer of onycholytic nails.[1,5] The nail plate is usually discolored green or black (Figure 31-6). Patients

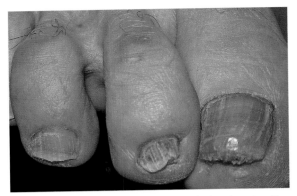

▲ **Figure 31-3.** Onychomycosis. Thick discolored nail plate and subungual hyperkeratosis.

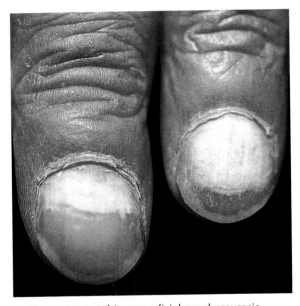

▲ **Figure 31-4.** White superficial onychomycosis. White chalky nail plate.

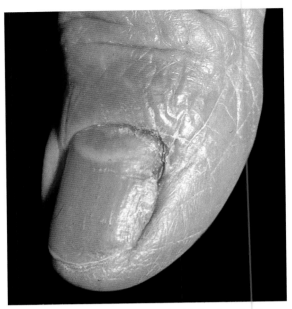

▲ **Figure 31-5.** Candia paronychial infection. Erythema and swelling of cuticle with small areas of leukonychia.

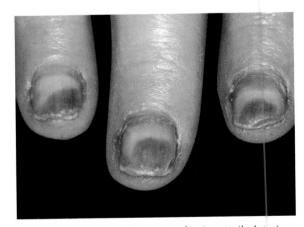

▲ **Figure 31-6.** Pseudomonas infection. Nail plate is green and thickened.

often have a history of wet-work. Bacterial cultures of pus or nail clippings can confirm the diagnosis. Treatment involves trimming the onycholytic portion of the nail and the use of one of the following topical therapies: Soaking affected nails two to three times a day in a dilute bleach solution (2% sodium hypochlorite) or half-strength vinegar, application of polymyxin B, chlorhexidine solution, 15% sulfacetamide, gentamicin or chloramphenicol ophthalmological solution or octenidine dihydrochloride 0.1% solution for 4 weeks or until resolved.[1,5] Systemic antibiotics should not be administered.

▼ PAPULOSQUAMOUS DISEASES

Psoriasis

Psoriasis is a common cause of nail disease. Patients often report a personal or family history of psoriasis. Of patients with known psoriasis, about 90% will experience some nail changes at some point over the course of their disease, and nail disease is more commonly seen in adults than children.[6] Patients with nail involvement are more likely to have psoriatic arthritis, so it is important to ask about a

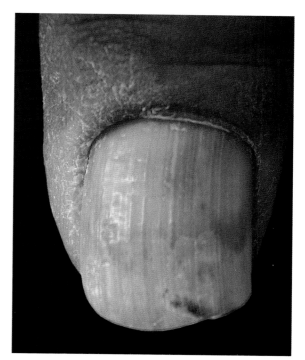

▲ **Figure 31-7.** Psoriasis. Nail pits, onycholysis, and "oil drop" like appearance with thin psoriatic plaque on nail folds.

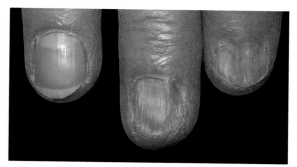

▲ **Figure 31-8.** Lichen planus. Longitudinal ridging and thinning of nail plate with early pterygium formation.

history of joint pain.[6,7] Nail psoriasis significantly impacts patients' quality of life with pain and negative impact on activities of daily living, professional activities, and housework. Severe nail psoriasis is associated with a higher risk of depression and anxiety. Psoriasis of the nails commonly presents with pitting, onycholysis, subungual debris, and discoloration (Figures 31-7). The nails will usually be negative for fungal elements with the examination of a potassium hydroxide (KOH) preparation; however, psoriatic nails can be secondarily infected with a dermatophyte. Punch biopsy of an involved area of the nail unit (nail bed or matrix) can confirm the diagnosis.[1,6]

Topical treatment of nail psoriasis is challenging. High-potency topical corticosteroids (betamethasone or clobetasol) with or without vitamin D analogs (calcitriol or calcipotriol) can be used. For nail matrix lesions, these medications should be applied to the proximal nail fold. For nail bed lesions, the onycholytic nail should be trimmed back and the medications should be applied to the nail bed. Tazarotene gel 0.1% applied at bedtime to involved nail plates may improve onycholysis and pitting.[6] Intralesional triamcinolone 5–10 mg/mL is also useful for nail psoriasis, although the injections may be painful for the patient. Typically, 0.1 mL is injected at the proximal nail fold every 4–8 weeks for up to 6 months.[1]

Patients with psoriasis who require systemic medications should be referred to a dermatologist who may use biologic medications (TNF alpha inhibitors, IL-17 inhibitors and IL-12/23 inhibitors) which are the most efficacious for nail psoriasis.[6] Methotrexate, cyclosporine, acitretin, apremilast, or tofacitinib may also be recommended.[1,6]

Lichen Planus

Nail lichen planus most commonly occurs in isolation without any evidence of skin or mucosal lichen planus, but about 10% of patients with mucosal membrane or skin lichen planus also have nail involvement.[1,7] Nail lichen planus usually has an abrupt onset with longitudinal ridging, thinning, and fissuring of the nail plate (Figure 31-8).[8] Pain may be present.[1] Biopsy may be necessary for diagnosis in the absence of skin or mucous membrane findings. Early treatment may avert the possibility of pterygium formation. Once present, a pterygium is permanent and will not respond to any treatment. First line treatment for nail lichen planus is systemic or intralesional corticosteroids.[1] Systemic retinoids can also be used.[8] There are reports of success with topical tacrolimus [8,9] and a combination of topical tazarotene and clobetasol under occlusion.[9]

SYSTEMIC DISEASES

Beau's Lines

Beau's lines appear after a disruption of nail formation in the matrix. They present as horizontal, depressed, white, non-blanching, bands of the nail plate (Figure 31-9). The depth of the line corresponds to the severity of damage, and the width corresponds to the length of exposure.[1] These lines can usually elicit a history of major systemic stress due to illness, surgery, accident or history of exposure to a causative medication. Associated medications include chemotherapeutic medications and systemic retinoids.[10] No treatment is necessary since the lines will resolve when

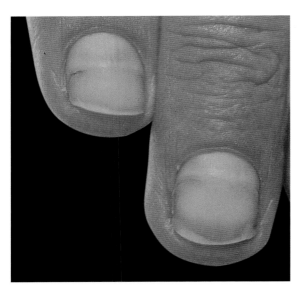

▲ **Figure 31-9.** Beau's lines. Horizontal, depressed white bands on fingernails.

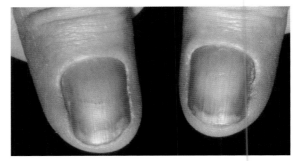

▲ **Figure 31-10.** Yellow nail syndrome. Nail plate is thickened and yellow.

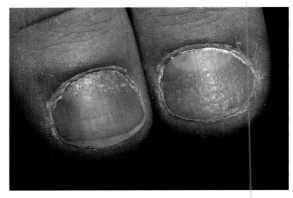

▲ **Figure 31-11.** Nail pits in alopecia areata. Superficial pitting in a geometric pattern.

the affected nail plate grows out. However, the lesions will continue to occur with repeated administration of causative medications or repeated illness.

Yellow Nail Syndrome

Yellow nail syndrome is commonly seen as part of a triad with lung disease and chronic lymphedema. Most patients are between the fourth and sixth decades of life, but cases have also been reported in children and infants.[11] It can also be associated with rheumatoid arthritis, chronic obstructive pulmonary disease, bronchiectasis, chronic bronchitis, sinusitis, carcinoma of the larynx and other malignancies, and thyroid disease. Yellow nail syndrome may be inherited or congenital.[1] Patients may have a history of associated conditions, or a family history of the syndrome. Examination shows diffuse yellow-colored, thickened nail plates with excessive curvature of the nails (Figure 31-10) or slowed rate of nail growth. All nails are affected.[1] Nail disease will sometimes resolve with treatment of the underlying condition.[1]

Alopecia Areata

Nail involvement in alopecia areata is present in up to 50% of children and 20% of adults.[1] Extensive nail involvement correlates with more severe hair loss, and has a worse prognosis.[1,12] The nail changes can precede, occur concomitantly or occur after hair loss. Rarely, nail changes can be the only finding in alopecia areata or may precede hair involvement.[1,12] Superficial, regular, geometric pitting is most common (Figure 31-11). This pitting is much more regular than pitting due to psoriasis.[13] Geometric punctate leukonychia can be seen as regularly spaced, small, and white spots on the nail plate.[13] Trachyonychia (sandpaper like nails) can occur. Non-specific findings may include Beau's lines, onychomadesis (shedding of nail plate), onychorrhexis (brittle nails), thinning or thickening of the nail plate, spoon nails, and red lunulae.[1,12] Biopsy of the matrix is usually not necessary, but if done will show spongiosis and a lymphocytic infiltrate of the proximal nail fold, nail matrix, nail bed, and/or hyponychium.[1,12] Oral or intralesional corticosteroids may improve the nail disease.[1,14] There is a report of successful treatment with topical tazarotene.[15] Case reports indicate that oral tofacitinib used to treat hair loss in alopecia areata may also be effective for improving associated nail disease. [15]

Trachyonychia (20 Nail Dystrophy)

Trachonychia (20-nail dystrophy) is most commonly caused by alopecia areata, and can affect 1–20 nails. It can also be caused by atopic dermatitis, ichthyosis vulgaris, lichen planus or psoriasis, and can be an isolated finding in childhood.[1,6,8] Nails have a roughened surface, with longitudinal ridging and thinning and are classically described as having a sandpaper appearance. There are no nail findings that distinguish trachyonychia due to alopecia areata, lichen planus, or psoriasis.[1] However, abnormalities suggestive of lichen planus, psoriasis, or alopecia areata may be present on the skin and help with diagnosis. Longitudinal nail biopsy can help determine the underlying disorder; however, it is not usually recommended for this relatively benign condition.[16] The condition usually resolves on its own in a few years when not associated with other skin diseases. Topical tazarotene has been reported to be useful.[17]

TRAUMA-INDUCED NAIL DISORDERS

Habit Tic

Habit tic deformity occurs with manipulation of the proximal nail fold. Patients may or may not admit to picking, rubbing, or scratching the proximal nail fold or cuticle, but often will absentmindedly pick at their cuticles during the office visit. The lesions are roughly parallel, horizontal depressions most often over the median nail plate (Figure 31-12). There may also be an absent cuticle, and a widening of the cuticular sulcus. Behavior modification is the most effective treatment. Manipulation of the nail fold should be minimized, by occluding with bandages, if necessary.[18] The condition may be successfully treated with selective serotonin reuptake inhibitors or other therapies used to treat obsessive compulsive disorders.[19] Cyanoacrylate adhesive (superglue) applied to the proximal nail fold 1–2 times weekly, to mimic the cuticle and seal the sulcus, has also been reported to be effective. This acts as a barrier to manipulation. Patients should be warned of the potential to develop allergic contact dermatitis to the adhesive.[18]

Onycholysis

Simple onycholysis is not due to any underlying medical disorder. The separation usually starts distally but can start proximally. The detached nail plate appears white due to air between the nail plate and nail bed (Figure 31-13). It is more common in women and adults. The longer the condition persists, the less likely it is to resolve. Patients may have a history of exposure to irritants (e.g., soaps), allergens (e.g., nail cosmetics or acrylates) or physical trauma.[20,21] The most common causes of toenail trauma are ill-fitting shoes, sports related trauma, long nails, and stubbing the toe.[20,21] Common causes of fingernail trauma include hitting the nail plate with a tool or squeezing the nail plate in a door, and vigorous cleaning under the nail. Onycholysis can also be associated with taxane chemotherapy and other oral medications.[20] Photo-onycholysis may be associated with the tetracyclines, particularly doxycycline and exposure to ultraviolet (UV) light.[20]

If a secondary infection with pseudomonas, mold or yeast is present the nail can appear green or brown. Candida is cultured more than 80% of the time, but is likely just a colonizer, as treatment with systemic antifungals does not cure onycholysis.[21] If reattachment does not occur, the nail bed will eventually cornify and produce dermatoglyphics like the rest of the digit. If this occurs, the nail plate will no longer attach to the nail bed.

Secondary onycholysis is caused by underlying nail disorders such as psoriasis, lichen planus, and onychomycosis

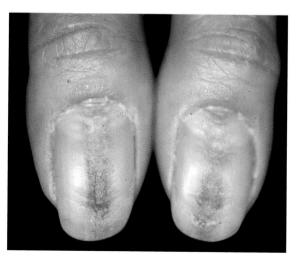

▲ **Figure 31-12.** Habit tic deformity. Parallel horizontal depressions over the medial nail plate caused by chronic rubbing of the cuticle.

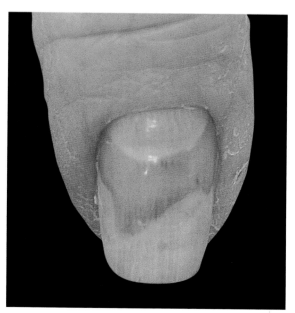

▲ **Figure 31-13.** Onycholysis. Distal nail plate appears white due to air in gap between the nail plate and nail bed.

or systemic diseases such as hyperthyroidism and porphyria. Tumors of the nail bed can also cause onycholysis.

Management involves minimizing nail trauma. The patient should be instructed to keep the detached portion of their nails trimmed back until the nail is reattached. They should not vigorously clean the area under the detached nail as this can cause further detachment. Patients should wear gloves for dry and wet work. They should not use any cosmetic nail products. Wearing shoes with low heels and a wide toe box is also recommended.

A topical antiseptic, such as thymol 4% solution, can be applied to the exposed nail bed to prevent infection.

AGING-RELATED NAIL CHANGES

Changes in the nails are a common part of the aging process. Changes to the texture, thickness and color of the nails are seen frequently, and can be very distressing to patients. As a person ages, the rate of nail plate growth slows and the nail plate morphology changes. The cause of this is not definitively known, but changes in microcirculation and cumulative effects of UV light exposure have been suggested as possible causes.[22]

Onychorrhexis

Onychorrhexis presents with exaggerated longitudinal ridging of the nails, sometimes accompanied by thinning or brittleness of the nail plate (Figure 31-14). This can be treated with hydration of the nail plate using emollients.[22] Ammonium lactate 12% lotion BID to the nail plate is often helpful. Caution should be used in applying nail

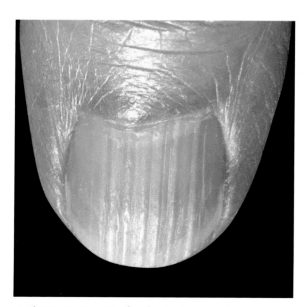

▲ **Figure 31-14.** Onychorrhexis. Exaggerated longitudinal ridging of the nail plate.

hardeners or lacquers. They can strengthen the nail plate temporarily, but the removal process can increase dehydration of the nail plate and increase problems with brittleness of the nails.[22] Biotin supplements are readily available and are a popular over the counter treatment of brittle nails. There is little evidence that biotin is effective for this purpose, so its use is generally not recommended. Patients and providers should be aware that biotin supplementation can lead to alterations in thyroid, prolactin, and pregnancy tests. Most alarmingly, it can result in falsely low troponin levels, which can lead to a missed diagnosis of myocardial infarction. If possible, patients should discontinue biotin supplements at least a week prior to any blood tests and inform their healthcare provider if they are taking biotin.

Onychauxis

Thickening of the nail plate, which can be associated with a change in color (typically yellowing) and increased opacity. Pain can sometimes result from thickened nails, particularly in the toenails while wearing shoes. 40% urea cream applied twice a day can be used to thin and soften the nail plate in order to allow trimming and debridement. If topical treatment fails and pain is significant, nail avulsion with matrixectomy in order to permanently prevent nail regrowth may be elected.[22]

Discoloration of Nail Plate

As mentioned earlier, yellow discoloration can be a consequence of a thickened nail plate related to the normal aging process. However, discoloration can also indicate the presence of infection, either bacterial or fungal. Onychomycosis is the most common disease of the nails, and typically involves discoloration of the nail plate. Onychomycosis prevalence increases with age.[22]

INDICATIONS FOR CONSULTATION

Patients should be referred to dermatology if they are not responding to therapy, or if the diagnosis is uncertain, or a biopsy of the nail unit is needed.

PATIENT INFORMATION

- MedlinePlus: www.nlm.nih.gov/medlineplus/naildiseases.html
- American Academy of Dermatology: www.aad.org/media-resources/stats-and-facts/prevention-and-care/nails/nails

REFERENCES

1. Rubin AI, Jellinek NJ, et al. *Scher and Daniel's Nails: Diagnosis, Surgery, Therapy.* 4rd ed. China : Springer; 2018.
2. Lipner SR, Scher RK. Onychomycosis, clinical overview and diagnosis *J Am Acad Dermatol.* 2019;580(4):835-851.

3. Welsh O, Vera-Cabrera L, Welsh E. Onychomycosis. *Clin Dermatol*. 2010; 28(2):151-159.
4. Daniel III CR, Jellinek NJ. Commentary: the illusory tinea unguium cure. *J Am Acad Dermat*. 2010;62(3):415-417.
5. Geizhals S, Lipner S. Retrospective case series on risk factors, diagnosis and treatment of pseudomonas aeruginosa nail infections. *Am J Clin Dermatol*. 2020;21(2): 297-302.
6. Bardazzi F, et al. Nail Psoriasis: An updated review and expert opinion on available treatments, including biologics. *Acta Derm Venereol*. 2019; 99: 516-523
7. Maddy AJ, Tosti A. What's new in nail disorders. *Dermatol Clin*. 2019;37(2):143-147.
8. Yesudian PD, de Berker D. Inflammatory nail conditions. Part 2: nail changes in lichen planus and alopecia areata. *Clin Exp Dermatol*. 2021;46(1):16-20.
9. Prevost NM, English III JC. Case Reports: Palliative treatment of fingernail lichen planus. *J Drugs Dermatol*. 2007; 6(2):202-4.
10. Piraccini BM, Iorizzo M, Starace M,Tosti A. Drug-induced nail diseases. *Dermatol Clin*. 2006; 24(3):387-91.
11. Al Hawsawi K, Pope E. Yellow nail syndrome. *Pediatric Dermatol*. 2010; 27(6): 675-6.
12. Chelizade K, Lipner S. Nail Changes in Alopecia Areata: an Update and Review. *Int J Dermatol*. 2018; 57(7):776-783
13. Vano-Galvan S, Aboin S, Bea-Ardebol S, Sanchez-Mateos J. Sudden hair loss associated with trachyonychia. *Cleve Clin J Med*.2008;75 (8):567-8.
14. Kar B, Handa S, Dogra S, Kumar B.Placebo-controlled oral pulse prednisolone therapy in alopecia areata. *J Am Acad Dermatol*.2005; (52)2: 287-90.
15. Dhayalan A, King BA. Tofacitinib citrate for the treatment of nail dystrophy associated with alopecia universalis. *JAMA Dermatol*. 2016;152(4):492-493.
16. Grover C, Khandpur S. Longitudinal nail biopsy: Utility in 20-Nail Dystrophy. *Dermatol Surg*. 2003; 29(11):1125-9.
17. Soda R, Diluvio L, Bianchi L, Chimenti S. Treatment of trachyonychia with tazarotene. *Clin Exper Dermatol*. 2005; 30(3) 301-2.
18. Ring DS. Inexpensive solution for habit-tic deformity. *Arch Dermatol*. 2010; 146(11):1222-3.
19. Vittorio CC, Phillips KA. Treatment of habit tic disorders with fluoxetine. *Arch Dermatol*. 1997;133(10): 1203-4.
20. Daniel III CR, Iorizzo M, Piraccini BM, Tosti A. Simple onycholysis. *Cutis*. 2011; 87: 226-8.
21. Zaias N, Escovar SX, Zaiac MN. Finger and toenail onycholysis. *J Eur Acad Dermatol Venereol*. 2015;29(5):848-853.
22. Abdullah L, Abbas O. Common nail changes and disorders in older people: diagnosis and management. *Canadian Family Physician*. 2011; 57: 173-81.

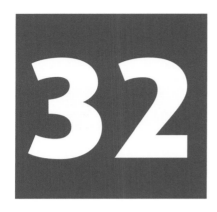

32

Skin Diseases of the Genitals and Perineum

Nora K. Shumway

▼ INTRODUCTION TO CHAPTER

A stroll down the pharmacy aisle is proof enough that genital symptoms plague our society. Many patients will go to great lengths to solve genital symptoms on their own, whether motivated by embarrassment, lack of access to medical care, or uncertainty as to which medical professional is best suited to treat the problem. This often leads to a delay in care and sometimes more than one cause of their symptoms by the time care is obtained. In fact, 1 in 6 women will experience an untreated vulvovaginal discomfort in their lifetime.[1] The following chapter will review the most common causes of genital complaints with some early intervention recommendations.

▼ ANATOMY

Prior to reviewing the main causes of symptoms and disease, it is important to review normal genital anatomy which is also highlighted in the figures below. Knowing normal genital anatomy can help the clinician identify abnormalities as well as communicate to other specialties the location of concern.

The external component of female genitalia is called the vulva (Figure 32-1). The labia majus extends bilaterally from the mons to the perineum at the fourchette and is a hair bearing area. Between the labia majus are two labia minus which extend from the clitoral hood to just anterior to the labia majus insertion. Between the labia majus and labia minus is the interlabial sulcus. The labia minora can vary significantly in size and whether it extends beyond the labia majora externally. The clitoral hood when retracted will expose the clitoris. The area inside the labia minora is called the vestibule within which one will find the urethral orifice, trigone area, and the vaginal opening.

Penile anatomy consists of two main sections: the shaft and then distally the glans (Figure 32-2). The cone like glans contains the slit like urethral opening. The glans is separated from the shaft by the corona which in uncircumcised men is covered by the prepuce or foreskin. The concavity between the corona and the shaft is the sulcus.

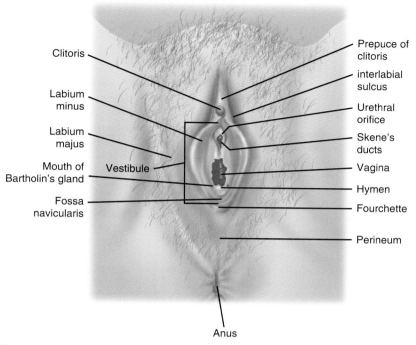

▲ **Figure 32-1.** Illustration of female external genitalia. Reproduced with permission from Jones HW, Rock JA: TeLinde's Operative Gynecology, 11th ed. Philadelphia, PA: Lippincott Williams & Wilkins; 2015.

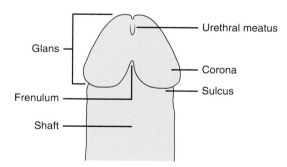

▲ **Figure 32-2.** Illustration of male external genitalia.

CATEGORIES OF DISEASE

Skin diseases of the genitals and perineum can be classified into five broad categories:

- Dermatitis
  - Irritant contact dermatitis and allergic contact dermatitis
  - Lichen simplex chronicus

- Papulosquamous disorders
  - Psoriasis
  - Lichen planus
  - Lichen sclerosus
- Infection
  - Fungal
    - Candidiasis
    - Tinea cruris
  - Bacterial
    - Erythrasma
    - Folliculitis
    - Hidradenitis
    - Perianal streptococcal disease
    - Syphilis
  - Viral
    - Herpes simplex
    - Molluscum
    - Human papillomavirus

- Cancerous and precancerous tumors
  - Squamous cell carcinoma
  - Melanoma
  - Extramammary paget's disease
- Dysesthesias/Genital pain syndromes
  - Vulvodynia
  - Scrotodynia
  - Perianal pruritus/anal pain

GENERAL MANAGEMENT GUIDELINES

One of the primary management strategies is to simplify the treatment regimen and remove the possibility of worsening symptoms from irritation or allergy. As noted previously, many patients experiment with various over-the-counter remedies before presenting to a clinician and develop extensive hygienic routines, which often may do more harm than good. Women should be instructed to wash with warm water only with of their hands. No other cleaning agents, soaps, or douches should be used in the vulva. Men should be instructed to wash with the mildest soap possible or just with water once or twice daily. If a woman is menstruating, they should use tampons if tolerated or cotton, unscented pads that are changed frequently, and not use any plastic liners on a regular basis unless absolutely necessary. If the patient is using plastic liners due to incontinence issues, the incontinence should be addressed so these can be stopped. Patients should refrain from applying anything to the genital region other than prescribed treatments.

Pure petroleum jelly should be applied for symptom control prior to and/or after urination or defecation if these cause discomfort.[2] If the patient is experiencing discomfort with cleaning after defecation the use of a "peri" bottle or other spray device such as a bidet or portable bidet can avoid unnecessary friction, help with cleansing and avoid use of any premoistened wipes. All premoistened or baby wipes should be avoided. If there is chronic irritation due to incontinence, or skin fold occlusion due to obesity, a barrier product may be indicated such as zinc oxide. However, the patient should use products with as few other ingredients as possible. Ointments are preferred over the use of creams or gels, which have greater potential to irritate the skin. Sometimes creams are preferred by men in the inguinal folds, but if any fissures are present creams can cause burning.

When prescribing a potent topical corticosteroid, such as clobetasol ointment, a clinician may preemptively treat fungal and yeast overgrowth with an agent such as oral fluconazole, particularly in women. A single oral dose of 150 mg to 200 mg fluconazole is often preferred over topical azole treatments due to the high incidence of irritation caused by the latter.[1] The mucosal surfaces of the genitals are relatively resistant to the adverse effects of topical steroid medications, whereas the keratinized skin, especially the skin folds and medial thighs, are prone to develop steroid atrophy and striae. When possible, the patient should be asked to demonstrate correct application of topical treatments, using a hand-held mirror and petroleum jelly. This will ensure that treatments are applied to the correct region, and in proper amounts. A very thin layer needs to be applied given the small surface area. This often amounts to the quantity you would imagine obtaining off of a tip of a pen for the vulva and less for the glans of the penis.

IRRITANT AND ALLERGIC CONTACT DERMATITIS

Introduction

Irritant (ICD) and allergic contact dermatitis (ACD) are a common occurrence in the genital region, often due to patient's attempts at self-treatments with the numerous over the counter products available. In general, when pruritus occurs in this area patients feel "unclean" and so start overzealous cleaning routines that usually worsen symptoms.[3] It is estimated that about 54% of women presenting to a vulvar clinic have a component of either irritant or allergic contact dermatitis. The most common irritants include bodily fluids such as feces, urine, blood and sweat, bathing products such as soaps, lubricants, menstrual products, worsening friction and components of topical preparations such as alcohol and propylene glycol.[4]

Pathogenesis

Irritant contact dermatitis develops from application of a chemical or substance that results in direct cytotoxic effects and is not immunologically caused. Irritant contact dermatitis can occur in anyone using a product that is inappropriate for the genital surface or used in a manner that exceeds the recommended application. Sometimes, given the nature of genital skin even very infrequent applications of "approved" over the counter products are enough to lead to significant symptoms.

Allergic contact dermatitis is a delayed hypersensitivity reaction that occurs in individuals who have been previously sensitized to the offending agent. Allergic contact dermatitis usually occurs 2–7 days after exposure.[4]

Clinical Presentation

▶ History

Irritant and allergic contact dermatitis symptoms are most often described as pruritus, but can also be burning/stinging, irritation or pain in the acute setting. Irritant and allergic contact dermatitis are more likely diagnosis if symptoms are acute since the history of product usage is more obvious. Chronic irritant or allergic contact dermatitis can often be more difficult as it can be subtle. It can be caused by products that have been used for many years

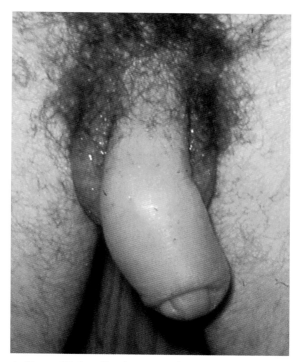

Figure 32-3. Allergic contact dermatitis due to lubricating jelly. Erythema and marked swelling of the penis and testicles.

and so suspected to not be the cause, intermittently used, "approved" for genital use or products transferred from other body sites.

Physical Examination

In the acute setting, irritant and allergic contact dermatitis can both result in marked edema, bulla, vesicles, erythema, and ulcerations (Figure 32-3). However, with milder irritants or weak allergens contact dermatitis may present with mild erythema or just stinging/burning or without any cutaneous changes. In patients with darker skin tones, erythema can appear more purple or hyperpigmented. Patients with chronic disease may present with lichen simplex chronicus, which will be discussed later. Sometimes patients will have even a combination of both irritant and allergic contact dermatitis.

Laboratory Findings

A skin biopsy could be considered, but usually is not necessary. It would show eczematous or spongiotic changes. Sometimes severe irritant contact dermatitis shows cytotoxic changes or necrosis if severe.

Diagnosis

Diagnosis is often made clinically based on the physical examination findings of erythema, without evidence of scarring or features of other dermatoses. Irritant and allergic contact dermatitis should be considered in any patient with genital complaints even if they have an alternative diagnosis if they are failing to respond to treatment as expected or develop sudden worsening of symptoms.

▶ Differential Diagnosis

✓ In the acute setting the differential includes: Herpes, candida, immunobullous dermatoses, erosive lichen planus, bullous fixed drug eruption, and extramammary Pagets disease.

✓ In the subacute to chronic setting: Tinea, candida, inverse psoriasis, and atopic dermatitis can be considered.

Management

The mainstay of treatment is avoidance of any irritant or allergen followed by the treatment of symptoms with topical corticosteroids and sedating antihistamines at bedtime, if needed. To ensure avoidance of all possible topical allergens or irritants, it is important to obtain an exhaustive history from the patient on what they are using in and near the affected area and cessation of all possible products. See earlier section in general management guidelines for basic recommendations for all patients. If the dermatitis is acute and severe, oral steroids or a strong topical steroid such as clobetasol 0.05% ointment daily for 1–2 weeks might be needed with tapering to a mid- or low-potency topical steroid. Otherwise, a low-potency topical steroid such as desonide 0.05% ointment or tacrolimus ointment, 0.03% or 0.1% twice a day for 2–4 weeks is often helpful.

For more information, see Chapter 8.

Clinical Course and Prognosis

Once the irritant or allergen is avoided, symptoms should improve and resolve within several weeks depending on the initial severity. However, treatment with a topical steroid is recommended to help speed up the symptom resolution process.

Indications for Consultation

One should consider consultation with dermatology if patients are not responding as expected or if other areas of the body are involved. Patch testing can be done by dermatology to evaluate further for possible allergens and to ensure no alternative diagnosis.[5]

Patient Information

National Eczema Society:
    www.eczema.org/information-and-advice/types-of-
eczema/female-genital-eczema/
    www.eczema.org/information-and-advice/types-of-
eczema/male-genital-eczema/

▼ LICHEN SIMPLEX CHRONICUS

Introduction

Lichen simplex chronicus is a response of the skin to repeated rubbing or scratching and is a description that does not indicate the cause. While it is a secondary reaction, it causes significant symptoms. Patients may have underlying atopic dermatitis, but lichen simplex chronicus can also be triggered initially by irritant or allergic contact dermatitis or even infectious causes.

Pathogenesis

Lichen simplex chronicus develops secondary to the itch/scratch cycle. This cycle is marked by a worsening itch sensation due to repeated scratching and therefore reducing each component of the cycle will subdue both symptoms.

Clinical Presentation

▶ History

The patient often reports significant pruritus which is often only relieved by scratching/rubbing sometimes until the point of pain is reached.

▶ Physical Examination

On physical examination, an area of lichenification or xerotic plaques with prominent skin markings is seen, which depending on the skin subtype, can be gray or hyperpigmented (Figure 32-4). This commonly occurs on labia majora, scrotum into inguinal fold, and perianal area.

Management

It is important to break the itch/scratch cycle.[6,7] The first step in treatment is eliminating all possible irritant/allergic topical products as recommended above in the general management guidelines. Due to the chronicity of this condition, it is recommended that the highest potency steroid possible be used; however, one needs to proceed with caution in areas at higher risk of atrophy due to accidental transfer to uninvolved skin particularly when used on the scrotum or inguinal folds. If there is a lower risk of atrophy such as on the mons pubis one could use clobetasol ointment 0.05% daily until resolved with follow-up at least monthly and tapering when possible. In higher risk areas for atrophy such as scrotum or inguinal fold triamcinolone

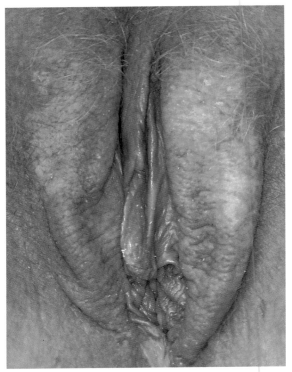

▲ **Figure 32-4.** Lichen simplex chronicus. Hypopigmented, pruritic plaques with epidermal thickening on the vulva due to chronic rubbing and scratching.

ointment 0.1% should be initially used with counseling patients on transfer risk and again tapering when able. Sometimes even in higher risk areas for atrophy, higher potency corticosteroids may be needed to gain relief, and break the itch/scratch cycle. Nighttime sedation with antihistamines can often be helpful.[1] For immediate symptom control, keeping the area cool and well ventilated is recommended as heat/sweat are common triggers for scratching. Cool compresses for a short duration can help with immediate short-term relief; however, caution is advised with direct application due to high risk of cold damage of genitals. For more information, see Chapter 8.

Clinical Course and Prognosis

Once lichen simplex chronicus develops it can often have a high rate of recurrence and immediate treatment of symptoms can be helpful in preventing thicker and therefore more treatment resistant lesions.

Indications for Consultation

Reasons for consultation include failure of first line therapy, concern for possible unidentified cause of coexisting contact dermatitis, significant pain, or bleeding.

Patient Information

▼ PSORIASIS

Introduction

Genital psoriasis occurs in approximately two-thirds of patients with psoriasis and may be the only psoriatic lesions present in 2–5% of patients. Despite this common occurrence, almost half of affected patients do not discuss their symptoms with their providers and therefore, it is important to specifically ask about genital involvement in all patients with known psoriasis.[8] Due to frequent lack of treatment, this type of psoriasis often has serious quality of life ramifications leading to poorer quality of life scores and higher rates of depression than patients with non-genital psoriasis. Patients also often have decreased sexual wellbeing because of their disease.[9]

Clinical Presentation

▶ History

Patients often describe their genital psoriasis as itchy, painful, and associated with dyspareunia and or worsen with sexual activity due to koebernization.[10]

▶ Physical Examination

Genital psoriasis can appear as well defined erythematous plaques, usually without scale (Figures 32-5, A and B); however, it can also present as more ill-defined erythema in the perianal or vulvar mucosal surfaces. In women, it is most commonly found on the labia majora and perineum. In men, it is commonly located on the shaft of the penis and scrotum and less commonly on the glans and does not depend on circumcision status. When attempting to make this diagnosis, it is helpful to evaluate other areas such as scalp, ears, elbows, knees, gluteal cleft, and nails for signs of psoriasis as this usually is not an isolated finding. As with all psoriasis, it is important to screen for psoriatic arthritis which results in morning joint stiffness usually lasting more than 30 minutes.

▶ Laboratory Findings

Usually, a biopsy is not needed as this is a clinical diagnosis; however, when performed will show a typical psoriasis pattern of inflammation. As psoriasis is often misdiagnosed or concomitant with candidiasis, a fungal culture can be helpful to rule this out.

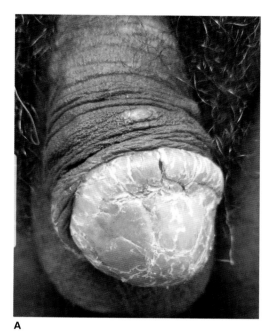

A

B

▲ **Figure 32-5.** Psoriasis **A.** Well demarcated scaly plaque on glans penis **B.** Erythematous scaley papules and plaques on scrotum, penis, suprapubic area and thighs.

Diagnosis

Genital psoriasis usually presents with erythematous plaques in conjunction with psoriasis in other areas of the body such as the scalp and extensor extremities.

▶ Differential Diagnosis

The most common differential diagnoses include the following:

✓ Allergic/irritant contact dermatitis, lichen simplex chronicus
✓ Candidiasis, tinea cruris
✓ Zoon's balanitis and extramammary Paget disease

Management

As for all inflammatory dermatoses of the genital region, a simplified hygiene routine is recommended to avoid any coexisting irritant or allergic contact as discussed in general guidelines. Otherwise, first-line therapy is the use of topical steroids. Depending on the location, different strengths of steroids are recommended. In general, a lower potency topical steroid such as desonide 0.05% ointment can be prescribed twice a day; however, a mid- to high potency steroid might be used with caution during the week with breaks on the weekend with close follow-up and tapering down as quickly as possible to a lower strength steroid. Discuss the risk of transfer to surrounding skin which can result in atrophy from higher strength topicals. Alternatively, calcineurin inhibitors such as tacrolimus 0.1% ointment or pimecrolimus 1% cream could be used and sometimes can be used for maintenance to prevent flares from keobernization.[8,9] Ointments are recommended if there is any break in skin to prevent burning sensation from alcohol present in cream formulations. Calcineurin inhibitors often can cause a burning sensation for the first couple of applications but then this symptom usually abates. It is important to address how genital psoriasis can affect the patient's sexual health either due to direct symptoms or concern that it is associated with an infectious disease. Addressing these concerns is important to improving patient's quality of life.[9]

For more information, see Chapter 9.

Clinical Course and Prognosis

As psoriasis is a chronic condition, long-term therapy is often required.

Indications for Consultation

Consultation to dermatology is recommended if there is failure of improvement with topical steroids and for evaluation for potential systemic medications. Other indications for referral include pain not improving or localized to just one area of involvement raising concern for malignancy, concern of coexisting unidentified allergic contact dermatitis, and widespread psoriatic disease in need of management. Recommend referral to rheumatology if concern for possible psoriatic arthritis.

Patient Information

American Academy of Dermatology:
https://www.aad.org/public/diseases/psoriasis

▼ LICHEN PLANUS

Introduction

Lichen planus occurs in approximately 1% of the population with involvement of genital, cutaneous, esophageal, and oral mucosal surfaces.[11] Involvement of genital and oral mucosal surfaces often occur in the same patient and can often be asymptomatic, so screening patients for disease is important if lichen planus is located elsewhere. In long-standing cases, there is a risk of malignant transformation, so this should always be considered if there is localized pain, an area not responding to treatment or an area clinically different than the rest of their disease.[1,11]

Pathogenesis

The precise pathophysiology of lichen planus is not clearly defined at this time. It is thought to be related to a T-cell mediated autoimmune reaction to antigens on keratinocytes in the basal cell layer resulting in apoptosis. It can be triggered by certain medications and hepatitis C.

Clinical Presentation

▶ History

Patients either are asymptomatic or can describe pruritus, pain, or burning sensation.

▶ Physical Examination

There are two main subtypes of genital lichen planus: classic and erosive. Classic genital lichen planus usually looks similar to lichen planus on other body sites with violaceous, polygonal flat-topped papules or areas of white coloration with lacy Wickham's striae (Figure 32-6 A and B). It is often found on the mons pubis and labia majora in women and the glans and shaft in men. The erosive subtype is more common in women and presents as erythematous erosions that affect the labium minora, introitus, and even the vagina; and in men affects the glans. Later stages of erosive subtype can result in scarring and eventual obliteration of normal architecture causing significant dysfunction.[1]

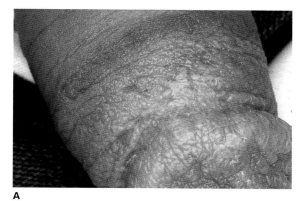

A

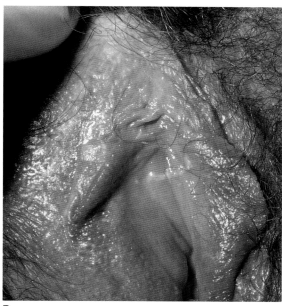

B

▲ **Figure 32-6.** Lichen planus. A. Polygonal flat-topped papules on shaft and corona of penis. B. White flat-topped small papules on labia minora and majora.

▶ **Laboratory Findings**

As this can commonly occur in the setting of hepatitis C, routine hepatitis screening is recommended. A skin biopsy will show a pattern of lichenoid inflammation.

Diagnosis

The diagnosis can be made clinically especially if it occurs in the setting of oral lichen planus, which usually has more typical findings, or cutaneous disease. A biopsy is often helpful particularly in the erosive

subtype. When evaluating an erosive lesion, taking a biopsy from the edge of the erosion is the most helpful, and will show a lichenoid dermatitis, which when combined with the clinical examination, can confirm the diagnosis.[12] If ruling out an autoimmune bullous disease, a perilesional biopsy for direct immunofluorescence is needed as well.

▶ **Differential Diagnosis**

The differential diagnosis includes the following:

✓ Lichen sclerosus, zoon's balanitis fixed drug reaction, erythema multiforme, condyloma

✓ Mucous membrane/cicatricial pemphigoid, pemphigus vulgaris

✓ Squamous cell carcinoma

Management

The first step in management is examination for oral, cutaneous, and genital involvement. As lesions can be asymptomatic, direct visualization is important. There are no official guidelines on how to screen for esophageal involvement, as it is rare and usually only associated with oral lichen planus; however, screening for dysphagia and/or odynophagia symptoms is helpful prior to any referral or evaluation.[13] Like all other genital concerns, a simplified hygiene routine as described in the general management section is recommended.

If disease is limited to just the genital mucosa, first-line therapy is topical steroids. For non-erosive disease low- or mid-potency topical steroids such as desonide 0.05% ointment or triamcinolone 0.1% cream/ointment (with caution) is often sufficient.[11] For erosive disease, a higher potency topical steroid such as clobetasol 0.05% ointment twice a day until erosions are healed is often needed with follow up every 6–8 weeks. When symptoms improve, tapering down to the lowest topical steroid or switching to tacrolimus ointment 0.1% is recommended. If vaginal involvement is present, then hydrocortisone acetate 200 mg or 300 mg compounded vaginal suppositories can be used nightly usually at least for a month and then tapered as able. To prevent obliteration of vagina, twice a week use of a dilator or vaginal intercourse is recommended when pain control is adequate. In addition, it is recommended to treat with weekly fluconazole 150–200mg to prevent candidiasis when using vaginal suppositories. If the woman is post-menopausal topical estrogen is often recommended.[1] Because of the often associated pain and effect on sexual health that comes along with particularly the erosive subtype, patients should be directed to counseling and sex therapy when appropriate.[11]

For more information, see Chapter 9.

Clinical Course and Prognosis

Classic forms of genital lichen planus tend to be more treatment sensitive whereas erosive lichen planus tends to be more treatment resistant and requires long-term management rather than cure.[11] Due to risk of squamous cell carcinoma development, particularly in the erosive subtype, monthly monitoring until symptoms are controlled and then evaluation every 6 months is recommended.[1] Aggressive therapy is recommended to avoid permanent scarring, dysfunction, and reduce risk of malignant transformation.

Indications for Consultation

Patients should be referred to dermatology or obstetrics/gynecology if there is concern for malignancy, or failure to respond to topical therapy or if the clinician is unable to evaluate for vaginal involvement. Referral to gastroenterology should be considered in patients with dysphagia and/or odynophagia particularly when seen with oral lichen planus.

Patient Information

LICHEN SCLEROSUS

Introduction

Lichen sclerosus is also referred to as lichen sclerosus et atrophicus or balanitis xerotica obliterans in men. Lichen sclerosus typically presents in prepubescent adolescents or in middle age or post-menopausal women and is more common in women than men. In men, it is exclusively found in uncircumcised men. It has been reported in about 10% of affected individuals family members.[11] There is an association with malignant transformation which is seen in about 5% of women and men with lichen sclerosus.[14] In children, it often can be a mimicker of sexual abuse due to associated bleeding.[12]

Pathogenesis

At this time, there is not clear evidence as to why lichen sclerosus develops in patients; however, autoimmunity is thought to play some part in the disease process.

Clinical Presentation

History

Women most often are present with significant pruritus, dyspareunia, dysuria, and/or constipation; however, lichen sclerosus can be asymptomatic. Men usually present due to the visual changes and sometimes difficulty with urination due to secondary phimosis. Symptoms in men tend to develop with increased severity of disease.[12]

Physical Examination

Lichen sclerosus presents as white patches often with fine cigarette paper-like appearance, fissures, purpura, or evidence of hemorrhage.[1] As this is a scarring process there will be loss of normal vulvar architecture (Figure 32-7A) and in men, a sclerotic-like ring on the prepuce/foreskin will be present which can progress and lead to phimosis, adhesions with the glans, painful erections, and even urinary retention (Figure 32-7B). Scarring is a key to physical examination finding. In women, lichen sclerosis usually presents around the clitoris, labia minora, perineum, and perianally in a "figure of 8 pattern" but can also be in just localized areas in this same distribution. In men, it is usually present on the prepuce and sometimes can involve the frenulum or urethral meatus.[14] Lichen sclerosus may also present on the non-genital skin (Figure 32-8).

Laboratory Findings

While not required to make the diagnosis, a biopsy can be helpful in early disease or atypical presentations.

Diagnosis

The key diagnostic findings include white atrophic plaques often with signs of purpura and scarring.

Differential Diagnosis

The differential diagnosis includes the following:
- ✓ Lichen planus, allergic contact dermatitis, lichen simplex chronicus
- ✓ Candidiasis and mucous membrane pemphigoid
- ✓ Vitiligo

Management

Lichen sclerosus requires high-potency steroid treatment with tapering down to either less frequent dosing or a lower topical steroid potency for control. A key component to treatment is that even when the patient is asymptomatic, continued maintenance therapy is required to keep symptoms at bay and prevent scarring. First-line treatment is the application of a high potency topical steroid like clobetasol 0.05% ointment twice a day until skin texture normalizes with follow up every 6–8 weeks.[1] In men, circumcision can often resolve symptoms, but this is not always the case. Surgical intervention has not shown to be of any benefit for women and so is not recommended, beyond what is needed to repair any result of scarring.[14] Once skin has

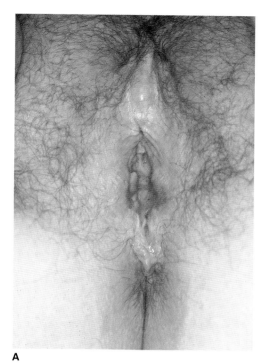

A

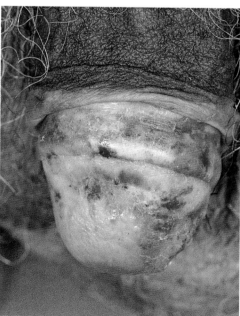

B

▲ **Figure 32-7.** Lichen sclerosus. A. White atrophic plaque with scarring and loss of labia minora. Extentsion on to perineum and perianal area forming a "figure of 8 pattern." B. White, sclerotic plaque with purpura on glans penis.

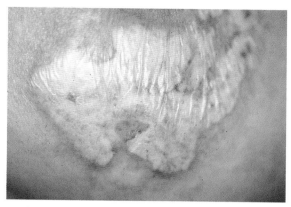

▲ **Figure 32-8.** Extragenital lichen sclerosus on breast. Atrophic plaque with thin "cigarette paper" like surface.

normalized in color and texture, topical steroid application with either clobetasol 0.05% ointment or a mid-potency topical steroid such as triamcinolone 0.1% ointment can be decreased from daily to every other day, or tacrolimus 0.1% ointment twice daily can be introduced. Additionally, estrogen cream can be helpful in post-menopausal women and sedating antihistamines may be helpful with night-time pruritus.[1] Like all other genital concerns, a simplified hygiene routine as described in the general management section is recommended as well.

Clinical Course and Prognosis

If untreated, lichen sclerosis is a progressive disease that leads to significant architecture changes which can lead to decreased sexual function due to loss of exposure of clitoral head, fusion of labia, phimosis, urinary retention, and about 5% chance of squamous cell carcinoma development. Treatment both prevents scarring and therefore dysfunction and reduces risk of malignancy development.[1] Lichen sclerosus is a chronic condition that requires maintenance treatment as discussed earlier and continued follow-up even when asymptomatic.

Indications for Consultation

Consultation to a dermatologist should be considered if the patient is not responding to first-line therapy, or has significant pain despite treatment, extragenital involvement, or atypical presentations. A referral to urology/urogynecology should be considered to discuss circumcision if failing treatment in men or having urinary retention concerns in both men and women.

Patient Information

National Organization for Rare Diseases:
    https://rarediseases.org/rare-diseases/lichen-sclerosus/

CANDIDIASIS

Introduction

Candidiasis results from overgrowth of *Candida* species which are part of the normal flora of the genital tract. However, when candida is a pathogen it causes inflammation, leading to symptoms. It is the second most common cause of vaginitis behind bacterial vaginosis in women.

Clinical Presentation

▶ History

Candidasis usually presents with symptoms of irritation, pruritus, and/or a burning sensation in the area of involvement. Obesity, incontinence, diabetes, immunosuppression, corticosteroid therapy, pregnancy, infected sexual partner, and antibiotic use predisposes patients to candida infections.

▶ Physical Examination

Candidiasis presents with brightly erythematous plaques sometimes with satellite lesions, fissuring, and white discharge or debris in areas of occlusion or increased moisture (Figure 32-9). In uncircumcised men, it most commonly occurs on the glans and corona; however, it can also involve the scrotum.

▶ Laboratory Findings

A fungal culture is only recommended in recalcitrant disease. Numerous spores and pseudohyphae can be seen with a potassium hydroxide (KOH) examination of skin scrapings.

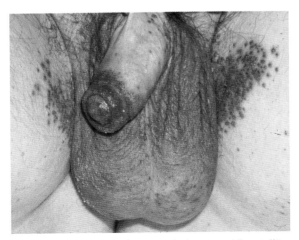

▲ **Figure 32-9.** Candidiasis. Red plaques with satellite pustules on inner thighs, scrotum and penis

Diagnosis

The key diagnostic findings are erythematous plaques which may have satellite lesions.

▶ Differential Diagnosis

✓ Contact dermatitis, psoriasis
✓ Tinea cruris, erythrasma

Management

About 90% of infections from *C. albicans* are sensitive to topical azoles. First-line treatment, if there are no erosions or mucosal surface damage, is nystatin or an azole cream or a suppository if there is vaginal involvement. Otherwise, oral fluconazole as either a single 150 or 200 mg dose or pulse weekly for 2–3 weeks or weekly for 6 months can be recommended. For severe acute infections, two or three doses of 150 or 200 mg of fluconazole every 3 days can be used.[15]

For more information, see Chapter 12.

Clinical Course and Prognosis

Although candidiasis can be a recurrent disease, it usually responds to topical therapy.

Indications for Consultation

Patients should be referred to dermatology if not responding or only partially responding to treatment.

Patient Information

National Organization for Rare Diseases:
https://rarediseases.org/rare-diseases/candidiasis/

TINEA CRURIS

Introduction

Tinea cruris is caused by a superficial infection with a dermatophyte such as the *Trichophyton* genera. It is more common in men than women.

Clinical Presentation

Tinea cruris typically presents as erythematous plaques that involve the inner proximal thigh
(Figure 32-10) and can spread to the buttocks and suprapubic area, but spares the scrotum, as compared to candidiasis which may affect the scrotum. It is often pruritic; however, it can sometimes be asymptomatic.

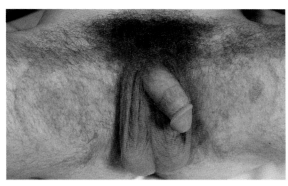

▲ **Figure 32-10.** Tinea cruris. Annular plaques with advancing scaly borders on upper medial thigh. The penis and scrotum are spared.

▶ Laboratory Findings

Diagnosis can be made clinically but a potassium hydroxide (KOH) examination of scale or fungal culture can be helpful if the diagnosis is in question.

Diagnosis

The key diagnostic findings are red/brown annular plaques in the inner proximal thighs.

▶ Differential Diagnosis

✓ Candida, erythrasma
✓ Psoriasis

Management

Treatment is primarily with topical therapies unless there is follicular involvement due to previous use of topical steroids. First-line treatment is usually terbinafine 1% cream for 2–4 weeks. Tinea cruris often spreads from the feet to the groin and therefore treatment of the patient's feet can sometimes help with recurrence.[16]

For more information, see Chapter 12.

Indications for Consultation

Severe or persistent disease that does not respond to therapy.

Patient Information

MedlinePlus :
    https://medlineplus.gov/ency/article/000876.htm

▼ ERYTHRASMA

Introduction

Erythrasma is a common bacterial infection that occurs in intertriginous warm, moist areas of the body including the crural and intergluteal folds.

Pathogenesis

Erythrasma is the superficial infection caused by *Corynebacterium minutissimum.*

Clinical Presentation

Erythrasma occurs often in the axilla and groin with an increased incidence in patients with obesity or hyperhidrosis due to increased growth in warm and humid environments. Erythrasma presents as an asymptomatic pink or tan plaques (Figure 32-11). It can be distinguished from tinea or candida by its bright coral-red fluorescence under a Wood's lamp. However, this can be falsely negative if patient has recently bathed.

Diagnosis

The bright coral-red fluorescence under a Wood's lamp and the distribution usually confirms the diagnosis.

▶ Differential Diagnosis

✓ Tinea cruris, candida
✓ Inverse psoriasis, lichen planus, contact dermatitis

▶ Laboratory Findings

Bacterial cultures or Gram stains may be done but are rarely needed.

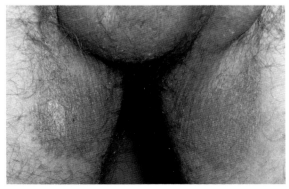

▲ **Figure 32-11.** Erythrasma. Well defined, rust colored thin plaques on medial thighs.

Management

Treatment focuses on decreasing moisture if possible and the use topical clindamycin or erythromycin or a topical azole antifungal agent such as ketoconazole.[17]

Clinical Course and Prognosis

Erythrasma usually responds to treatment but can recur.

Indications for consultation

Severe or persistent disease that does not respond to therapy.

Patient Information

SkinSight:
   https://www.skinsight.com/skin-conditions/adult/erythrasma

▼ HIDRADENITIS SUPPURATIVA

Introduction

Hidradenitis Suppurativa is a chronic inflammatory condition that can affect the groin, labia, scrotum, suprapubic area, and buttocks as well as axilla and inframammary area.

Clinical Presentation

Patients with hidradenitis suppurativa can present with a wide spectrum of clinical signs including erythematous follicular-based papules, comedones, painful nodules, scarring, and draining sinuses. Hidradenitis suppurativa is most often seen in reproductive aged women but can also occur in men. Patients are often misdiagnosed with recalcitrant folliculitis or recurrent abscesses. A helpful diagnostic tip is the distribution of symptoms, presence of scarring, and recurrence.[18] For more information, see Chapter 10.

▼ PERIANAL STREPTOCOCCAL DISEASE

Introduction

Perianal streptococcal disease is an uncommon superficial infection of the perianal area. It is more common in children than adults. The true incidence is unknown.

Pathogenesis

Group-A beta hemolytic streptococci infection is the most common cause; however, other bacteria have been reported as causes for perianal infections.

Clinical Presentation

Perianal strep presents as sharply demarcated perianal erythema which may have fissures and erosions (Figure 32- 12).

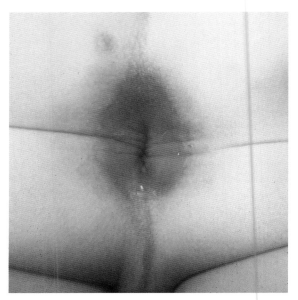

▲ Figure 32-12. Perianal streptococcal disease. Sharply demarcated perianal erythema in a child.

A characteristic foul odor may be present. Perianal pruritus, pain with defecation, and blood in the stool may be present.

   Culture swabs are usually positive for group-A beta hemolytic streptococci.

Diagnosis

Bacterial culture and clinical findings support the diagnosis.

▶ Differential Diagnosis

✓ Candida infection
✓ Psoriasis and dermatitis

Management

Treatment is focused on oral antibiotics based on associated sensitivities.[19]

Indications for Consultation

Severe or persistent disease that does not respond to therapy.

Patient Information

StatPearls:
   https://www.ncbi.nlm.nih.gov/books/NBK547663/

Syphilis is a sexually transmitted infection caused by *Treponema pallidum* of which the incidence is increasing in the United States in all sexual orientations. It initially presents as a primary, usually single, painless ulcer that appears within 3 weeks of exposure (Figure 32-13). It often occurs on the glans or the vulva. The secondary manifestations of syphilis are not confined to the genitalia but can include condylomata lata which are soft pink papules and nodules on the genitals.[20] For further information, see Chapter 11.

Introduction

Herpes simplex virus (HSV) is the most common cause of genital erosions and blisters. In the United States, almost 1 in 5 people have been infected with this virus. However, about 90% of patients with genital herpes simplex virus are unaware of their infection and asymptomatic shedding is common. The most common subtype of genital herpes is from HSV-2; however, HSV-1 infection is possible as well due to oral-genital contact.

Clinical Presentation

▶ History

There is usually a prodrome of tingling or burning prior to the onset of painful vesicles and erosions. The primary episode occurs 2–7 days after exposure and recurrences are common and are usually milder.

▶ Physical Examination

Herpes simplex presents as grouped small 1–3 mm vesicles or ulcerations on an erythematous base (Figure 32-14). It is most common on the genitals, perianal area or buttocks, and proximal thighs. Herpes simplex on the buttocks or proximal thighs can have a pustular appearance with surrounding erythema.[21]

▶ Laboratory Findings

When herpes simplex is suspected, it is recommended a swab be obtained for polymerase chain reaction (PCR) in the acute setting when vesicles or open erosions are present. Antibody testing does not help diagnose an acute infection as it only suggests past exposure.

Diagnosis

The key diagnostic clinical features of herpes simplex are painful, grouped vesicles, or erosions.

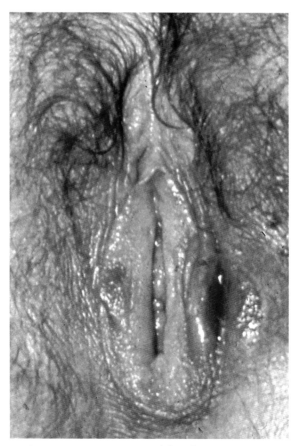

▲ **Figure 32-13.** Primary syphilis. Chancre presenting as an asymptomatic ulcer on the intralabial sulcus.

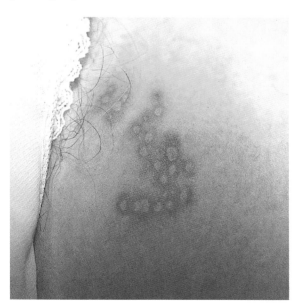

▲ **Figure 32-14.** Herpes simplex. Grouped vesicles on an erythematous base on medial thigh.

▶ Differential Diagnosis

✓ Syphilitic chancre
✓ Other: Trauma, aphthae, chancroid, lymphogranuloma venereum, and granuloma inguinale

Management

The recommended treatment for the primary episode is valacyclovir 1 gram by mouth every 12 hours for 7–10 days or acyclovir 400 mg by mouth three times a day for 7–10 days. For recurrences valacyclovir 500 mg by mouth every 12 hours for 3 days or acyclovir 800 mg by mouth three times a day for 2 days is recommended. One could consider suppressive therapy with acyclovir 400 mg twice a day or valacyclovir 1 gram daily.[22]

For more information, see Chapter 13.

Clinical Course and Prognosis

Herpes simplex infections can be recurrent; however, this can vary significantly from patient to patient with some people needing suppressive therapy to control outbreaks and others having very rare occurrences.

Indications for Consultation

Consultation to dermatology should be considered if not responding to typical treatment regimens.

Patient Information

Centers for Disease Control and Prevention:
  www.cdc.gov/std/herpes/default.htm

MOLLUSCUM CONTAGIOSUM

Introduction

Molluscum primarily occur in children less than 15 years old or in young adults as a sexually transmitted infection.[23] They are transmitted from direct skin-to-skin contact or through fomites.

Pathogenesis

Molluscum contagiosum is caused by a member of the poxvirus group, which contain double- stranded DNA and replicate within the cytoplasm of epithelial cells.

Clinical Presentation

Molluscum contagiosum presents with small 2–4 mm firm, smooth, flesh colored, umbilicated papules which can exhibit the Koebner phenomenon. They are often asymptomatic but can sometimes be pruritic. They can also be painful when resolving and be associated with significant inflammation and appear like a boil.

▶ Laboratory Findings

The diagnosis can be confirmed by incising a lesion with a needle and squeezing out the core with gloved fingers or with a small curette. The core should be squashed between two glass slides to flatten the specimen. The specimen can be stained with Giemsa stain and examined for the presence of large, purple, oval bodies which are the viral inclusion bodies within the cytoplasm of keratinocytes. These inclusion bodies can also be seen in skin biopsy specimens.

Diagnosis

The key diagnostic clinical features of molluscum are small skin-colored papules with central umbilication.

Differential Diagnosis

- Folliculitis
- Milia

Management

Treatment options include observance, cryotherapy, curettage, in office application of cantharidin, or intralesional candida antigen.[24] It is recommended that patients avoid shaving involved areas to prevent spread of the virus.

For more information, see Chapter 13.

Clinical Course and Prognosis

Molluscum usually eventually self-resolve, but this can take up to 4 years with continued spread in the meantime.

Indications for Consultation

Severe or persistent disease that does not respond to therapy.

Patient Information

American Academy of Dermatology:
  www.aad.org/public/diseases/a-z/molluscum-contagiosum-overview

GENITAL WARTS (CONDYLOMA ACUMINATUM)

Introduction

Genital warts are caused by the human papillomavirus (HPV) and are spread by direct skin to skin contact.

Pathogenesis

The most prevalent benign genital warts are usually caused by HPV types 6 and 11. HPV genotypes, such as 16, 18,

31, and 33 may be oncogenic, inducing malignant transformation to squamous cell carcinoma in the anogenital and oropharyngeal areas.

Clinical Presentation

▶ History

Genital warts are most often asymptomatic, but can cause pruritus, pain, bleeding, burning, or if large can cause difficulty with hygiene after voiding.

▶ Physical Examination

Genital warts can be found anywhere along the genital skin including both mucosal and keratinized skin. They present as pink, brown, red, black, or skin-colored papules and plaques (Figure 32-15. A and B).

Diagnosis

The key diagnostic features of genital warts are discrete or grouped papules and plaques on the genitals or perineum.

Differential Diagnosis

- Pearly penile papules which can be distinguished by their specific circumferential location on the rim of the glans.
- Enlarged sebaceous glands on the vulva.

Management

Crucial to treatment is avoiding genital hair grooming to prevent further spread of the virus. The main treatments all are focused on causing enough inflammation so that the virus is destroyed by the patient's immune system. Treatments include cryotherapy every 4–6 weeks or imiquimod cream 5% applied at night three times a week for 16 weeks.[25]

Human papillomavirus infection is not only is a very common sexually transmitted infection but has been linked to genital and anal cancer and so prevention of HPV with vaccination is important. The current recommendation is for everyone aged 9–26 years virus to receive the current human papillomavirus vaccination; however, it is encouraged that this be done at the youngest age possible in an attempt to gain immunity prior to HPV exposure.[26] It is estimated that if all children were vaccinated this would eliminate over 90% of cervical, oropharyngeal, anal, vaginal, vulvar, and penile cancers caused by human papillomavirus.[27]

HPV infections can be more severe in patients who are immunosuppressed such as patients with human immunodeficiency virus (HIV).

For more information, see Chapter 13.

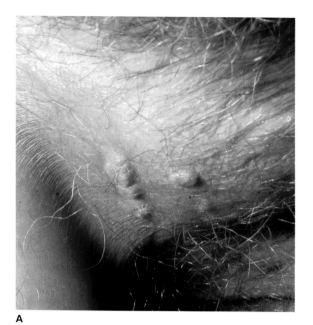

A

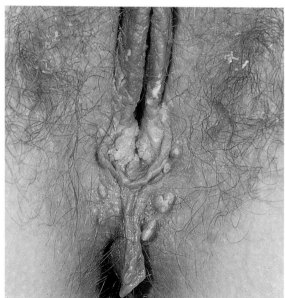

B

▲ **Figure 32-15** Genital warts (condyloma acuminatum). **A.** Skin colored verrucous papules on side of scrotum **B.** Pink to skin-colored verrucous papules on the fourchette and perineal body.

Clinical Course and Prognosis

Multiple repeat treatments are often needed for resolution and recurrences are common.

Indications for Consultation

Patients should be referred to either dermatology, obstetrics/gynecology, urology, or general surgery depending on the location of involvement for recalcitrant lesions. Lesions that have any associated pain or bleeding or significantly large lesions that might require surgical debulking may require a team approach for successful treatment outcomes. Consultation should also be considered in patients with a history of genital or perianal malignancies.

Patient Information

Centers for Disease Control and Prevention:
   www.cdc.gov/std/hpv

GENITAL MALIGNANT AND PREMALIGNANT LESIONS

Introduction

The most common type of genital malignancy is squamous cell carcinoma which has several names depending on if it occurs in a male or female and its relationship to HPV or an underlying dermatosis.

Clinical Presentation

The clinical appearance of genital squamous cell carcinoma can vary from a subtle erythematous macule to a large exophytic verrucous nodule with white coloration and hemorrhage (Figure 32-16 A and B). Color can vary from white or gray to red or brown. The lesions can either be asymptomatic or have pain out of proportion to findings on examination. Skin biopsies are usually diagnostic.

Clinical Course and Prognosis

In women, there are two main categories of squamous cell carcinoma separated by their relationship to HPV.

When HPV related, it is classified as either low-grade squamous *intraepithelial lesion of the vulva (vulvar LSIL)* which is not considered a premalignant state and was previously called a condyloma or *high-grade squamous intraepithelial lesion of the vulva (vulvar HSIL)* which is a premalignant condition.

If related to vulvar dermatoses such as lichen planus or lichen sclerosis and not to HPV, it is classified as *differentiated vulvar intraepithelial neoplasia (dVIN)* (Figure 32-17), which has a higher chance of recurrence, more uncommon than HPV premalignant forms and has a decreased disease-specific survival compared to a vulvar low-grade squamous intraepithelial lesion.[28]

When vulvar cancer is invasive, it is then called vulvar *squamous cell carcinoma.* Less than 5% of vulvar low-grade squamous intraepithelial lesions progress to invasive

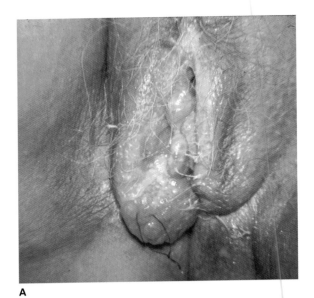

A

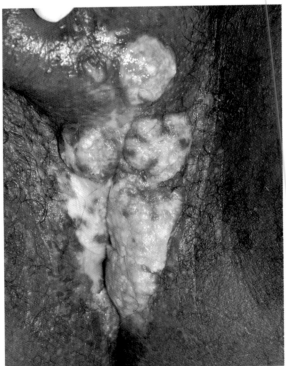

B

▲ **Figure 32-16.** Genital squamous cell carcinoma. **A.** Exophytic nodule on labia majora. **B.** Pink, hypopigmented indurated plaque with superficial erosion on perineum and base of the scrotum.

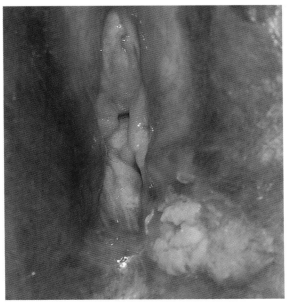

Figure 32-17. Differentiated vulvar intraepithelial neoplasia (dVIN). White hyperkeratotic plaque on labium majus.

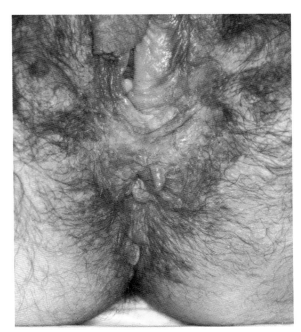

Figure 32-18. Bowenoid papulosis. Multiple dark brown, verrucous plaques on labia and perineum.

squamous cell carcinoma however it accounts for 40% of all vulvar squamous cell carcinoma.[29]

Premalignant lesions are separated by their relationship with human papilloma virus subtype.

- High risk HPV subtypes are associated with *Bowen's disease, bowenoid papulosis*
- (Figure 32-18), *erythroplasia of Queyrat* (Figure 32-19).
- Low risk HPV subtypes are associated with condyloma acuminata and Buschke-Lowenstein tumors.

Non-HPV related lesions result from inflammatory conditions such as lichen sclerosus and balanitis related to lack of circumcision.[30]

An increased risk of genital squamous cell carcinoma has been associated with lack of circumcision, phimosis, balanitis, obesity, lichen sclerosus, smoking, low socioeconomic status, HPV, and a history of psoralen plus ultraviolet A light exposure.[30]

Penile cancer typically appears in the 7th decade. Around 40% of all penile cancers are associated with HPV and tend to have a better disease-specific survival rate than cancers not related to HPV; however, there is debate in the literature on this topic.[31]

Diagnosis

A skin biopsy is needed to confirm the diagnosis of a pre-malignant or malignant lesion in the genital and perineal

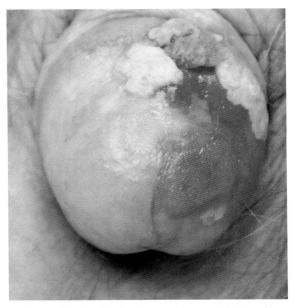

Figure 32-19. Erythroplasia of Queyrat. Red and white hyperkeratotic plaques on the glans penis.

areas. The presence of any persistent lesion(s) that does not respond to therapy should alert the clinician to the possibility of a neoplasm especially in high-risk individuals.

▶ Differential Diagnosis

✓ Genital warts (condyloma accuminata)
✓ Underlying dermatosis such as lichen sclerosus or infection such as candidiasis

Management

To help improve outcomes for patients with genital malignancies, it is crucial that the clinician maintains a high level of suspicion and does not hesitate to perform a biopsy when needed. Signs of concern are lesions failing to respond to treatment, rapidly growing lesion(s) with or without symptoms or bleeding lesions.

There are multiple ways to perform a biopsy depending on the location. In general, on the penile shaft a shave biopsy is recommended while on the vulva, a punch or snip removal, using a suture placed through the area of concern to provide tension and to tent up the area of biopsy, is the most useful. To help with the increased level of pain with biopsy in the genitals the area can be pre-treated with lidocaine 2.5% and prilocaine 2.5% cream (EMLA) or lidocaine gel. For punch biopsies gel foam or an absorbable suture can be used. If using suture, try to keep the tails long to prevent discomfort. In all cases of genital malignancy, a biopsy is required for diagnosis.

Indications for Consultation

A patient should be referred if a clinician is not comfortable with performing a biopsy and when there is suspicion for possible malignancy. Once the diagnosis has been made, further consultation with obstetrics/gynecology is needed. A Mohs micrographic surgery consult may be needed depending on the consulting provider's scope of practice and availability.

Other Genital Malignancies

Two less common genital malignancies include melanoma and extramammary Paget disease. Melanoma is rare and accounts for up to 10% of all genital malignancies and can be amelanotic in about 25% of the cases. These usually present as an asymptomatic tan to black papule or plaque with asymmetry, irregular color, and indistinct borders and may be ulcerated. Extramammary Paget disease is an intraepidermal adenocarcinoma that can be a primary malignancy or secondary to an underlying genitourinary or gastrointestinal cancer which can be distinguished by pathologic staining. These more often occur in females who are in their 60s. They frequently are asymptomatic; however, these lesions can metastasize and have high rates of recurrence due to subclinical spread. Extramammary Paget disease presents as a well demarcated pink scaly plaque with white epithelium or so called "strawberry and cream appearance" (Figure 32-20).[29]

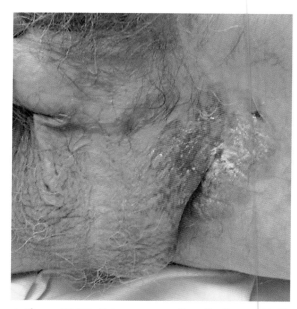

▲ **Figure 32-20.** Extramammary Paget's disease. Well demarcated pink - white plaque on scrotum extending into the inguinal fold.

Patient Information

- American Society of Clinical Oncology:
  https://www.cancer.net/cancer-types/vulvar-cancer/introduction
- American Cancer Society:
  https://www.cancer.org/cancer/vulvar-cancer/treating/by-stage.html

▼ DYSESTHESIAS/GENITAL PAIN SYNDROMES

Genital dysesthesias have many names depending on the location, such as vulvodynia, scrotodynia, and idiopathic perianal pruritus, to name a few. Patients often report pruritus, burning sensations and/or pain with no visible external changes noted.

Genital dysesthesias can be seen in isolation with no cutaneous changes, or they can occur in the setting of primary chronic dermatoses. So, they should be considered when patients are clinically improving but symptoms persist.

There are many theories as to the etiology of these symptoms, but the overarching theory is that there are abnormalities in the peripheral nervous system contributing to the abnormal sensations patients experience. Because these are a diagnosis of exclusion, it is recommended that all suspected patients have a second opinion by dermatology and as needed by gynecology, urology or general surgery depending on the exact distribution and the consulting clinician's scope of practice. The main treatments are focused on reducing abnormal nerve signaling with medications such as oral gabapentin or topical lidocaine, and relieving musculoskeletal imbalance with physical therapy, and dealing with the psychological consequences of persistent symptoms and their effect on sexual health.[1,2,32]

REFERENCES

1. Mauskar MM, Marathe K, Venkatesan A, Schlosser BJ, Edwards L. Vulvar Diseases: Conditions in adults and children. *J Am Acad Dermatol.* 2020; 82:1287-98.
2. Mauskar MM, Marathe K, Venkatesan A, Schlosser BJ, Edwards L. Vulvar Diseases: Approach to the patient. *J Am Acad Dermatol.* 2020; 82:1277-84
3. Ansari P. Pruritus Ani. *Clin Colon Rectal Surg.* 2016; 29:38-42
4. Woodruff CM, Trivedi BS, Botto N, Kornik R. Allergic contact dermatitis of the vulva. *Contact Dermatitis.* 2018;29(5):233-43.
5. Warshaw EM, Kimyon RS, Silverberg JI, et al. Evaluation of patch test findings in patients with anogenital dermatitis. *JAMA Dermatol.* 2019;156(1):85-91.
6. Savas JA, Pichardo RO. Female genital itch. *Dermatol Clin.* 2018; 36:225-243
7. Lynch P. Lichen simplex chronicus (atopic/neurodermatitis) of the anogenital region. *Dermatol Ther.* 2004;17(1):8-19.
8. Beck KM, Yang EJ, Sanchez IM, Liao W. Treatment of genital psoriasis: a systematic review. *Dermatol Ther.* 2018; 8:509-525.
9. Kelly A, Ryan C. Genital Psoriasis: impact on quality of life and treatment options. *Am J Clin Dermatol.* 2019;20(5):639-646.
10. Watchorn RE, Bunker CB. Genital diseases in the mature man. *Clin Dermatol.* 2018; 36:197-207.
11. Moyal-Barracco M, Edward L. Diagnosis and therapy of anogenital lichen planus. *Dermatol Ther.* 2004;17:38-46
12. Andreassi L, Bilenchi R. Non-infectious inflammatory genital lesions. *Clin Dermatol.* 2014;32:307-314.
13. Lu CY, Hsieh MS, Wei KC, Ezmerli M, Kuo CH, Chen W. Gastrointestinal involvement of primary skin diseases. *J Eur Acad Dermatol Venereol.* 2020.
14. Charlton OA, Smith SD. Balanitis xerotica obliterans: a review of diagnosis and management. *Int J Dermatol.* 2019;58:777-781.
15. Vaginitis in Nonpregnant Patients: ACOG Practice Bulletin, Number 215. *Obstet Gynecol.* 2020;135(1):e1-e17.
16. Ely JW, Rosenfeld S, Seabury Stone M. Diagnosis and management of tinea infections. *Am Fam Physician.* 2014;90(10):702-710.
17. Chen D, Ferringer R. Red-brown patches in the groin. *Cutis.* 2018;101(6):416-420.
18. Goldburg SR, Strober BE, Payette MJ. Hidradenitis suppurativa: Epidemiology, clinical presentation, and pathogenesis. *J Am Acad Dermatol.* 2020;82(5):1045-1058.
19. Kahlke V, Jongen J, Peleikis HG, Herbst RA. Perianal streptococcal dermatitis in adults: its association with pruritic anorectal diseases is mainly caused by group B Streptococci. *Colorectal Dis.* 2013;15(5):602-607.
20. Centers for Disease Control and Prevention. 2015 sexually transmitted disease treatment guidelines. Available at: https://www.cdc.gov/std/tg2015/syphilis.htm
21. Groves MJ. Genital Herpes: A Review. *Am Fam Physician.* 2016;93(11):928-934.
22. Centers for Disease Control and Prevention. 2015 Sexually transmitted diseases treatment guidelines, genital HSV infections. Available at https://www.cdc.gov/std/tg2015/herpes.htm
23. Becker TM, Blount JH, Douglas J, Judson FN. Trends in molluscum contagiosum in the United States, 1966-1983. *Sex Transm Dis.* 1986;13(2):88-92. PMID: 3715678
24. van der Wouden JC, van der Sande R, Kruithof EJ, Sollie A, van Suijlekon-Smit LWA, Koning S. Interventions for cutaneous molluscum contagiosum. *Cochrane Database Syst Rev.* 2009;(4):CD004767. Published 2009 Oct 7.
25. Park IU, Introcaso C, Dunne EF. Human Papillomavirus and Genital Warts: A Review for the Evidence for the 2015 Centers for Disease Control and Prevention Sexually Transmitted Disease Treatment Guidelines. *Clin Infect Dis.* 2015;61 Suppl 8:S849-S855.
26. Centers for Disease Control and Prevention. Vaccines and Preventable Diseases. HPV vaccine Recommendations. Available at http://www.cdc.gov/vaccines/vpd/hpv/hcp/recommendations.html
27. Saslow D, Andrews KS, Manassaram-Baptiste D, Smith RA, Fontham ETH; American Cancer Society Guideline Development Group. Human papillomavirus vaccination 2020 guideline update: American Cancer Society guideline adaptation [published online ahead of print, 2020 Jul 8]. *CA Cancer J Clin.* 2020;10.3322/caac.21616.
28. Committee Opinion No. 675 Summary: Management of Vulvar Intraepithelial Neoplasia. *Obstet Gynecol.* 2016;128(4):937-938.
29. Weinberg D, Gomez-Martinez RA. Vulvar Cancer. *Obstet Gynecol Clin North Am.* 2019;46(1):125-135.
30. Douglawi A, Masterson TA. Penile cancer epidemiology and risk factors: a contemporary review. *Curr Opin Urol.* 2019;29(2):145-149.
31. Stratton KL, Culkin DJ. A contemporary review of HPV and Penile Cancer. *Oncology.* 2016;30(3):245-249.
32. Cohen AD, Vander T, Medvendovsky E, et al. Neuropathic scrotal pruritus: Anogenital pruritus is a symptom of lumbosacral radiculopathy. *J Am Acad Dermatol.* 2005; 52:61-6.

Diseases of the Oral Cavity

Ioannis G. Koutlas

INTRODUCTION TO CHAPTER

Many dermatologic conditions, inflammatory, immuno-logic, infectious, or neoplastic can also occur in the oral mucosa, with essentially similar clinicopathologic features. Occasionally, the mouth is the sole manifestation of a dermatologic condition as in the case with lichen planus, pemphigoid or erythema multiforme. There are also common conditions which are unique to the oral mucosa, such as recurrent aphthous stomatitis (canker sores) and geographic tongue. In this chapter, the reader will be introduced to the clinical characteristics, differential diagnosis, and management of common oral conditions.

ANATOMY OF THE ORAL CAVITY

The oral cavity consists of two parts, an outer vestibule, bounded by the lips and cheeks, and the oral cavity proper that includes the maxillary and mandibular alveoli and the gingiva, the hard and soft palate, floor of mouth, and tongue (Figure 33-1). The posterior aspect of the oral cavity proper is bounded by the faucial pillars and the tonsils. With the exception of the posterior one-third of the tongue, which is of endodermal origin, the epithelium that lines the oral mucosa derives from ectoderm. In contrast to

the skin, the oral epithelium exhibits different patterns of keratinization. For example:

- The masticatory mucosa (hard palate, gingiva, and alve-olar mucosa) has keratinized (also referred to as ortho-keratinized; no nuclei in the stratum corneum) or parakeratinized (retained nuclei in the stratum corneum) squamous epithelium.

- The tongue has parakeratinized, non-keratinized, and specialized epithelia (papillae).

- The buccal mucosa and vestibule have non-keratinized stratified or parakeratinized squamous epithelia, respectively.

- The lips feature non-keratinized stratified squamous epithelium in their inner aspect, while the lip vermilion is orthokeratinized stratified with the intermediate area between the inner lip and the lip vermilion being surfaced by parakeratinizing stratified squamous epithelium.

The supporting connective tissue is of ectomesenchymal origin. Adnexal elements are not present in the connective tissue of the oral mucosa, with the exception of sebaceous glands, known as Fordyce granules/spots (Figure 33-2), which are present in 70–90% of individuals. However, the

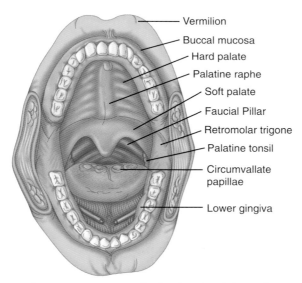

△ Figure 33-1. Topographic landmarks of the oral mucosa. Reproduced with permission from Brunicardi FC, Andersen DK, Billiar TR, et al: Schwartz's Principles of Surgery, 11th ed. New York, NY: McGraw Hill; 2019.

Vermilion
Buccal mucosa
Hard palate
Palatine raphe
Soft palate
Faucial Pillar
Retromolar trigone
Palatine tonsil
Circumvallate papillae
Lower gingiva

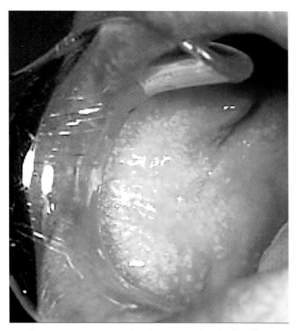

△ Figure 33-2. Intraoral sebaceous glands (Fordyce granules). Small yellow papules on the vestibule and buccal mucosa.

mouth has 800–1000 lobules of minor salivary glands, with the exception of the gingiva and the anterior aspect of the hard palate where salivary glands are not present.

CATEGORIES OF ORAL DISEASES

Clinically, oral lesions can be categorized as the following.

- **Ulcerated:** Traumatic ulcers, recurrent aphthous stomatitis.
- **Vesiculobullous:** Herpes simplex, herpes zoster, varicella, mucous membrane pemphigoid, pemphigus vulgaris, erythema multiforme, Stevens Johnson syndrome/toxic epidermolysis.
- **Maculopapular:** Geographic tongue, candidiasis, oral lichen planus, leukoplakia, erythroplakia, and oral squamous cell carcinoma.
- **Exophytic, papillary or fungating:** Oral papilloma, intraoral verruca vulgaris, multifocal viral hyperplasia (Heck's disease).
- **Nodular or polypoid:** Fibromas, mucocele, epulides.
- **Pigmented:** Oral pigmentation, oral melanocytic macules, intraoral melanocytic nevi, oral melanoma, melanoacanthoma, smoker's melanosis, metallic oral pigmentation, and other exogenous pigmentations.

Special attention should be given to lesions that are white (leukoplakic), or red (erythroplakic) or a mixture of the two (erythroleukoplakic) and lesions that are gray, black or brown, as these lesions may represent oral potentially malignant conditions.

ULCERATED LESIONS

Oral ulcers have various etiologies which include trauma, immunologic diseases, infections (bacterial, deep fungal, or viral), and neoplasms (squamous cell carcinoma, lymphoma, malignant salivary gland tumors, etc.). They are generally painful, except for squamous cell carcinoma which may be asymptomatic, when it presents as an ulcer.

Traumatic Ulcers

▶ Introduction

Traumatic ulcers are usually the result of physical injury (e.g., accidental biting during mastication, contact with sharp or broken cusps of teeth, sharp food), and less often, thermal or chemical burn (e.g., chemicals used during dental or surgical procedures, aspirin, alcohol, peroxide, other acidic substances).

▶ Clinical Presentation

Traumatic ulcers frequently affect the tongue (Figures 33-3 and 33-4), lips (Figure 33-5), and buccal mucosa and in cases of vigorous tooth brushing, small and often multiple ulcerations can occur on the gingiva. In general, traumatic ulcers present as round, ovoid or irregular, erythematous lesions usually covered by a pseudomembrane and surrounded by a white border which represents reactive epithelial regeneration.

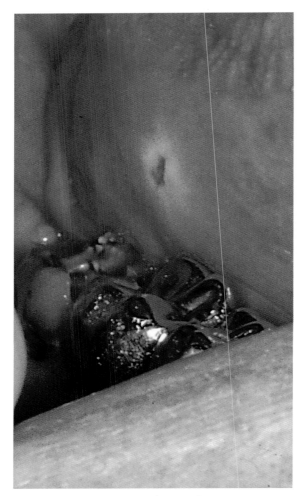

▲ **Figure 33-3.** Traumatic ulcer on the tongue. Trauma due to adjacent broken molar cusp.

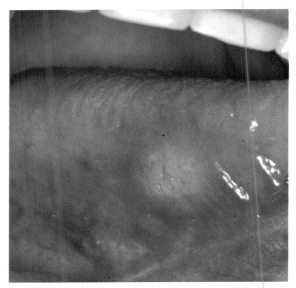

▲ **Figure 33-4.** Traumatic ulcer on the tongue covered by pseudomembrane. Round white rim indicating epithelial hyperplasia and regeneration.

▶ **Management**

Traumatic ulcers heal after removal of the cause and depending on the size and the location; they usually heal within 1–2 weeks. Over the counter topical dyclonine hydrochloride, hydroxypropyl cellulose, lidocaine, or benzocaine can relieve the pain associated with ulcerations. Treatment with topical corticosteroids (gels are preferred over creams and ointments since they adhere better to the oral soft tissues) can be used in some instances. Ulcers of the tongue may take more time to resolve due to the unique nature and composition of the tongue, which is a movable muscle. Ulcerated lesions that last longer than 3 weeks without an obvious etiology should raise a clinician's suspicion of neoplasia and these lesions should be biopsied with incisional or excisional techniques.

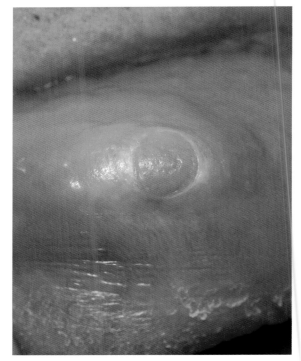

▲ **Figure 33-5.** Traumatic ulcer of the lower lip with reactive hyperplasia of the epithelium.

Recurrent aphthous stomatitis (RAS)

▶ Introduction

Recurrent aphthous stomatitis (canker sores) is one of the most common oral mucosal lesions presenting with one or multiple ulcers NOT preceded by vesicles or bullae.[1] RAS affects between 5% and 60% (mean 20%) of people with a predilection for females, White individuals, and children of higher socioeconomic status.

Many predisposing factors have been implicated with the development of RAS. In some patients, there is genetic predisposition with certain human leukocyte antigen (HLA) types. Hypersensitivity to certain foods such as citrus fruits, chocolate, coffee, gluten, nuts, strawberries, tomatoes, medications (e.g., non-steroidal anti-inflammatory drugs (NSAIDs), beta blockers), sodium lauryl sulfate in toothpastes, smoking cessation, stress, trauma, infectious agents (e.g., *Helicobacter pylori*, herpes simplex, and streptococci), and female hormonal changes have been associated with development of RAS.

Systemic diseases presenting with oral ulcers similar to RAS include nutritional deficiencies (iron, folate, vitamin B complex), immunoglobulin (Ig)A deficiency, Behçet's disease, Sweet's syndrome (acute neutrophilic dermatosis), PFAPA syndrome (periodic fever, aphthae, pharyngitis and cervical adenitis), inflammatory bowel disease, reactive arthritis (previously known as Reiter syndrome), cyclic neutropenia, and Acquired Immunodeficiency syndrome (AIDS). Very recently, it has been proposed that RAS, PFAPA, and Behçet's disease represent a spectrum with different HLA alleles influencing the phenotype.[2]

▶ Clinical Presentation

RAS ulcers are mostly round or ovoid and generally painful. They are usually covered by a pseudomembrane and surrounded by an erythematous halo. There are three types of aphthae: minor, major, and herpetiform.

- Minor aphthae (Figure 33-6), are the most common form of RAS and typically present with recurring episodes of 1–5 small ulcers, less than 1 cm in greatest diameter. They predominantly affect the non-masticatory mucosa and are usually seen in the anterior part of the mouth. They last 7–14 days, if left untreated.

- Major aphthae (Figure 33-7) are larger, deeper, last longer (2–6 weeks) and are very painful. Major aphthae are most frequently seen on the lips and the posterior oropharynx.

- Herpetiform RAS (Figure 33-8) is characterized by as many as 50–100 small ulcers and may clinically resemble ulcers of primary herpes simplex, thus the confusing term "herpetiform." Recurrences are usually closely spaced in time and location and lesions although favoring the non-masticatory mucosa, can be seen throughout the mouth.

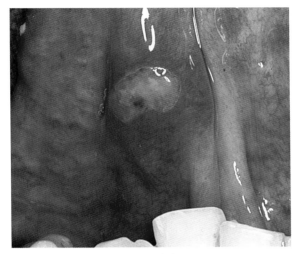

▲ **Figure 33-6.** Recurrent aphthous stomatitis, minor aphtha.

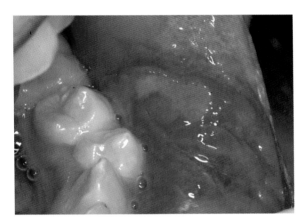

▲ **Figure 33-7.** Recurrent aphthous stomatitis, major aphtha of the lower lip.

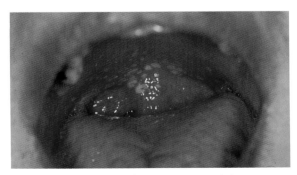

▲ **Figure 33-8.** Herpetiform recurrent aphthous stomatitis of the soft palate extending to the oropharynx.

Management

The treatment for RAS depends on the extent and degree of pain of the lesions. Some patients can tolerate the lesions and associated pain, but other patients have difficulty eating during episodes. Over the counter topical anesthetics or protective bio-adhesive products such as Orajel, Orabase, and Zilactin may be of some benefit. Fluocinonide or betamethasone diproprionate 0.05% gels can be used topically 2–3 times a day. They should be applied to early lesions at the onset of prodromal pain and tingling. Steroid solutions, such as dexamethasone 0.5 mg/5 mL and prednisolone or betamethasone syrups may be used in patients who have widespread lesions. In hard to reach areas, such as tonsillar pillars, beclomethasone diproprionate aerosol sprays are used.

Systemic steroids can be used in patients with very painful major aphthae and in herpetiform lesions. Occasionally, systemic steroids are used in conjunction with topical steroids. RAS that does not respond to steroids should be referred to specialists who may prescribe dapsone, tacrolimus, thalidomide, tetracycline, levamisole, and other medications as alternatives to steroids. Cauterization with silver nitrate and laser ablation are not recommended. Besides using medications to treat RAS, the clinician should review the eating habits of patients which may be contributing to RAS. If indicated, an evaluation should be done for systemic diseases which could be related to RAS.

VESICULOBULLOUS LESIONS

Vesiculobullous lesions of the oral mucosa may be due to trauma, allergic reactions (Figure 33-9), infections (herpes simplex or zoster) or immune-mediated disease (pemphigus vulgaris, mucous membrane pemphigoid). Intact vesicles are rarely identified and generally the lesions manifest as erosions and ulcerations since most blisters rupture spontaneously. Therefore, a clinician should specifically ask about the presence or absence of oral blisters when evaluating a patient with oral erosions and ulcerations.

Primary and Secondary Herpes Simplex (HSV)

Introduction

Oral HSV is generally due to HSV type I.[3] In rare cases, HSV type II, may be the cause due to oral–genital sexual contact. Primary infection by herpes simplex presents as gingivostomatitis (Figure 33-10). However, the vast majority of individuals without antibodies against HSV type I, when infected, do not have clinical symptoms or signs. Direct contact with an asymptomatic individual shedding the virus in saliva, or with a person with recurrent infection such as herpes labialis are modes of transmission. After the primary infection, the virus is transported to sensory or autonomic ganglia where it remains in a latent state.

Reactivation of the HSV virus is responsible for recurrent disease which usually affects the lip (herpes labialis or cold sore) (Figure 33-11) or intraorally on the masticatory mucosa of the hard palate or gingiva (Figure 33-12). Perioral lesions may also occur on the skin of the nose, cheek, or chin. Triggering factors include immunosuppression, menstruation, stress, ultraviolet light, and local trauma. Intraoral lesions may occur shortly after dental appointments and prolonged dental procedures. Prodromal symptoms such as burning, itching, or tingling are common. Intraoral recurrent herpes of the masticatory mucosa is generally very painful although the lesions are small and superficial.

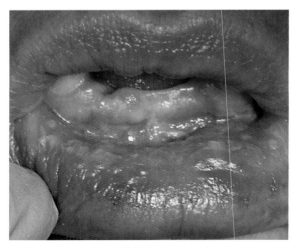

▲ **Figure 33-9.** Vesiculobullous contact hypersensitivity. Reaction to impression material used during dental work.

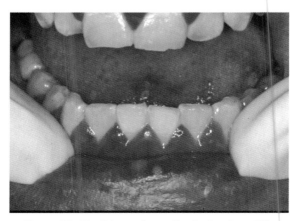

▲ **Figure 33-10.** Primary herpetic gingivostomatitis. Small ulcers on the lower lip and tongue in association with erythematous and edematous gingiva.

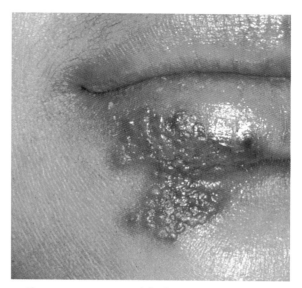

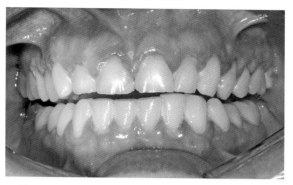

▲ Figure 33-13. Herpetic gingivostomatitis. Adult female with lesions characterized by ulcers affecting the gingiva

▲ Figure 33-11. Herpes labialis. Grouped vesicles on an erythematous base.

that rapidly rupture to form multiple small red, white, or yellow ulcerations throughout the mouth (Figure 33-10). The lips of the patients become crusted with serum and blood and the gingiva are edematous and erythematous and covered with small ulcers. Patients may also have anterior cervical lymphadenopathy, chills, high fever (103° to 105°F), nausea and irritability. Self-inoculation to the fingers, eyes, and genitals can occur. Older patients with primary disease may also present with gingivostomatitis (Figure 33-13) or pharyngotonsillitis.

Recurrent herpes labialis presents as coalescing vesicles that rupture and subsequently crust. Without treatment complete healing occurs after 1–2 weeks. Intraoral recurrent herpes presents as small shallow and coalescing yellow-white or erythematous ulcers preceded by vesicles which heal within 1–2 weeks.

Reactivation in immunocompromised patients such as HIV-positive and transplant patients may lead to a chronic herpetic infection that is persistent and characterized by atypical lesions that can mimic major aphthae or necrotizing stomatitis. In some patients, these atypical ulcers also harbor cytomegalovirus co-infection. These patients should be referred to specialists for oral biopsies to confirm the diagnosis and to specialists for management.

▶ Management

Pediatric primary infections can be treated with palliative topical rinsing with 0.5–1% dyclonine hydrochloride and if needed with acyclovir suspension during the first 3 symptomatic days in a rinse-and-swallow mode. If needed, oral medications for primary and recurrent herpes simplex can be used. Table 33-1 lists selected treatment options for adolescents and adults. Topical medications are also available (Table 33-2). Diphenhydramine elixir mixed 1:1 with Kaopectate (bismuth subsalicylate) can also be used as rinse and expectorate for symptomatic relief of pain, especially prior to meals to help nutrition maintenance.

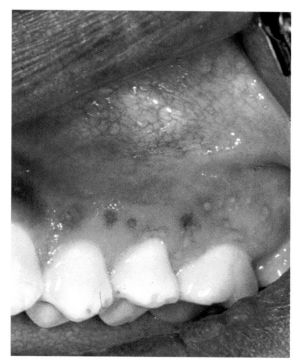

▲ Figure 33-12. Recurrent intraoral herpes of the maxillary gingiva.

▶ Clinical Presentation

Primary HSV infection presents as acute gingivostomatitis in children and adolescents with multiple, 1–2 mm vesicles

Table 33-1. Oral medications for primary and recurrent oral-labial herpes simplex in adults and adolescents.

Medication	Selected Dosing Options	Duration
Acyclovir	Primary: 400 mg 3 times a day.	7–10 days.
	Recurrent: 800 mg twice a day.	5 days.
Famciclovir	Primary: 250 mg 3 times a day.	7–10 days.
	Recurrent: 1,500 mg one dose.	1 day.
Valacyclovir	Primary: 1,000 mg twice a day.	7–10 days.
	Recurrent: 2,000 mg every 12 hours.	1 day.

Table 33-2. Topical medications for recurrent oral-labial herpes simplex.

Medication	Dosage	Duration
Acyclovir 5% ointment	Apply every 3 hours, 6 times a day.	7 days.
Docosanol 10% cream nonprescription	5 times a day.	Up to 10 days.
Penciclovir 1% cream	Every 2 hours while awake.	4 days.

Varicella (Chickenpox) and Herpes Zoster (Shingles)

▶ Introduction

Varicella and herpes zoster are caused by the varicella-zoster virus (VZV). Varicella is the primary infection and patients present primarily with cutaneous lesions; however, oral lesions are not uncommon (Figure 33-14) and may precede the skin lesions. Vesicular lesions usually appear on the lips and the palate and in contrast to primary herpes are generally painless.

Herpes zoster is due to reactivation of latent VZV in the dorsal spinal ganglia. The prevalence increases with age and occurs in 10–20% of individuals who had varicella. Most affected patients have a single episode. Predisposing factors include stress, immunosuppression, treatment with cytotoxic medications, presence of malignancies, and older age. For head and neck cases, dental manipulation may be the trigger.

▶ Clinical Presentation

The lesions of herpes zoster can affect the face and oral mucosa unilaterally and follow the path of the involved nerve (Figure 33-15). Since affected nerve endings can cross the midline, a few lesions can be seen on the other side of the midline. Patients present with very small vesicles which

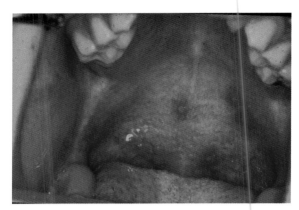

▲ **Figure 33-14.** Chicken pox. Shallow small ulcers on the palate in a child.

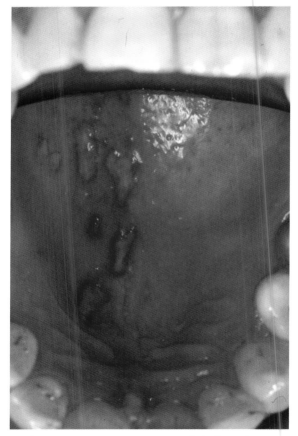

▲ **Figure 33-15.** Herpes zoster. Oral shallow ulcers distributed on only side of the mouth.

rupture and leave behind shallow painful ulcerations. Occasionally, if the maxilla is involved, tooth necrosis and in rare cases bone necrosis can occur.

Management

Treatment for herpes zoster should begin as soon as the diagnosis is established. Acyclovir at a dose of 800 mg five times daily orally for 7–10 days, valacyclovir 1 gram three times a day orally for 7 days, or famciclovir 500 mg 3 times a day orally for 7 days, are the drugs of choice. Analgesics and antiepileptics (gabapentin, carbamazepine) and tricyclic antidepressants can be used for pain relief. Also, oral corticosteroids are sometimes prescribed to older, immunocompetent patients (with no contraindications to steroids) to decrease the incidence of postherpetic neuralgia.

Mucous Membrane Pemphigoid (MMP) and Pemphigus Vulgaris (PV)

Introduction

Mucous membrane pemphigoid (MMP)[4] and pemphigus vulgaris (PV)[5] are uncommon immunologic vesiculobullous diseases that can have oral manifestations. MMP (Figure 33-16), also known as cicatricial pemphigoid, generally involves only the mouth which is in contrast to bullous pemphigoid (the most common type of cutaneous pemphigoid) rarely presents with oral manifestations.

Clinical Presentation

In PV (Figure 33-17), oral lesions may be the "first to show and last to go" and oral mucosal involvement is seen in almost all cases. Lesions present as painful erosions or ulcerations preceded by vesicles. If intact vesicles are seen, MMP is more likely the diagnosis. This is because the

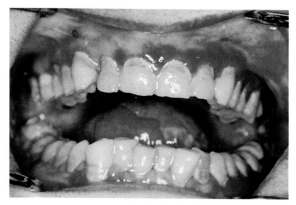

Figure 33-17. Pemphigus vulgaris. Widespread oral lesions affecting the gingiva presenting as desquamative gingivitis on the tongue and buccal mucosa.

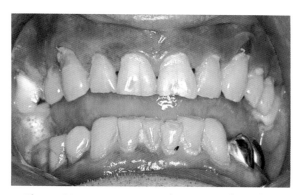

Figure 33-18. Mucous membrane pemphigoid presenting as desquamative gingivitis.

vesicles in MMP are subepithelial and thus deeper seated, in contrast to the vesiculobullous lesions in PV which are intraepithelial. Patients with PV present, only infrequently, with intact vesicles. It is important for the clinician to question the patient about formation of vesicles or bullae when multiple shallow ulcerations are identified in the mouth. Also, in patients presenting with PV, but more importantly with MMP, synchronous or metachronous ocular involvement may occur leading to scarring of the conjunctiva.

When the gingiva is involved in MMP and PV, mucosal sloughing and erosions are the primary clinical features. This is referred to as desquamative gingivitis and diffuse erythematous lesions covering most, if not all of the gingiva can occur (Figure 33-18). Desquamative gingivitis is a clinical descriptive term and not a diagnosis. The term has been misused to refer to erythematous gingiva without evidence of a vesiculobullous process. In order of frequency, the underlying condition of desquamative gingivitis can be MMP, atrophic or bullous lichen planus or pemphigus.[6]

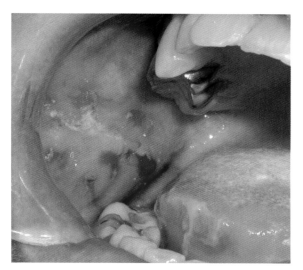

Figure 33-16. Benign mucous membrane pemphigoid affecting the tongue, buccal mucosa, and palate.

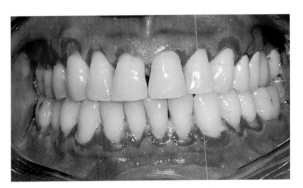

▲ **Figure 33-19.** Pemphigus vulgaris. Erosive lesions on the free gingiva.

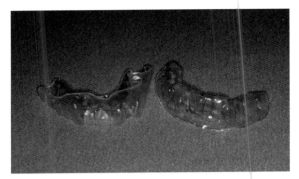

▲ **Figure 33-20.** Fabricated customized trays that can be used as a vehicle for topical treatment of widespread gingival lesions.

Patients with oral PV can present occasionally with multiple shallow ulcerations of the free gingiva (Figure 33-19). Such lesions can persist after successful treatment of all other mucocutaneous lesions and achieving resolution is problematic.

In the differential diagnosis of immunologically mediated oral vesiculobullous and ulcerative processes one should include erythema multiforme, hypersensitivity reactions, angina bullosa hemorrhagica, linear IgA disease and, bullous lichen planus, the latter being an infrequent form of oral lichen planus.

▶ Management

Treatment for MMP depends on the severity of lesions and the areas affected. Topical steroids including fluocinonide, betamethasone dipropionate, or clobetasol propionate 0.05% gels may be used for mild disease. For widely distributed lesions, dexamethasone 0.5/5 mL rinse may be prescribed. Secondary candidiasis may develop as a side effect to topical corticosteroid treatment and can be treated with oral antifungal medications.

Systemic therapy is typically required and is usually managed by a team approach with clinicians in oral pathology, dermatology, and ophthalmology. These specialists often use systemic treatment with prednisone in more severe cases. Other systemic medications for the treatment of MMP include azathioprine, dapsone and mycophenolate mofetil. Combination treatment for MMP with tetracycline 1–2 grams a day and nicotinamide 1–2 grams a day has been used as an alternative to corticosteroids and other immunosuppressive agents. For patients with gingival manifestations, excellent dental hygiene is important for good results. Also, the fabrication of customized trays by the patient's dentist as a vehicle for better delivery is recommended (Figure 33-20).

Treatment for oral lesions of PV is more complicated since the disease is systemic. Systemic treatment should start immediately after the diagnosis is established by a specialist. Ideally, a patient with pemphigus should be treated by a physician with expertise in immunosuppressive therapy. A combination of systemic corticosteroids and immunosuppressive drugs such as azathioprine is chosen in many cases. Topical steroids may be used for persistent oral lesions.

Erythema Multiforme (EM), Stevens Johnson Syndrome/Toxic Epidermal Necrolysis (SJS/TEN)

▶ Introduction

EM and SJ/TEN present with oral and cutaneous lesions.[7] EM usually affects teenagers and young adults and is typically triggered by a herpes simplex infection or it may be caused by medications including antibiotics or anticonvulsants. SJS/TEN is commonly caused by medications and less commonly by infections. For further information, see Chapter 18.

▶ Clinical Presen tation

Oral lesions may precede or be concomitant with skin lesions, which present as erythematous papules and macules frequently having a target or targetoid appearance. EM and SJS/TEN have an acute onset and may be accompanied by malaise, fever, headache, and sore throat. EM usually does not affect the oral cavity but can result in significant erosions and crusting on the lips.

In most patients with SJS/TEN the lesions usually occur in the non-masticatory mucosa with the gingiva and hard palate being relatively spared. Oral lesions (Figures 33-21) usually start as erythematous patches, with or without vesicle formation, which ulcerate leaving extensive and painful erosions and ulcerations covered by pseudomembrane, as well as areas of necrosis. Many patients present with blood-crusted lips which is a useful clinical sign (Figure 33-22). Besides oral and cutaneous lesions, patients can have genital, pharyngolaryngeal, esophageal, and bronchial lesions.

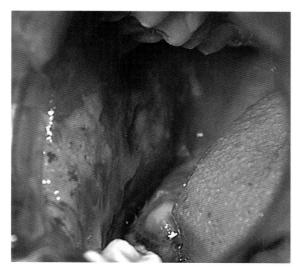

▲ **Figure 33-21.** Erythema multiforme. Oral ulcerations.

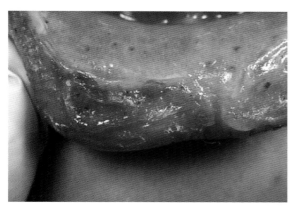

▲ **Figure 33-22.** Erythema multiforme. Crusted lips with ulcerated areas can be a useful clinical sign for the diagnosis of oral erythema multiforme.

▶ Management

It is important to identify any potential medication causes and treat any infection that may have caused EM or SJS/TEN. The causative medication should be immediately discontinued. The treatment of oral EM has been controversial. Some clinicians advocate supportive care; however, in widespread and severe lesions systemic prednisone is indicated. Patients with suspected SJS/TEN should be referred for specialty care. Extensive oral and cutaneous involvement should be managed in a hospital setting, and patients with TEN should be preferably managed in a burn unit. Patients with EM can usually be managed as outpatients with supportive care. For further information, see Chapter 18.

▼ MACULOPAPULAR LESIONS

There is a wide variety of oral lesions that can present intraorally as macules or papules. Lesions with such patterns include geographic tongue, candidiasis, lichen planus/lichenoid lesions, leukoplakia, erythroplakia, and squamous cell carcinoma.

Geographic tongue (migratory glossitis, migratory stomatitis)

▶ Introduction

Geographic tongue[8] is a common inflammatory disorder of primarily the tongue occurring in approximately 1–3% of the population and often discovered during routine evaluation of the mouth. Some studies have shown an increased prevalence in women. There is a genetic predisposition, and, in some patients, there is a family history. Lesions of geographic tongue may be encountered in patients with psoriasis and, according to studies, patients with psoriasis are up to four times more frequently affected than otherwise healthy patients.[9] The topic remains controversial with some authors considering geographic tongue an oral manifestation of psoriasis,[10] while others have not confirmed this association.[11] One should note here that patients with psoriasis may present rarely with oral lesions (Figure 33-23) that can be painful and vary from plaques to ulcers that tend to flare up with the patients' cutaneous lesions.[12] Other conditions that have shown an increased prevalence of geographic tongue include diabetes mellitus, reactive arthritis, and Down syndrome. Allergies, hormonal

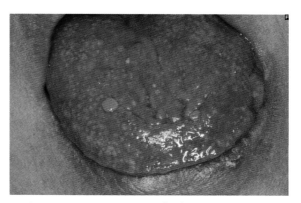

▲ **Figure 33-23.** Psoriasis. Multiple symptomatic white erosive lesions on the tongue and crusted lesions on the lips. Additional unrelated findings on the tongue include fissures in the middle of the dorsal surface, as well as, two fibrous polyps. The patient had also lesions on the gingiva and palate.

disturbances, and stress have also been associated with an increased prevalence of geographic tongue.

▶ Clinical Presentation

Geographic tongue is characterized by a single or frequently several erythematous lesions occasionally surrounded by a white or yellow line representing epithelial hyperplasia (Figure 33-24). Lesion size may vary and change shape and size, sometimes within hours. Lesions typically occur on the dorsum and ventral surfaces of the tongue, extending occasionally to the lateral aspects. When the dorsum of the tongue is affected, there is loss of lingual papillae. Symptomatic depapillation of the tongue may also be seen in anemia (e.g., iron deficiency, pernicious), candidiasis, or diabetes mellitus. Thus, such conditions should be excluded in symptomatic cases that have clinically the appearance of geographic tongue.

In rare occasions lesions can be found in other parts of the mouth such as the buccal mucosa and the palate (Figure 33-25). However, these patients almost always have lesions on the tongue. In addition, lesions of migratory glossitis are often seen in conjunction with deep fissures on the tongue dorsum (fissured tongue) (Figure 33-26). Occasionally, patients report lesion-free periods.

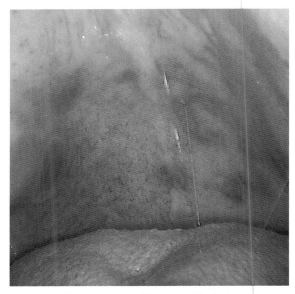

▲ **Figure 33-25.** Geographic stomatitis (migratory stomatitis). Erythematous lesions on the posterior hard palate extending to the soft palate.

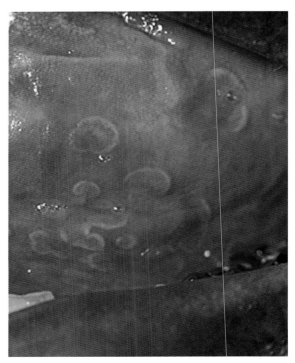

▲ **Figure 33-24.** Geographic tongue (migratory glossitis). Multiple areas of erythema with a white border on the ventral surface of the tongue.

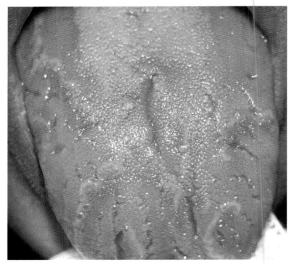

▲ **Figure 33-26.** Geographic and fissured tongue. Dorsum of the tongue featuring multiple areas of erythematous areas surrounded by white lines and present of linear fissures in the middle and anterior aspect of the tongue.

▶ Management

The lesions of geographic tongue are generally asymptomatic; however, tingling or burning sensation may be reported in association with spicy or acidic foods or brushing of the tongue with toothpaste. Other than reassuring the patient on the benign nature of geographic tongue, treatment is not necessary. For symptomatic patients, especially those who complain of burning sensation or pain, topical fluocinonide 0.05% gel may be used. Also, there are case reports advocating the use of zinc sulfate 200 mg 3 times a day or vitamin B complex supplementations. A diagnostic biopsy may be performed in cases of inability to exclude geographic tongue from other conditions that may share similar clinical features including erythroleukoplakia (see below).

Candidiasis

▶ Introduction

Candidiasis of the oral mucosa is caused by *Candida albicans* which presents in two forms, yeast and hyphae, the former being generally innocuous while the latter invades the host tissue.[13,14] Other forms of *Candida* that can be identified in the mouth; however, far less frequently, include *C. glabrata, C. tropicalis, C. krusei, C. parapsilosis,* and *C. dubliniensis.* Among all oral fungal infections, candidiasis is by far the most common. The organism is present in the mouth of 30–50% of individuals without causing disease and its presence in the mouth increases with age. Factors that have been associated with the development of clinical disease include the immune status of the host, the strain of *Candida* and the environment of the mouth. For example, patients with iron deficiency or pernicious anemia, on long-term antibiotics and steroids (topical, inhaled, or systemic), those with human immunodeficiency virus (HIV) infection or acquired immunodeficiency syndrome (AIDS), or dry mouth can develop candidiasis. Smoking has also been related to the hyperplastic form of candidiasis. However, healthy individuals can also be affected.

▶ Clinical Presentation

Clinically, there are four forms of candidiasis: pseudomembranous, erythematous, hyperplastic, and mucocutaneous.

- *Pseudomembranous candidiasis (thrush)* is a common form and it is usually acute. It affects approximately 5% of infants and 10% of debilitated older adults as well as patients on long-term antibiotics or those with dry mouth or immunocompromised patients. The term pseudomembranous is misleading since there is no pseudomembrane present. Instead, creamy white or yellow, easily detached aggregates of yeast and desquamated epithelial cells are seen on the oral soft tissues (Figure 33-27) of the palate, buccal mucosa, and tongue. They are easily removed with a tongue blade, cotton swab, or dry gauze leaving behind normal or erythematous oral mucosa. If bleeding occurs during this procedure, an underlying disease such as lichen planus/lichenoid mucositis or a neoplastic epithelial process, should be suspected and excluded by biopsy. In most

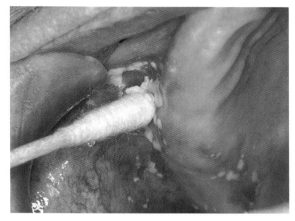

▲ **Figure 33-27.** Pseudomembranous candidiasis (thrush). Thick white plaques easily removed by a cotton-tipped applicator.

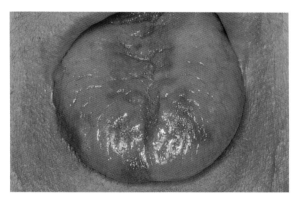

▲ **Figure 33-28.** Atrophic candidiasis. Atrophy of the tongue papillae in a patient with pernicious anemia.

cases of thrush there are no symptoms; however, burning sensations, pain, and altered taste have been reported.

- *Erythematous candidiasis* is characterized by red patchy areas with minimal or no white plaques of fungal aggregates. Erythematous candidiasis can have several clinical presentations that include acute atrophic candidiasis, central papillary atrophy of the tongue (median rhomboid glossitis), angular cheilitis, and denture stomatitis.

- Acute atrophic candidiasis (Figure 33-28) is usually seen in patients on long-term antibiotic treatment, with xerostomia, blood dyscrasias, or immunosuppression. Patients usually complain of a burning sensation (scalded mouth). When the tongue is affected, there is loss of the filiform papillae (bald tongue).

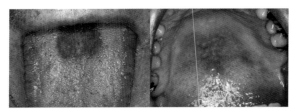

▲ **Figure 33-29.** Candidiasis. Central papillary atrophy of the tongue and candidiasis of the palate ("kissing effect").

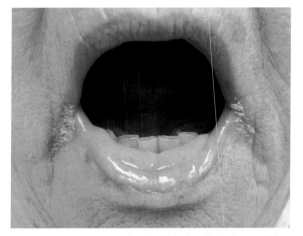

▲ **Figure 33-30.** Angular cheilitis (perlèche). Candida infection of oral commissures.

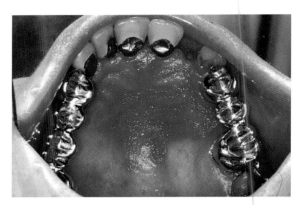

▲ **Figure 33-31.** Denture stomatitis caused by candida in a patient wearing a "flipper" (temporary removable denture to replace a missing tooth).

- *Central papillary atrophy of the tongue,* also referred to as rhomboid glossitis is a mostly asymptomatic, chronic form of candidiasis, presenting as a depapillated, usually symmetrical area on the middle and posterior central aspect of the tongue which appears smooth or, less frequently, lobulated. Lesions may also occur on the palate ("kissing" effect) or the buccal mucosa (Figure 33-29). This is referred to as chronic multifocal candidiasis.

- *Angular cheilitis (perlèche)* presents with fissures and cracks in the commissures of the lip (Figure 33-30). Typically, it is seen in older patients with reduced vertical occlusal dimension (superior–inferior relationship of the maxilla to the mandible when the teeth are fully occluded), usually denture wearers, as well as patients with multifocal candidiasis. While in some instances only candida is present, the majority of lesions harbor also *Staphylococcus aureus,* while some are caused only by this bacterium. Candida in angular cheilitis can spread to lips and perioral tissues.

- *Denture stomatitis* refers to erythematous lesions in the areas covered by the dentures, or other removable dental prosthetic appliances, especially if they are continuously worn (Figure 33-31). These lesions are generally asymptomatic. Interestingly, a biopsy most often does not feature any evidence of fungus. In such cases, candida is found in the pores of the dentures; however, similar lesions can be caused by bacteria or they can be the result of allergic response to the denture base or inadequate curing of the acrylic used for the fabrication of the dental prosthesis.

- *Hyperplastic candidiasis* is an unusual form seen primarily in smokers. It is most commonly seen on the buccal mucosa or the tongue (Figure 33-32). In this form of candidiasis, non-removable white plaques are present. Although it is known that candida can induce epithelial proliferation, it is not entirely clear if some lesions of hyperplastic candidiasis represent leukoplakias superinfected by candida. Occasionally, lesions disappear after antifungal treatment thus confirming the cause and effect role of candida in their development. Leukoplakias superinfected with candida can also have a speckled appearance, that is, speckled mixed white and red lesions (speckled leukoplakia). In such instances, antifungal treatment may improve the appearance of the leukoplakia to a smoother, more homogenous white lesion.

- *Mucocutaneous candidiasis*[15] is a relatively rare immunologic disorder in which patients develop lesions affecting the mouth (hyperplastic candidiasis and other forms), nails, skin, and other mucosal surfaces. In some patients, mutations in the autoimmune regulator gene (*AIRE*) have been identified. Lesions appear early in life and persist. However, they are not invasive, and they can be controlled with continuous antifungal treatment. There is also association of mucocutaneous candidiasis with endocrinopathies and rarely there is associated ectodermal dysplasia. Associated endocrinopathies include hypothyroidism, primary Addison's disease,

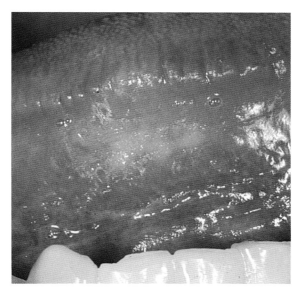

▲ **Figure 33-32.** Hyperplastic candidiasis. Non-removable white lesion diagnosed on cytologic smear. The patient was a heavy smoker.

diabetes mellitus, and hypoparathyroidism. In these patients, there is increased risk for the development of oral or esophageal carcinoma.

Management

The treatment of oral candidiasis involves elimination of factors, if possible, that contribute to persistent infection. It is important for patients to maintain high level oral hygiene. Topical treatments include the following:

- Clotrimazole troches (imidazole agent) one 10 mg troche slowly dissolved in the mouth 5 times per day for 10–14 days.
- Nystatin oral suspension (polyene agent) 1 or 2 pastilles 200,000–400,000 IU dissolved slowly in the mouth 4 to 5 times per day for 10–14 days.
- Itraconazole oral solution (triazole agent) 10 mL vigorously swished and swallowed twice daily for 1–2 weeks.

When systemic treatment is needed fluconazole (triazole agent) 200 mg tablets the first day and then 100 mg per day for 1–2 weeks should be the first choice.

Oral Lichen Planus

Introduction

Oral lichen planus (OLP)[16,17] is a relatively common chronic T cell-mediated autoimmune disease affecting 1–2% of the population. In contrast to cutaneous lichen planus which is usually self-limiting, OLP is generally a chronic disease

which may be difficult to palliate and rarely spontaneously resolves. Also, and more importantly, lesions of OLP may infrequently undergo neoplastic transformation thus causing morbidity and mortality. The malignant potential varies in studies between 0.4% to over 5%. However, a recent study presenting meta-analysis of reported studies on the malignant potential of lichen planus has shown a very low rate for malignant transformation.[18]

Patients with OLP may have concomitant extraoral manifestations and 15% of patients with OLP develop subsequently extraoral disease. The severity of OLP does not, in general, correlate with the extent of cutaneous disease. Also known is the association of OLP of the gingiva with vulvovaginal or penile LP.

Clinical Presentation

OLP is seen primarily in the fifth and sixth decades of life and it is twice more common in females than males. Lesions of OLP can also be seen in children and adolescents. Patients with OLP have higher levels of anxiety and those with atrophic (erosive) forms have higher depression scores. Occasionally, symptoms can be debilitating to patients leading to anxiety and depression.[19] Association of OLP with hepatitis C has been established.[16]

There are three well recognized forms: reticular, atrophic, and erosive. Reticular OLP (Figure 33-33) is the most common form and is characterized by multiple papules or plaques that coalesce forming striations (Wickham striae). Interestingly, lesions of reticular OLP rarely cause symptoms and frequently patients are unaware of their existence. Atrophic and erosive forms (Figure 33-34) are less common. However, these forms are the most frequently encountered in the clinical practice because they cause varying degrees of discomfort. The erosive form is mostly

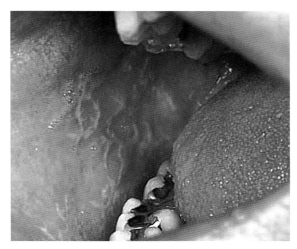

▲ **Figure 33-33.** Lichen planus. Reticular form (Wickham striae) on the buccal mucosa.

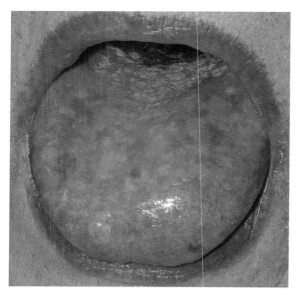

▲ **Figure 33-34.** Lichen planus. Atrophic and ulcerated areas on the tongue.

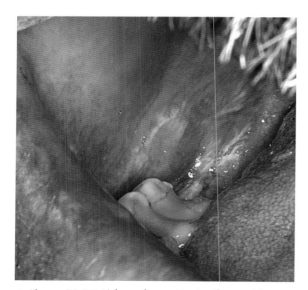

▲ **Figure 33.35** Lichen planus. Erosive form with areas of Wickham striae.

used as a clinical term when ulcerated lesions are encountered. The term erosive may be incorrect since erosions are extremely rare, histopathologically, with lesions being covered by atrophic epithelium or ulcerated. These forms may be associated with reticular lesions (Figure 33-35) and occasionally erythematous, atrophic, and ulcerated lesions feature radiating white striations. Rarely, vesicles, and bullae (bullous LP) may be seen.

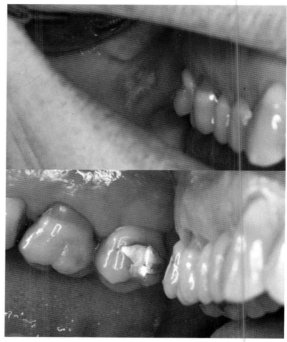

▲ **Figure 33-36.** Lichenoid lesions due to contact allergy on the buccal mucosa (upper part) due to dental restoration. These lesions are mostly asymptomatic.

The most frequent sites of OLP are the posterior buccal mucosa bilaterally, dorsolateral tongue, gingiva, palate, and lip vermillion. Occasionally, lesions of OLP are associated with candidiasis which alters their clinical appearance especially those of the reticular form. In cases of candida superinfection in reticular OLP, patients may complain of burning sensation. The characteristic striations of OLP are seen after the candida infection is treated.

The diagnosis of lichen planus is established clinically and histopathologically. The differential diagnosis includes the following:

- Lichenoid hypersensitivity reactions due to contact hypersensitivity to dental materials (Figure 33-36) and flavoring food agents such as cinnamon or mints (Figure 33-37) although in the latter, characteristic Wickham striae are not encountered.

- Lichenoid drug reaction (Figure 33-38), graft versus host disease (GVHD), and oral lesions of lupus erythematosus (Figure 33-39) may have similar or indistinguishable clinicopathologic features. Therefore, the clinician should exclude such possibilities prior to establishing the diagnosis of OLP.

- Chronic ulcerative stomatitis (Figure 33-40) and vesiculobullous diseases.

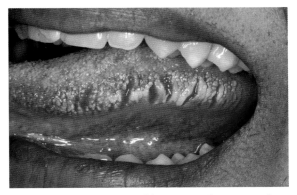

▲ **Figure 33-37.** Lichenoid lesions on the tongue due to cinnamon-related contact hypersensitivity.

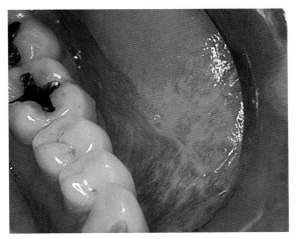

▲ **Figure 33-38.** Lichenoid lesions on lower buccal mucosa due to medication.

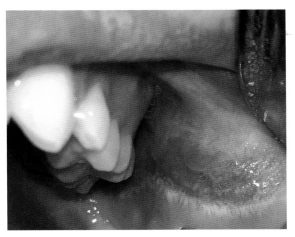

▲ **Figure 33-39.** Lichenoid lesion of the buccal mucosa in a patient with systemic lupus erythematosus. Radiating striations surround the lesion.

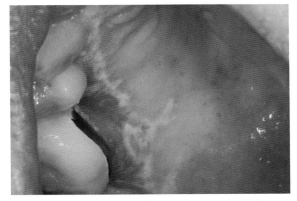

▲ **Figure 33-40.** Chronic ulcerative stomatitis, left maxillary gingiva (intraoral mirror). Erythematous lesion with white striations on the periphery. Reproduced with permission from Indraneel Bhattacharyya, DDS, MS.

▶ Management

Treatment of OLP is needed for the symptomatic atrophic and erosive forms. Patients with reticular OLP may be followed every 6–12 months. If patients are symptomatic, they may have candida superinfection and antifungal medications should resolve the symptoms. Because of the autoimmune nature of LP and depending on the severity of lesions, topical, and/or systemic corticosteroids may be indicated. Topical steroids include fluocinonide, betamethasone dipropionate, or clobetasol propionate 0.05% gels. For widely distributed lesions, dexamethasone 0.5 mg/5mL rinse may be used. For widespread lesions customized trays fabricated by the patient's dentist can be used as a vehicle for the application of steroid gels. Secondary candidiasis which may develop as a side effect to topical corticosteroid treatment can be eliminated by antifungal agents (see Management of Candidiasis). Topical tacrolimus ointment has been used in recalcitrant cases. Systemic treatment with prednisone may be needed in severe cases of erosive OLP. Other systemic medications that have been used by specialists for the treatment of OLP include azathioprine, dapsone, levamisole, and thalidomide.

Leukoplakia

▶ Introduction

Leukoplakia is defined by the World Health Organization (WHO) as "a white patch or plaque that cannot be characterized clinically or pathologically as any other disease." It is a term that does not define a specific entity but excludes a wide variety of white lesions that present distinct clinical and/or histopathologic characteristics. It is a strictly clinical term that should be used by clinicians to communicate the

Table 33-3. Lesions included and excluded from the term leukoplakia.

Includes: Erythroleukoplakia and proliferative verrucous leukoplakia.
Excludes: Lichen planus, frictional keratosis, tobacco pouch keratosis, nicotine stomatitis, linea alba, leukoedema, actinic cheilitis, hypertrophic candidiasis, hairy leukoplakia, white sponge nevus, and squamous cell carcinoma.

presence of a white lesion, the specific type of which they are uncertain of. Table 33-3 includes lesions that should be included and excluded from the term leukoplakia.

Note among those excluded lesions is the entity referred to as hairy leukoplakia (Figure 33-41), which is a type of white lesion exhibiting specific clinicopathologic features and is caused by Epstein-Barr virus (EBV). It is frequently superinfected by candida and seen mostly in immunosuppressed patients and those with HIV/AIDS. Examples of hairy leukoplakia are encountered in patients using steroidal aerosol sprays for chronic obstructive pulmonary disease[20] or in older individuals as the result of immunosenescence (Figure 33-42). This is but an example of the confusion that the term leukoplakia can cause.

Etiologic factors for the development of leukoplakic lesions include all forms of tobacco, alcohol abuse, ultraviolet light (for labial lesions), Candida *albicans*, and sanguinaria (bloodroot, a plant used in some nonprescription dental hygiene products). Among those factors, tobacco appears most closely associated with the development of leukoplakia. It is known that around 80% of patients with leukoplakia are smokers and that heavier smokers have greater numbers of lesions and larger lesions compared to light smokers. Also, smoking cessation leads to decrease in size or disappearance of leukoplakias in many patients. However, one should note that some patients with

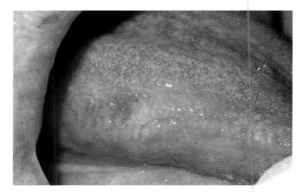

▲ **Figure 33-42.** Hairy leukoplakia. HIV negative female and without history of chronic obstructive pulmonary disease.

leukoplakia never smoked and that non-smokers with leukoplakia have higher risk for the development of squamous cell carcinoma compared to smokers.

Leukoplakia is considered an oral potentially malignant disorder (OPMD). However, in only 5–25% of the cases are definite histopathologic criteria to support cytologic and architectural changes consistent with intraepithelial neoplasia. The nature of leukoplakia as an OPMD has been established by clinical investigations and long-term monitoring of lesions. These studies have confirmed a malignant transformation potential of about 4–5%, which increases in certain subtypes of leukoplakia (erythroleukoplakia, proliferative verrucous leukoplakia) to up to 47%. The progression and time of the development of histologically recognizable dysplasia in leukoplakic lesions are uncertain and occasionally invasive squamous cell carcinoma can occur without evidence of recognizable dysplasia.

The estimated prevalence of leukoplakia is between 1% and 4% and, recently, there appears to be gender parity although in past years approximately 70% of the patients were males. The most frequent sites of occurrence are the vestibule and buccal mucosa followed by the palate, alveolar ridge, lower lip, tongue, and floor of mouth. The sites in the mouth in which leukoplakias present high risk for the development of dysplasia and squamous cell carcinoma are, in descending order, the floor of mouth, ventrolateral tongue, lower lip, palate, buccal mucosa, vestibule, and retromolar mucosa.

▶ Clinical Presentation

Clinically, leukoplakic lesions vary in clinical appearance from thin and homogeneous to thick irregular, leathery patches that may have distinct borders or blend with the surrounding tissues (Figures 33-43, 33-44, and 33-45). Variations within the same lesion also occur. Occasionally, an erythematous component is present (erythroleukoplakia) (Figure 33-46). Such lesions have a higher risk for being dysplastic or invasive squamous cell carcinoma at

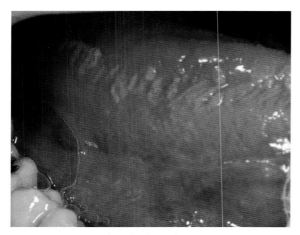

▲ **Figure 33-41.** Hairy leukoplakia. Vertical white popular lesions on the lateral border of the tongue in a HIV+ patient.

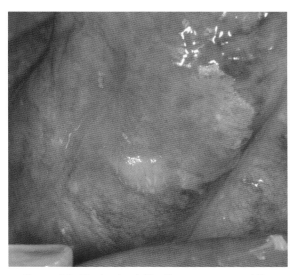

▲ **Figure 33-43.** Leukoplakia. Homogeneous white plaque on the ventral surface of the tongue.

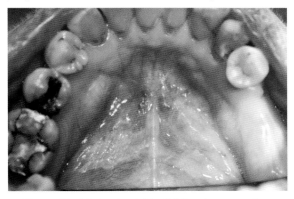

▲ **Figure 33-44.** Leukoplakia. White plaque on the floor of the mouth. The right side of the lesion is thin and homogeneous, the left side is thickened.

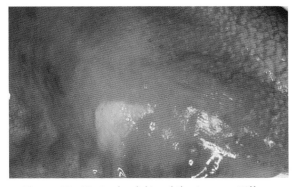

▲ **Figure 33-45.** Leukoplakia of the tongue. Diffuse, thin area on the right lateral border of the tongue with triangular thick plaque in the center.

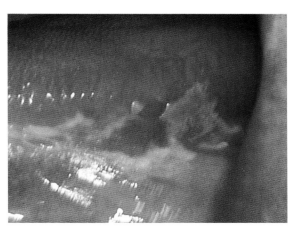

▲ **Figure 33-46.** Erythroleukoplakia of the left ventrolateral aspect of the tongue.

the time of diagnosis. Proliferative verrucous leukoplakia (PVL),[21] a subtype of leukoplakia, is characterized by the development of more than one lesion that exhibit various patterns of maturation even within the same patient (Figure 33-47A,B). Lesions of PVL have a very high risk for the development of verrucous or squamous cell carcinoma. They occur more frequently in women and less than one-third of the patients are smokers.

In the concept of OPMD/squamous cell carcinoma one should include erythroplakia. This is defined as a red patch that cannot be clinically or pathologically diagnosed as any other condition. However, this definition is misleading, because at the time of biopsy lesions of erythroplakia show severe dysplasia, carcinoma in situ, or invasive squamous cell carcinoma. Erythroplakia is less common than leukoplakia. It occurs in middle-aged to older adults and the sites of predilection are the floor of mouth, tongue, and soft palate (Figure 33-48).

▶ Management

The following algorithm is suggested for specialists when dealing with patients with oral potential malignant disorder. The gold standard for the diagnosis of clinically identified suspicious oral lesions is a surgical biopsy (excisional or incisional) and a photograph.

The histopathologic report of the oral biopsy could include two of the following possibilities:

1. Low-risk lesion with mild dysplasia or just epithelial hyperplasia
2. High-risk lesion with moderate or severe dysplasia.

If the oral biopsy reports a low risk lesion with mild dysplasia or just epithelial hyperplasia the patient should be referred for resection (scalpel or laser) to a specialist

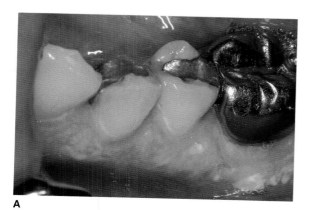

A

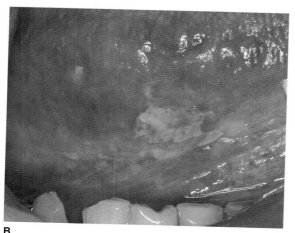

B

▲ **Figure 33-47.** A: Proliferative verrucous leukoplakia. Leukoplakic lesion on the mandibular alveolus. B: Proliferative verrucous leukoplakia on the tongue in the same patient.

such as an oral or an ears nose and throat (ENT) surgeon if there are clinical concerns such as the following.

- The lesion is not homogeneous.
- The lesion is greater than 200 square millimeters.
- The lesion is on the tongue or floor of mouth.
- The lesion has an erythematous component.
- The patient is a smoker.

Follow-up specialty visits should include close monitoring of the patient (e.g., 1 month after the procedure, then every 3 months for the first year, every 6 months the second year, and then yearly for at least 5 years to life). Clinical photography is highly recommended at every appointment. A repeat biopsy may be indicated in cases of non-homogeneous lesions.

If there are no clinical concerns as listed earlier, these lesions should be monitored every 4–6 months or resected

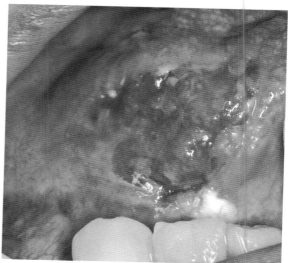

▲ **Figure 33-48.** Erythroplakia. Erythroplakic lesion on the left posterior hard and soft palate

followed by monitoring as above. If there are changes in the appearance of the lesions and/or enlargement, rebiopsy and/or resection should be performed.

If the oral biopsy reports a high-risk lesion with moderate or severe dysplasia, the lesions should be completely excised by a specialist and monitored as above.

Photodynamic therapy[22] using 5-aminolevulinic acid is a promising alternative for treatment of dysplastic lesions. Administration of oral 13-*cis*-retinoic acid have been used with some studies presenting encouraging results[23] although toxic side effects[24] may limit their use. Lastly, cryosurgery[25] has been utilized as an alternative to conventional surgery and laser ablation.

Oral squamous cell carcinoma

▷ Introduction

Oral cancer accounts for less than 3% of all cancers in the United States. Over 20,000 cases are diagnosed per year with more than 5,000 patients dying of this disease annually. Oral squamous cell carcinoma represents approximately 95% of all types of malignancy affecting the oral cavity. Most patients are older than 60 years. However, there is an alarming increase in the number of younger patients without the traditional risk factors. Based on incidence rates less than 1% of men and women will be diagnosed with oral squamous cell carcinoma during their lifetime. Male to female ratio is approximately 2.5:1.

The major etiologic factors include tobacco and alcohol. All forms of smoked tobacco have been associated with increased risk. However, in smokeless tobacco, the association with the development of oral squamous cell carcinoma remains weak and controversial. In contrast, chewing of betel quid (paan, pan supari combination of tobacco, areca nut, and slaked lime) is a major cause for oral squamous cell carcinoma in the Indian subcontinent and Southeast Asia. Also, combination of heavy smoking and alcohol abuse results in a synergistic effect and increases the risk further.

Besides smoking and alcohol abuse, human papillomavirus (HPV) has been implicated in many cases of oropharyngeal and tonsillar carcinoma. However, although presence of HPV can be observed in some cases of oral squamous carcinoma, association of HPV with the development of squamous cell carcinoma of the oral mucosa proper has not been determined. Oropharyngeal squamous cell carcinoma associated with HPV has apparently a better prognosis.[26] However, smokers with HPV-related oropharyngeal cancer, have the same prognosis as patients with non-HPV oropharyngeal cancer.

Recently the Food and Drug Administration has expanded the indication for HPV vaccine (Gardasil 9) for oropharyngeal cancer with a confirmatory trial being underway by the NIH (NCT04199689). Although currently infrequently encountered, patients with severe iron deficiency (Plummer-Vinson syndrome) have an elevated risk for development of esophageal and oropharyngeal squamous cell carcinoma.

▶ Clinical Presentation

There is a variety of clinical appearances of oral squamous cell carcinoma. Tumors can be ulcerated (Figure 33-49), endophytic, exophytic (Figure 33-50), leukoplakic, or erythroleukoplakic. While some tumors are clinically obvious, there are occasions where lesions are small (Figure 33-51), painless, and mimicking

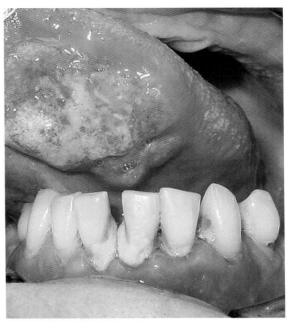

▲ **Figure 33-50.** Exophytic squamous cell carcinoma of the ventral surface of the tongue.

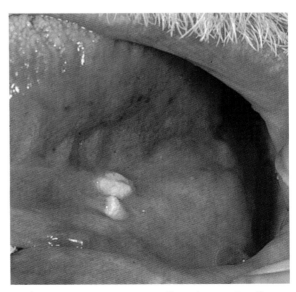

▲ **Figure 33-51.** Squamous cell carcinoma. Small white plaque on the ventral surface of the tongue.

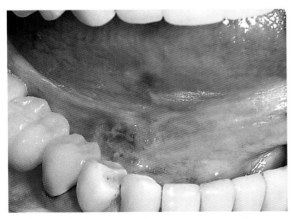

▲ **Figure 33-49.** Ulcerated squamous cell carcinoma of the floor of the mouth.

inflammatory processes (Figure 33-52). Such is the case of lesions seen in association with dental prostheses or presenting as "inflamed" gingiva (Figure 33-53). In such cases, consultation with dental professionals is necessary.

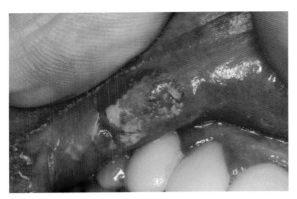

Figure 33-52. Squamous cell carcinoma. Ulcerated lesion on the upper lip thought to be traumatic in origin.

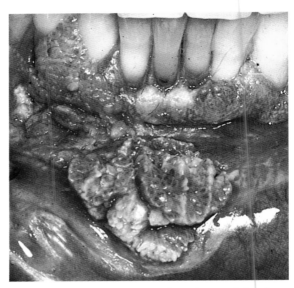

Figure 33-54. Squamous cell carcinoma. Extensive papillary lesion affecting the mandibular vestibule, inner lip and mandibular gingiva.

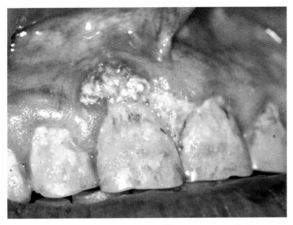

Figure 33-53. Squamous cell carcinoma of the maxillary gingiva mimicking an inflammatory lesion.

Management

Diagnostic biopsies should be obtained of all suspicious lesions that present with the aforementioned characteristics. Treatment of oral cancer involves a team of physicians that include ear nose and throat/oral surgery and maxillofacial specialists, oncologists, and prosthodontists.

PAPILLARY, EXOPHYTIC, OR FUNGATING LESIONS

Papillary, exophytic, or fungating lesions occurring in the oral mucosa include papilloma verruca vulgaris, condyloma accuminatum, lesions of multifocal viral epithelial hyperplasia (focal epithelial hyperplasia; Heck's disease), papillary and verrucoid dysplasia as seen in proliferative verrucous leukoplakia, and papillary, verrucoid, or fungating variants of squamous cell carcinoma (Figure 33-54).

Oral Papilloma

It is a common benign epithelial proliferation similar to common warts of the skin. It is presumed that most, if not all, papillomas are induced by HPV. HPV 6 and 11 have been identified in almost half of oral papillomas. Children and young adults are most frequently affected and there is no gender predilection. Generally, papillomas present as solitary epithelial proliferations exhibiting finger-like projections (Figure 33-55) or a cauliflower-like pattern. The most frequent sites are the tongue, palate and lips. Occasionally, more than one site can be simultaneously affected (papillomatosis).

Intraoral verruca vulgaris

It is uncommon. Occasionally, patients with cutaneous lesions also develop oral lesions (Figure 33-56).

Condyloma Acuminatum

It can occur in the oral mucosa (Figure 33-57) and has similar clinical and histopathologic characteristics as of genital lesions. When identified in the mouth of children, sexual abuse is a concern and should be investigated.

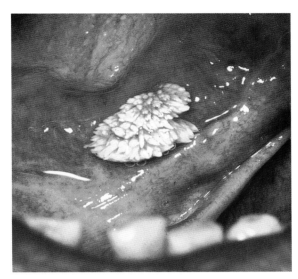

Figure 33-55. Papilloma. Well defined white plaque with finger-like projections often caused by human papilloma virus (HPV)

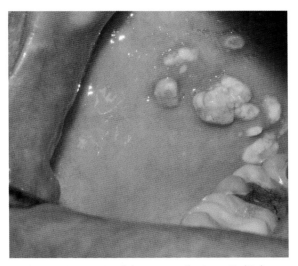

Figure 33-57. Condyloma acuminatum. Multiple papular lesions on the right buccal mucosa

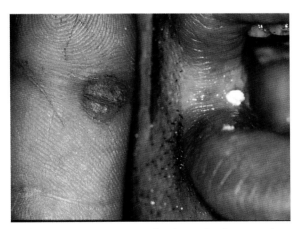

Figure 33-56. Verruca vulgaris on the finger and the commissure.

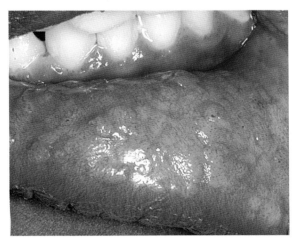

Figure 33-58. Multifocal epithelial hyperplasia (Heck's disease). Multiple papules forming cobblestone pattern on the inner lower lip caused by human papillomavirus (HPV) 13 or 32.

Multifocal Epithelial Hyperplasia

It is an HPV-related proliferation (HPV 13 and 32) characterized by multiple papular or nodular epithelial proliferations that occasionally coalesce forming a cobblestone pattern (Figure 33-58). Patients may have 20–100 lesions that rarely reach 1.0 cm in size. Lesions are seen more frequently in children. However, adults can also develop lesions also, especially if there is contact with affected children. Frequent sites of involvement include the lips, tongue, and buccal mucosa. The diagnosis can be made clinically and microscopically.

NODULAR OR POLYPOID LESIONS

The most common nodular or polypoid lesions of the oral mucosa are fibrous polyps (fibromas), mucoceles, and epulides.

Fibromas (fibrous hyperplastic lesions)

It present as sessile or pedunculated, rubbery, solitary tumors covered by normal colored or hyperkeratotic (white) mucosa (Figure 33-59). Although trauma has been

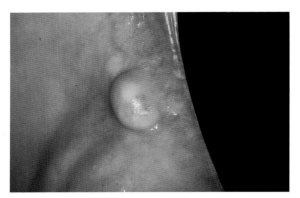

▲ **Figure 33-59.** Fibroma. Smooth papule on the buccal mucosa.

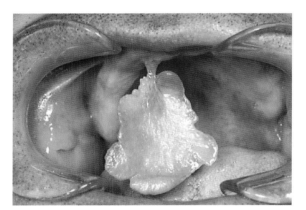

▲ **Figure 33-60.** Epulis fissuratum.

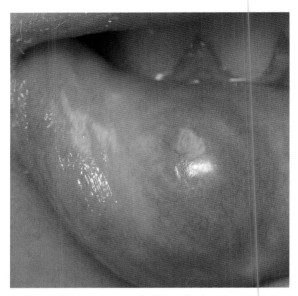

▲ **Figure 33-61.** Mucocele. Clear fluctuant cyst on the lower lip.

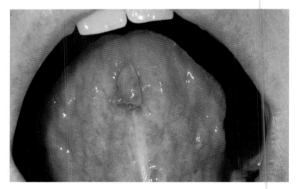

▲ **Figure 33-62.** Mucocele. Fluctuant cyst on ventral tongue.

traditionally regarded as the cause of oral fibrous overgrowths, the etiology is unknown. Most lesions arise on the buccal mucosa, tongue and lips, and their size rarely exceeds 1.5 cm. Most fibromas are asymptomatic, unless there is ulceration due to trauma. Most cases are seen in the 4th to 6th decades of life and females are twice as frequently affected as males. The observed higher frequency in females may be due to the fact that women are more concerned about their oral health compared to males. Also, fibrous hyperplastic lesions may be seen on the alveolus of patients with ill-fitting dentures referred to as epulis fissuratum or denture injury tumor (Figure 33-60). Surgical excisional biopsy to confirm the diagnosis and to exclude other soft tissue tumors is recommended.

Mucocele

Mucocele refers to a clinically fluctuant nodular mass containing salivary mucus.[27] It is either of extravasation type due to severing of a salivary gland excretory duct and spillage of mucus in the connective tissue, or retention type, resulting from obstruction of a salivary duct, the latter being less common. Extravasation type mucoceles (Figure 33-61) are most frequently seen on the lower lip and less frequently the ventral surface of the tongue of children or young adults (Figure 33-62), or the palate and retromolar mucosa of older individuals. Retention type mucoceles are seen in older adults on the upper lip, floor of mouth, and buccal mucosa. Thus, if a fluctuant lesion is on the lower lip of a child or young adult, the diagnosis is most likely that of a mucocele until proven histopathologically otherwise. However, a fluctuant lesion of the upper lip in an adult is not an extravasation mucocele until proven otherwise. These upper lip lesions are typically retention mucoceles, or benign or malignant cystic salivary gland tumors.

There is an uncommon variant referred to as superficial mucocele seen on the posterior palate and buccal mucosa.

They appear as single or multiple small translucent vesicles filled with clear saliva. The collection of mucus occurs in the surface epithelium. Multiple lesions, clustered or not, may be encountered in association with lichenoid disorders. In such cases, the differential diagnosis includes an immunologically mediated vesiculobullous disorder such as mucous membrane pemphigoid. Rarely, lymphangiectatic lesions may clinically mimic superficial mucoceles.[28]

Although mucoceles are indolent lesions, they should be excised and submitted for histopathologic evaluation to exclude the possibility of a cystic salivary gland tumor. Recurrence is infrequent, except those occurring on the ventral surface of the tongue which have an approximately 20–25% recurrence rate (personal experience of the author).

Epulides

Epulides are nodular soft tissue lesions typically of the gingiva and the alveolar mucosa. They include those characterized by the following:

- Fibrous hyperplasia (fibromas).
- Fibrovascular inflammatory hyperplasia or pyogenic granulomas (Figure 33-63).
- Fibroblastic proliferation with ossification (peripheral ossifying fibromas) (Figure 33-64).
- Collection of multinucleated giant cells in association with proliferating mesenchymal cells in a hemorrhagic stroma (peripheral giant cell granuloma) (Figure 33-65). Combination of the last two can occur.

As a rule, fibrovascular inflammatory hyperplasias and peripheral giant cell granulomas are usually erythematous and hemorrhagic. Fibrous proliferations and peripheral

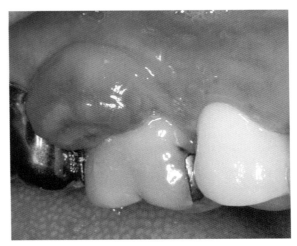
▲ **Figure 33-64.** Peripheral ossifying fibroma. Erythematous nodule on the maxillary gingiva.

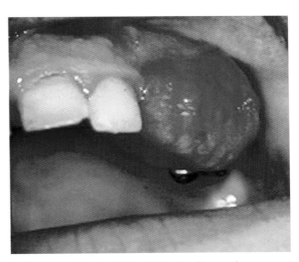
▲ **Figure 33-65.** Peripheral giant cell granuloma. Erythematous nodule on the maxillary gingiva.

ossifying fibromas have normal mucosal color, except if they are traumatized and ulcerated. Excision of epulides is recommended and recurrence is not uncommon in peripheral ossifying fibromas (about 15%)[29] and peripheral giant cell granulomas (10%)[30]. An infrequent gingival tumor, compared to other epulides, called peripheral odontogenic fibroma can be clinically indistinguishable from the lesions above and has a 50% recurrence rate.

PIGMENTED LESIONS

Pigmented lesions of the oral mucosa[31] are of two types: those related to melanin and those caused by other pigments, endogenous, or exogenous, the latter mostly metallic

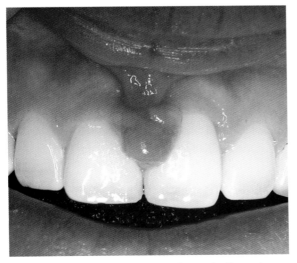
▲ **Figure 33-63.** Pyogenic granuloma. Erythematous smooth papule on the maxillary gingiva.

in origin. Also, certain systemic medications may cause pigmented lesions in the oral mucosa either by increase in melanin pigment or deposition of medication metabolites in the soft tissues. All oral pigmented lesions that cannot be related to a specific cause should be surgically excised for diagnosis.

Melanocytic Lesions

- **Oral (or ethnic) pigmentation** seen in darker-skinned individuals, varies in patterns, but is usually diffuse and bilateral with the color ranging from light to dark brown. The lesions are generally seen on the gingiva, buccal mucosa (Figure 33-66), lips, and tongue. Pinhead brown discolorations can be seen on the tips of the lingual fungiform papillae (Figure 33-67).
- **Oral melanotic macules** are the most common melanocytic lesions. They usually appear as single or multiple, well demarcated, less than 1 cm, light or dark brown lesions usually on the buccal and masticatory mucosa or on sun exposed areas of the vermilion border of the lower lip (Figure 33-68). There is a female predilection.
- **Intraoral melanocytic nevi** are uncommon. They are mostly acquired and present as pigmented and less frequently as nonpigmented macular, papular, or less frequently, nodular lesions (Figure 33-69). They are generally small with most lesions being less than 1 cm, although larger nevi have been described. Two-thirds of the patients are women and the average age is 35 years. Most lesions occur on the hard palate, buccal mucosa, and gingiva. As is the case on the skin, there are three common histologic types, junctional, compound, and intramucosal, the latter being the most frequent

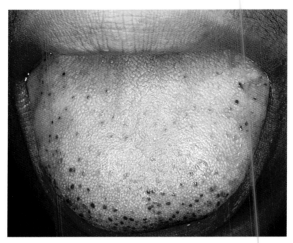

▲ **Figure 33-67.** Melanin pigmentation presenting as pin-point brown spots on the tips of the fungiform papillae in an African American individual.

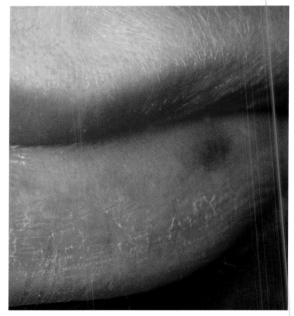

▲ **Figure 33-68.** Ephelis (freckle) on the lower lip.

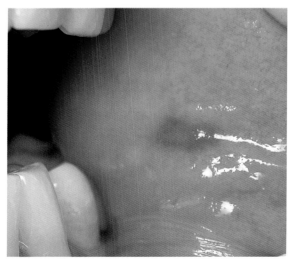

▲ **Figure 33-66.** Light brown macule on the buccal mucosa.

intraoral type. Intraoral blue nevi have been also described, predominantly in the palate (Figure 33-70). Other rare forms, for example, Spitz, halo, combined, and congenital nevi have also been reported. Although there is demographic epidemiologic correlation between oral nevi and oral melanoma, there is no proof that intraoral nevi are a marker for the development of oral melanoma.

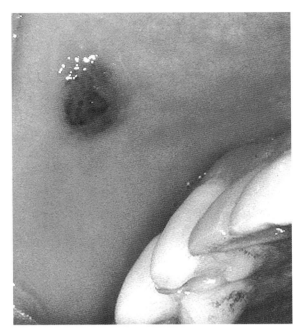

Figure 33-69. Intramucosal nevus of the inner aspect of the upper lip.

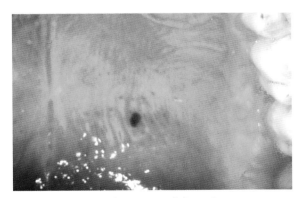

Figure 33-70. Blue nevus of the palate

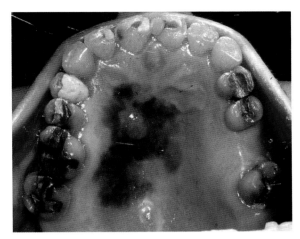

Figure 33-71. Melanoma of the palate. Black irregular pigmented lesion with central pink nodule as part of vertical growth of the tumor.

- **Oral melanomas** are very rare. They are usually macular, papular, or nodular and are most frequently pigmented (Figure 33-71), black, brown or gray, and rarely red or non-pigmented. The most frequent site is the masticatory mucosa and most patients are men. Most oral melanomas are clinically and histologically similar to acral lentiginous or nodular melanomas of the skin and combination of the two.
- **Melanoacanthoma** is a rare, apparently reactive, and in most instances self-limiting solitary or less frequently bilateral or multifocal process seen predominantly on the buccal mucosa of almost exclusively black individuals, primarily women.
- **Smoker's and post-inflammatory melanosis** are reactive lesions. Smoker's melanosis is seen in heavy smokers and is considered a protective response by the epithelium to the harmful substances of tobacco. Post-inflammatory melanosis is seen in chronic inflammatory diseases such as lichen planus, lichenoid mucositis, mucous membrane pemphigoid or pemphigus vulgaris. Hyperpigmentation occurs because of disruption of the basal cell layer leading to melanin accumulation in the connective tissue and within macrophages or stimulation of the epithelial melanocytes by inflammatory products (prostaglandins, leukotrienes, etc.) leading to an increase in melanin synthesis. Any site of the oral mucosa may be involved.
- **Systemic conditions** such as Peutz-Jeghers syndrome (Figure 33-72), PTEN hamartoma tumor syndromes, Addison's disease, may have oral and/or perioral melanin hyperpigmented lesions. In most instances the patients are aware of their condition and its clinical manifestations. Among such conditions one should also include Laugier-Hunziker (Laugier-Hunziker-Baran) syndrome seen more frequently in females, in which patients develop multiple oral melanocytic macules and less frequently nail (linear melanonychia) and vaginal lesions

Medication-Related Oral Pigmentation

Many therapeutic agents have been implicated with the development of oral mucosal pigmentations or discolorations either through deposition of metabolites, including iron-chelated metabolites, or stimulation of melanin

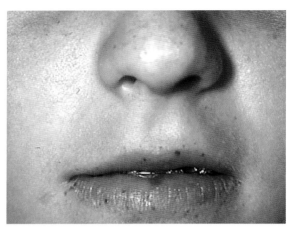

▲ **Figure 33-72.** Peutz-Jeghers syndrome. Multiple brown-black macules on the lips.

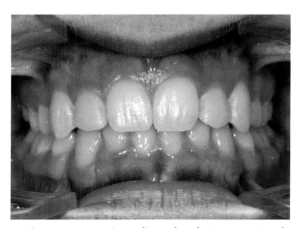

▲ **Figure 33-73.** Minocycline related pigmentation of the upper part of the maxillary and mandibular gingiva and the alveolar mucosa in a female patient treated with minocycline for acne.

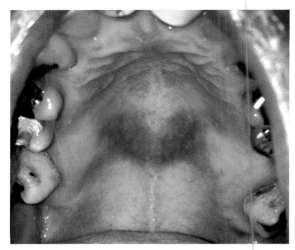

▲ **Figure 33-74.** Imatinib related oral pigmentation. Gray /blue pigmented macular lesion of the palate in a patient treated with imatinib for leukemia.

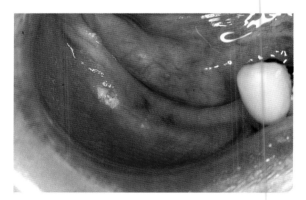

▲ **Figure 33-75.** Exogenous metallic pigmentation (amalgam tattoo). Pigmented lesion on the mandibular alveolar mucosa.

production. Examples of medications include minocycline (Figure 33-73), chloroquine, and other quinine derivatives, phenolphthalein, estrogen, AIDS-related medications, chemotherapeutic agents (Figure 33-74), but the list is expanding.

Metallic Oral Pigmentations and Other Exogenous Oral Pigmentations

These lesions are caused by either exogenous or endogenous pigments. Exogenous hyperpigmentation is mostly related to amalgam restorations (Figure 33-75). Lesions are usually located on the gingiva, alveolar mucosa, buccal mucosa, floor of mouth, and less often the tongue. The color is light to dark gray or even black depending on the amount and depth of the metal within the tissues. The size varies from a few millimeters to 2 cm. The cause can be iatrogenic or traumatic. Particles of amalgam may be embedded within the tissues during restorative procedures. Occasionally, metallic particles can be identified in dental radiographs as small radiopaque particles. Similar discolorations can occur from incidental or voluntary introduction of other metals such as graphite from pencil tips, tattoo ink, and chronic contact with charcoal toothpaste.

Heavy metals may also cause discoloration of the oral mucosa. Chronic exposure to heavy metals such as bismuth, lead, gold, or silver can cause oral hyperpigmented lesions, but these days, such cases are rare.

Extrinsic staining of the oral tissues may also occur in smokers or coffee or tea drinkers (Figure 33-76). Lastly,

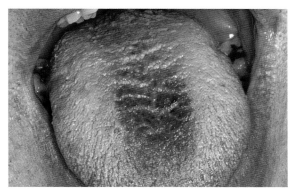

▲ **Figure 33-76.** Brown-black discoloration of the tongue in a heavy smoker and coffee drinker.

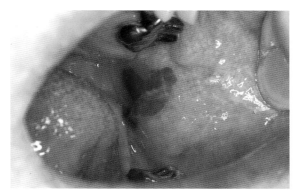

▲ **Figure 33-78.** Oral ecchymosis Patient with thrombocytopenia.

breakdown products of bacteria may stain the gingiva. This usually occurs in children.

Endogenous oral pigmentations

Lesions caused by endogenous pigments are usually related to blood extravasation (petechiae, ecchymoses, and hematomas) and products of hemoglobin degradation, that is, bilirubin and biliverdin. Trauma is the most common cause (Figure 33-77). The most frequently affected sites include the buccal mucosa, tongue and palate. Direct trauma to a tooth or teeth may lead to pulpal necrosis and discoloration of affected teeth. Also, patients with hemorrhagic diathesis related to bleeding disorders may develop multiple hemorrhagic lesions throughout the mouth. In such cases, thrombocytopenia is a frequent cause and should be excluded (Figure 33-78). Patients with congenital vascular lesions, that is, hemangiomas may present with red to purple lesions which are often tumorous (Figure 33-79). Rare systemic conditions associated with non-melanin associated hyperpigmented lesions of teeth and soft tissues

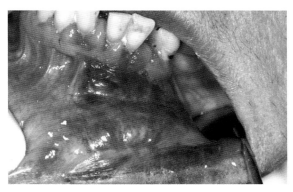

▲ **Figure 33-79.** Congenital hemangioma of the mandibular vestibular mucosa.

include hemochromatosis, erythroblastosis fetalis and biliary atresia associated hyperbilirubinemia, beta thalassemia, and erythropoietic porphyria.

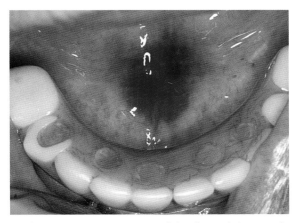

▲ **Figure 33-77.** Hematoma of the floor of the mouth.

▼ REFERENCES

1. Junge S, Kuffer R, Scully C, Porter SR. Mucosal disease series. Number VI. Recurrent aphthous stomatitis. *Oral Dis.* 2006;12:1-21.
2. Manthiram K, Preite S, Dedeoglu F, et al. Common genetic susceptibility loci link PFAPA syndrome, Behçet's disease, and recurrent aphthous stomatitis. *Proc Natl Acad Sci USA.* 2020;117:14405-14411.
3. Arduino PG, Porter SR. Oral and perioral herpes simplex virus type 1 (HSV-1) infection: review of its management. *Oral Dis.* 2006;12:254-70. PMID:16700734
4. Carey B, Setterfield J. Mucous membrane pemphigoid and oral blistering diseases. *Clin Exp Dermatol.* 2019;44:732-9.
5. Schmidt E, Kasperkiewicz M, Joly P. Pemphigus. *Lancet.* 2019;394:882-94.
6. Sklavounou A, Laskaris G. Frequency of Desquamative gingivitis in skin diseases. *Oral Surg Oral Med Oral Pathol Oral Radiol Endod.* 1983;56:141-4.

7. Grünwald P, Mockenhaupt M, Panzer R, Emmert S. Erythema multiforme, Stevens-Johnson syndrome/toxic epidermal necrolysis - diagnosis and treatment. *J Dtsch Dermatol Ges.* 2020;18:547-53.

8. Assimakopoulos D, Patrinakos G, Fotika C, Elisaf M. Benign migratory glossitis or geographic tongue: an enigmatic oral lesion. *Am J Med.* 2002;15:751-5.

9. Zargari O. The prevalence and significance of fissured tongue and geographic and psoriatic patients. *Clin Exp Dermatol.* 2006;31:192-5. PMID:16487088

10. González-Álvarez L, García-Martín J, García-Pola MJ. Association between geographic tongue and psoriasis: A systematic review and meta-analyses. *J Oral Pathol Med.* 2019;48:365-72.

11. Hietanen J, Salo OP, Kanerva L, Juvakoski T. Study of the oral mucosa in 200 consecutive patients with psoriasis. *Scand J Dent Res.* 1984;92:50-4.

12. Brooks JK, Kleinman JW, Modly CE, Basile JR. Resolution of psoriatic lesions on the gingiva and hard palate following administration of adalimumab for cutaneous psoriasis. *Cutis.* 2017;99:139-42.

13. Vila T, Sultan AS, Montelongo-Jauregui D, Jabra-Rizk MA. Oral candidiasis: a disease of opportunity. *J Fungi (Basel).* 2020;16:15.

14. Giannini P J, Shetty K V. Diagnosis and management of oral candidiasis. *Otolaryngol Clin North Am.* 2011;44:231-40.

15. Eyerich K, Eyerich S, Hiller J, Behrendt H, Traidl-Hoffmann C. Chronic mucocutaneous candidiasis, from bench to bedside. *Eur J Dermatol.* 2010;20:260-5.

16. Carrozzo M, Porter S, Mercadante V, Fedele S. Oral lichen planus: A disease or a spectrum of tissue reactions? Types, causes, diagnostic algorithms prognosis, management strategies. *Periodontol 2000.* 2019;80:105-25.

17. Cheng Y-SL, Gould A, Kurago Z, Fantasia J, Muller S. Diagnosis of oral lichen planus: a position paper of the American Academy of Oral and Maxillofacial Pathology. *Oral Surg Oral Med Oral Pathol Oral Radiol.* 2016;122:332-54.

18. Idrees M, Kujan O, Shearston K, Farah CS. Oral lichen planus has a very low malignant transformation rate: A systematic review and meta-analysis using strict diagnostic and inclusion criteria. *J Oral Pathol Med.* Published online January 25, 2020.

19. Wiriyakijja P, Porter S, Fedele S, et al. Health-related quality of life and its associated predictors in patients with oral lichen planus: a cross-sectional study. *Int Dent J.* Published online September 1, 2020.

20. Piperi E, Omlie J, Koutlas IG, Pambuccian S. Oral hairy leukoplakia in HIV-negative patients : report of 10 cases. *Int J Surg Pathol* 2010;18:177-83.

21. Hansen LS, Olson JA, Silverman S Jr. Proliferative verrucous leukoplakia. A long-term study of thirty patients. *Oral Surg Oral Med Oral Pathol.* 1985;60:285-98.

22. Jerjes W, Upile T, Hamdoo Z, et al. Photodynamic therapy outcome for oral dysplasia. *Lasers Surg Med.* 2011;43:192-9.

23. Lippman null. Head and Neck Chemoprevention: Recent Advances. *Cancer Control.* 1997;4:128-135.

24. Klaassen I, Braakhuis BJM. Anticancer activity and mechanism of action of retinoids in oral and pharyngeal cancer. *Oral Oncol.* 2002;38:532-42.

25. Prasad M, Kale TP, Halli R, Kotrashetti SM, Baliga SD. Liquid nitrogen cryotherapy in the management of oral lesions: a retrospective clinical study. *J Maxillofac Oral Surg.* 2009;8:40-42.

26. Ang KK, Harris J, Wheeler R, et al. Human papillomavirus and survival of patients with oropharyngeal cancer. *N Engl J Med.* 2010;363:24-35.

27. Chi AC, Lambert PR 3rd, Richardson MS, Neville BW. Oral mucoceles: a clinicopathologic review of 1,824 cases, including unusual variants. *J Oral Maxillofac Surg.* 2011;69:1086-93.

28. Koutlas IG, Dace B. Multifocal intraoral acquired lymphangiectases after surgical and radiation treatment for oral squamous cell carcinoma. *J Oral Maxillofac Surg.* 2006;64:528-30.

29. Buchner A, Hansen LS. The histomorphologic spectrum of peripheral ossifying fibroma. *Oral Surg Oral Med Oral Pathol Oral Radiol Endod.* 1987;63:452-61.

30. Katsikeris N, Kakarantza-Angelopoulou E, Angelopoulos AP. Peripheral giant cell granuloma. Clinicopathologic study of 224 new cases and review of 956 reported cases. *Int J Oral Maxillofac Surg.* 1988;17:94-9.

31. Meleti M, Vescovi P, Mooi WJ, van der Waal I. Pigmented lesions of the oral mucosa and perioral tissues: a flow chart for the diagnosis and some recommendations for the management. *Oral Surg Oral Med Oral Pathol Oral Radiol Endod.* 2008;105:606-16.

Cosmetic Dermatology

Christopher B. Zachary
Gretchen Bellefeuille
Hadley Johnson
Tiana Kazemi
Ronda Farah

INTRODUCTION TO CHAPTER

With regard to aesthetic issues, dermatologists have an important role in guiding their patients and can offer a wide variety of treatment modalities for skin rejuvenation and restoration. Furthermore, many patients with diseases of the skin are understandably concerned about the potential long-lasting effects on their appearance. Understanding the range of options available and the potential treatment outcomes is an important component of helping these patients reach a desired outcome. Moreover, cosmetic treatments can improve a person's self-image and, by extension, quality of life. When our patients feel comfortable with their bodies, they project self-confidence that others pick up on, which may lead to social and economic benefits.

Although many treatments are available, we present below favored treatment strategies. A more comprehensive list of treatment options for specific conditions is summarized in Tables 34-1 and 34-2.

EVALUATION OF THE COSMETIC PATIENT

The patient seeking advice and treatment for cosmetic concerns generally has a desired outcome in mind. The experienced clinician will help the patient identify these goals and accordingly choose an appropriate procedure. As part of this process, the astute physician will be realistic about the potential to achieve the patient's primary cosmetic goals.

The available literature examining the impact of cosmetic procedures on psychosocial well-being shows an overall positive trend with increased self-worth, self-esteem, quality of life, and decreased distress and shyness.[1] However, a small subset may have an outcome in mind that cannot realistically be achieved with any of the physician's treatment modalities. Such patients are more likely to be dissatisfied with their treatment and, by extension, their healthcare professional.

Identifying these patients can be challenging. Some studies show that male gender, younger age, and

Table 34-1. Non-surgical and minimally invasive treatment modalities for cosmetic disorders. On and off-label treatment options are reviewed.

Modality	Cosmetic Disorders	Notable Adverse Effects
Topical Products		
Retinoids	Fine and deep wrinkles, lax skin, lentigines, melasma, depressed scars	Irritation
Sunscreen	Facial erythema and telangiectasias, lentigines, melasma	Irritation (chemical sunscreens)
Tyrosinase Inhibitors	Lentigines, melasma	Irritation
Silicone Gel Sheeting	Elevated scars	None
Eflornithine	Hair reduction	Irritation
Minoxidil	Hair restoration	Irritation, hypertrichosis
Bimatoprost	Eyelash growth	Irritation, hypertrichosis
Oral Medications		
5-alpha Reductase Inhibitors	Hair restoration	Sexual dysfunction (males), gynecomastia (males), breast tenderness (females), irregular menstrual spotting (females) teratogenic (hypospadias), suicidal ideation
Minimally Invasive		
Botulinum Toxin	Fine and deep wrinkles, ptosis, hyperhidrosis	Asymmetry, brow/lid ptosis
Fillers	Fine and deep wrinkles, lax skin, depressed scars, volumetric reduction	Asymmetry, allergy, granulomatous reaction, bruising, vascular occlusion, blindness and stoke.
Autologous Fat Transfer	Fine and deep wrinkles, lax skin, depressed scars, volumetric reduction	Asymmetry, variable take
Mesotherapy Deoxycholic acid	Excess body fat	Bruising, discomfort, numbness, rare temporary nerve injury (marginal mandibular branch of facial nerve)
Subcision	Depressed scars	Pain, bruising
Sclerotherapy	Spider and varicose veins	Post inflammatory hyper-pigmentation, coagulum
Intralesional 5-Fluorouracil	Elevated scars, keloids	Necrosis, post inflammatory hyper- or hypo-pigmentation
Intralesional Corticosteroid	Elevated scars, keloids	Atrophy, hypopigmentation
Physical Treatments		
Chemical Peels	Fine and deep wrinkles, lentigines, melasma, depressed scars	Irritation, erythema, scar, post inflammatory hyper- or hypo-pigmentation
Dermabrasion	Fine and deep wrinkles, lentigines, melasma, depressed scars	Irritation, erythema, scar, post inflammatory hyper- or hypo-pigmentation
Cryotherapy	Lentigines, elevated scars	Blister, scar, post inflammatory hyper- or hypo-pigmentation
TCA CROSS technique	Depressed scars	Scar, post inflammatory hyper- or hypo-pigmentation
Pressure	Elevated scars	None
Compression Stockings	Spider veins	None

Trichloroacetic acid chemical reconstruction of skin scars, TCA CROSS

Table 34-2. Surgical and devices/laser treatment modalities for cosmetic disorders.

Modality	Cosmetic Disorders	Potential Adverse Effects
Surgical		
Facelift	Deeper wrinkles, lax skin	Scar, infection, hematoma, asymmetry, and nerve damage.
Suture Suspension Lift	Deep wrinkles, lax skin	Scar, infection, hematoma, asymmetry, and nerve damage.
Blepharoplasty	Lax skin	Scar, infection, hematoma, asymmetry, and nerve damage.
Liposuction	Excess body fat	Scar, infection, hematoma, asymmetry, and nerve damage.
Abdominoplasty	Lax skin	Scar, infection, hematoma, asymmetry, and nerve damage.
Punch Excision	Depressed scars	Scar
Surgical Excision	Elevated scars, tattoo removal	Scar, infection, hematoma, asymmetry, and nerve damage.
Hair Transplantation	Hair restoration	Infection, scarring, poor outcomes
Devices/Lasers		
KTP Laser[a]	Facial erythema and telangiectasia, spider veins, lentigines, tattoo removal	Blister, scar, post inflammatory hyper- or hypo-pigmentation
Pulsed-Dye Laser	Facial erythema and telangiectasia, spider veins, lentigines, elevated scars, facial rejuvenation	Blister, scar, post inflammatory hyper- or hypo-pigmentation
Ruby[a]	Lentigines, hair removal, tattoo removal	Blister, scar, post inflammatory hyper- or hypo-pigmentation
Alexandrite[a]	Facial erythema and telangiectasia, spider veins, lentigines, hair removal, tattoo removal	Blister, scar, post inflammatory hyper- or hypo-pigmentation
Diode	Facial erythema and telangiectasia, spider veins, hair removal	Blister, scar, post inflammatory hyper- or hypo-pigmentation
Nd:YAG[a]	Facial erythema and telangiectasia, spider veins, lentigines, melasma, hair removal, tattoo removal	Blister, scar, post inflammatory hyper- or hypo-pigmentation
Intense-Pulsed Light (IPL)	Facial erythema and telangiectasia, lentigines, melasma, hair removal	Blister, scar, post inflammatory hyper- or hypo-pigmentation
Non-Ablative Lasers (Fractionated)	Lentigines, melasma, depressed scars, elevated scars, facial rejuvenation	Erythema, blister, scar, post inflammatory hyper- or hypo-pigmentation
Ablative Resurfacing Lasers	Fine and deep wrinkles, lax skin, lentigines, melasma, depressed scars, elevated scars, facial rejuvenation	Erythema, blister, scar, post inflammatory hyper- or hypo-pigmentation
Cryolipolysis	Excess body fat	Asymmetry, pain
Photobiomodulation	Hair restoration	Erythema, tingling, no serious adverse events reported.
Radiofrequency	Lax skin, excess body fat	Asymmetry, pain
High-Intensity Ultrasound	Lax skin, excess body fat	Asymmetry, pain
Microfocused Ultrasound	Lax skin	Asymmetry, pain
Electrolysis	Hair removal	Scar, post inflammatory hyper- or hypo-pigmentation

[a] Continuous wave versus Q-switched.
KTP, Potassium-titanyl-phosphate.

psychological co-morbidities (i.e., depression, anxiety, personality disorders) are more commonly associated with decreased patient satisfaction even with an objectively successful outcome.[1,2] Additionally, the nature and degree of the procedure itself may play a role, with "restorative" procedures such as face lifts and neurotoxins, resulting in less body-image disturbance than "type-change" procedures such as rhinoplasty or breast augmentation.[1,3]

A special subset of cosmetic patients with unattainable expectations that every provider should be aware of are those suffering from body dysmorphic disorder.[4,5] Body dysmorphic disorder is a psychiatric condition that manifests as an unhealthy preoccupation with minor or imagined defects and may be exacerbated by cosmetic surgery as the underlying issue is primarily psychiatric.[6] While it can be difficult to elucidate mild cases of body dysmorphic disorder based solely on an initial consultation, ultimately the cosmetic dermatologist is responsible for his/her patients' health and should develop a sense of when a procedure is unlikely to satisfy the patients' needs or lead to poor outcomes.[4,5]

SKIN TONE AND TEXTURE

Easy and effective preventive strategies to combat photoaging include diligent sun protection with sun protective clothing, hats, and sunscreens. In particular, physical blockers with zinc oxide and titanium dioxide are often recommended. Consistent topical retinoid use remains the mainstay for aesthetic topicals.[7] These may lead to skin irritation including erythema, scale, or even dermatitis and therefore, may not be tolerated by all patients. Furthermore, many retinoids are deactivated by sunlight, therefore nighttime application in small amounts is recommended. The addition of other cosmeceuticals such as vitamins C, E, ferulic, lactic acid, kojic acid, alpha hydroxy acids, and glycolic acids may also improve skin appearance.[8-12]

Once the topical regiment has been optimized, procedures impacting the epidermis and superficial dermis can be considered. Numerous options exist on the market and reviewing all of them are beyond the scope of this chapter. We will review commonly used modalities within this section. Microdermabrasion (MDA) is a minimally invasive epidermal procedure that can treat uneven skin texture and tone that removes the very top layer of the epidermis (stratum corneum) via gentle mechanical abrasion.[13] Other options include hydradermabrasion, which involves the use of vortexed water to abrade the superficial layer of the skin (HydraFacial, Edge Systems LLC, Signal Hill, CA), superficial chemical peels, microneedling, and low intensity low density non-ablative fractional laser resurfacing.

FACIAL REDNESS

Facial erythema in both photodamaged skin and rosacea is related to dilation of blood vessels or the creation of new ones. Consistent sunscreen use is important for both prevention and maintenance. Avoiding triggers such as alcoholic beverages, caffeine, spicy foods, and stress can also be helpful. Topical alpha agonists such as brimonidine (Mirvaso®, Galderma, Fort Worth, TX) reduce facial erythema, especially in rosacea; however, the effects generally only last for a few hours and rebound erythema along with facial irritation have been reported.[14] Oxymetazoline hydrochloride 1% cream (Rhofade, EPI Health LLC,

Charleston, SC), another topical alpha agonist, may also help to reduce erythema with relatively few adverse effects.[15] For a non-pharmacologic option, cosmetics with green pigmentation can also counter and reduce the redness associated with rosacea.[16]

Sunscreen use can mitigate the erythema associated with photoaging and rosacea and is also an adjunct to the vascular lasers. A variety of vascular lasers can be used, including the 595 nm pulsed-dye laser (PDL) and the 532 nm KTP laser are very effective and commonly used.[17,18]

Intense-Pulsed Light (IPL) is another excellent option. IPL is a non-laser flashlamp device that uses filtered broadband light at 510–1,200 nm. This is effectively absorbed by reds and browns, and thus treats lentigines and telangiectasias on the face, neck, and chest.[17]

Risks of vascular lasers and intense-pulsed light include blistering, scarring, bruising, hypopigmentation, and hyperpigmentation. All laser surgeons, their staff, and patients must wear wavelength appropriate eye protection to avoid damage to the iris and retina. The patient must also be counseled on the need for multiple treatments and touch-up sessions. Additionally, it is the authors' experience that these treatments are not routinely covered by insurance.

LENTIGINES

Lentigines, commonly referred to as liver, sun, or age spots, are epidermal lesions indicative of photodamage. Medical evaluation of these lesions to rule out any possibility of melanoma must be performed prior to any treatment and biopsy may be indicated. They can be treated with a variety of agents. Often, a combination of physical and topical treatments is used. As with many conditions in dermatology, diligent sun protection is advised for both primary prevention and to prolong treatment effects. Topical treatment options include skin lightening agents such as hydroquinone often combined with regiments which may include retinoids and/or kojic acid. Common physical treatments include gentle cryotherapy, 532 nm green light laser, intense pulse light (IPL), very short pulsed nano- and pico-second lasers, and both fractional ablative and non-ablative laser resurfacing. Chemical peels remain some of the most versatile treatments for these issues. Dermatologic assessment including skin type, lesion size, number of lesions, location, pregnancy status, and lesion distribution are all necessary to determine the optimal treatment regimen.

MELASMA

Melasma is a common disorder of facial dyspigmentation that is exacerbated by ultraviolet (UV) radiation and hormonal influences (such as pregnancy and oral contraceptive use). Treatment of melasma can be very difficult, particularly due to the frustrating ease with which it recurs. Therapy aims to address pigmentation and vascularity.

Topical options include retinoids, hydroquinone, corti-costeroids, azelaic acid, and kojic acid. Patients should be advised that chronic hydroquinone use can lead to permanent dyspigmentation, called exogenous ochronosis. Procedural options include chemical peels, micro-needling (to enhance transdermal drug delivery), and lasers (QS Nd:YAG, non-ablative fractional lasers). Recently, oral tranexamic acid has been shown to be an effective adjunct therapy for refractory melasma.[19] Its use is probably contraindicated in those with a history of thrombotic disease.[19] Epidermal melasma is much easier to treat than dermal melasma.[20–22] Avoidance of all pigmentary triggers should be stressed, including regular sunscreen use and sun avoidance.[20–22]

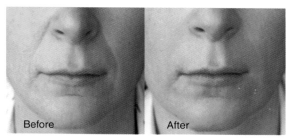

▲ **Figure 34-1.** Filler before and after. The nasolabial folds and pre-jowl sulcus before (left) and after (right) injection of a hyaluronic acid filler. Note how the profile of the folds is significantly reduced, giving the central and lower face a rejuvenated, more youthful appearance.

POST INFLAMMATORY HYPERPIGMENTATION

Post inflammatory hyperpigmentation is a very common occurrence after any inflammatory insult to the skin, including acne and trauma. It is typically macular in nature and due to reactive hypermelanosis. While post inflammatory hyperpigmentation will gradually self-improve over months to years, patients often seek treatment for faster resolution, especially on cosmetically sensitive areas such as the face. The treatment for post inflammatory hyperpigmentation is similar to that of lentigines and melasma, as they all share a similar underlying pathophysiology. Topical retinoids and hydroquinone, salicylic, or glycolic acid peels in combination with tretinoin or hydroquinone, and QS Nd:YAG laser are some of the effective options. Diligent sun protection should also be advised.[23,24]

FINE AND DEEP WRINKLES

Fine wrinkles (rhytides), particularly around the eyes and mouth, are a common patient concern. They are related to natural aging, use of musculature, and chronic sun exposure within the superficial dermis and epidermis. The development of these early rhytides can often be prevented by the new concept of *prejuvenation*, a process that treats the skin before the clinical signs of aging starts. Minimally invasive combination procedures play a remarkable preventative role. These include botulinum toxins which will prevent the formation of permanent rhytides and will soften those that already exist. These commonly occur on the forehead, glabella, crows feet, chin, nasalis region, and neck.[25] Fine perioral and crow's feet rhytides generally respond well to a combination of botulinum toxin, laser resurfacing, and dermal fillers. Additional treatment options include chemical peels, manual dermabrasion, and radiofrequency (RF) microneedling, used singly or in combination.

Deep rhytides, often referred to as dynamic rhytides, are multifactorial and caused by years of underlying muscle movement, age-related soft-tissue volume loss, gravitational force, and deeper structural changes due to facial bone resorption. Deeper rhytides, particularly in the nasolabial folds, and the pre-jowl sulcus, can be softened to become less prominent with dermal fillers alone (Figure 34-1). More recent trends to revolumize the lip, malar and zygomatic regions of the face have gained in popularity (Figure 34-2 A, B). Use of dermal fillers within the pyriform fossa, nasolabial fold, mental crease, and chin are also available. Patients with HAART related fat atrophy can be dramatically improved with Sculptra (Galderma, Fort Worth, TX). Laser resurfacing remains the gold standard for skin rejuvenation and skin tightening, almost exclusively with the CO2 and Er:YAG lasers. The newer fractionated lasers, both ablative and non-ablative, remain popular and are quite effective for skin rejuvenation.[26] Other energy-based options include radiofrequency skin tightening (Thermage, Solta Medical, Bothell, WA) and ultrasound, either microfocused (Ulthera, Merz Aesthetics, Raleigh, NC) or unfocused (SofWave, SofWave Medical, Israel). None of these replace a facelift, but might be indicated to stave off such a procedure. Non-energy based treatments have also been developed including absorbable thread lifts such as Poly (Glycolide/L-Lactide Surgical Suture, CPT Sutures Co., Ltd, Ho Chi Minh City, Vietnam) and Silhouette InstaLift (Suneva Medical, San Diego, CA), marketed for the repositioning of facial tissue.[27]

SPIDER VEINS

Commonly found on the legs, these superficial dilated blood vessels are typically multifactorial in origin. Some influences include genetics, prolonged standing, pregnancy, and hormonal factors. Patients typically require a skilled cutaneous and vascular assessment prior to treatment; those with saphenous vein reflux will not benefit from treatment of superficial vascular lesions alone, but will need saphenofemoral endovenous ablation.[28–31] Otherwise, sclerotherapy with foam or liquid sclerosing agents are the preferred treatments for these smaller leg veins. Some prefer to treat these with vascular lasers.

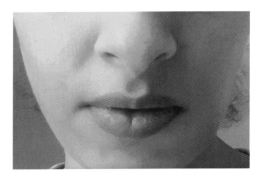

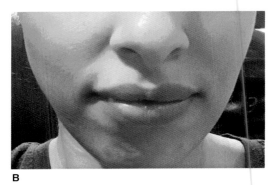

A

B

▲ **Figure 34-2.** Filler revolumization of the upper lip utilizing a hyaluronic acid filler. A. Prior to treatment. B. Immediately following post filler revolumization of the cheeks and upper lip. Reproduced with permission from Ronda Farah, MD.

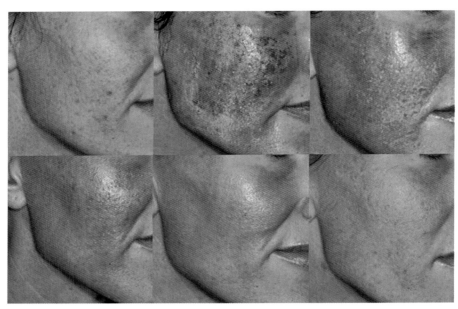

▲ **Figure 34-3.** Predictable wound healing and treatment response of a fractionated ablative laser. A patient with acne scarring and lentigines. 6 consecutive images are shown, demonstrating the predictable healing sequence of the fractionated CO_2 ablative laser. From left to right (top row) are: pre-operative, post-operative, and 3-day follow-up pictures. Note the pinpoint bleeding immediately after the procedure and how the skin has healed with only residual erythema by day 3. At 1 week (lower left), most of the erythema has resolved. At 1 month (lower middle), the patient has notable improvement in texture, tone, and color, which is maintained 3 months post-procedure (lower right).

SCARS

Multiple modalities exist for treatment of scars; location, skin type, symptomatology, dyspigmentation, age, and presence of hypertrophy are all factors that should be considered prior to treatment. Silicone gel sheets are favored by some as a painless adjunct, but have limited benefit. Darker scars may benefit from use of topical hydroquinone.

Macular post-surgical scars or other traumatic scars without contractures often improve over time. Combination use of pulsed dye laser and fractional resurfacing with technologies such as the 1550 nm non-ablative fractional laser or the 10,600 CO_2 fractional ablative resurfacing laser have demonstrated improvement in patient populations (Figure 34-3).[32,33] Radiofrequency (RF) microneedling may also have a role in improving scars, though large

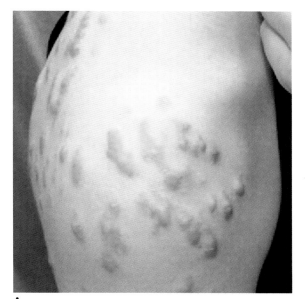

A

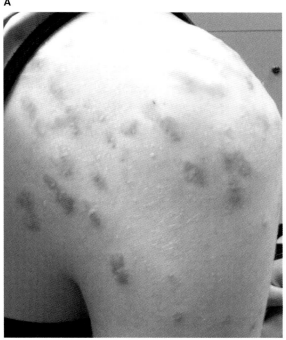

B

Figure 34-4. Patient with history of hypertrophic acneiform scars that has undergone series of pulsed dye laser and intralesional triamcinolone acetonide injections. A Before treatment B. After treatment. Reproduced with permission from Ronda Farah, MD.

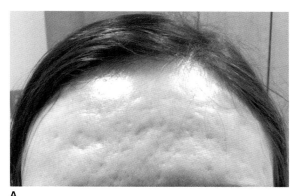

A

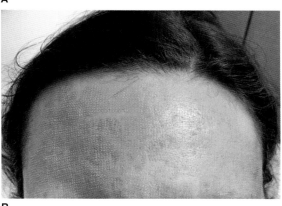

B

Figure 34-5. Acne scarring on the forehead. A. Acneiform scarring prior to treatment. B. Acneiform scarring immediately post treatment with a fractional ablative CO2 laser. Reproduced with permission from Ronda Farah, MD.

randomized studies are needed to clarify the amount of improvement and longevity of results.[34]

Raised scars can present a more challenging clinical treatment path. Hypertrophic scars are typically limited to the injured skin. Keloids generally expand beyond the injured region. Intralesional steroid injections, with or without 5-fluorouracil, are routinely used for the management of hypertrophic scars and keloids. Pulsed dye lasers have also been utilized to reduce vascularity for hypertrophic scars and keloids (Figure 34-4) [35] Surgical intervention is typically reserved for non-responsive keloidal scars. Fractionated lasers are also commonly used to improve the appearance of these scars. The combination with laser-assisted drug delivery of topical steroids also is a promising new field.[36] However, laser-assisted drug delivery is not without risks which include introduction of non-sterile product and granulomas.[37]

Acne scars such as ice pick, rolling and box scars, are now routinely treated with fractional laser resurfacing (Figure 34-5 A, B). These include the use of ablative and

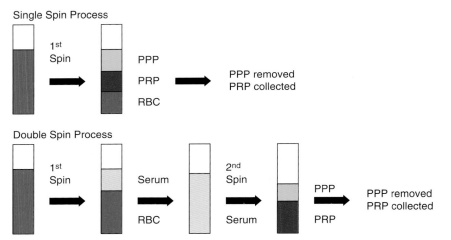

Single Spin Process

1st Spin

PPP
PRP
RBC

PPP removed
PRP collected

Double Spin Process

1st Spin

Serum
RBC

2nd Spin

Serum

PPP
PRP

PPP removed
PRP collected

▲ **Figure 34-6.** Platelet rich plasma (PRP) spin processes. Platelet poor plasma (PPP) is drawn off the top of the specimen in each example after the final spin. Reproduced with permission from Ronda Farah, MD and Gretchen Bellefeuille, BS.

non-ablative lasers and results are quite impressive, particularly after a series of treatments. Some remain resistant to treatment. More recently, radiofrequency (RF) microneedling is being touted as a possible treatment option, especially for darker skin types. Alternatively the CROSS (chemical reconstruction of skin scars) technique and or subcision have been demonstrated to be rather useful.

LASER HAIR REMOVAL

Permanent hair reduction can be achieved with various lasers and is most efficacious in fair-skinned patients with dark coarse hairs. This is due to the increased contrast between the darkly pigmented hair follicle and the less pigmented surrounding skin cells, which allows for laser and light devices to more selectively target hair follicles. The 810-nm-diode and 755-nm Alexandrite lasers are most commonly used, while the 1064-nm Nd:YAG laser is safer in patients with darker skin tones.[38] Sequential treatments, usually spaced 6–8 weeks apart, are commonly needed. Laser hair removal requires firm knowledge of laser-based devices and treatment settings. Scarring, discoloration, blisters, hives, blindness, and even paradoxical hypertrichosis of treated areas have been reported.[39] Factory settings are not always optimal for patient scenarios. In addition, those using hair removal devices need to understand how to manage complications from laser treatments, especially when providing laser hair removal services.[40] In this regard, IPL hair removal is the most common cause for litigious action.[41]

ALOPECIA-RELATED PROCEDURES

Minimally invasive procedures for hair loss include platelet rich plasma (PRP) and hair transplantation. Platelet rich plasma is an autologous concentrate of platelets suspended

in plasma that contains a high saturation of platelets and growth factors that are reported to promote cell proliferation and healing (Figure 34-6). Platelet rich plasma is trending in the literature, primarily as a treatment of androgenetic alopecia. However, this is not an FDA-cleared indication and its use is not first line.[42,43] Platelet-rich plasma is typically offered by dermatologists after failure of standard of care including options such as topical minoxidil, finasteride, and spironolactone, depending on the patient's clinical situation. Typically, platelet rich plasma requires a series of injections, followed by a prolonged maintenance.[44] Risks of platelet rich plasma include pain, swelling, infection, clot, no improvement, bruising, bleeding, and hematoma at site of blood draw.[45]

Hair transplantation may yield the best natural-appearing outcome, although not all patients may be eligible candidates.[46] Methods of transplantation include follicular unit transplantation; (also known as strip harvesting), follicular unit extraction, and donor elliptical harvesting. These procedures can be done in an outpatient setting with local anesthesia.[47]

TATTOO REMOVAL

The mainstay of tattoo removal are light-based devices.[48] Based on the principles of selective photothermolysis, lasers with the correct wavelength and very short pulse durations are necessary to achieve tattoo particle destruction. Short pulses are achieved with so called Q-switching (QS), a process which applies to both nanosecond and picosecond devices. The QS 532 nm, 694 nm, 755 nm, and 1064 nm can all target tattoo pigments of different colors. QS lasers traditionally generate pulse widths in the order of nanoseconds (ns), and are therefore referred to as ns-devices.

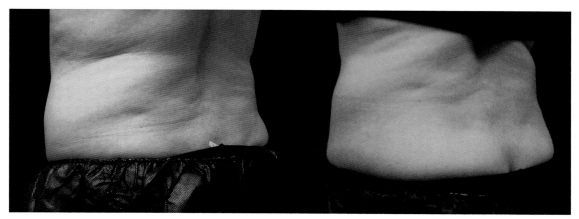

▲ **Figure 34-7.** Cryolipolysis. Before (left) and after (right) photographs of a patient who had undergone cryolipolysis. With this modality, the superficial fat layers can be induced to apoptose. Commonly treated areas include the upper and lower abdomen and flanks, as in this patient.

Pico-second (ps) lasers are the newest Q-switched devices and generate a pulse in the order of picoseconds. Currently available ps-devices include PicoSure (Cynosure, Westford, MA) (755 nm), enLIGHTen (Cutera, Brisbane, CA) (1064 nm), and PicoWay (Candela Medical, Wayland, MA) (1064 nm, 785 nm, and 532 nm). Ps-devices are now offered with full field or fractionated handpieces, which can also improve texture and tone of the skin.[49]

Caution should be taken in the treatment of white, red, orange, yellow, turquoise, lavender, pink, tan, and brown tattoos as they may contain either titanium dioxide or ferric oxide.[48] Laser treatment of these two metal oxides can result in immediate and permanent pigment tissue darkening.[50]

Fractionated ablative lasers are non-selective (i.e., do not target a specific pigment), but may allow transepidermal elimination of pigment through generation of columns of epidermal and dermal injury, particularly after treatment with a Q-switched laser.[51] Traditional laser ablation with CO_2 or Er:YAG lasers, while not generally recommended, can often remove a tattoo in one session, though second intention healing *always results in scarring*. Finally, surgical excision and closures may be used to physically remove the tattoo. These latter two treatments can be helpful in those cases of hypersensitivity to tattoo particles, as treatment with the QS lasers can result in anaphylaxis in a sensitized individual.[48,51]

CONSIDERATIONS IN SKIN OF COLOR

Patients with darker skin phototypes are at a higher risk for developing post inflammatory hyperpigmentation and dyspigmentation after cosmetic procedures where energy and inflammation is introduced into the epidermis/dermis. This particularly includes chemical peels and lasers/light

device treatments. Any procedure that causes epidermal injury carries the risk of dyspigmentation and scarring; physicians should choose devices and parameters accordingly and have a proper understanding of wound healing and laser tissue interaction.

BODY SCULPTING

Liposuction remains the treatment of choice for extensive body sculpting.[52] However, during the past decade, noninvasive devices have been developed that target fat and induce lipolysis. These modalities include bulk cooling (cryolipolysis) (Figure 34-7), bulk heating (long pulse 1064 nm and radiofrequency), and to a lesser extent focused ultrasound.[53,54] Mesotherapy is an injectable approach to treating medical and esthetics problems, but has a checkered history. However, injections of deoxycholate (Kybella, Allergan Aesthetics, Irvine, CA) into the fat provides safe, predictable, and efficacious reduction in localized submental fat.[55,56]

CELLULITE

Cellulite affects up to 80% of postpubertal women and is a common reason for cosmetic consultation.[57] It is characterized by large, metabolically stable adipocytes predominantly in the lower body that result in distinct skin texture change resembling an orange peel. The literature proposes that approximately 85% and 98% of all women will experience cellulite in their lifetime.[58] Women across all ethnicities and races may be affected, although it is less common in Asian women when compared to Caucasian women.[58] Women can experience cellulite as early as 15 years of age, but it typically presents between the ages of 20 and 30.[58]

Treatment is challenging, especially as the pathophysiology of this condition is still incompletely understood. Current options include topicals (methylxanthine and retinoids, energy-based devices, acoustic wave therapy, subcision, fillers, and collagenases (Qwo, Endo Esthetics LLC, Malvern, PA). The most promising new treatment is Rapid Acoustic Pulse (RAP) ReSound technology by Soliton. This very high intensity ultra short-wave acoustic energy induces the shearing stress to the tethering fibers which cause cellulite in the first place. A combination approach with multiple synergistic treatment modalities yields the best results.[59]

REFERENCES

1. Castle DJ, Honigman RJ, Phillips KA. Does cosmetic surgery improve psychosocial wellbeing? *Med J Aust.* 2002; 176(12): 601-4.
2. Castle, DJ.; Phillips, KA. Disorders of body image. Hampshire, UK: Wrightson Biomedical; 2002.
3. Sarwer DB, Wadden TA, Pertschuk MJ, Whitaker LA. The psychology of cosmetic surgery: a review and reconceptualization. *Clin Psychol Rev.* 1998;18:1–22.
4. Greenberg JL, Weingarden H, Wilhelm S. A practical guide to managing body dysmorphic disorder in the cosmetic surgery setting. *JAMA Facial Plast Surg.* 2019;21(3):181-182.
5. Krebs G, Fernández de la Cruz L, Mataix-Cols D. Recent advances in understanding and managing body dysmorphic disorder. *Evid Based Mental Health.* 2017;20(3):71-75.
6. Phillips KA, Dufresne RG. Body dysmorphic disorder. A guide for dermatologists and cosmetic surgeons. *Am J Clin Dermatol.* 2000;1(4):235-43.
7. McCook JP. Topical Products for the Aging Face. *Clin Plast Surg.* 2016;43(3):597-604.
8. Murray JC, Burch JA, Streilein RD, Iannacchione MA, Hall RP, Pinnell SR. A topical antioxidant solution containing vitamins C and E stabilized by ferulic acid provides protection for human skin against damage caused by ultraviolet irradiation. *J Am Acad Dermatol.* 2008;59(3):418-25.
9. Draelos ZD, Hall S, Munsick C. A 14-day Controlled study assessing qualitative improvement with 15% lactic acid and ceramides in skin moisturization and desquamation. *J Clin Aesthet Dermatol.* 2020;13(8):E54-E58.
10. Saeedi M, Eslamifar M, Khezri K. Kojic acid applications in cosmetic and pharmaceutical preparations. *Biomed Pharmacother.* 2019;110:582-593.
11. Ditre CM, Griffin TD, Murphy GF, Sueki H, Telegan B, Johnson WC, Yu RJ, Van Scott EJ. Effects of alpha-hydroxy acids on photoaged skin: a pilot clinical, histologic, and ultrastructural study. *J Am Acad Dermatol.* 1996;34(2 Pt 1): 187-95.
12. Narda M, Trullas C, Brown A, Piquero-Casals J, Granger C, Fabbrocini G. Glycolic acid adjusted to pH 4 stimulates collagen production and epidermal renewal without affecting levels of proinflammatory TNF-alpha in human skin explants. *J Cosmet Dermatol.* 2021 Feb;20(2):513-521.
13. El-Domyati M, Hosam W, Abdel-Azim E, Abdel-Wahab H, Mohamed E. Microdermabrasion: a clinical, histometric, and histopathologic study. *J Cosmet Dermatol.* 2016;15(4):503-513.
14. Anderson MS, Nadkarni A, Cardwell LA, Alinia H, Feldman SR. Spotlight on brimonidine topical gel 0.33% for facial erythema of rosacea: safety, efficacy, and patient acceptability. *Patient Prefer Adherence.* 2017 6;11:1143-1150.
15. Garcia C, Birch M. Oxymetazoline hydrochloride 1% cream (Rhofade) for persistent facial erythema associated with Rosacea. *Am Fam Physician.* 2018;97(12):808-810.
16. Rivero AL, Whitfeld M. An update on the treatment of rosacea. *Aust Prescr.* 2018;41(1):20-24.
17. Neuhaus IM, Zane LT, Tope WD. Comparative efficacy of nonpurpuragenic pulsed dye laser and intense pulsed light for erythematotelangiectatic rosacea. *Dermatol Surg.* 2009; 35 (6): 920-928.
18. Tierney E, Hanke CW. Randomized controlled trial: comparative efficacy for the treatment of facial telangiectasias with 532 nm versus 940nm diode laser. *Lasers Surg Med.* 2009; 41 (8): 555-62.
19. Lee HC, Thng TG, Goh CL. Oral tranexamic acid (TA) in the treatment of melasma: A retrospective analysis. *J Am Acad Dermatol.* 2016;75(2):385-92.
20. Polder KD, Landau JM, Vergilis-Kalner IJ, Goldberg LH, Friedman PM, Bruce S. Laser eradication of pigmented lesions: a review. *Dermatol Surg.* 2011; 37 (5): 572-595.
21. Spierings NMK. Melasma: A critical analysis of clinical trials investigating treatment modalities published in the past 10 years. *J Cosmet Dermatol.* 2020;19(6):1284-1289.
22. Ogbechie-Godec OA, Elbuluk N. Melasma: an Up-to-Date Comprehensive Review. *Dermatol Ther (Heidelb).* 2017;7(3): 305-318.
23. Shenoy A, Madan R. Post-inflammatory hyperpigmentation: a review of treatment strategies. *J Drugs Dermatol.* 2020;19(8): 763-768.
24. Fatima S, Braunberger T, Mohammad TF, Kohli I, Hamzavi IH. The role of sunscreen in melasma and postinflammatory hyperpigmentation. *Indian J Dermatol.* 2020;65(1):5-10.
25. Humphrey S. Neurotoxins: evidence for prevention. *J Drugs Dermatol.* 2017 1;16(6):s87-s90.
26. Alexiades-Armenakas M, Newman J, Willey A, Kilmer S, Goldberg D, Garden J, Berman D, Stridde B, Renton B, Berube D, Hantash BM. Prospective multicenter clinical trial of a minimally invasive temperature-controlled bipolar fractional radiofrequency system for rhytid and laxity treatment. *Dermatol Surg.* 2013;39(2):263-73.
27. Suneva Medical. 2021. Retrieved from https://www.suneva-medical.com/products/silhouette-instalift/
28. Nijsten T, van den Bos RR, Goldman MP, Kockaert MA, Proebstle TM, Rabe E, Sadick NS, Weiss RA, Neumann MH. Minimally invasive techniques in the treatment of saphenous varicose veins. *J Am Acad Dermatol.* 2009;60(1):110-9.
29. Mann MW. Sclerotherapy: It is back and better. *Clin Plast Surg.* 2011; 38 (3): 475-487.
30. Duffy DM. Sclerosants: a comparative review. *Dermatol Surg.* 2010; 36 Suppl 2: 1010-25.
31. McCoppin HH, Hovenic WW, Wheeland RG. Laser treatment of superficial leg veins: a review. *Dermatol Surg.* 2011; 37 (6): 729-41.
32. Cohen JL, Geronemus R. Safety and efficacy evaluation of pulsed dye laser treatment, co2 ablative fractional resurfacing, and combined treatment for surgical scar clearance. *J Drugs Dermatol.* 2016;15(11):1315-1319.
33. Cho S, Jung JY, Shin JU, Lee JH. Non-ablative 1550 nm erbium-glass and ablative 10,600 nm carbon dioxide fractional lasers for various types of scars in Asian people: evaluation of 100 patients. *Photomed Laser Surg.* 2014;32(1): 42-6.

34. Boen M, Jacob C. A review and update of treatment options using the acne scar classification system. *Dermatol Surg.* 2019;45(3):411-422.

35. Oosterhoff TCH, Beekman VK, van der List JP, Niessen FB. Laser treatment of specific scar characteristics in hypertrophic scars and keloid: A systematic review. *J Plast Reconstr Aesthet Surg.* 2021;74(1):48-64.

36. Al Janahi S, Lee M, Lam C, Chung HJ. Laser-assisted drug delivery in the treatment of keloids: A case of extensive refractory keloids successfully treated with fractional carbon dioxide laser followed by topical application and intralesional injection of steroid suspension. *JAAD Case Rep.* 2019;5(10):840-843.

37. Soltani-Arabshahi R, Wong JW, Duffy KL, Powell DL. Facial allergic granulomatous reaction and systemic hypersensitivity associated with microneedle therapy for skin rejuvenation. *JAMA Dermatol.* 2014;150(1):68-72.

38. Ibrahimi OA, Avram MM, Hanke CW, Kilmer SL, Anderson RR. Laser hair removal. *Dermatol Ther.* 2011; 24 (1): 94-107.

39. Lim SP, Lanigan SW. A review of the adverse effects of laser hair removal. *Lasers Med Sci.* 2006;21(3):121-5.

40. Ginsberg BA. Dermatologic care of the transgender patient. *Int J Womens Dermatol.* 2016;3(1):65-67.

41. Jalian HR, Jalian CA, Avram MM. Common causes of injury and legal action in laser surgery. *JAMA Dermatol.* 2013;149(2):188–193.

42. Stevens J, Khetarpal S. Platelet-rich plasma for androgenetic alopecia: A review of the literature and proposed treatment protocol. *Int J Womens Dermatol.* 2018;21;5(1):46-51.

43. Khatu SS, More YE, Gokhale NR, Chavhan DC, Bendsure N. Platelet-rich plasma in androgenic alopecia: myth or an effective tool. *J Cutan Aesthet Surg.* 2014;7(2):107-10.

44. Hausauer AK, Jones DH. Evaluating the efficacy of different platelet-rich plasma regimens for management of androgenetic alopecia: a single-center, blinded, randomized clinical trial. *Dermatol Surg.* 2018;44(9):1191-1200.

45. Garg S, Manchanda S. Platelet-rich plasma-an 'Elixir' for treatment of alopecia: personal experience on 117 patients with review of literature. *Stem Cell Investig.* 2017; 4:64.

46. Barrera A. The use of micrografts and minigrafts in the esthetics reconstruction of the face and scalp. *Plast Reconsts Surg.* 2003; 112 (3): 883-90.

47. Avram MR, Watkins S. Robotic hair transplantation. *Facial Plast Surg Clin North Am.* 2020;28(2):189-196.

48. Choudhary S, Elsaie ML, Leiva A, Nouri K. Lasers for tattoo removal: a review. *Lasers Med Sci.* 2010; 25 (5): 619-627.

49. Torbeck RL, Schilling L, Khorasani H, Dover JS, Arndt KA, Saedi N. Evolution of the picosecond laser: A review of literature. *Dermatol Surg.* 2019;45(2):183-194.

50. Kasai K. Picosecond laser treatment for tattoos and benign cutaneous pigmented lesions (secondary publication). *Laser Ther.* 2017;26(4):274-281.

51. Ibrahimi OA, Syed, Sakamoto FH, Avram MM, Anderson RR. Treatment of tattoo allergy with ablative fractional resurfacing: a novel paradigm for tattoo removal. *J Am Acad Dermatol.* 2011; 64 (6): 1111-14.

52. Tierney EP, Kouba DJ, Hanke CW. Safety of tumescent and laser-assisted liposuction: review of the literature. *J Drugs Dermatol.* 2011; 10 (12): 1363-69.

53. Alizadeh Z, Halabchi F, Mazaheri R, Abolhasani M, Tabesh M. Review of the mechanisms and effects of noninvasive body contouring devices on cellulite and subcutaneous fat. *Int J Endocrinol Metab.* 2016; 14(4), e36727.

54. Mulholland RD, Paul MD, Chalfoun C. Noninvasive body contouring with radiofrequency, ultrasound, cryolipolysis, and low-level laser therapy. *Clin Plast Surg.* 2011; 38 (3): 503-20.

55. Shridharani SM. Early Experience in 100 Consecutive patients with injection adipocytolysis for neck contouring with ATX-101 (Deoxycholic Acid). *Dermatol Surg.* 2017;43(7):950-958.

56. Duncan D, Rotunda AM. Injectable therapies for localized fat loss: state of the art. *Clin Plast Surg.* 2011; 38 (3): 489-501.

57. Sadick N. Treatment for cellulite. *Int J Womens Dermatol.* 2018;5(1):68-72.

58. Council ML. Guide to Minimally Invasive Aesthetic Procedures. Lippincott Williams & Wilkins; 2020 Sep 8.

59. Davis DS, Boen M, Fabi SG. Cellulite: Patient selection and combination treatments for optimal results-a review and our experience. *Dermatol Surg.* 2019;45(9):1171-1184.

Skin Diseases of the Scalp

Maria K. Hordinsky

INTRODUCTION TO CHAPTER

The scalp is characterized by a high density of sweat glands and pilosebaceous units consisting of hair follicles, sebaceous glands, and arrector pili muscles. It is estimated that there are some 100,000 follicles on the scalp, so this also means that there are about 100,000 sebaceous glands and associated arrector pili muscles.

Hair on the scalp protects the skin from ultraviolet light and if absent or decreased, predisposes balding individuals to sunburns, photo damage, and photosensitivity. Likewise, the presence of hair may make cleaning the scalp surface with shampoos challenging permitting the development of scalp conditions such as dandruff and seborrheic dermatitis related to colonization of commensal *Malassezia* yeasts.

APPROACH TO DIAGNOSIS

Skin diseases involving the scalp can be broadly classified into the following categories (Table 35-1).

- Inflammatory dermatoses
- Cicatricial alopecias
- Infections/infestations
- Neoplasia

Lesions on the scalp can also be related to photo damage or systemic diseases such as dermatomyositis or to bullous conditions such as pemphigus vulgaris or pemphigus erythematosus.

EVALUATION

Most skin diseases of the scalp are diagnosed clinically based on the patient's history and physical findings. Scalp biopsy or additional tests may be needed to confirm the diagnosis. Some of these additional tests include:

- A potassium hydroxide (KOH) examination and/or fungal cultures when tinea capitis is suspected.
- Bacterial if there is a primary or secondary skin infection.
- Polymerase chain reaction (PCR) for varicella zoster virus (VZV), herpes simplex virus (HSV)-1, HSV-2 is the preferred test to confirm the diagnosis of herpes zoster or simplex. Viral culture and Tzanck smear can also be utilized.
- Patch testing if allergic contact dermatitis is a consideration.
- Biopsy for direct immunofluorescence if a bullous disorder is suspected.

Table 35-1. Skin Diseases of the Scalp.

Disease	Features
Inflammatory Dermatoses	

Allergic contact dermatitis 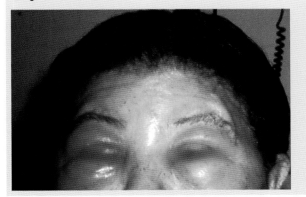	Epidemiology:
	  Uncommon.
	  F > M
	  Any age.
	History:
	  Pruritic. Onset is within hours or days after contact with the allergen.
	Physical Exam:
	  Usually presents with erythema, edema and pruritus of the forehead, eyelids, ears, and less so, the scalp.
	  (See chapter 8)

Atopic dermatitis 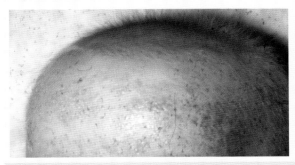	Epidemiology:
	  Common.
	  M > F.
	  More common in infants.
	History:
	  Pruritic.
	Physical Exam:
	  Scalp involvement more commonly seen in infants. Usually presents as scaly erythematous plaques with crust and excoriations.
	  (See chapter 8)

Psoriasis 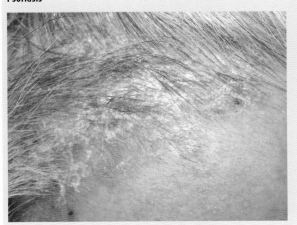	Epidemiology:
	  Common.
	  M > F.
	History:
	  Asymptomatic to pruritic.
	Physical Exam:
	  Red papules and plaques with silvery, thick, adherent scale can be present.
	  (See chapter 9)

(continued)

Table 35-1. Skin Diseases of the Scalp. (Continued)

Disease	Features

Seborrheic dermatitis 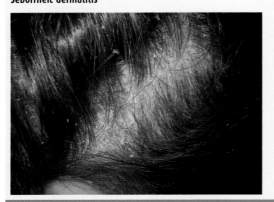	Epidemiology:
	  Common.
	  M > F.
	History:
	  Dry, scaly, and itchy scalp.
	Physical Exam:
	  Presents with "dandruff", white flakes with no erythema. Moderate to severe seborrheic dermatitis is characterized by erythematous plaques with white greasy scales.
	  (See chapter 9)

Cicatricial Alopecias	

Acne keloidalis nuchae 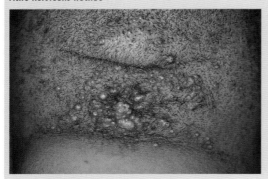	Epidemiology:
	  Common.
	  M > F.
	  Black men with Afro-textured hair are the predominate population at risk.
	History:
	  May be associated with scalp injury.
	Physical Exam:
	  Presents with inflamed papules or pustules and keloid-like scarring on the posterior lower scalp and nape of the neck.
	  (See chapter 10)

Central centrifugal cicatricial alopecia 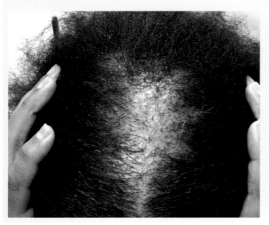	Epidemiology:
	  Uncommon.
	  Predominantly affects middle-aged women of African ancestry. F > M with prevalence reported to range from 2.7% to 5.6%.
	History:
	  Usually presents with asymptomatic hair loss over the crown of the scalp, sometimes symptomatic and with signs of inflammation.
	Physical Exam:
	  Hair thinning on the vertex region followed by progressive hair loss that extends peripherally in a centrifugal, symmetric manner; perifollicular erythema, and scale are found at the periphery of areas of alopecia.
	  (See chapter 30)

(continued)

Table 35-1. Skin Diseases of the Scalp. (Continued)

Disease	Features
Discoid lupus erythematosus 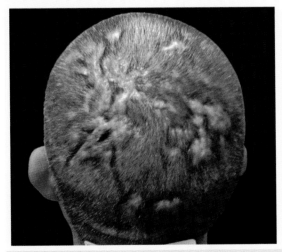	**Epidemiology:** Uncommon. F > M. 15–30% of patients with systemic lupus erythematosus (SLE) develop discoid lupus erythematosus (DLE). Five to 28% of patients with DLE may develop concurrent SLE. **History:** Mild pruritus, pain or burning may be present. **Physical Exam:** Discrete, erythematous, indurated plaques with follicular plugging in association with depressed central scars, atrophy, telangiectasias, and hyperpigmentation and/or hypopigmentation. (See chapter 30)
Dissecting cellulitis 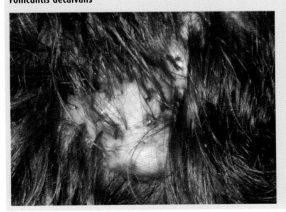	**Epidemiology:** Uncommon. M > F. Males between the ages of 18–40, more common in Black men; may be part of a follicular triad which includes acne conglobata and hidradenitis suppurativa. **History:** Drainage, pruritus and pain may all be present. **Physical Exam:** Recurrent pustules, scarring alopecia, boggy plaques with sinus tract formation are present, *Staphylococcus aureus* is commonly isolated. (See chapter 30)
Folliculitis decalvans	**Epidemiology:** Uncommon. M > F. **History:** Spontaneous bleeding, pain, pruritus, and/or burning may be present. **Physical Exam:** Multifocal scalp involvement with pustules with or without inflammatory papules, at the periphery of areas of alopecia. (See chapter 30)

(continued)

Table 35-1. Skin Diseases of the Scalp. (Continued)

Disease	Features
Frontal fibrosing alopecia 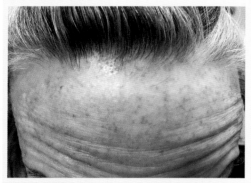	Epidemiology: Uncommon F > M. History: Characterized by the development of frontotemporal loss of terminal fibers. Physical Exam: Hair loss in a band-like distribution with perifollicular erythema and scale at the periphery of areas of alopecia. Associated with facial papules and loss of eyebrows. (See chapter 30)
Lichen planopilaris 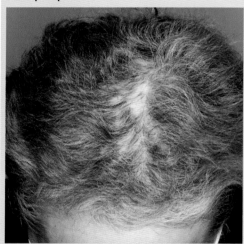	Epidemiology: Uncommon. F > M. History: Pruritus, burning and scalp tenderness are common. Presents with single or multiple areas of scalp hair loss; may present with lichen planus on other body sites. Physical Exam: Perifollicular erythema and follicular hyperkeratosis on the vertex and parietal areas of the scalp. (See chapter 30)
Infectious/Infestations	
Folliculitis 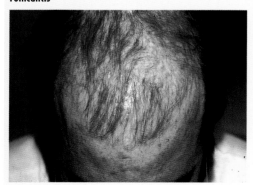	Epidemiology: Common. M:F dependent upon etiology which may include occlusion, heat, humidity, immunosuppression, medications, disease such as diabetes. History: May be pruritic. Physical Exam: Characterized by follicular 1–3 mm pustules and/or inflammatory papules. (See chapter 10)

(continued)

Table 35-1. Skin Diseases of the Scalp. (Continued)

Disease	Features

Head lice
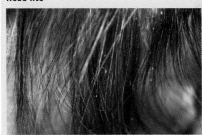
	Epidemiology:
	    Common.
	    F > M.
	    School children ages 3–11, especially girls with long hair; black children are less commonly affected.
	History:
	    Pruritus.
	Physical Exam:
	    The occipital scalp, posterior ears and neck are the most common affected sites; pyoderma and regional lymphadenopathy may be present.
	    (See chapter 14)

Herpes zoster
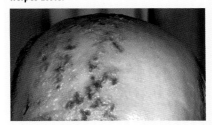
	Epidemiology:
	    Common.
	    F > M.
	    Primarily older individuals.
	History:
	    Painful in prodromal period, during and after infection.
	Physical Exam:
	    Vesicles on a red base in a dermatomal pattern.
	    (See chapter13)

Kerion
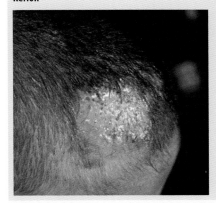
	Epidemiology:
	    Uncommon.
	    Children are more affected than adults; animals can be the source of infection.
	History:
	    Very tender.
	Physical Exam:
	    Characterized by inflammation and suppurative lesions on the scalp, there may be sinus formation and rarely mycetoma like grains.
	    (See chapter 12)

Tinea capitis
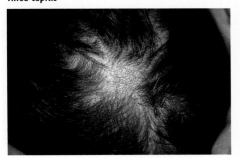
	Epidemiology:
	    Common.
	    F > M.
	    Most common in children 3–7 years old and relatively uncommon after puberty.
	History:
	    May be asymptomatic or pruritic.
	Physical Exam:
	    Characterized by adherent scale with no alopecia or with areas of alopecia that have broken hair fibers which appear like black dots.
	    (See chapter 12)

(continued)

Table 35-1. Skin Diseases of the Scalp. (Continued)

Disease	Features
Neoplasia	

Actinic keratosis 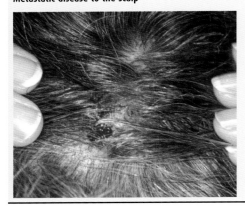	Epidemiology:
	  Common.
	  M > F.
	  Age>50 years.
	History:
	  May be tender and persist for months to years. History of excessive sun exposure and balding. When numerous, patients may mistake these as "rash."
	Physical Exam:
	  Skin-colored, yellow-brown, or pink gritty papules and plaques with adherent hyperkeratotic scale.
	  (See chapter 21)

Metastatic disease to the scalp	Epidemiology:
	  Uncommon as a primary presentation.
	  Cutaneous metastasis from a primary visceral malignancy is relatively uncommon (0.22% to 10% in different series); scalp accounts for 4% to 6.9%.
	History:
	  May be the first sign of a visceral malignancy.
	Physical Exam:
	  May appear as pigmented, skin-colored, pink, or red nodules.

Skin Diseases of the Face

Brittney Schultz
Noah Goldfarb

INTRODUCTION

The face is the area of the body most exposed to sunlight and therefore at highest risk for ultraviolet (UV) light induced dermatoses (photodermatoses), photoaging, and skin cancers. The face also has the highest density of sebaceous glands, predisposing this area to conditions such as acne, rosacea, and seborrheic dermatitis. Inflammation around the hair follicles may lead to skin diseases such as folliculitis and pseudofolliculitis barbae. In addition, skin diseases involving mucous membranes will typically affect the eyes, nose, and mouth. Since the face is so critical to non-verbal communication and social interactions, skin diseases involving this area can cause a significant degree of emotional distress.

APPROACH TO DIAGNOSIS

Skin diseases involving the face can be broadly placed into the following categories starting with the most common diseases (Table 36-1):

- Pilosebaceous disorders
- Inflammatory dermatoses
- Infectious diseases
- Pigment disorders
- Ultraviolet induced photodermatoses
- Connective tissue diseases

Papules and pustules can be seen in several conditions such as acne, rosacea, perioral dermatitis, folliculitis, pseudofolliculitis barbae, impetigo, and acute contact dermatitis. Acne can be distinguished by the presence of its hallmark lesions, comedones. Rosacea can sometimes be difficult to distinguish from acne. Patients with rosacea classically have central facial erythema, flushing, telangiectasias, and lack comedones.

Facial inflammatory dermatoses also have a broad differential, but the most common causes of eczematous eruptions on the face are atopic dermatitis in children and contact and seborrheic dermatitis in adults. Connective tissue diseases, such as dermatomyositis and lupus erythematosus, should be considered in the differential for eczematous facial eruptions not responding to standard therapy, particularly when photodistributed. Annular scaly plaques should raise suspicion for tinea faciei, honey-colored crust suggests impetigo, and unilateral dermatomal involvement is classic for herpes zoster (shingles).

For some diagnoses, the absence of facial involvement can be quite helpful. For example, in adult patients, scabies classically does NOT affect the face.

EVALUATION

- Most inflammatory and pilosebaceous skin diseases and pigment disorders on the face are diagnosed clinically based on the patient's history and physical findings and usually do not require diagnostic testing for confirmation of the diagnosis.

- A potassium hydroxide (KOH) examination and/or fungal culture should be for any annular scaly plaque.
- Polymerase chain reaction (PCR) for herpes simplex virus (HSV)-1, HSV-2, and varicella zoster virus (VZV) is the preferred test to confirm the diagnosis of herpes

simplex or zoster. Viral culture and Tzanck smear can also be utilized.

- A skin biopsy should be done if discoid or acute cutaneous lupus is suspected.
- Patch testing can be done for recalcitrant rashes in which allergic contact dermatitis is suspected.

Table 36-1. Differential diagnosis for diseases of the face.

Disease	Epidemiology, History, and Physical Examination
Pilosebaceous Disorders	

Acne vulgaris
 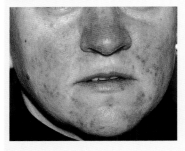
	Epidemiology:
	   Common.
	   Teens: M > F.
	   Adults: F > M.
	   Age: Adolescents and young adulthood.
	 History:
	   Asymptomatic, may be pruritic or tender.
	   Individual lesions last weeks to months.
	   Fluctuating course.
	   Menstrual flares common.
	 Physical Exam:
	   Open (black heads) and closed (white heads) comedones, erythematous papules, pustules, cysts, and nodules.
	   Distinguish from rosacea by the presence of comedones.
	   (see Chapter 10)

Rosacea
 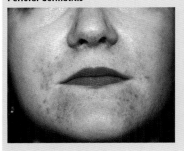
	Epidemiology:
	   Common.
	   F > M.
	   Age: 30–50 years.
	 History:
	   Facial flushing, stinging, or burning.
	   Eye dryness, itching, stinging, or burning.
	   Chronic course.
	 Physical Exam:
	   Flushing (transient erythema), non-transient erythema, papules, pustules and telangiectasias on central face. Blepharitis and conjunctivitis may be present.
	   Distinguish from malar rash of SLE by history.
	   (see Chapter 10)

Perioral dermatitis	Epidemiology:
	   Common.
	   F >> M.
	   Age: 20–45 years of age.
	 History:
	   Asymptomatic, or pruritic or burning.
	   Duration: Weeks to months.
	   May be triggered by topical corticosteroid use.
	 Physical Exam:
	   Grouped, monomorphic follicular erythematous papules, vesicles, and pustules in the perioral region Spares lips.
	   Can extend to the periocular region.
	   Distinguish from contact dermatitis by lack of lip involvement.
	   (see Chapter 10)

(continued)

Table 36-1. Differential diagnosis for diseases of the face. (Continued)

Disease	Epidemiology, History, and Physical Examination

Pseudofolliculitis barbae 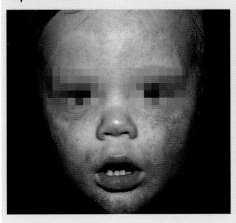	Epidemiology:
	  Common.
	  M >> F.
	  Age: Teenagers and young adults, predominately skin of color.
	History:
	  Asymptomatic or tender. Chronic course. Flares with shaving.
	Physical Exam:
	  Papules and pustules in the beard distribution, posterior neck, cheeks, mandibular area, and chin.
	  Distinguish from acne by absence of comedones and predominant involvement of beard distribution.
	  (see Chapter 10)

Inflammatory Dermatoses

Disease	Epidemiology, History, and Physical Examination

Atopic dermatitis 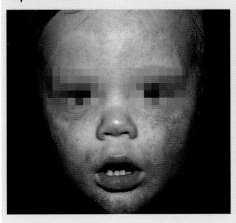	Epidemiology:
	  Common.
	  F > M.
	  Age: Can occur at any age, but most commonly occurs in infancy and childhood. Adult onset can occur.
	History:
	  Pruritus. Chronic course with exacerbations.
	  Bacterial superinfection is common.
	  Usually worse in winter. Personal and family history of atopy (asthma, seasonal allergies, allergic rhinitis, atopic dermatitis).
	Physical Exam:
	  Infants: Ill-defined red papules, scaly plaques, and excoriations on cheeks. Also commonly presents on trunk and extensor extremities. Fissuring common. May have accentuated creases under the eyes (Dennie-Morgan fold).
	  Children & Adults: Ill-defined red lichenified plaques on cheeks and eyelids (if facial involvement present). More commonly presents with hand, foot, and flexural involvement. May have associated keratosis pilaris.
	  Distinguish from other forms of dermatitis by involvement of classic distribution, as well as history of atopy. Distinguish from psoriasis based on morphology (psoriasis more well-demarcated, thicker scale) and distribution.
	  (see Chapter 8)

Allergic contact dermatitis (ACD) 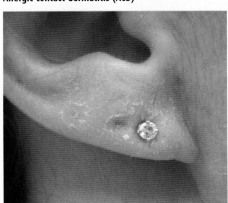	Epidemiology:
	  Common.
	  F > M.
	  Age: Any age, may be more common in adults due to increased product usage.
	History:
	  Pruritic. Onset is hours to days after contact with allergen.
	Physical Exam:
	  Geometric or linear configuration as well as a sharply demarcated distribution are clues to an external cause.
	  Acute: Pink to red, edematous papules and plaques with vesiculation. Frequent sites of involvement include eyelids and lips. Earlobes frequently involved with nickel allergy.
	  Chronic: Xerosis, fissuring, hyperpigmentation, and lichenification at sites of direct contact with allergen.
	  Distribution will be a clue to culprit allergen.
	  Distinguish from other types of dermatitis due to a sharply demarcated distribution and geometric/linear configuration. Patch testing required to distinguish allergic from irritant contact dermatitis. Distinguish from atopic dermatitis due to history of atopy and additional classic areas of involvement of atopic dermatitis.
	  (see Chapter 8)

(continued)

Table 36-1. Differential diagnosis for diseases of the face. (Continued)

Disease	Epidemiology, History, and Physical Examination

Irritant contact dermatitis (ICD)
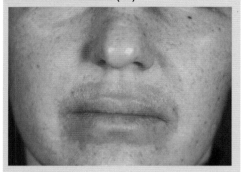
	Epidemiology:
	    Common.
	    F > M.
	    Age: Any age.
	History:
	    Pruritic, painful, or burning. May have history of atopy.
	    Variable onset depending on frequency of exposure and strength of irritant.
	    More common in occupations that require frequent hand washing and exposure to water/soap such as health care workers, janitorial services, and food industry employees.
	    Patients with atopic dermatitis are at increased risk.
	Physical Exam:
	    Well-demarcated plaque with a "glazed" appearance.
	    Eyelids are a frequent site of involvement as chemical may transfer from hands to eyelids inadvertently.
	    May appear identical to allergic contact dermatitis. Need patch testing to differentiate.
	    (see Chapter 8)

Seborrheic dermatitis
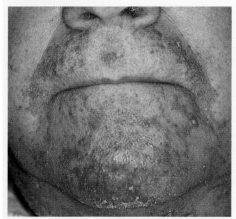
	Epidemiology:
	    Common.
	    M > F.
	    Age: Bimodal age distribution with peaks in infancy and adulthood.
	History:
	    Asymptomatic or mildly pruritic.
	    Waxing and waning course with seasonal variations.
	Physical Exam:
	    Infants: Scalp, diaper involvement common.
	    Adults: Greasy scale and underlying erythema on the eyebrows, nasolabial folds, lateral aspects of the nose, retro-auricular areas and ears, often symmetric.
	    Concurrent flaking of scalp common.
	    Distinguish from malar rash of systemic lupus erythematosus (SLE) by nasolabial and melolabial fold involvement (both spared in SLE).
	    (see Chapter 9)

Sarcoidosis
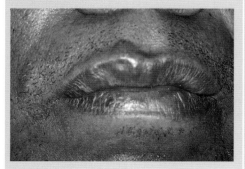
	Epidemiology:
	    Uncommon.
	    F > M.
	    Age: Onset most common in 3rd decade of life.
	History:
	    Typically, asymptomatic.
	    Chronic course, remissions can occur.
	    May have concurrent systemic involvement, most commonly pulmonary and ocular organ systems.
	Physical Exam:
	    Many clinical presentations, known as "the great mimicker."
	    Classically have reddish-brown "apple jelly" papules and plaques with or without scale. Frequently with periocular/perioral and nasal involvement. Can also involve the trunk and extremities.
	    Can preferentially develop within scars and tattoos. Alopecia and nail changes can occur.
	    Nasal ala involvement can be a sign of pulmonary involvement.
	    Can develop associated erythema nodosum.
	    Sarcoidosis is a diagnosis of exclusion. When occurring on the face, distinguish from acne by lack of comedones and characteristic reddish-brown nature.
	    (see Chapter 15)

(continued)

Table 36-1. Differential diagnosis for diseases of the face. (Continued)

Disease	Epidemiology, History, and Physical Examination
Infectious Diseases	

Herpes simplex labialis (HSV)

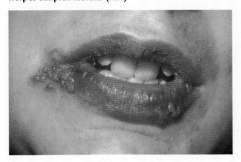

Epidemiology:
  Common.
  M:F unknown.
  Age: Primary infection is in childhood, recurrence at any age.
  Usually caused by HSV1 >> HSV2, but can be either.
History:
  Lesions may be preceded by pain/tingling.
  Fever and pharyngitis may be present with primary infection.
  Lesions last 1–2 weeks.
  Can be triggered by fever, sun exposure, stress.
Physical Exam:
  Grouped vesicles, usually on lips or perioral area.
  Primary infection can present as gingivostomatitis with vesicles on lips, tongue, gingiva, buccal mucosa, and oropharynx.
  May be difficult to distinguish from bullous impetigo. Distinguishing feature: vesicles on erythematous base.
  (see Chapter 13)

Herpes zoster (shingles)

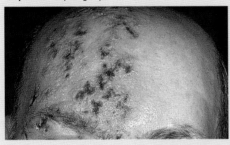

Epidemiology:
  Common
  F > M.
  Age: Any age, but usually >50 years.
History:
  Severe pain, pruritus, or paresthesias may precede eruption. Lasts 3–4 weeks.
  Can have longer lasting pain (post-herpetic neuralgia).
  Increased risk with immunosuppression.
Physical Exam:
  Grouped vesicles on an erythematous base that form crusts in a unilateral dermatome.
  Most commonly affected dermatome on the face is innervated by the trigeminal nerve, particularly the ophthalmic division.
  Dermatomal distribution helps to distinguish herpes zoster from herpes simplex.
  (see Chapter 13)

Impetigo

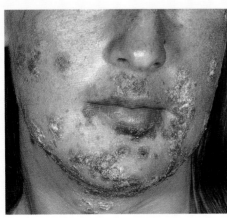

Epidemiology:
  Common.
  M = F.
  Age: Young children.
History:
  May be pruritic.
  Lasts days to weeks. Frequently spreads through schools and day care centers.
Physical Exam:
  Non-bullous impetigo: Honey-colored crusts with erosions on central face, particularly around the nares and lips.
  Bullous impetigo: Starts as a superficial vesicle, which rapidly enlarges into a flaccid bulla. Most commonly affects the face, groin, and extremities.
  When occurring on the face, may be difficult to distinguish from herpes simplex labialis. Distinguishing feature: honey-colored crusting.
  (see Chapter 11)

(continued)

Table 36-1. Differential diagnosis for diseases of the face. (Continued)

Disease	Epidemiology, History, and Physical Examination
Tinea faciei 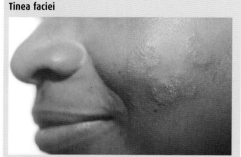	Epidemiology: Uncommon. F > M. Age: Any age, with peaks in childhood and between 20-40 years of age. History: Asymptomatic or pruritic. More common in children in contact with domestic pets and livestock. Physical Exam: Starts as a scaly annular plaque that develops a raised border that advances peripherally and may develop papules and pustules. Most commonly occurs on the cheeks. Distinguish from atopic dermatitis by annular morphology and peripheral scale. (see Chapter 12)
Pigmentation Disorders	
Melasma 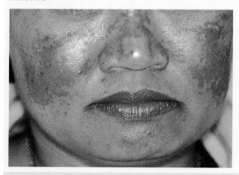	Epidemiology: Common. F >> M. Age: Young adulthood. History: Asymptomatic. Last months to years. May have history of sunlight exposure, pregnancy, or exogenous hormone exposure. Physical Exam: Symmetric patches of hyperpigmentation on the forehead, cheeks, nose, upper lip, chin, and jawline. Distinguishing feature: symmetric nature, "moth-eaten" appearance of hyperpigmented patches. (see Chapter 23) (Reproduced with permission from Charles E.Crutchfield III, MD).
Vitiligo 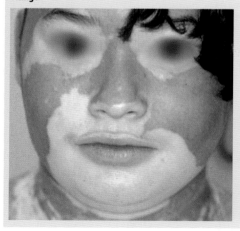	Epidemiology: Common. M = F. Age: Typically 10–30 years of age. If new onset > 50 years of age, consider melanoma-associated leukoderma and perform full-body skin exam. History: Asymptomatic. Chronic course. May be progressive. Personal or family history of autoimmune disease. Physical Exam: Well-demarcated white depigmented macules and patches in symmetric distribution. Accentuated with Wood's lamp. When occurring on the face, favors the perioral and periocular regions. Other commonly affected areas include dorsal hands, ventral wrists, extensor forearms, and genitals. Distinguish from pityriasis alba by well-demarcated nature and depigmentation on Wood's lamp. (see Chapter 23) (Reproduced with permission from Charles E. Crutchfield III, MD).

(continued)

Table 36-1. Differential diagnosis for diseases of the face. (Continued)

Disease	Epidemiology, History, and Physical Examination

Alopecia

Alopecia Areata

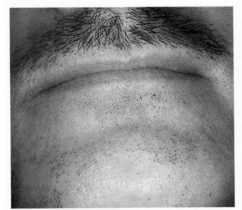

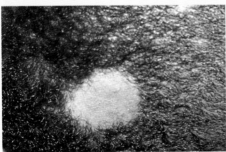

Epidemiology:
  Common.
  M = F
  Age: All ages.
History:
  Usually asymptomatic.
  Last months to years.
Physical Exam:
  Non-scarring patchy or complete loss of eyebrow, eyelash, beard or facial hair fibers. Scalp is commonly affected.
  (see Chapter 30)

Photodermatoses

Photoaging

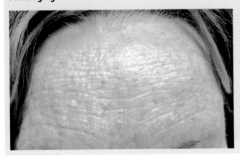

Epidemiology:
  Common.
  M:F unknown.
  Age >40 years.
History:
  Asymptomatic.
  Cigarette smoking hastens skin aging.
  Risk is inversely related to skin pigmentation.
Physical Exam:
  Dyspigmentation, wrinkling, telangiectasias, atrophy, and leathery thickening on the face, lateral neck, central upper chest, extensor forearms, and dorsal hands.
  Distinguishing feature: more prominent in chronically photo-exposed locations.
  (see Chapter 34)

(continued)

Table 36-1. Differential diagnosis for diseases of the face. (Continued)

Disease	Epidemiology, History, and Physical Examination
Phototoxicity 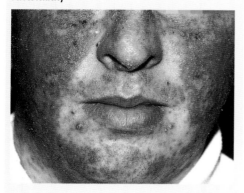	Epidemiology: 　Common. 　M:F unknown. 　Age: Any age. History: 　Pain, burning and pruritus. Worse in summer. Several medications, chronic porphyrias, and photosensitive dermatoses can cause exaggerated response to UV exposure. 　Risk is inversely related to skin pigmentation. Physical Exam: 　Bright red patches with edema and blistering that heal with desquamation and hyperpigmentation on sun-exposed areas including the forehead, nose, and malar cheeks. 　Other commonly affected areas include neck and upper chest, upper back, extensor forearms, and dorsal hands. 　Distinguishing feature: classically spares photoprotected locations such as periorbital and perioral areas as well as nasolabial folds.

Connective Tissue Diseases

Disease	Epidemiology, History, and Physical Examination
Discoid lupus erythematosus 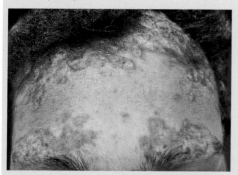	Epidemiology: 　Uncommon. 　F > M. 　Age: 20–45 years of age. History: 　Asymptomatic or mildly pruritic. 　Sunlight may precipitate flares. 　5–10% develop SLE. 　May resolve spontaneously. Physical Exam: 　Red or purple patch with superficial scale that enlarges into a plaque with central scarring and dyspigmentation. 　Commonly involves scalp (60%), face, and ears. Can have associated alopecia. 　Other commonly affected locations include upper chest, neck, and extensor surfaces of the arms and hands. 　Distinguishing feature: dyspigmentation and conchal bowl involvement characteristic. (see Chapter 15)
Acute cutaneous lupus erythematous (ACLE) 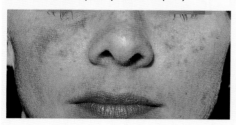	Epidemiology: 　Uncommon. 　F > M. 　Age: Any age, but most commonly 30–40 years of age. History: 　Always associated with systemic lupus erythematosus (SLE). 　Pruritus or burning. Exacerbated by sun exposure. Associated with diffuse hair loss, arthritis, fatigue, oral ulcers, and other systemic findings consistent with SLE. Physical Exam: 　Pink to red edematous papules, plaques, and patchy erythema with variable scale. 　Typically in photosensitive distribution, involving the forehead, malar cheeks, and bridge of the nose (i.e., malar or butterfly rash). 　Classically spares nasolabial/melolabial folds. 　Other commonly affected locations include the neck, upper chest, and dorsal arms/hands. 　Classically spares the skin overlying the joints of the hand. 　Distinguished from dermatomyositis by typically sparing the nasolabial/melolabial folds and dorsal joints of the hands, areas which are classically involved in dermatomyositis. (see Chapter 15)

(continued)

Table 36-1. Differential diagnosis for diseases of the face. (Continued)

Disease	Epidemiology, History, and Physical Examination

Dermatomyositis	Epidemiology:
	  Uncommon.
	  F > M.
	  Age: Bimodal; peaks at ages 5–10 and greater than 50 years of age.
	History:
	  Typically, very pruritic, but may be asymptomatic. Chronic course.
	  Associated with photosensitivity, scalp pruritus/burning, and symmetric proximal muscle weakness.
	  Associated with malignancy in older adults (>60 years of age) and male sex.
	Physical Exam:
	  Pink-violet patches in affected areas. Commonly on scalp and periocular region (heliotrope rash). Can have centrofacial erythema that classically involves the melolabial folds.
	  Distinguished from acute cutaneous lupus erythematosus (ACLE) in SLE by involvement of nasolabial/melolabial folds and skin overlying joints, which are classically spared in ACLE.
	  (see Chapter 15)

DM, dermatomyositis; F, female; M, male; SLE , Systemic lupus erythematosus; UV, ultraviolet

37

Skin Diseases of the Arms

Noah Goldfarb
Brittney Schultz

INTRODUCTION

Many skin conditions that affect the arms result from their direct exposure to sunlight, contact with allergens or irritants, trauma, bug bites, and other environmental insults. The arms are within close reach of the contralateral hand, so patients can easily scratch pruritic dermatoses. Scratching or trauma may produce a linear streak of papules (Koebner phenomenon) in certain diseases such as psoriasis and lichen planus. Some skin diseases have a predilection for specific locations on the arms. While it is unknown why many dermatoses tend to localize to certain anatomical locations, lesion distribution is frequently a very important clue to establish diagnosis.

APPROACH TO DIAGNOSIS

Skin diseases involving the arms can be broadly placed into the following categories starting with the most common diseases (Table 37-1).

- Inflammatory Dermatoses
- Infectious Diseases
- Infestations and bites
- Immunobullous Diseases
- Autoimmune Diseases
- Neoplastic

The distribution of skin lesions is often helpful in diagnosing skin diseases located on the arms. For example,

psoriasis, nummular dermatitis, and dermatitis herpetiformis usually favor the extensor surface especially the elbows. Photodermatoses, including lupus erythematosus and dermatomyositis, affect areas exposed to light. Keratosis pilaris is typically seen on the proximal dorsal arms, and atopic dermatitis generally affects the extensor surface in infants and flexural surface in children and adults. Lichen planus and scabies are commonly located on the volar wrist and flexural surfaces.

EVALUATION

- Most inflammatory skin diseases on the arm are diagnosed clinically based on the patient's history and physical findings and usually do not require diagnostic testing for confirmation of the diagnosis.
- A potassium hydroxide (KOH) examination and/or fungal cultures should be done for any rash with annular scaly plaques.
- Bacterial cultures can be done if primary or secondary infections are suspected.
- Polymerase chain reaction (PCR) for herpes simplex virus (HSV)-1, HSV-2, and varicella zoster virus (VZV) is the preferred test to confirm the diagnosis of herpes simplex or zoster. Viral culture and Tzanck smear can also be utilized.
- Skin biopsies can be done if the clinical presentation is equivocal.
- Patch testing should be done if allergic contact dermatitis is suspected.

Table 37-1. Skin Disease on the Arms.

Disease	Features
Inflammatory Dermatoses	
Atopic dermatitis 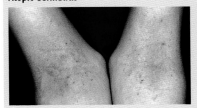	**Epidemiology:** Common. F > M. Age: Can occur at any age, but most commonly occurs in infancy and childhood. Adult onset can occur. **History:** Very pruritic. Chronic course with exacerbations. Bacterial superinfection common. Usually worse in winter. Personal and family history of atopy (asthma, seasonal allergies, allergic rhinitis, and atopic dermatitis). **Physical Exam:** *Infants:* Red papules, scaly poorly demarcated plaques, excoriations, and crusting on extensor arms and legs, cheeks, and trunk. *Children/Adults:* Red lichenified poorly demarcated plaques and excoriations on flexor arms and legs, especially antecubital and popliteal fossae. Distinguish from other forms of dermatitis by classic distribution, as well as history of atopy. Distinguish from psoriasis based on morphology (psoriasis more well-demarcated, thicker scale) and classic distribution. (see Chapter 8).
Lichen simplex chronicus (LSC) 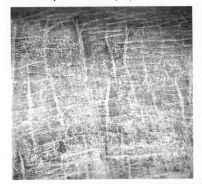	**Epidemiology:** Common. F > M. Age: >20 years of age. **History:** More common in atopic patients. Paroxysmal episodes of pruritus disproportionate to external stimuli, for example, changing clothes. Emotional stress may exacerbate eruption. **Physical Exam:** Sharply defined plaque(s) with accentuated skin lines. May appear, pink, shiny, dyspigmented, or sometimes mildly scaly. Distinguished from lichen planus or psoriasis by morphology (accentuation of skin lines in LSC) and usually limited to only a few unilateral locations, unlike psoriasis or lichen planus which involve classic areas with symmetric distribution. (see Chapter 8).
Prurigo nodularis 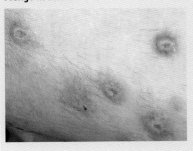	**Epidemiology:** Common. F > M. Age: Any age, but more common in older adults. **History:** Pruritic. Persists for months to years. Variable patient insight. May admit to picking and/or scratching lesions. Can be idiopathic or secondary to other underlying conditions, for example, atopic dermatitis, HIV, hypothyroidism, renal or liver disease, lymphoma. Some cases related to anxiety or other psychiatric disorders. Bug bites and folliculitis may exacerbate. **Physical Exam:** Solitary or multiple discrete, well-demarcated, dome-shaped, hyperpigmented papules, or nodules, often in variable stages of healing. Sparing on central back where patient unable to reach is referred to as butterfly sign. Typical location involving extensor extremities. Distinguished from other causes of epidermal hyperplasia, for example, seborrheic keratoses, squamous cell carcinoma, lichen planus based on morphology (rubbery, symmetric, hyperkeratotic, centrally eroded) and easy to reach location of lesions. (see Chapter 8).

(continued)

Table 37-1. Skin Disease on the Arms. (Continued)

Disease	Features

Nummular dermatitis
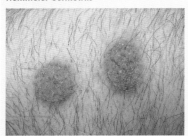
	Epidemiology:
	  Common.
	  M > F.
	  Age: Bimodal; peaks in young and older adults.
	History:
	  Pruritus is common.
	  Chronic, waxing and waning course.
	  Worse in fall and winter.
	Physical Exam:
	  Round, light pink, scaly, thin, 1–3 cm plaques, most commonly located on the extensor extremities, but can occur anywhere on the body. Sometimes they can be more moist and indurated or more xerotic with reticular fissuring. Can have overlying crusting and impetiginization.
	  Distinguish from psoriasis by fine scale, reticular fissuring, less well-demarcated borders, and lack of involvement of classic psoriasis areas, for example, scalp, elbows, knees, supragluteal cleft.
	  (see Chapter 8).

Allergic contact dermatitis (ACD)
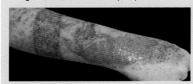
	Epidemiology:
	  Common.
	  F > M.
	  Age: Any age, may be more common in adults due to increased product usage.
	History:
	  Pruritus, sometimes with blisters. Onset is hours to days after contact with allergen.
	Physical Exam:
	  Geometric or linear configuration as well as a sharply demarcated distribution are clues to an external cause
	  Acute: Pink to red, edematous, plaques with papules and vesicles, sometimes bullae.
	  Chronic: Xerosis, fissuring, hyperpigmentation and lichenification at sites of direct contact with allergen.
	  Distinguish from other types of dermatitis due to a sharply demarcated distribution and geometric/linear configuration. Location is an important clue to the cause. For example, on the arm and axilla, ACD is more likely due to preservatives, fragrances and clothing.
	  (see Chapter 8).

Keratosis pilaris
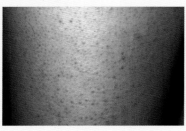
	Epidemiology:
	  Common.
	  F > M.
	  Age: Starts in childhood and typically worsens in adolescents
	History:
	  Usually asymptomatic, rarely mild pruritus.
	  Often seen associated with atopy.
	Physical Exam:
	  Follicular-based, keratotic, monomorphic papules with peripheral erythema. Stippled or "gooseflesh" appearance on proximal extensor surfaces.
	  Distinguish from folliculitis or other pilosebaceous conditions by the diffuse symmetric distribution on the bilateral proximal extremities.
	  (see Chapter 8).

(continued)

Table 37-1. Skin Disease on the Arms. (Continued)

Disease	Features

Psoriasis vulgaris (chronic plaque psoriasis) 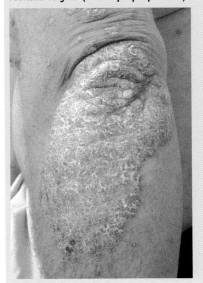	Epidemiology:
	  Common.
	  M = F.
	  Age: Any age but bimodal distribution peaks in 20s and 50s.
	History:
	  Asymptomatic or mildly pruritic. Chronic. Associated with inflammatory arthritis and cardiovascular comorbidities (e.g., obesity, diabetes mellitus type II, hyperlipidemia, hypertension, as well as atherosclerotic cardiovascular and cerebrovascular disease). Family history of psoriasis.
	Physical Exam:
	  Well-demarcated, salmon pink to red papules and plaques with overlying silvery, thick, adherent scale.
	  Typically located on elbows and extensor extremities, as well as scalp, knees, genitals, umbilicus, lower back, and retro-auricular area.
	  Distinguished from dermatitis by the very well-demarcated borders, symmetric distribution, thick white scale, and involvement of other classic areas (scalp, ears, elbows, knees, gluteal cleft, umbilicus).
	  (see Chapter 9).

Lichen planus 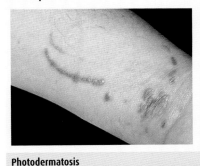	Epidemiology:
	  Uncommon.
	  M = F.
	  Age: Any age, but most commonly between 30 and 60 years of age.
	History:
	  Pruritic. Lasts months to years. May be drug-induced or associated with Hepatitis C.
	Physical Exam:
	  Multiple variants exist. Classically flat-topped, well-defined, polygonal, violaceous, and shiny papules. Can see overlying reticular fine white lines (Wickham striae) Typical locations include volar wrists, ankles, glans penis, and lower back. Can have associated mucosal and nail involvement.
	  Distinguishing feature: extremely pruritic, purple papules in classic locations.
	  (see Chapter 9).

Photodermatosis	(see Chapter 36).
Infectious Diseases	

Tinea Corporis 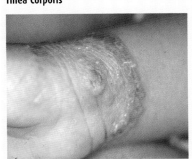	Epidemiology:
	  Uncommon.
	  M = F.
	  Age: All ages, but more common in children.
	History:
	  Asymptomatic or mildly pruritic.
	  Associated with hot/humid weather, farming, and crowded living conditions.
	Physical Exam:
	  Annular plaque(s) with a scaly, raised well-demarcated border and central clearing.
	  Most commonly located on extremities and trunk including buttocks.
	  May be difficult to distinguish from psoriasis or dermatitis, when it does not present as the classic annular plaque with central clearing and edge of scale. For scaly plaques that do not fit a classic psoriasis distribution or do not fit a clear type of dermatitis, a KOH exam may be needed to solidify the diagnosis.
	  (see Chapter 12).

(continued)

Table 37-1. Skin Disease on the Arms. (Continued)

Disease	Features
Infestations and Bug Bites	
Scabies 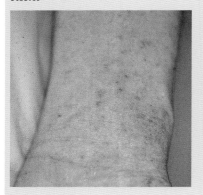	**Epidemiology:** Common. M = F. Age: Any age, but more common in children. **History:** Intense pruritus. Chronic symptoms until treated. **Physical Exam:** Multiple excoriated papules and occasionally small (<1 cm), white, linear, serpiginous tracks, or thread-like lesions referred to as burrows. Typical locations include web spaces of fingers and toes, volar wrist, elbows, axillae, areola, navel, waistline, and genitals. Palm and sole involvement more common in infants. Spares the head and neck. Sometimes difficult to distinguish from other diffuse papular eruptions. The classic involvement of web spaces, navel and genitals can usually help distinguish from other rashes. Itchy papules on male scrotum are almost pathognomonic for scabies and burrows are always pathognomonic for scabies. (see Chapter 14).
Bug bites 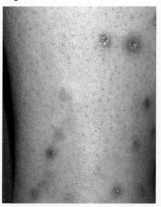	**Epidemiology:** Common. M = F. Age: Any age, but usually in childhood, adolescents, and young adulthood. **History:** Acute onset. Pruritic. Due to bites from insects, for example, mosquito, bedbug, flea, and mite. Most are aware of bug bites, but when the reaction is delayed or occurs during sleep, patients may not know they were bitten. Patients with chronic lymphocytic leukemia may demonstrate an exaggerated response. **Physical exam:** Clustered, pink papules or vesicles. May have a central hemorrhagic punctum. Bedbugs and fleas may demonstrate the "breakfast, lunch and dinner" sign, which involves three or more papules in a linear distribution, a few centimeters apart. Typically involving exposed areas of the body, most commonly extensor extremities. Distinguish from urticaria by more localized and clustered appearance of papules or vesicles with central punctum and duration > 24 hours (see Chapter 14).
Immunobullous Diseases	
Dermatitis herpetiformis (DH) 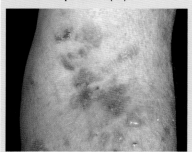	**Epidemiology:** Uncommon. F > M. Age: Any age, but most common between 20 and 60 years of age. **History:** Severe episodic pruritus. Almost all patients have an associated gluten-sensitive enteropathy (celiac disease). DH also associated with several other cell-mediated autoimmune diseases including type I diabetes mellitus, vitiligo, alopecia areata, autoimmune thyroid disease, and pernicious anemia. **Physical Exam:** Grouped, pink, crusted papules, and erosions. Vesicles rarely seen due to excoriation. Typical locations include extensor extremities, elbows, knees, back, buttocks, scalp, and neck in a symmetric distribution. Distinguished from widespread dermatitis by morphology of grouped eroded papules and involvement of classic areas, for example, post-auricular scalp, elbows, and buttocks. Gastrointestinal symptoms can also be a clue. (see Chapter 19)

(continued)

Table 37-1. Skin Disease on the Arms. (Continued)

Disease	Features
Autoimmune Diseases	

Acute cutaneous lupus erythematosus (ACLE)

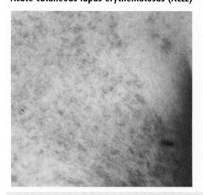

Epidemiology:
  Uncommon.
  F > M.
  Age: Any age, but most commonly 30–40 years of age.
History:
  Always associated with systemic lupus erythematosus (SLE).
  Pruritus or burning. Exacerbated by sun exposure. Associated with hair loss, arthritis, fatigue, oral ulcers, and other systemic findings consistent with SLE.
Physical Exam:
  Pink to red edematous papules, plaques, and patchy erythema with variable scale. Typically, in photosensitive distribution, including the dorsal arms/hands. Classically sparing the skin overlying the joints.
  Distinguished from dermatomyositis by typically sparing the nasolabial/melolabial folds and dorsal joints of the hands, areas which are classically involved in dermatomyositis. (see Chapter 15).

Subacute cutaneous lupus erythematosus (SCLE)

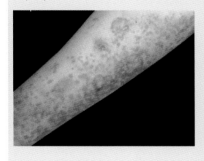

Epidemiology:
  Uncommon.
  M > F.
  Age: Any age, but most commonly ages 15–70 years of age.
History:
  Lesions may be asymptomatic or mildly pruritic. May be drug-related, associated with Sjogren Syndrome or SLE, or idiopathic.
Physical Exam:
  Pink to red, well-demarcated, annular and polycyclic plaques with edge of scale. Many of the plaques develop central clearing and may develop hypopigmentation. Unlike discoid lesions, SCLE does not resolve with atrophy or scarring.
  Typically located in photo-distributed sites, including shoulders and extensor arms. Classically sparing the face.
  Distinguished from psoriasis and other papulosquamous eruptions due to its photo-distribution. Distinguished from discoid lupus erythematosus by the lack of atrophy or scarring.
  (see Chapter 15).

Dermatomyositis (DM)

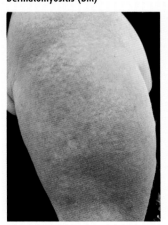

Epidemiology:
  Uncommon.
  F > M.
  Age: Bimodal; peaks at ages 5–10 and greater than 50 years of age.
History:
  Typically very pruritic, but may be asymptomatic. Chronic course.
  Associated with photosensitivity, scalp pruritus/burning, and symmetric proximal muscle weakness.
  Associated with malignancy in older adults (>60 years of age) and male sex.
Physical Exam:
  Pink-violet patches located in photo-distributed sites, including the shoulders, proximal upper arms and upper back, referred to as the shawl sign.
  Distinguished from acute cutaneous lupus erythematosus (ACLE) in SLE by involvement of nasolabial/melolabial folds and skin overlying joints, which are classically spared in ACLE. (see Chapter 15).

(continued)

Table 37-1. Skin Disease on the Arms. (Continued)

Disease	Features
Neoplasia	
Actinic keratoses 	Epidemiology: Common. M > F. Age: > 50 years. History: Persists for months-years, can wax/wane. Asymptomatic or tender. Risk Factors: Advancing age, cumulative sun exposure, outdoor occupation, fair skin type. Physical Exam: Skin-colored, to pink, rough/gritty papules and plaques with adherent hyperkeratotic scale. May be easier to palpate than visualize. Most commonly located on dorsal forearms/hands as well as scalp, forehead, temples, cheeks, nose, ears, and posterior/lateral neck. Distinguished from various other dermatoses involving the dorsal arms by the rough/gritty texture on palpation. (see Chapter 21).

ACLE, acute cutaneous lupus erythematosus; ACD, allergic contact dermatitis; DH, dermatitis herpetiformis; F, female; LSC, lichen simplex chronicus; M, male; SCLE; subacute cutaneous lupus erythematosus; SLE, systemic lupus erythematosus

Skin Diseases of the Hands

Noah Goldfarb
Brittney Schultz

INTRODUCTION

Hands have structures with many unique structural and functional features. As such, they are prone to developing specific dermatologic diseases. Structurally, the palms have a thick keratin layer, a high concentration of sweat glands, Meissner's corpuscles, and other mechanoreceptors. Functionally, we use our hands to explore the world. Therefore, hands are subject to physical injury. Hands are often the first body part to come into contact with objects and substances in our environment. As a result, they are frequently the site of exposure to allergens, irritants, and infectious agents. This concept is central to the transmission of pathogens and development of certain dermatologic conditions such as contact dermatitis. Given their distal location, the neurovascular supply of hands (particularly the digits) can also predispose to neuropathies and ischemic insults. The dorsal hands tend to get more sun exposure than centrally located anatomical structures thereby subjecting them to photodermatoses and actinic damage. Hands may also manifest cutaneous signs of internal disease.

APPROACH TO DIAGNOSIS

Skin diseases involving the hands can be broadly placed into the following categories starting with the most common diseases (Table 38-1):

- Inflammatory dermatoses
- Infectious Diseases
- Infestations
- Systemic and autoimmune diseases
- Pigment disorders
- Neoplasia

For dermatoses affecting the hands, the specific location of involvement on the hand can be an important clue for the diagnosis. The dorsal hands are highly exposed to sunlight, and therefore are commonly affected by skin conditions aggravated by sunlight, including photodermatoses, connective tissue diseases such as lupus erythematosus and dermatomyositis, as well as neoplasia related to excessive ultraviolet (UV) exposure. Several dermatoses commonly affect the palms including tinea manuum (fine scaling), palmoplantar pustulosis (pustules), hand-foot-mouth disease (vesicles), and secondary syphilis (macules and papules, sometimes with overlying scale). Classically, dyshidrotic dermatitis affects the lateral digits, whereas irritant contact dermatitis and scabies, present in the finger web spaces.

EVALUATION

- Most inflammatory hand dermatoses including dyshidrotic dermatitis, atopic dermatitis, psoriasis, and irritant contact dermatitis are diagnosed based on the patient's history and clinical findings and usually do not require diagnostic testing.
- A potassium hydroxide (KOH) examination and/or fungal cultures should be done in most scaly hand

rashes. Tinea manuum may be clinically indistinguish-able from inflammatory dermatoses such as dermatitis and psoriasis.

- Patch testing should be done if allergic contact dermatitis is a likely diagnosis.
- Skin biopsies can be done to exclude other diagnoses if otherwise clinically equivocal.
- Bacterial cultures can be done if primary or secondary infections are suspected.

- Polymerase chain reaction (PCR) for herpes simplex virus (HSV)-1, HSV-2, and varicella zoster virus (VZV) is the preferred test to confirm the diagnosis of herpes simplex or zoster. Viral culture and Tzanck smear can also be utilized.
- A thorough history with review of systems and physical exam are very important for cutaneous manifestations of internal disease and connective tissue disorders. Suspicion for these diseases may prompt further evaluation with appropriate laboratory studies

Table 38-1. Skin diseases of the hands.

Disease	Features
Inflammatory dermatoses	
Allergic contact dermatitis (ACD) 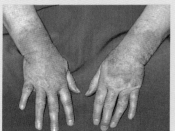	Epidemiology: Common. F > M. Age: Any age, more common in adults due to increased topical product usage. History: Itchy rash, sometimes with blisters and painful fissures. Onset is hours to days after contact with allergen. Physical Exam: Geometric or linear configuration as well as a sharply demarcated distribution are clues to an external cause. *Acute*: Pink to red, edematous papules and plaques with vesiculation. *Chronic*: Xerosis, fissuring, hyperpigmentation, and lichenification at sites of direct contact with allergen. Distribution will be a clue to culprit allergen. Distinguish from other types of dermatitis due to a sharply demarcated distribution and geometric/linear configuration. Can be very difficult to differentiate from irritant contact dermatitis and atopic hand dermatitis, without patch testing. Distinguish from atopic dermatitis due to history of atopy and additional classic areas of involvement of atopic dermatitis. (see Chapter 8).
Irritant contact dermatitis (ICD) 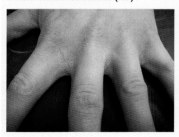	Epidemiology: Common. F > M. Age: More common in adults. History: Pruritic, burning, or painful. Variable onset depending on frequency of exposure and strength of irritant (e.g., cleansers, soaps, detergents, repetitive friction, wet work, or frequent hand washing). Patients with atopic dermatitis are at increased risk. Physical Exam: Well-demarcated with a "glazed" appearance. Erythema, fissures, blistering and scaling, usually in finger web spaces, or dorsum of hands. Distinguished from allergic contact dermatitis by patch testing. ICD more common than ACD. Distinguish from atopic dermatitis due to history of atopy and classic areas of involvement of atopic dermatitis. (see Chapter 8).

(continued)

Table 38-1. Skin diseases of the hands. (Continued)

Disease	Features

Atopic hand dermatitis 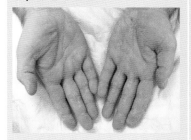	Epidemiology:
	  Common.
	  F > M.
	  Age: Atopic dermatitis can occur at any age, but most commonly begins in infancy and childhood. Atopic hand dermatitis is more common in adults.
	History:
	  Pruritus. Chronic course with exacerbations.
	  Bacterial superinfection common.
	  Usually worse in winter. Worsens with frequent exposure to irritants or water.
	  Family or personal history of atopy (asthma, seasonal allergies, allergic rhinitis, atopic dermatitis). Hand dermatitis may be only presentation in adults.
	Physical Exam:
	  Pink to hyperpigmented, fissured, mildly scaly, lichenified, poorly demarcated plaques, most commonly on dorsal hands. Scaling and painful fissuring sometimes more prominent on the palms and fingers.
	  Distinguish from other forms of hand dermatitis by history of atopy. Distinguish from psoriasis which has well-demarcated plaques compared to the poorly demarcated ones in atopic dermatitis.
	  (see Chapter 8).

Dyshidrotic dermatitis (pompholyx) 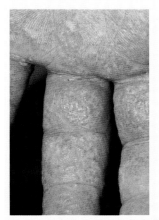	Epidemiology:
	  Common.
	  F > M.
	  Age: Young adults, 20–40 years of age.
	History:
	  Severely pruritic. Chronic and recurrent with attacks lasting 2–4 weeks. Exacerbated by stress and exposure to allergens or irritants.
	  Associated with atopic dermatitis.
	Physical Exam:
	  Multiple, grouped, tapioca colored, non-inflammatory vesicles, and bullae located on lateral surface of fingers and palms.
	  Distinguished from allergic contact dermatitis by the recurrent crops of blisters most prominent on lateral aspects of digits.
	  (see Chapter 8).

Psoriasis vulgaris (plaque psoriasis) 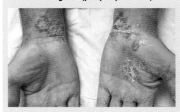	Epidemiology:
	  Common.
	  M = F.
	  Age: Any age but bimodal distribution peaks in 20s and 50s.
	History:
	  Asymptomatic to mildly pruritic. Chronic course. Associated with inflammatory arthritis and cardiovascular comorbidities (e.g., obesity, diabetes mellitus type II, hyperlipidemia, hypertension, as well as atherosclerotic cardiovascular and cerebrovascular disease).
	  Family history of psoriasis.
	Physical Exam:
	  Symmetric, well-demarcated, plaques with hyperkeratotic, adherent white or yellow scale and underlying pink inflammatory base. May be associated with painful fissures. More classic, well-demarcated, salmon plaques with overlying white/silvery scale may be present on the dorsal hands and overlying joints. Hand involvement may be only manifestation of psoriasis. Nails are also frequently affected.
	  Distinguished from dermatitis by the very well-demarcated borders, symmetric distribution, thick white/silvery scale, and involvement of other classic areas (scalp, ears, elbows, knees, gluteal cleft, umbilicus).
	  (see Chapter 9).

(continued)

Table 38-1. Skin diseases of the hands. (Continued)

Disease	Features
Palmoplantar pustulosis (PPP) 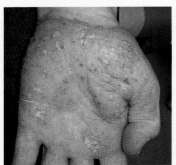	Epidemiology: Uncommon. F > M. Age: Onset typically 50–60 years of age. History: Pruritus, burning, or pain. Lasts years. Waxing and waning course. Strongly associated with tobacco use. May be localized variant of psoriasis limited to palms and soles. Physical Exam: Scattered creamy yellow pustules and dusky red macules on palms and soles. Distinguished from vesicular tinea manuum/pedis by the deep-seated creamy yellow pustules in PPP compared with clear vesicles/bullae in tinea. (see Chapter 9).
Granuloma annulare 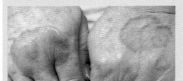	Epidemiology: Uncommon F > M. Age: Localized type: Children and young adults. Generalized type: bimodal distribution, age <10 and 30–60 years of age. History: Typically asymptomatic. Lasts months to years. Recurrence is common. Physical Exam: Skin-colored or pink papules or annular plaques generally without surface change. Can be localized or generalized. Typical Locations: Localized type: dorsal hands/feet, and extensor extremities. Generalized type: trunk and extremities. Distinguished from tinea corporis due to absent scale or surface change. Distinguish from sarcoidosis clinically by localized involvement of dorsal hands/feet. Would typically require a biopsy to differentiate from sarcoidosis for the generalized type.

Infectious Diseases

Disease	Features
Tinea manuum 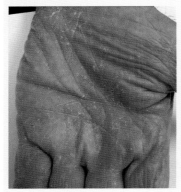	Epidemiology Uncommon. M > F. Age: Occurs after puberty. Increasing prevalence with age. History: Asymptomatic or pruritic. Lasts months to years. Can occur from contact with infected person or animal or autoinoculation (e.g., from foot or groin). Usually associated with tinea pedis, with either two hands and one foot involved or one hand and two feet involved. Physical Exam: On palm, presents with diffuse fine scaling. Unilateral in ~50%. On dorsum of hand presents with annular red plaque with peripheral scale at leading edge and central clearing. Nails may be affected. Typically associated with tinea pedis. Distinguished from palmar psoriasis by poor demarcation and fine scale. Distinguishing from dermatitis may be more difficult and may require KOH exam. Association with "moccasin-like" tinea pedis can help differentiate from other hand rashes. (see Chapter 12).

(continued)

Table 38-1. Skin diseases of the hands. (Continued)

Disease	Features

Herpetic whitlow 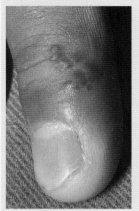	Epidemiology:
	  Rare.
	  M = F.
	  Age: Young children and adults (medical professionals, especially dentists).
	History:
	  Painful.
	  Increased risk from finger-sucking behavior in young children.
	Physical exam:
	  Grouped and confluent vesicles on red edematous base on a distal digit.
	  (see Chapter 13).

Warts (Verruca vulgaris) 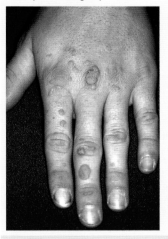	Epidemiology:
	  Common.
	  M > F.
	  Age: More common in children and young adults.
	History:
	  Asymptomatic or painful. May persist for years.
	Physical Exam:
	  Discrete or confluent hyperkeratotic, verrucous skin colored to brown papules or plaques on palms or dorsal hand with loss of skin lines. May have black or brown dots within the lesions created by thrombosed capillaries. Flat warts may be more difficult to diagnose, as they lack the typical hyperkeratotic/verrucous appearance. Flat warts present as homogenous, shiny, smooth, flat-topped pink to light brown papules, typically presenting in clusters.
	  Distinguished from callus by interruption of dermatoglyphics.
	  (see Chapter 13)

Secondary syphilis 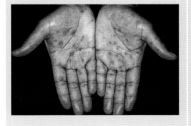	Epidemiology:
	  Common.
	  M > F.
	  Age: 15–40 years of age.
	History:
	  Most commonly manifested by diffuse eruption on trunk, palms, and soles that develops 2–10 weeks after primary chancre, typically on genitals, and self-resolves within 3–12 weeks. May recur. Systemic symptoms may be present or shortly precede onset of eruption (fever, malaise, myalgia, headache).
	  Risk factors: HIV increases the risk of acquiring syphilis and vice versa.
	Physical Exam:
	  Can manifest in many ways including red-brown or ham colored macules or papules +/- scale on the palms and soles.
	  Palm/sole involvement is an important feature that can help differentiate secondary syphilis from other papulosquamous eruptions like pityriasis rosea. Have a low threshold for checking teponema pallidum serology in any patient with a pityriasis rosea-like eruption.
	  (see Chapter 11).

(continued)

Table 38-1. Skin diseases of the hands. (Continued)

Disease	Features
Infestation	

Scabies 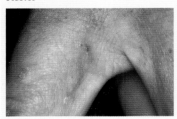	Epidemiology:
	    Common.
	    M = F.
	    Age: Any age, but more common in children.
	History:
	    Intense pruritus. Chronic symptoms until treated.
	Physical Exam:
	    Multiple excoriated papules and occasionally small (<1 cm), white, linear, serpiginous tracks, or thread-like lesions, referred to as burrows.
	    Typical locations include web spaces of fingers and toes, volar wrists, elbows, axillae, areola, navel, waistline, and genitals. Palm and sole involvement more common in infants. Spares the head and neck.
	    Sometimes difficult to distinguish from other diffuse papular eruptions. The classic involvement of web spaces and flexor wrists, navel and genitals can usually help distinguish from other rashes. Itchy papules on male scrotum are almost pathognomonic for scabies and burrows are always pathognomonic for scabies.
	    (see Chapter 14).

Systemic & Autoimmune Diseases	

Raynaud phenomenon 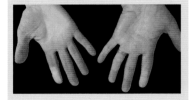	Epidemiology:
	    Common.
	    F > M.
	    Age: Onset in 2nd decade of life.
	History:
	    Triggered by cold and stress.
	    No underlying condition.
	Physical Exam:
	    Classic triphasic sequence of 1) vasoconstriction leading to pallor (white), 2) venous stasis leading to cyanosis (blue), and 3) compensatory reperfusion leading to erythema (red).
	    Can be difficult to distinguish from secondary Raynaud's phenomenon which is associated with underlying systemic conditions, most commonly connective tissue diseases such as systemic sclerosis or systemic lupus erythematosus as well as medications and vibratory trauma. Nail fold capillary changes can help differentiate primary Raynaud's disease versus secondary Raynaud's phenomenon.
	    Ulceration, scarring and necrosis occur with secondary Raynaud's phenomenon and not primary Raynaud's disease.
	    (see Chapter 15).

Acute cutaneous lupus erythematosus 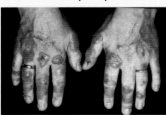	Epidemiology:
	    Uncommon.
	    F > M.
	    Age: Any age, but most commonly 30–40 years of age.
	History:
	    Always associated with systemic lupus erythematosus (SLE).
	    Pruritus or burning. Exacerbated by sun exposure. Associated with diffuse hair loss, arthritis, fatigue, oral ulcers, and other systemic findings consistent with SLE.
	Physical Exam:
	    Pink to red edematous papules, plaques and patchy erythema with variable scale, most notable in photosensitive distribution, including involving dorsal arms/hands, as well as forehead, malar cheeks, bridge of the nose, neck, upper chest, and back.
	    Classically spares the skin overlying the joints of the hand and nasolabial/melolabial folds.
	    Distinguished from dermatomyositis by typically sparing the nasolabial/melolabial folds and dorsal joints of the hands, areas which are classically involved in dermatomyositis.
	    (see Chapter 15).

(continued)

Table 38-1. Skin diseases of the hands. (Continued)

Disease	Features

Dermatomyositis 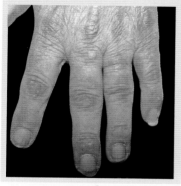	Epidemiology:
	   Uncommon.
	   F > M.
	   Age: Bimodal; peaks at ages 5–10 and greater than 50 years of age.
	 History:
	   Typically very pruritic, but may be asymptomatic. Chronic course.
	   Associated with photosensitivity, scalp pruritus/burning, and symmetric proximal muscle weakness.
	   Associated with malignancy in older adults (>60 years of age) and male sex.
	 Physical Exam:
	   Pink-violet patches overlying joints, especially joints of the hands, as well as elbows, and knees (Gottron's sign). Also flat-topped violaceous papules overlying knuckles and interphalangeal joints (Gottron's papules). Periungual erythema and ragged cuticles with cuticular overgrowth. Distinguished from acute cutaneous lupus erythematosus (ACLE) in SLE by involvement of nasolabial/melolabial folds and skin overlying joints, which are classically spared in ACLE. (see Chapter 15).

Systemic sclerosis (SSc or scleroderma) 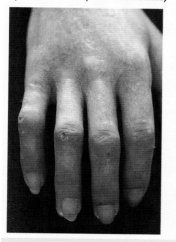	Epidemiology:
	   Uncommon.
	   F > M.
	   Age: Onset typically 30–50 years of age.
	 History:
	   Raynaud's phenomenon, especially with ulceration. Swelling of fingers. Other symptoms include dyspnea on exertion (caused by pulmonary fibrosis in diffuse cutaneous SSc or pulmonary hypertension in limited cutaneous SSc), dysphagia, weight loss, gastrointestinal distress, and pruritus.
	   Positive antibodies: ANA (90%), anti-centromere (limited cutaneous SSc), anti-SCL 70 (diffuse cutaneous SSc), anti-RNA polymerase III (diffuse cutaneous SSc associated with malignancy)
	 Physical exam:
	   Early: Swelling/edema of hands and feet. Digital ulceration and pitted scarring.
	   Late: Shiny, hardening and tightening of the skin involving the skin distal to the elbow and knees (both diffuse and limited cutaneous SSc) and proximal to the elbows and knees (diffuse cutaneous SSc).
	   Other findings to help distinguish systemic sclerosis include calcinosis cutis, matted telangiectasias on face, trunk and hands, hyperpigmentation with perifollicular hypopigmentation, and nail fold capillary dilation and drop out.
	   (see Chapter 15).

Porphyria Cutanea Tarda (PCT) 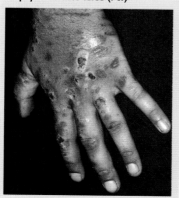	Epidemiology:
	   Rare.
	   M = F.
	   Age: Adults 30–50 years of age.
	 History:
	   Hereditary (20%), acquired (80%).
	   Drugs/toxins: ethanol, hexachlorobenzene, estrogen. Several drugs can cause an eruption that mimics PCT (pseudo-porphyria) including NSAIDs, especially naproxen, as well as several antibiotics, retinoids and diuretics.
	   Other predisposing factors: diabetes mellitus, liver disease (alcoholic liver disease, hemochromatosis, hepatitis C).
	   Onset is gradual.
	   Pain from erosions. Patients may complain of "fragile skin" on hands.
	 Physical Exam:
	   Erosions and tense vesicles/bullae with normal appearing surrounding skin (non-inflammatory). Atrophic, white-pink scars, and milia on dorsal hands.
	   Pseudo-PCT caused by drugs is indistinguishable from PCT and can only be differentiated by normal porphyrin levels.
	   (see Chapter 15).

(continued)

Table 38-1. Skin diseases of the hands. (Continued)

Disease	Features
Pigment Disorders	
Vitiligo 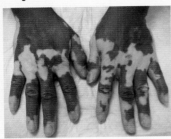	Epidemiology: Common. M = F. Age: Typically, 10–30 years of age. If new onset > 50 years of age, consider melanoma-associated leukoderma and perform full-body skin exam. History: Asymptomatic. Chronic course and progressive. Personal or family history of autoimmune disease. Physical Exam: Well-demarcated depigmented, stark white macules and patches in symmetric distribution. Accentuated with Wood's lamp. Typically located on dorsal hands, ventral wrists, extensor forearms, genitals, and face, favoring the perioral and periocular regions. Distinguish from post inflammatory hypopigmentation by well-demarcated nature, symmetric distribution and depigmentation on Wood's lamp. (see Chapter 23).
Neoplasia	
Actinic keratoses 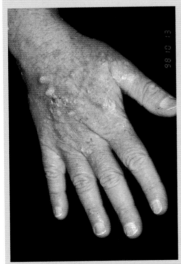	Epidemiology: Common. M > F. Age: > 50 years. History: Persists for months-years, can wax/wane. Asymptomatic or tender. Risk Factors: Advancing age, cumulative sun exposure, outdoor occupation, fair skin type. Physical Exam: Skin-colored, yellow-brown, pink ill-defined rough/gritty papules and plaques with adherent hyperkeratotic scale May be easier to palpate than visualize. Most commonly located on scalp, forehead, temples, cheeks, nose, ears, neck, posterior/lateral neck, and dorsal forearms/hands. Distinguished from various other dermatoses involving the dorsal arms by the rough/gritty texture on palpation of actinic keratoses. (see Chapter 21).

ACD, allergic contact dermatitis; ACLE, acute cutaneous lupus erythematosus; F, female; HSV, herpes simplex virus; ICD, irritant contact dermatitis; M, male; PCT, porphyria cutanea tarda; PPP, palmoplantar pustulosis; SSc, scleroderma; SLE, systemic lupus erythematosus.

Skin Diseases of the Legs

Brittney Schultz
Noah Goldfarb

INTRODUCTION

The legs are predisposed to dermatoses that are gravity-dependent, including stasis dermatitis and vascular conditions such as leukocytoclastic vasculitis, the pigmented purpuric dermatoses, and livedo reticularis. Legs are also the site of frequent trauma and thus are susceptible to conditions that may be induced by trauma including superficial thrombophlebitis, pyoderma gangrenosum, necrobiosis lipoidica, chronic ulcers, and cellulitis. In patients with pre-existing vascular conditions affecting the lower extremities, including diabetes mellitus, venous insufficiency, and peripheral vascular disease, traumatic wounds may take longer to heal with an increased risk of infection.

APPROACH TO DIAGNOSIS

Skin diseases involving the arms can be broadly placed into the following categories starting with the most common diseases (Table 39-1):

- Inflammatory Dermatoses
- Infectious Diseases
- Neoplasia
- Systemic Diseases
- Vascular Diseases

Differentiating between these conditions can usually be done accurately based on an appropriate history and physical examination. Skin biopsies are uncommonly required to make a diagnosis of a rash on the legs, except to confirm the diagnosis of vasculitis, rule out pyoderma gangrenosum, or in recalcitrant eruptions. Occasionally, dermatitis on the lower extremities may be difficult to distinguish from cellulitis. Cellulitis involving the lower extremities tends to present unilaterally compared with a dermatitis, which usually involves both extremities. Widespread stucco keratosis on the legs are also included because sometimes they are misdiagnosed as a "rash."

EVALUATION

- Most leg rashes including stasis dermatitis, nummular dermatitis, asteatotic dermatitis, cellulitis, diabetic dermopathy, pretibial myxedema, superficial thrombophlebitis, pigmented purpuric dermatoses, and livedo reticularis are diagnosed clinically based on the patient's history and physical findings and usually do not require diagnostic testing for confirmation of the diagnosis.

- The diagnosis for erythema nodosum and necrobiosis lipoidica can be made from the history and physical examination alone, but many clinicians obtain a skin biopsy to confirm the clinical diagnosis. Additional evaluation for the underlying cause of erythema nodosum is also recommended.

- In all patients with suspected leukocytoclastic vasculitis, skin biopsies for routine histology, and direct immunofluorescence should be done to confirm the diagnosis and evaluate for IgA deposition. Basic laboratory tests should also be done to evaluate for renal or liver involvement.

- In patients with suspected pyoderma gangrenosum, skin biopsy for routine histology and tissue culture to rule out bacterial, deep fungal, and atypical mycobacterium infections should be performed. While the skin biopsy is non-specific in pyoderma gangrenosum, a biopsy is required to exclude other diagnoses, since pyoderma gangrenosum is a diagnosis of exclusion.
- Skin biopsies on the lower extremity should be done with caution because wounds in this area heal slower and get infected more often. This is especially pertinent to patients with pre-existing vascular conditions affecting the lower extremities, including diabetes mellitus, venous insufficiency, or peripheral vascular disease.

When possible, an attempt should be made to biopsy lesions that are located most proximally.
- A potassium hydroxide (KOH) examination and/or fungal cultures should be done for any annular scaly plaques.
- Bacterial cultures can be performed if primary or secondary infection is suspected.
- Polymerase chain reaction (PCR) for herpes simplex virus (HSV)-1, HSV-2, and varicella zoster virus (VZV) is the preferred test to confirm the diagnosis of herpes simplex or zoster. Viral culture and Tzanck smear can also be utilized.
- Patch testing should be done if allergic contact dermatitis is suspected.

Table 39-1. Differential diagnosis for skin diseases of the legs.

Disease	Epidemiology, History, and Physical Examination
Inflammatory Dermatoses	

Asteatotic dermatitis (eczema craquelé, xerotic dermatitis) 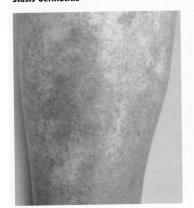	Epidemiology:
	    Common.
	    M > F
	    Age: Typically > 60 years.
	History:
	    Pruritus and dry skin.
	    Waxing and waning course.
	    Worse in winter and low humidity climates. May be exacerbated by excessive bathing in absence of moisturization and use of harsh soaps.
	Physical Exam:
	    Poorly-demarcated, erythematous or hyperpigmented, fissued/cracked, mildly scaly plaques on bilateral anterior lower legs. May have a shiny/glazed appearance.
	    Distinguishing feature: cracked, "dry riverbed" appearance.
	    (see Chapter 8 Dermatitis)

Stasis dermatitis	Epidemiology:
	    Common.
	    F > M.
	    Age: Middle-aged and elderly adults.
	History:
	    Asymptomatic or pruritic.
	    Associated with leg swelling.
	    May have history of varicose veins and thrombophlebitis.
	Physical Exam:
	    Erythematous, scaly plaques on bilateral anterior lower legs, especially medial ankles.
	    Plaques may also be hyperpigmented, lichenified, or sclerotic.
	    Distinguish from cellulitis by bilateral distribution and lack of systemic symptoms.
	    (see Chapter 28).

(continued)

Table 39-1. Differential diagnosis for skin diseases of the legs. (Continued)

Disease	Epidemiology, History, and Physical Examination

Nummular eczema
 	
	Epidemiology:
	  Common.
	  M > F.
	  Age: Bimodal; peaks in young and older adults.
	History:
	  Pruritus is common.
	  Chronic, waxing and waning course.
	  Worse in fall and winter.
	Physical Exam:
	  Round, light pink, scaly, thin, 1–3 cm plaques, most commonly located on the extremities, especially on the legs, but can occur anywhere on the body. Sometimes they can be more moist and indurated and sometimes more xerotic with reticular fissuring. Can have overlying crusting and impetiginization.
	  Distinguish from psoriasis by fine scale, reticular fissuring, less well-demarcated borders, and lack of involvement of classic psoriasis areas (scalp, ears, elbows, knees, gluteal cleft, umbilicus).
	  (see Chapter 8).

Psoriasis vulgaris (chronic plaque psoriasis)
 	
	Epidemiology:
	  Common.
	  M = F.
	  Age: Any age but bimodal distribution peaks in 20s and 50s.
	History:
	  Asymptomatic to mildly pruritic. Chronic course.
	  Associated with inflammatory arthritis and cardiovascular comorbidities (e.g., obesity, diabetes mellitus type II, hyperlipidemia, hypertension, as well as atherosclerotic cardiovascular and cerebrovascular disease).
	  Family history of psoriasis.
	Physical Exam:
	  Well-demarcated, salmon pink to red papules and plaques with overlying white/silvery, thick, adherent scale. Most common on knees, usually symmetric. Other commonly affected areas include scalp, ears, elbows, gluteal cleft, and umbilicus.
	  Distinguish from nummular eczema by the very well-demarcated borders, symmetric distribution, thick white/silvery scale, and involvement of other classic areas.
	  (see Chapter 9).

Erythema nodosum
 	
	Epidemiology:
	  Uncommon.
	  F > M.
	  Age: 20–40 years of age.
	History:
	  Tender lesions.
	  Variable course.
	  May be associated with fevers and arthralgias.
	  Can be idiopathic or triggered by infections (streptococcus), medications (estrogens and OCPs, sulfonamides, iodides, penicillin), autoimmune diseases (sarcoidosis, inflammatory bowel disease), and malignancies.
	Physical Exam:
	  Indurated, tender, red, deep, poorly defined nodules, usually on bilateral shins.
	  Distinguish from cellulitis by bilateral and more multifocal papulonodular nature.

(continued)

Table 39-1. Differential diagnosis for skin diseases of the legs. (Continued)

Disease	Epidemiology, History, and Physical Examination

Pyoderma gangrenosum 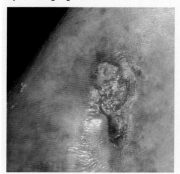	Epidemiology:
	  Rare.
	  F > M.
	  Age: All ages, but typically 30–40 years of age.
	History:
	  Painful. May last months to years.
	  Spontaneous healing may occur.
	  Can worsen after trauma (such as biopsy).
	  Can be associated with systemic disease – most often inflammatory bowel disease, arthritis, or hematologic disorder.
	Physical Exam:
	  Initially, a hemorrhagic pustule with surrounding erythema.
	  Later, ulceration with a dusky red/purple and undermined border. Base of ulcer with granulation tissue, eschar, and purulent material.
	  Most commonly occurs on pretibial region.
	  (see Chapter 28).
	  Pyoderma gangrenosum is a diagnosis of exclusion and other causes of ulceration including infection must be ruled out. A distinguishing feature of pyoderma gangrenosum is exquisite pain.

Infectious Diseases	

Cellulitis 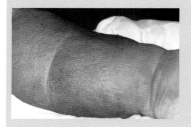	Epidemiology:
	  Common.
	  M = F.
	  Age: Any age. More common in adults.
	History:
	  Acute onset of pain and swelling, fever, malaise, and chills.
	  More common in lymphedema and areas of skin breakdown.
	  Risk increased with obesity, prior surgical site intervention, hepatic or renal disease, connective tissue disease, and malignancy.
	Physical Exam:
	  Localized, warm, red, tender plaque with ill-defined borders, usually on lower leg.
	  Distinguish from stasis dermatitis by unilateral distribution and systemic symptoms.
	  (see Chapter 11).

Tinea corporis 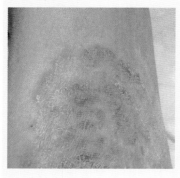	Epidemiology:
	  Common.
	  M = F.
	  Age: Any age, but more common in children.
	History:
	  Asymptomatic or mildly pruritic.
	  Associated with hot/humid weather, farming, and crowded living conditions.
	  History of concomitant tinea pedis.
	Physical Exam:
	  Solitary or grouped, well-demarcated, red, annular plaques with a raised border and peripheral scale. Sometimes peripheral vesicles, pustules, or follicular papules. Typically located on trunk or limbs. When occurring on lower legs, may be an extension of concomitant tinea pedis.
	  Distinguish from nummular eczema by central clearing and concomitant tinea pedis.
	  May be difficult to distinguish from psoriasis or dermatitis, when it does not present as the classic annular plaque with central clearing and edge of scale. For scaly plaques that do not fit a classic psoriasis distribution or do not fit a clear type of dermatitis, an in-office KOH exam may be needed to solidify the diagnosis.
	  (see Chapter 12).

(continued)

Table 39-1. Differential diagnosis for skin diseases of the legs. (Continued)

Disease	Epidemiology, History, and Physical Examination
Benign Neoplasia	
Stucco keratoses 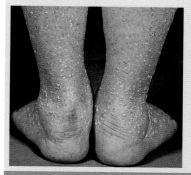	**Epidemiology:** Common. M > F. Age: Older adults. **History:** Asymptomatic and usually unnoticed. **Physical Exam:** Keratotic, stuck-on appearing, whitish-gray papules bilaterally on extensor surface. Distinguish from verruca by "stuck-on" appearance, location on lower legs and dorsum of feet rather than plantar feet, and lack of any black dots within lesion.
Systemic Diseases	
Diabetic dermopathy (Reproduced with permission from Wolff K, Johnson RA, Suurmond D: Fitzpatrick's Color Atlas & Synopsis of Clinical Dermatology, 5th ed. New York, NY: McGraw Hill; 2005.) 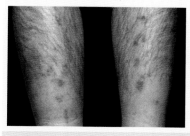	**Epidemiology:** Uncommon. M:F unknown. Age: Usually >50 years. **History:** Asymptomatic. Appears in crops. Slowly resolves with scarring. **Physical Exam:** Well-circumscribed, round, atrophic, and hyperpigmented plaques that heal with scarring on bilateral shins. Distinguish from stasis dermatitis by lack of erythema. (see Chapter 15).
Pretibial myxedema 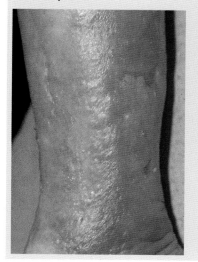	**Epidemiology:** Rare. F > M. Age: Older adults. **History:** Can be asymptomatic, painful, or pruritic. Often associated with hyperthyroidism (most commonly Graves). Can appear after treatment of thyroid disease. **Physical Exam:** Non-pitting edema or pink, waxy indurated nodules and plaques on shins with peau d'orange appearance. Distinguish from cellulitis by bilateral distribution and more subacute to chronic presentation. (see Chapter 15).

(continued)

Table 39-1. Differential diagnosis for skin diseases of the legs. (Continued)

Disease	Epidemiology, History, and Physical Examination

Necrobiosis lipoidica
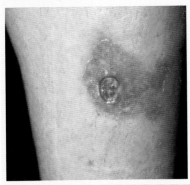
	Epidemiology:
	  Uncommon.
	  F > M.
	  Age: Young adults.
	History:
	  Usually asymptomatic but may ulcerate and become painful. Gradual onset. May last years.
	  One-third have history of diabetes or minor trauma.
	Physical Exam:
	  Well-demarcated, shiny plaques with a mildly elevated, erythematous border and an atrophic, yellowish, waxy center on bilateral shins.
	  Differentiate from stasis dermatitis and cellulitis by more well-demarcated appearance, yellowish hue, and chronic presentation.
	  (see Chapter 15).

Thrombocytopenic purpura (TP)
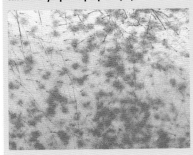
	Epidemiology:
	  Uncommon.
	  M = F.
	  Age: Any age, depending on etiology.
	History:
	  Asymptomatic.
	  Onset over hours.
	  Associated with low platelets due to HIV, TTP, ITP, DIC, drugs, infections, bone marrow dyscrasias, splenic sequestration, etc.
	Physical Exam:
	  Petechiae presenting as non-blanching, non-palpable bright red macules.
	  Ecchymosis with larger red macules and black-and-blue patches.
	  Later these acquire a yellowish-green appearance.
	  Commonly present on shins.
	  Differentiate from leukocytoclastic vasculitis by macular non-palpable presentation and low platelets.
	  (see Chapter 24).

Vascular Diseases	

Superficial thrombophlebitis
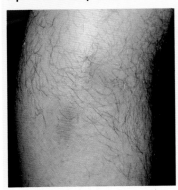
	Epidemiology:
	  Common.
	  M = F.
	  Age: Young- to middle-aged adults.
	History:
	  Asymptomatic or tender.
	  Idiopathic or due to trauma, infection, IV extravasation, or migratory thrombophlebitis.
	  Can be associated with deep vein thrombosis.
	Physical Exam:
	  Red and tender subcutaneous cord with swelling along the course of a vein.
	  Can occur on the trunk or extremities, but most commonly occurs on the legs.
	  Distinguish from cellulitis by palpable cord along the course of a vein.

(continued)

Table 39-1. Differential diagnosis for skin diseases of the legs. (Continued)

Disease	Epidemiology, History, and Physical Examination

Leukocytoclastic vasculitis
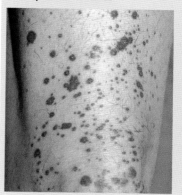
	Epidemiology:
	    Common.
	    M = F.
	    Age: All ages.
	History:
	    Asymptomatic, pruritic, or tender.
	    Can last days to years depending on etiology. Idiopathic or due to drugs, underlying CVD, infections, or malignancy.
	Physical Exam:
	    Palpable purpura/petechiae with bright red well-defined macules and scattered red papules on lower legs (shins) and ankles. May have associated pustules and bullae. Distinguishing feature is "palpable purpura" but the differential for the underlying etiology can be broad.
	    (see Chapter 24).

Pigmented purpuric dermatosis (Schamberg's disease)
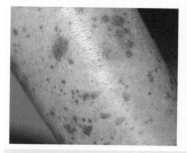
	Epidemiology:
	    Common.
	    M > F.
	    Age: Typically 30–60 years.
	History:
	    Asymptomatic or mildly pruritic. Slowly evolving over months. Chronic, persistent.
	Physical Exam:
	    Characteristic purpuric, speckled, "cayenne pepper–like" macules or less commonly annular plaques and lichenoid papules on lower legs.
	    Distinguish from stasis dermatitis by more macular appearance and reddish-brown or orangish color.
	    (see Chapter 24).

Livedo reticularis
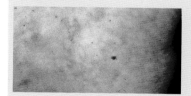
	Physiologic (cutis marmorata)
	Epidemiology:
	    Common.
	    M:F unknown.
	    Age: More apparent in neonates, infants and children.
	History:
	    Asymptomatic.
	    A physiologic phenomenon that occurs in the cold.
	Physical Exam:
	    Purple discoloration of the skin in a netlike distribution on the lower extremities that resolves with warming.
	Primary/idiopathic/pathologic livedo reticularis
	Epidemiology:
	    Uncommon.
	    F > M.
	    Age: 20–50 years old.
	History:
	    Asymptomatic or mild pain/numbness.
	    No underlying systemic diseases.
	Physical Exam:
	    Purple discoloration of the skin in a netlike distribution on the lower extremities that does not improve or resolve with warming.

(continued)

Table 39-1. Differential diagnosis for skin diseases of the legs. (Continued)

Disease	Epidemiology, History, and Physical Examination

	Secondary pathologic livedo reticularis
	Epidemiology:
	  Depends on underlying cause.
	History:
	  Asymptomatic or symptoms related to underlying cause.
	  Associated with conditions that cause vasospasm, increased blood viscosity, vasculitis, or intravascular obstruction.
	Physical Exam:
	  Purple discoloration of the skin in a netlike distribution on the lower extremities that persists after rewarming. When it has a more retiform appearance it is referred to as livedo racemosa.
	  Distinguishing feature: "netlike" appearance.
	  (see Chapter 24).

CVD, collagen vascular disorder; DIC, disseminated intravascular coagulation; F, female; HIV, human immunodeficiency virus; ITP, idiopathic thrombocytopenic purpura; IV, intravenous; M, male; OCP, oral contraceptive pills; TTP, thrombotic thrombocytopenic purpura.

Skin Diseases of the Feet

Brittney Schultz
Noah Goldfarb

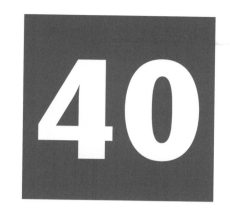

INTRODUCTION

Acral surfaces, such as the feet, have unique characteristics that make them prone to certain dermatologic conditions. The plantar surface of the foot has the thickest keratin layer, a high concentration of eccrine sweat glands as well as sensory nerves, Pacinian corpuscles and other mechanoreceptors. The combination of abundant keratin and sweat creates an ideal environment for fungal infections. Friction and contact with footwear also make the feet susceptible to contact dermatitis. In addition, the feet are disproportionately affected by vascular disorders, due to their gravity-dependent anatomical location, and by peripheral small fiber sensory neuropathies. Since the feet are a site of frequent injury, vascular disorders and sensory neuropathies predispose this area to recurrent and difficult to manage wounds.

APPROACH TO DIAGNOSIS

Skin diseases involving the feet can be broadly placed into the following categories starting with the most common diseases (Table 40-1).

- Inflammatory Dermatoses
- Infectious Diseases
- Ulcers

The most common causes of skin diseases on the feet are dermatophyte infections and inflammatory dermatoses. Clinically these two categories of disease are often indistinguishable from one another. The presence of fissures and/ or scale in the toe web space and nail dystrophy is more suggestive of a dermatophyte infection, but nail dystrophy can also occur in psoriasis. History is often most helpful for vascular disorders affecting the feet.

EVALUATION

- Inflammatory skin diseases, such as dyshidrotic dermatitis, atopic dermatitis, psoriasis, and warts, are typically diagnosed clinically based on the patient's history and physical findings and usually do not require diagnostic testing.
- Potassium hydroxide (KOH) examination and/or fungal cultures should be done for almost all foot rashes as fungal infections may be indistinguishable from inflammatory dermatoses.
- Bacterial culture should be done if a bacterial toe web infection or cellulitis is suspected.
- Polymerase chain reaction (PCR) for herpes simplex virus (HSV)-1, HSV-2, and varicella zoster virus (VZV) is the preferred test to confirm the diagnosis of herpes simplex or zoster. Viral culture and Tzanck smear can also be utilized.
- Skin biopsy could be considered if psoriasis is a likely diagnosis; however, the histopathologic changes of psoriasis on the foot are often nonspecific.
- Patch testing can be considered for any rash in which allergic contact dermatitis is suspected.
- Diagnosis of ulcers is often based on the history and clinical examination.

Table 40-1. Differential diagnosis for skin diseases of the feet

Disease	Epidemiology, History, and Physical Examination
Infectious Diseases	

Tinea pedis

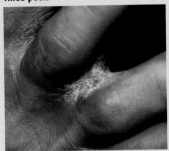
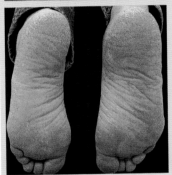

Epidemiology:
  Common.
  M > F.
  Age: Occurs after puberty. Increasing prevalence with age.
History:
  Asymptomatic or pruritic. Lasts months to years. Can occur from contact with infected person or animal or autoinoculation (e.g., from groin). Associated with onychomycosis. Can be associated with tinea manuum, with either two hands and one foot involved or one hand and two feet involved.
Physical Exam:
  Interdigital type: Dry scaling and/ or maceration, peeling, fissuring in toe webs.
  Moccasin type: Well-demarcated erythematous patch with fine, white uniform scale on soles and sides of feet.
  Inflammatory/bullous type: Vesicles or bullae containing clear fluid, erosions on the soles.
  Distinguished from plantar psoriasis by poor demarcation and fine scale. Distinguishing from dermatitis may be more difficult and may require KOH exam. Presence of onychomycosis or hand involvement of one hand can be a helpful clue.
  (see Chapter 12)

Cellulitis

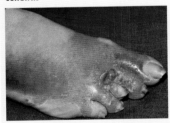

Epidemiology:
  Common.
  M = F
  Age: Any age. When occurring on feet, more common in adults.
History:
  Acute onset of pain and swelling, fever, malaise, and chills.
  More common in lymphedema and areas of skin breakdown.
  Risk increased with obesity, prior surgical site intervention, hepatic or renal disease, connective tissue disease, and malignancy.
Physical Exam:
  Localized warm, red, tender plaque with ill-defined borders.
  Concurrent tinea pedis/onychomycosis can be portal of entry.
  Distinguish from stasis dermatitis by unilateral nature and systemic symptoms.
  (see Chapter 11)

Warts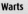

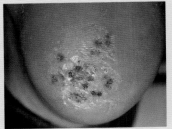

Epidemiology:
  Common.
  M > F.
  More common in children and young adults.
History:
  Asymptomatic or painful. May persist for years.
Physical Exam:
  Discrete or confluent hyperkeratotic papules or plaques on soles. May have black or brown dots within the lesions created by thrombosed capillaries.
  Distinguish from callus by interruption of dermatoglyphics.
  (see Chapter 13)

(continued)

Table 40-1. Differential diagnosis for skin diseases of the feet (Continued)

Inflammatory Dermatoses

Allergic contact dermatitis

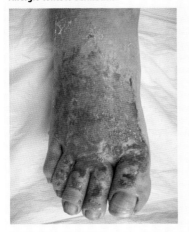

Epidemiology:
    Common.
    F > M.
    Age: Any age, may be more common in adults due to increased topical product usage.
History:
    Pruritic and painful fissures and vesicles.
    Onset is hours to days after contact with allergen. Shoes are a frequent culprit.
Physical Exam:
    Geometric or linear configuration as well as a sharply demarcated distribution are clues to an external cause.
    Acute: Pink to red, edematous papules, and plaques with vesiculation.
    Chronic: Xerosis, fissuring, hyperpigmentation, and lichenification at sites of direct contact with allergen.
    Distribution of involvement may give you clues to allergen. Dorsal toes commonly affected in allergic contact dermatitis caused by materials in shoes.
    Compared to other types of dermatitis, the well-demarcated and often geometric involvement can be clues to allergic contact dermatitis. Patch testing required to distinguish allergic from irritant contact dermatitis. Distinguish from atopic dermatitis due to history of atopy and additional classic areas of involvement of atopic dermatitis.
    (see Chapter 8)

Atopic dermatitis

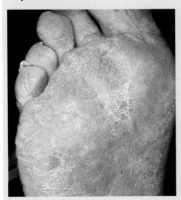

Epidemiology:
    Common
    F > M.
    Age: Can occur at any age, but most commonly occurs in infancy and childhood. Adult onset can occur.
History:
    Pruritus. Chronic course with exacerbations.
    Superinfection common.
    Usually worse in winter. Personal and family history of atopy (asthma, seasonal allergies, allergic rhinitis, atopic dermatitis).
Physical Exam:
    Presents with swelling, xerosis, fissuring, erythema, and lichenification on the dorsal feet and soles.
    Distinguish from other forms of dermatitis by involvement of classic distribution, as well as history of atopy. Distinguish from psoriasis by more common dorsal involvement rather than plantar involvement. Additionally, distinguish from psoriasis based on morphology (psoriasis more well-demarcated, thicker scale), distribution (psoriasis frequently involves extensor surfaces, scalp, and ears).
    (see Chapter 9)

Dyshidrotic dermatitis (pompholyx)

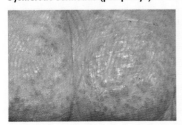

Epidemiology:
    Common.
    F > M.
    Age: Young adults, 20–40 years of age.
History:
    Severely pruritic. Chronic and recurrent with attacks lasting 2–4 weeks. Exacerbated by stress and exposure to allergens or irritants.
    Associated with atopic dermatitis.
Physical Exam:
    Multiple, grouped "tapioca-like" vesicles and erosions on a non-inflammatory base located on the soles.
    Differentiate from bullous tinea pedis by lack of toe web maceration and no nail involvement. If still in doubt, perform KOH.
    (see Chapter 8).

(continued)

Table 40-1. Differential diagnosis for skin diseases of the feet (Continued)

Psoriasis vulgaris (chronic plaque psoriasis) 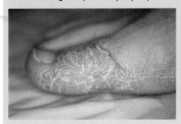	**Epidemiology:** Common. M = F. Age: Any age, but bimodal distribution peaks in 20s and 50s. **History:** Asymptomatic or mildly pruritic. Chronic. Associated with inflammatory arthritis and cardiovascular comorbidities (e.g., obesity, diabetes mellitus type II, hyperlipidemia, hypertension, as well as atherosclerotic cardiovascular and cerebrovascular disease). Family history of psoriasis. **Physical Exam:** Well-demarcated plaques with adherent, thick scale on an erythematous base. Less commonly presents with pustules over pressure-bearing regions of the soles. Distinguished from dermatitis by the very well-demarcated borders, symmetric distribution, thick white scale, and involvement of other classic areas (scalp, ears, elbows, knees, gluteal cleft, and umbilicus). (see Chapter 9).
Palmoplantar pustulosis (PPP) 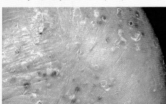	**Epidemiology:** Uncommon. F > M. Age: Onset typically 50–60 years of age. **History:** Pruritus, burning or pain. Lasts years. Chronic waxing and waning course. Strongly associated with tobacco use. May be localized variant of psoriasis limited to palms/soles. **Physical Exam:** Scattered creamy yellow pustules and dusky red macules on soles, with a tendency to affect the heel and instep of the foot; may be bilateral or unilateral. Distinguished from bullous tinea pedis by the deep-seated creamy yellow colored pustules in PPP compared with clear vesicles/bullae in tinea. (see Chapter 9).

Ulcers

Venous ulcer 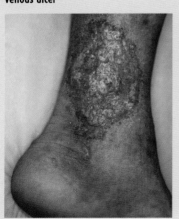	**Epidemiology:** Common. M:F unknown. Age: More common in adults. **History:** Painful ulceration ranging from mild to severe. Associated with venous stasis. **Physical Exam:** Ulceration with background edema. May have associated varicosities. Frequently occurs over or proximal to medial malleolus. Distinguish from arterial ulcer by background lower extremity edema, more proximal involvement, and less often evidence of PAD. (see Chapter 28).

(continued)

Table 40-1. Differential diagnosis for skin diseases of the feet (Continued)

Arterial ulcer

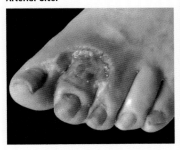

Epidemiology:
  Uncommon manifestation of peripheral arterial disease (PAD).
  M > F.
  Age: PAD more common after 65 years of age.
History:
  Very painful (although pain may be lessened if concurrent diabetic neuropathy).
  Often starts at tips of toes or heel.
Physical Exam:
  Painful ulceration with irregular borders in distal location with pale base. Can become gangrenous with superimposed infection.
  May have other signs of PAD – cool extremities, hair loss, dependent rubor, pallor with elevation, decreased/absent peripheral pulses.
  Distinguish from venous ulcer by more distal involvement and evidence of PAD.
  (see Chapter 28).

Neuropathic ulcer

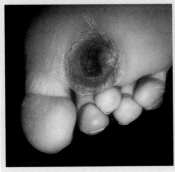

Epidemiology:
  Uncommon.
  M:F unknown.
  Age: More common in adults.
History:
  Painless ulcer.
  May have associated symptoms of neuropathy.
  Most commonly associated with diabetes.
Physical Exam:
  Ulceration over a pressure point of the plantar foot.
  Frequently has surrounding callus.
  Can have exposed bone or tendon.
  Distinguish from venous and arterial ulcers by painless nature and location on pressure point. History of diabetes also helpful.
  (see Chapter 28).

F, females; M, males; PAD, peripheral arterial disease.

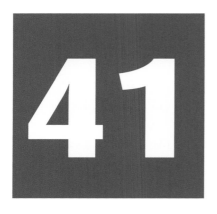

41

Skin Diseases of the Trunk

Noah Goldfarb
Brittney Schultz

INTRODUCTION

The trunk is a general term for the core body region including the chest, abdomen, flanks, and back. Excluding the V-neck and upper back, most of the trunk is covered by clothing, and thus is less exposed to sunlight. Therefore, photo-aggravated or photo-induced dermatoses can frequently be seen on the upper chest and upper back, but typically spare the rest of the trunk. On the other hand, the lower trunk is more commonly involved with dermatoses related to clothing. Clothing may incite rashes due to allergic contact dermatitis from chemicals in the clothing, soaps, dryer sheets, and laundry detergents. Clothing also may create a warmer, humid environment ideal for the development of diseases such as folliculitis, acne, and tinea versicolor.

A high density of sebaceous glands in the presternal area may provide an ideal location for malassezia yeast proliferation, making this a common location for seborrheic dermatitis.

Skin folds are also prominent on the trunk including the axilla as well as the infra-mammary and infra-abdominal regions. Skin folds are unique environments with increased moisture, due to sweat retention, and warmth, that breeds overgrowth of specific microbial flora, especially yeasts, and can lead to maceration. In addition, the occlusive environment increases various inflammatory pathways and can result in friction between tissues that can result in irritation. Finally, the umbilicus is unique in that it has a high density of apocrine glands. Interestingly, some conditions including psoriasis and scabies often favor this site.

APPROACH TO DIAGNOSIS

Skin diseases involving the trunk can be broadly placed into the following categories starting with the most common diseases (Table 41-1):

- Inflammatory Dermatoses
- Infectious Diseases
- Pilosebaceous Disorders
- Autoimmune Diseases
- Other

Inflammatory diseases are the most common cause of skin disease on the trunk, such as morbilliform drug rashes, guttate psoriasis, and pityriasis rosea.

EVALUATION

- Most skin diseases on the trunk are diagnosed clinically based on the patient's history and physical examination findings and usually do not require diagnostic testing for confirmation of the diagnosis.
- A potassium hydroxide (KOH) examination and/or fungal culture should be done for any annular scaly plaques or scaly macules with variable color.
- Bacterial cultures can be done if primary or secondary infections are suspected.
- Polymerase chain reaction (PCR) for herpes simplex virus (HSV)-1, HSV-2, and varicella zoster virus (VZV) is the preferred test to confirm the diagnosis of herpes

simplex or zoster. Viral culture and Tzanck smear can also be utilized.

- A rapid plasma reagin (RPR) or treponema pallidum serology should be done if secondary syphilis is suspected and in pityriasis rosea-like rashes in high risk groups.

- Skin biopsies can be done if the clinical presentation is equivocal
- Patch testing should be done if allergic contact dermatitis is suspected.

Table 41-1. Skin diseases of the trunk.

Disease	Features
Inflammatory Dermatoses	
Allergic contact dermatitis (ACD)	Epidemiology: Common. F > M. Age: Any age, may be more common in adults due to increased product usage. History: Itchy rash, sometimes with blisters and painful fissures. Onset is hours to days after contact with allergen. Physical Exam: Geometric or linear configuration as well as a sharply demarcated distribution are clues to an external cause *Acute*: Pink to red, edematous, plaques with papules and vesicles. *Chronic*: Xerosis, fissuring, hyperpigmentation and lichenification at sites of direct contact with allergen. Distinguish from other types of dermatitis due to a sharply demarcated distribution and geometric/linear configuration. Location is an important clue to the cause of ACD involving the axilla (e.g., preservatives, fragrances and clothing) or navel/lower abdomen (nickel). (see Chapter 8).
Psoriasis vulgaris (chronic plaque psoriasis)	Epidemiology: Common. M = F. Age: Any age but bimodal distribution peaks in 20s and 50s. History: Asymptomatic to mildly pruritic. Chronic course. Associated with inflammatory arthritis and cardiovascular comorbidities (e.g., obesity, diabetes mellitus type II, hyperlipidemia, hypertension, as well as atherosclerotic cardiovascular and cerebrovascular disease) Family history of psoriasis. Exacerbated by HIV and several medications (e.g. beta-blockers, hydroxychloroquine) Physical exam: Well-demarcated, salmon pink to red papules and plaques with overlying white/silvery, thick, adherent scale. Typically located on lower back, umbilicus, scalp, extensor extremities, elbows, knees, genitals, and retro-auricular area. Distinguished from dermatitis by the very well-demarcated borders, symmetric distribution, thick white/silvery scale, and involvement of other classic areas (scalp, ears, elbows, knees, gluteal cleft, umbilicus). (see Chapter 9).

(continued)

Table 41-1. Skin diseases of the trunk. (Continued)

Disease	Features

Guttate psoriasis
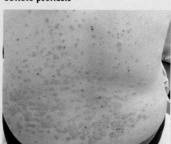
	Epidemiology:
	  Uncommon.
	  M = F.
	  Age: Usually <30 years of age.
	History:
	  Acute onset, self-limited. May be recurrent.
	  Some patients have associated chronic plaque psoriasis or develop it later.
	  Associated with group A hemolytic streptococci infections, typically of the upper respiratory tract, but has also been reported in children with perianal infections.
	  Associated drugs: lithium, beta-blockers.
	Physical exam:
	  Small (<1 cm), circular, well-demarcated, pink to salmon colored papules and plaques with minimal scale. Typically located on trunk and proximal extremities.
	  Distinguished from pityriasis rosea by absent "trailing edge of scale". Distinguished from syphilis due to lack of palm/sole involvement but have low threshold to check treponema pallidum serology. The well-demarcated edge with scale seen with guttate psoriasis helps to place it in the papulosquamous category, distinguishing it from viral or drug exanthems.
	  (see Chapter 9).

Seborrheic dermatitis
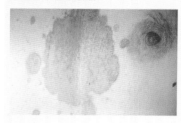
	Epidemiology:
	  Common.
	  M > F.
	  Age: Bimodal age distribution with peaks in infancy and adulthood.
	History:
	  Asymptomatic or mildly pruritic.
	  Waxing and waning course with seasonal variations.
	Physical Exam:
	  Infants: Typically scalp and diaper area involvement
	  Adults: Greasy scale and underlying erythema on the central chest, eyebrows, nasolabial folds, lateral aspects of the nose, retro-auricular areas and ears, often symmetric. Concurrent flaking of scalp common.
	  Distinguish from malar rash of SLE by nasolabial and melolabial fold involvement (both classically spared in SLE).
	  (see Chapter 9).

Pityriasis rosea
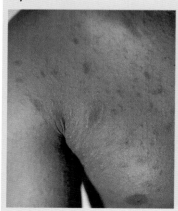
	Epidemiology:
	  Common.
	  F > M.
	  Age: Children and young adults.
	History:
	  Seen in fall or spring.
	  Variable pruritus, sometimes preceding non-specific "flu-like" symptoms.
	  Spontaneous remission in 6–12 weeks.
	Physical Exam:
	  Begins with a herald patch, an oval, slightly elevated, salmon pink, 2–5 cm plaque with trailing collarette of scale. Later dull pink oval papules and plaques with fine scale develop symmetrically on trunk in "Christmas tree-like" distribution.
	  Pityriasis rosacea is distinguished from secondary syphilis which has palmoplantar involvement and no "trailing edge of scale". Presence of preceding genital ulcer favors syphilis and presence of preceding herald patch favors pityriasis rosea. Would have a low threshold to check treponema pallidum serology.
	  (see Chapter 9).

(continued)

Table 41-1. Skin diseases of the trunk. (Continued)

Disease	Features

Drug exanthem 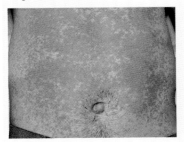	Epidemiology:
	  Common.
	  F > M.
	  Age: Any age, but increased prevalence in older adults.
	History:
	  Asymptomatic or pruritic. Rarely painful.
	  Symptoms, onset, and duration variable, depending on offending agent. History of recent changes or adjustments to medications typically within 2 weeks. Hepatitis, acute kidney injury and eosinophilia can occur with more severe drug eruptions with internal involvement, also referred to drug-induced hypersensitivity syndrome.
	  Risk factors: Elderly, concomitant viral infections, especially HIV (trimethoprim-sulfamethoxazole), and EBV/CMV (amoxicillin or ampicillin).
	Physical exam:
	  Symmetric eruptions, often starting on the trunk and pressure-bearing areas and may generalize. Wide variation in morphologies with morbilliform (pink macules and papules) and urticarial-like most common. Other presentations include scarlatiniform (diffuse erythema) and petechial eruptions. Exanthematous drug eruptions may resolve with desquamation.
	  Facial involvement with swelling, especially ears, mucosal involvement, blisters, purpura, and pain, rather than pruritus, may signify more severe drug rashes with systemic involvement. Can be difficult to distinguish from viral exanthem. Recently initiated new medication would favor drug exanthem.
	  (see Chapter 17)

Grover's disease (transient acantholytic dermatosis) 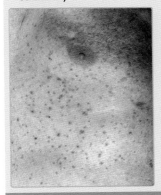	Epidemiology:
	  Common.
	  M > F.
	  Age: ≥ 50 years of age.
	History:
	  Variable pruritus.
	  Abrupt onset with chronic course. Exacerbated by heat, sweat, sunlight, fever, and bedridden status.
	Physical Exam:
	  Discrete, scattered, and/or confluent red hyperkeratotic scaly papules sometimes with crust and erosion on central trunk and proximal extremities.
	  Distinguished from folliculitis by lack of hair follicle involvement. Papules also have overlying central hyperkeratotic scale, and absent pustules.
	  Reproduced with permission from Kang S, Amagai M, Bruckner AL, et al: Fitzpatrick's Dermatology, 9th ed. New York, NY: McGraw Hill; 2019

Infectious Diseases

Disease	Features

Cutaneous candidiasis 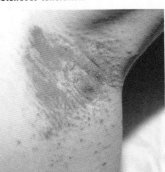	Epidemiology:
	  Common.
	  M = F.
	  Age: Infants and older adults at increased risk.
	History:
	  Pruritus, tenderness.
	  Risk factors include pregnancy, immunodeficiency, obesity, diabetes, antibiotics and glucocorticoid use.
	Physical Exam:
	  Moist, macerated, poorly demarcated red plaques with satellite papules and pustules at periphery located in inframammary, axillary, abdominal and inguinal skin folds as well as on genitals.
	  Distinguished from inverse psoriasis due to the poor-demarcation of the plaques. Distinguished from other types of intertriginous plaques due to the satellite lesions.
	  (see Chapter 12).

(continued)

Table 41-1. Skin diseases of the trunk. (Continued)

Disease	Features

Tinea versicolor 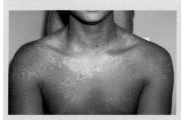	Epidemiology:
	    Common.
	    M = F.
	    Age: Typically adolescents and young adults.
	History:
	    Asymptomatic, rarely mild pruritus.
	    Duration of months to years. More common in summer and warm humid environments.
	Physical exam:
	    Tan to reddish brown oval macules and patches with fine powdery scale that appear after scratching. Variable amounts of hyper- or hypopigmentation. Typically located on central back/chest, neck, and proximal upper extremities.
	    (see Chapter 12).

Tinea corporis 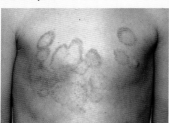	Epidemiology:
	    Common.
	    M = F.
	    Age: All ages, but more common in children.
	History:
	    Asymptomatic or mildly pruritic.
	    Associated with hot/humid weather, farming, and crowded living conditions.
	Physical Exam:
	    Annular plaque(s) with a scaly, raised well-demarcated border and central clearing.
	    Typically located on trunk or limbs. Bathing suit distribution and buttocks is common.
	    May be difficult to distinguish from psoriasis or dermatitis, when it does not present as the classic annular plaque with central clearing and edge of scale. For scaly plaques that do not fit a classic psoriasis distribution or do not fit a clear type of dermatitis, a KOH exam may be needed to clarify the diagnosis.
	    (see Chapter 12).

Infectious exanthems 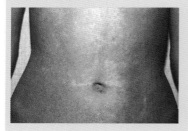	Epidemiology:
	    Common.
	    M: F Unknown.
	    Age: Most common in people younger than 20 years of age.
	History:
	    Viral pathogens are most common, but can be bacterial (e.g., group A streptococcus, mycoplasma spp. rickettsial spp.).
	    Prodromal symptoms including malaise, fever, sore throat, nausea, vomiting, diarrhea
	    Typically self-limiting, 1–2 weeks.
	Physical exam:
	    Multiple presentations including scarlatiniform (generalized erythema), morbilliform (generalized pink macules and papules), or vesicular.
	    Often accompanied by oral mucous membrane involvement (vesicles, ulcers, petechiae), lymphadenopathy, hepatomegaly, splenomegaly.
	    Distinguished from drug eruption due to prodromal symptoms, and lack of any new culprit medications.
	    (see Chapter 26).

Herpes zoster (shingles) 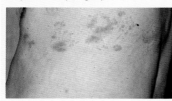	Epidemiology:
	    Common.
	    F > M.
	    Age: Any age but usually >50 years of age.
	History:
	    Severe pain, pruritus, or paresthesias may precede eruption. Lasts 3–4 weeks.
	    Can have longer lasting pain (post-herpetic neuralgia).
	    Increased risk with immunosuppression.
	Physical Exam:
	    Grouped vesicles on an erythematous base that forms crusts in a unilateral dermatome. More rarely presenting with well-demarcated superficial reticulate and punched out ulcers. Most commonly located on thorax.
	    Dermatomal distribution helps to distinguish herpes zoster from herpes simplex.
	    (see Chapter 13).

(continued)

Table 41-1. Skin diseases of the trunk. (Continued)

Disease	Features

Secondary syphilis 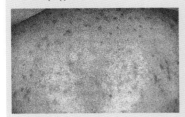	Epidemiology:
	  Uncommon
	  M > F.
	  Age: 15–40 years.
	History:
	  Most commonly manifested by diffuse itchy eruption on trunk, palms and soles that develops 2–10 weeks after primary chancre and self-resolves within 3–12 weeks but may recur. Systemic symptoms may be present or shortly precede onset of eruption (fever, malaise, myalgia, headache).
	  Risk factors: HIV increases the risk of acquiring syphilis and vice versa.
	Physical Exam:
	  Palms/Soles: Red-brown or ham colored macules or papules +/- scale.
	  Trunk: Multiple diffuse, pink, macules or scattered, discrete, firm, red, scaly, well-defined papules in symmetrical distribution. Sometimes with blisters and painful fissures (see Chapter 11)

Pilosebaceous Disorders

Disease	Features

Acne vulgaris 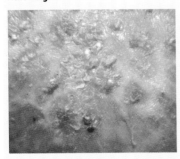	Epidemiology:
	  Common.
	  Teens: M > F.
	  Adults: F > M.
	  Age: Adolescents and young adulthood.
	History:
	  Asymptomatic or may be pruritic or tender.
	  Individual lesions last weeks to months.
	  Fluctuating course. Peri-menstrual flares common.
	Physical Exam:
	  Open (black heads) and closed (white heads) comedones, erythematous papules, pustules, cysts, and nodules.
	  Distinguished from rosacea by the presence of comedones.
	  (see Chapter 10).

Folliculitis 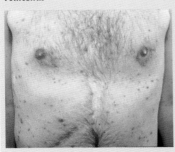	Epidemiology:
	  Common.
	  M > F.
	  Age: All ages, typically after puberty.
	History:
	  Variable pruritus. Can be caused by bacteria (e.g., *Staphylococcus auerus, Pseudomonas aerginosa*), fungi (*Malassezia* spp.), shaving, or occlusion. More common in obese and diabetic patients. Can be recurrent or chronic.
	Physical Exam:
	  Multiple small inflammatory follicular papules and/or pustules. Location typically differs depending on the underlying etiology. Folliculitis due to *P. aeruginosa* is most commonly located on the lower trunk and buttocks when due to contaminated whirlpools (hot tub folliculitis). Folliculitis due to Malassezia spp. is more common on the upper back/chest, proximal upper arms, neck, and hairline. *S. aureus* folliculitis has more variable distribution. Distinguished from acne by lack of comedones and scarring. Concomitant facial involvement is not as common as in acne.
	  (see Chapter 10).

(continued)

Table 41-1. Skin diseases of the trunk. (Continued)

Disease	Features

Hidradenitis suppurativa 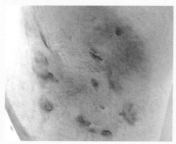	Epidemiology:
	  Uncommon.
	  F > M.
	  Age: Typically presents between ages 11–50. Rarely occurs before puberty or after menopause.
	History:
	  Chronic (>6 months) with recurrent, intermittent flares of painful abscesses and drainage.
	Physical exam:
	  Characteristic lesions include inflammatory, tender nodules, abscesses and tunnels with or without drainage, that heal with hypertrophic scarring. May have large open comedones and comedones with multiple openings.
	  Typically located in intertriginous folds including axilla, inframammary folds, lower abdominal fold, inguinal folds, and buttocks.
	  Differentiated from acne vulgaris by involvement of intertriginous folds and buttocks.
	  Differentiated from staphylococcal folliculitis/furunculosis due to chronic and recurrent nature of characteristic lesions.
	  (see Chapter 10).

Autoimmune Diseases

Disease	Features

Acute cutaneous lupus erythematosus (ACLE) 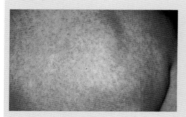	Epidemiology:
	  Uncommon.
	  F > M.
	  Age: Any age, but most commonly 30–40 years of age.
	History:
	  Always associated with systemic lupus erythematosus (SLE).
	  Pruritus or burning. Weeks to months duration. Exacerbated by sun exposure. Associated with hair loss, arthritis, fatigue, oral ulcers, and other systemic findings consistent with SLE.
	Physical Exam:
	  Pink to red edematous papules, plaques, and patchy erythema with variable scale.
	  Typically in photosensitive distribution, including the upper chest and back.
	  Distinguished from dermatomyositis by typically sparing the nasolabial/melolabial folds and dorsal joints of the hands, areas which are also involved in dermatomyositis.
	  (see Chapter 15).

Subacute cutaneous lupus erythematosus (SCLE) 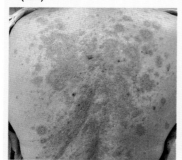	Epidemiology:
	  Uncommon.
	  F > M.
	  Age: Any age, but most commonly ages 15–70 years of age.
	History:
	  Lesions may be asymptomatic or mildly pruritic. May be drug-related, associated with Sjogren syndrome or SLE, or idiopathic.
	Physical Exam:
	  Pink to red, well-demarcated, annular and polycyclic plaques with edge of scale. Many of the plaques develop central clearing and may develop hypopigmentation. Unlike discoid lesions, SCLE does not resolve with atrophy or scarring.
	  Typically located in photo-distributed sites, including neck, upper chest and back, shoulders, and extensor arms classically. Classically sparing the face.
	  Distinguished from psoriasis and other papulosquamous eruptions due to its photo-distribution.
	  Distinguished from discoid lupus erythematosus by the lack of atrophy or scarring.
	  (see Chapter 15).

(continued)

Table 41-1. Skin diseases of the trunk. (Continued)

Disease	Features

Dermatomyositis 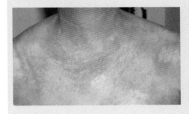	Epidemiology:
	  Uncommon.
	  F > M.
	  Age: Bimodal; peaks at ages 5–10 and greater than 50 years of age.
	History:
	  Typically very pruritic, but may be asymptomatic. Chronic course.
	  Associated with photosensitivity, scalp pruritus/burning, and symmetric proximal muscle weakness.
	  Associated with malignancy in older adults (>60 years of age) and male sex.
	Physical Exam:
	  Pink-violet patches located in photo-distributed sites, including the upper chest (V-sign) and shoulders, proximal upper arms and upper back (shawl sign).
	  Distinguished from acute cutaneous lupus erythematosus (ACLE) in SLE by involvement of nasolabial/melolabial folds and skin overlying joints, which are classically spared in ACLE. (see Chapter 15).

Other	

Acanthosis nigricans (AN) 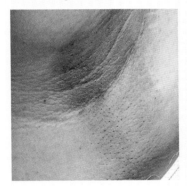	Epidemiology:
	  Common.
	  M = F.
	  Increased in people with darker skin.
	History:
	  Asymptomatic.
	  Associated with obesity and type 2 diabetes mellitus. Rare cases associated with medications and internal malignancy.
	Physical Exam:
	  Symmetric, velvety, hyperpigmented plaques with accentuated skin lines. Associated with skin tags (acrochordons).
	  AN associated with malignancy is indistinguishable from benign AN, but typically involves more unusual sites (palms or mucous membranes). (see Chapter 15).

ACD, allergic contact dermatitis; ACLE, acute cutaneous lupus erythematosus; AN, acanthosis nigricans; F, female; M, male; SCLE, subacute cutaneous lupus erythematosus.

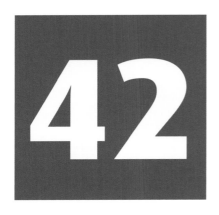

Skin Diseases Involving Multiple Body Regions

Brittney Schultz
Noah Goldfarb

INTRODUCTION

Many common diseases such as atopic dermatitis, psoriasis, drug rashes, urticaria, viral exanthems, bug bites, and vitiligo present with lesions in multiple body regions. Less common disorders such as syphilis, erythema multiforme, Stevens–Johnson syndrome/toxic epidermal necrolysis (SJS/TEN), immunobullous diseases, cutaneous T-cell lymphomas, and connective tissue disorders also present in multiple body locations. The presence or absence of mucosal involvement can be a helpful clue.

APPROACH TO DIAGNOSIS

Skin diseases involving multiple body sites can be broadly placed into the following categories starting with the most common (Table 42-1):

- Inflammatory Dermatoses
- Infectious Diseases
- Infestations and bites
- Drug rashes and urticaria
- Connective tissue diseases
- Autoimmune bullous diseases
- Pigment disorders
- Neoplastic

Lesion distribution is frequently a very important clue to the diagnosis. For example, atopic dermatitis typically involves the flexor extremities, specifically the popliteal and antecubital fossae, whereas psoriasis vulgaris usually involves the elbows, knees, and extensor surfaces. Cutaneous T-cell lymphoma characteristically involves the "bathing-suit" distribution. Erythema multiforme has an acral predilection of "targetoid" lesions and may involve mucosal surfaces. It is still unclear why certain diseases have a predilection for specific anatomic locations.

Diffuse maculopapular (morbilliform) or erythematous patchy (scarlatiniform) exanthems that often involve the trunk are typically due to a medication reaction or viral exanthem. Clinically these conditions may appear indistinguishable, but a thorough history, especially a recent initiation of a medication within 2-3 weeks, is often helpful in differentiating them. SJS/TEN can initially present similarly to a morbilliform eruption, but lesions are often painful and duskier with an "atypical targetoid" morphology and subsequent progression to blisters and erosions. Furthermore, there is usually mucosal involvement in SJS/TEN and Nikolsky sign is positive given fragility of blisters.

The presence or absence of scale can also be helpful in narrowing your diagnosis. Inflammatory disorders such as atopic dermatitis, contact dermatitis, and psoriasis typically have more epidermal changes with scaling as opposed to morbilliform eruptions. Additionally, they usually have accentuation in specific characteristic locations as discussed above.

Bullae and vesicles are the primary lesions associated with immunobullous dermatoses. These dermatoses are a group of antibody-mediated conditions that present with either flaccid or tense bullae depending on whether the autoantigens are located within the epidermis (e.g., pemphigus

554

vulgaris) or at the junction of the epidermis and the dermis (e.g., bullous pemphigoid, dermatitis herpetiformis), respectively. As flaccid bullae are fragile, patients who would otherwise present with flaccid bullae may not present with any bullae and instead may present with erosions and a surrounding edge of scale. Nikolsky sign is positive in conditions with flaccid bullae (e.g., pemphigus, SJS/TEN). In dermatitis herpetiformis, bullae would be tense due to location of auto-antigen but are rarely seen due to intense pruritus and frequent excoriation.

▼ EVALUATION

- Most inflammatory skin diseases, such as atopic dermatitis, nummular dermatitis and psoriasis, can be diagnosed clinically, but any inflammatory dermatoses that has an atypical presentation or does not respond to appropriate treatment may require serial biopsies to verify the correct diagnosis and exclude the diagnosis of cutaneous T-cell lymphoma.

- Potassium hydroxide (KOH) examination and/or fungal cultures should be performed for annular scaly plaques with central clearing.
- Skin biopsy should be performed on any patient with erythroderma (> 80% body surface area with erythema and scaling).
- Skin biopsy should be performed for any bullous dermatoses at the edge of the bullae for routine histopathlogic examination and from adjacent perilesional skin for direct immunofluorescence studies.
- Skin biopsy should be performed urgently in any patient with suspected SJS/TEN to verify diagnosis.
- Polymerase chain reaction (PCR) for varicella zoster virus (VSZ) and herpes simplex virus (HSV)-1 and HSV-2 is the preferred test to confirm the diagnosis of herpes zoster or simplex. Skin biopsy, viral culture, and Tzanck smear can also be utilized.
- Patch testing can be considered for any rash in which allergic contact dermatitis is suspected.

Table 42-1. Differential diagnosis of skin diseases involving multiple body regions.

Disease	Epidemiology, History, and Physical Examination
Inflammatory Dermatoses	

Allergic contact dermatitis 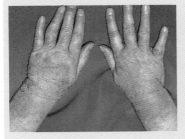	Epidemiology:
	  Common.
	  F > M.
	  Age: Any age, may be more common in adults due to increased product usage.
	History:
	  Pruritus.
	  Onset is hours to days after contact with allergen.
	Physical Exam:
	  Geometric or linear configuration as well as a sharply demarcated distribution are clues to an external cause.
	  Acute: Pink to red, edematous papules and plaques with vesiculation.
	  Chronic: Xerosis, fissuring, hyperpigmentation, and lichenification at sites of direct contact with allergen.
	  Typical Locations: Scalp, face, eyelids, earlobes, neck, hands, wrists, or feet.
	  Distribution can be a clue to culprit allergen.
	  Distinguish from other types of dermatitis due to a sharply demarcated distribution and geometric/linear configuration. Patch testing required to distinguish allergic from irritant contact dermatitis. Distinguish from atopic dermatitis due to history of atopy and additional classic areas of involvement of atopic dermatitis.
	  (see Chapter 8).

Irritant contact dermatitis 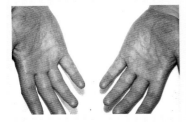	Epidemiology:
	  Common.
	  F > M.
	  Age: Any age.
	History:
	  Pruritic, painful, or burning. May have history of atopy.
	  Variable onset depending on frequency of exposure and strength of irritant.
	  More common in occupations that require frequent hand washing and exposure to water/soap such as health care workers, janitorial services, and food industry employees.
	  Patients with atopic dermatitis are at increased risk.
	Physical Exam:
	  Well-demarcated plaque with a "glazed" appearance.
	  Typical Locations: Eyelids, hands, forearms, and face.
	  May appear identical to allergic contact dermatitis. Need patch testing to differentiate.
	  (see Chapter 8).

(continued)

Table 42-1. Differential diagnosis of skin diseases involving multiple body regions. (Continued)

Disease	Epidemiology, History, and Physical Examination

Atopic dermatitis (AD)
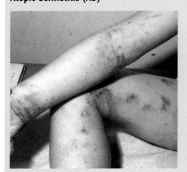
	Epidemiology:
	  Common.
	  F > M.
	  Age: Can occur at any age, but most commonly occurs in infancy and childhood. Adult onset can occur.
	History:
	  Pruritus. Chronic course with exacerbations.
	  Superinfection common.
	  Usually worse in winter. Personal and family history of atopy (asthma, seasonal allergies, allergic rhinitis, atopic dermatitis).
	Physical Exam:
	  Red papules, scaly plaques, lichenification, and excoriations.
	  Typical Locations:
	  Infants: Cheeks, trunk, and extensor extremities.
	  Children & Adults: Neck, wrists, hands, ankles, feet, and flexor extremities, especially antecubital and popliteal fossae.
	  Distinguish from psoriasis based on morphology (psoriasis more well-demarcated, thicker scale), and distribution (psoriasis frequently involves extensor surfaces, umbilicus, scalp, ears, diaper region), and history of atopy in AD, but not in psoriasis.
	  (see Chapter 8).

Nummular dermatitis
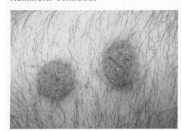
	Epidemiology:
	  Common.
	  M > F.
	  Age: Bimodal; peaks in young and older adults.
	History:
	  Pruritus is common.
	  Chronic, waxing and waning course.
	  Worse in fall and winter.
	Physical Exam:
	  Round, light pink, scaly, thin, 1–3 cm plaques, most commonly located on the extremities, especially on the legs, but can occur anywhere on the body. Occasionally lesions can be more moist and indurated, and sometimes more xerotic with reticular fissuring. Can have overlying crusting and impetiginization.
	  Typical Locations: Trunk and extremities.
	  Distinguish from psoriasis by fine scale, reticular fissuring, less well-demarcated borders, and lack of involvement of classic psoriasis areas (e.g., scalp, elbows, knees, and supragluteal cleft).
	  (see Chapter 8).

Prurigo nodularis
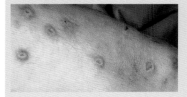
	Epidemiology:
	  Common.
	  F > M.
	  Age: Any age, but more common in older adults.
	History:
	  Pruritic. Persists for months to years. Variable patient insight. May admit to picking and/or scratching lesions. Can be idiopathic or secondary to other underlying etiology (e.g., hyperthyroidism, renal or liver disease, lymphoma, and iron-deficiency).
	Physical Exam:
	  Solitary or multiple discrete, well-demarcated, dome-shaped hyperpigmented papules or nodules often in variable stages of healing.
	  Sparing on central back where patient is unable to reach referred to as the butterfly sign.
	  Typical Locations: Extensor extremities.
	  When limited to a single lesion, prurigo nodules can be difficult to distinguish from other causes of epidermal hyperplasia, including benign lesions, such as seborrheic keratoses, or malignant lesions, such as squamous cell carcinoma (SCC).

(continued)

Table 42-1. Differential diagnosis of skin diseases involving multiple body regions. (Continued)

Disease	Epidemiology, History, and Physical Examination
Psoriasis vulgaris 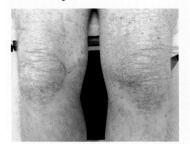	Epidemiology: Common. M = F. Age: Any age but bimodal distribution peaks in 20s and 50s. History: Asymptomatic to mildly pruritic. Chronic course. Associated with inflammatory arthritis and cardiovascular comorbidities (e.g., obesity, diabetes mellitus type II, hyperlipidemia, hypertension, as well as atherosclerotic cardiovascular and cerebrovascular disease). Family history of psoriasis. Associated drugs: lithium, beta-blockers. Physical Exam: Well-demarcated, salmon pink to red papules and plaques with overlying silvery, thick, adherent scale. Often symmetric. Nail pitting/dystrophy. Typical Locations: Scalp, extensor extremities, elbows, knees, genitals, umbilicus, lower back, and retroauricular area. Distinguished from dermatitis by the very well-demarcated borders, symmetric distribution, thick white/silvery scale, and involvement of other classic areas. (see Chapter 9).
Guttate psoriasis 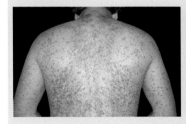	Epidemiology: Uncommon. M = F. Age: Usually <30 years of age History: Acute onset, self-limited. May be recurrent. Some patients have associated chronic plaque psoriasis or develop plaque psoriasis later. Associated with group A hemolytic streptococcal infections, typically of the upper respiratory tract, but has also been reported in children with perianal infections. Physical exam: Small (<1 cm), circular, well-demarcated, pink- to salmon-colored papules and plaques with minimal scale. Typical Locations: Trunk and proximal extremities. Distinguished from pityriasis rosea by absent "trailing edge of scale." Distinguished from syphilis due to lack of palm/sole involvement but have low threshold to check treponema pallidum serology. The well-demarcated edge +/− scale seen with guttate psoriasis helps to place it in the papulosquamous category, distinguishing it from viral or drug exanthems. (see Chapter 9).
Lichen planus 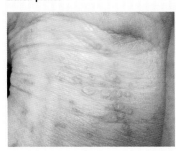	Epidemiology: Uncommon. M = F. Age: Any age, but most commonly between 30 and 60 years of age. History: Pruritic. Lasts months to years. May be drug-induced or associated with Hepatitis C. Physical Exam: Multiple variants exist. Classically flat-topped, well-defined, polygonal, violaceous, shiny papules. May have overlying fine white lines (Wickham striae). Can have associated mucosal involvement, most classically with reticular white lines (Wickham striae) on bilateral buccal mucosa. Erosive disease on mucosal surfaces carries higher risk for squamous cell carcinoma. Nail involvement with dorsal pterygium may also be seen. Typical Locations: Volar wrists, ankles, glans penis, lower back, and buccal mucosa in a symmetric distribution. Distinguishing feature: extremely pruritic, purple papules in classic locations. (see Chapter 9).

(continued)

Table 42-1. Differential diagnosis of skin diseases involving multiple body regions. (Continued)

Disease	Epidemiology, History, and Physical Examination

Erythroderma (exfoliative dermatitis) 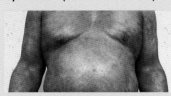	Epidemiology:
	  Rare.
	  M > F.
	  Age: Dependent on underlying cause. Usually older than 40 years of age.
	History:
	  Pruritic. Can develop acutely or chronically.
	  May have associated systemic signs/symptoms (chills, tachycardia, peripheral edema).
	  Several conditions can present with erythroderma, most commonly psoriasis, atopic dermatitis, drug reactions, and cutaneous T-cell lymphoma. Can also be idiopathic.
	  Can occur in children in setting of a hereditary ichthyosis.
	Physical Exam:
	  Erythema and scaling involving >90% of body surface area.
	  May have nail changes.
	  Typical Locations: Entire body affected.
	  May be difficult to discern underlying cause for erythroderma. History of pre-existing dermatosis such as psoriasis or atopic dermatitis or initiation of a new medication can be helpful clues.

Erythema multiforme 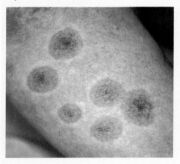	Epidemiology:
	  Uncommon.
	  M > F.
	  Age: Usually in children, adolescents, and young adults.
	History:
	  Asymptomatic or pruritic. May have associated fevers.
	  Most often triggered by infections, usually HSV.
	Physical Exam:
	  Typical target lesions consisting of papules or plaques with three concentric zones of color (dusky purpuric macule or vesicle in center; pale edematous intermediate zone; dark red periphery). May have mucosal involvement with erosions on lips.
	  Typical Locations: Palms, soles, dorsal hands/feet, forearms, face, genitals. Typically, symmetric.
	  Distinguished from secondary syphilis with the presence of classic target lesions and more erosions on lips.
	  (see Chapter 18)

Sarcoidosis 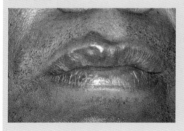	Epidemiology:
	  Uncommon.
	  F > M.
	  Age: Onset most common in 3rd decade of life.
	History:
	  Skin lesions are typically asymptomatic.
	  Chronic course, remissions can occur.
	  May have concurrent systemic involvement, most commonly pulmonary and ocular organ systems.
	Physical Exam:
	  Many clinical presentations, known as "the great mimicker".
	  Classically have reddish-brown "apple jelly" papules and plaques with or without scale. Can preferentially develop within scars and tattoos. Alopecia and nail changes can occur.
	  Nasal ala involvement can be a sign of respiratory involvement.
	  May be associated with erythema nodosum.
	  Typical Locations: Dependent on manifestation. Classic papules and plaques often with perioral/periocular and nasal involvement. Can also involve the trunk, extremities, tattoos, and scars.
	  Sarcoidosis is a diagnosis of exclusion. Distinguish from granuloma annulare by predilection for head/neck involvement.
	  (see Chapter 15).

(continued)

Table 42-1. Differential diagnosis of skin diseases involving multiple body regions. (Continued)

Disease	Epidemiology, History, and Physical Examination

Granuloma annulare
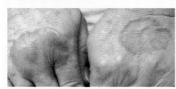
	Epidemiology:
	  Uncommon.
	  F > M.
	  Age:
	  Localized type: Children and young adults.
	  Generalized type: bimodal distribution, age
	  <10 and 30–60 years of age.
	History:
	  Typically asymptomatic.
	  Lasts months to years. Recurrence is common.
	Physical Exam:
	  Skin-colored papules or annular plaques generally without surface change or scale. Can be localized or generalized.
	  Typical Locations:
	  Localized type: dorsal hands/feet, and extensor extremities.
	  Generalized type: trunk and extremities.
	  Distinguish from tinea corporis due to absent scale or surface change. Distinguish from sarcoidosis by less predilection for head/neck involvement.
	  (see Chapter 15)

Infectious Diseases

Disease	Epidemiology, History, and Physical Examination

Herpes zoster (shingles)
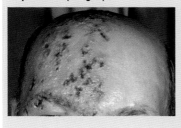
	Epidemiology:
	  Common.
	  F > M.
	  Age: Any age, but usually older than 50 years of age.
	History:
	  Severe pain, pruritus, or paresthesias preceding eruption. Lasts 3–4 weeks.
	  Can have longer lasting pain (post-herpetic neuralgia).
	  Increased risk with immunosuppression.
	Physical Exam:
	  Grouped vesicles on an erythematous base in a unilateral dermatome.
	  Typical Locations: Face and thorax (unilateral).
	  Dermatomal distribution helps to distinguish herpes zoster from herpes simplex.
	  (see Chapter 13)

Viral exanthem
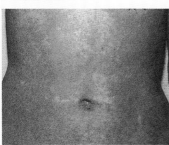
	Epidemiology:
	  Common.
	  M:F unknown.
	  Age: Usually in children less than 20 years of age.
	  Enterovirus infections are more common in the summer months.
	History:
	  Asymptomatic or associated with a prodrome of fever, malaise, rhinitis, sore throat, nausea, vomiting, diarrhea, or headache.
	  Typically self-limiting, 1–2 weeks.
	Physical Exam:
	  Multiple presentations including scarlatiniform (generalized erythema), morbilliform (generalized pink macules and papules, or vesicular.
	  Often accompanied by oral mucous membrane involvement (vesicles, ulcers, petechiae), lymphadenopathy, hepatomegaly, splenomegaly.
	  Typical Locations: Head, neck, trunk, and proximal extremities.
	  Can be difficult to distinguish from drug rash. Lack of new medication would favor viral exanthem.
	  (see Chapter 26)

(continued)

Table 42-1. Differential diagnosis of skin diseases involving multiple body regions. (Continued)

Disease	Epidemiology, History, and Physical Examination
Tinea corporis 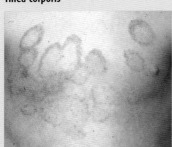	Epidemiology: Uncommon. M = F. Age: All ages, but more common in children. History: Asymptomatic or mildly pruritic. Associated with hot/humid weather, farming, and crowded living conditions. Physical Exam: Annular plaque(s) with a scaly, raised well-demarcated border and central clearing. Typical Locations: Trunk or limbs. May be difficult to distinguish from psoriasis or dermatitis, when it does not present as the classic annular plaque with central clearing and edge of scale. For scaly plaques that do not fit a classic psoriasis distribution or do not fit a clear type of dermatitis, an in-office KOH exam may be needed to solidify the diagnosis. (See Chapter 12)
Syphilis 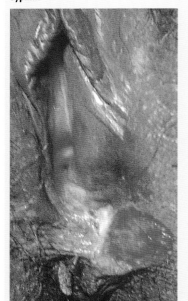 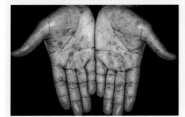	Epidemiology: Common. M > F. Age: 15–40 years. History: *Primary syphilis*: Asymptomatic ulcer (primary chancre), usually on glans penis or vulva, that develops ~3 weeks after infection. Lesion self-resolves in 2–10 weeks. *Secondary syphilis*: Most commonly manifested by diffuse eruption on trunk, palms, and soles that develops 2–10 weeks after primary chancre. Self resolves in 3–12 weeks but may recur. Systemic symptoms may be present at time of, or shortly preceding, onset of eruption (fever, malaise, myalgia, headache). Risk factors: HIV infection increases the risk of acquiring syphilis and vice versa. Physical Exam: *Primary syphilis*: Non-tender firm ulcer with raised border at site of entry. May have associated lymphadenopathy. *Secondary syphilis*: Can manifest in many ways including: Palms/soles: Red-brown or tan-colored macules or papules +/- scale Trunk: Multiple diffuse, pink, macules or scattered, discrete, firm, red, scaly, well-defined papules in symmetrical distribution Scalp: Patchy or diffuse alopecia. Oral mucosa: Mucous patches and fissured papules adjacent to the nose or mouth (split papules). Anogenital region: Moist warty papule (condylomata lata). Distinguished from pityriasis rosea by palmoplantar involvement and absent "trailing edge of scale". Presence of preceding genital ulcer favors syphilis and presence of preceding herald patch favors pityriasis rosea. (see Chapter 11)

(continued)

Table 42-1. Differential diagnosis of skin diseases involving multiple body regions. (Continued)

Disease	Epidemiology, History, and Physical Examination
Bites and Infestations	

Bug bites

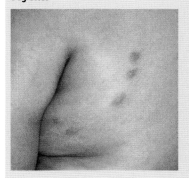

Epidemiology:
  Common.
  M = F.
  Age: Any age, but usually in childhood, adolescents, and young adulthood.
History:
  Acute onset. Pruritic.
  Due to bites from insect (e.g., mosquito, bedbug, flea, mite).
  Most are aware of bug bites, but when the reaction is delayed or occurs during sleep, patients may not know they were bitten.
  Patients with chronic lymphocytic leukemia may demonstrate an exaggerated response.
Physical Exam:
  Clustered, erythematous papules, or vesicles. May have a central hemorrhagic punctum.
  Bedbugs and fleas may demonstrate the "breakfast, lunch and dinner" sign, which involves three or more papules in a linear distribution, a few centimeters apart.
  Typical Locations: Exposed sites such as the head, neck, lower legs, and arms.
  Distinguish from urticaria by more localized and clustered appearance of papules or vesicles with central punctum and duration > 24 hours
    (see Chapter 14).

Scabies

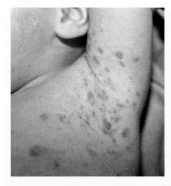

Epidemiology:
  Common.
  M = F.
  Age: Any age, but more common in children.
History:
  Intense pruritus. Chronic symptoms until treated.
Physical Exam:
  Multiple excoriated papules and occasionally small (<1 cm), white, linear, serpiginous tracks or thread-like lesions referred to as burrows. Can be nodular.
  Typical Locations: Finger webs, volar wrists, flexural areas, elbows, axillae, areola, navel, waistline, and genitals. Palm and sole involvement more common in infants. Spares the head and neck.
  Sometimes difficult to distinguish from other diffuse papular eruptions. The classic involvement of web spaces, navel, and genitals can usually help distinguish scabies from other rashes. Itchy papules on male scrotum are almost pathognomonic for scabies and burrows are always pathognomonic for scabies.
  (see Chapter 14).

| **Urticaria and Drug Rashes** | |

Urticaria

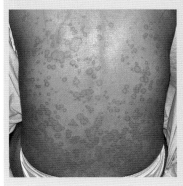

Epidemiology:
  Common.
  M = F.
  Age: Any age, but chronic urticaria is more common in adults.
History:
  Pruritic, sudden onset.
  Individual lesions last less than 24 hours. Acute urticaria may last up to 6 weeks.
  Often idiopathic. When cause identified, most commonly infections (upper respiratory infections), medications (antibiotics, NSAIDs), or food (children > adults). Rarely associated with autoimmune disease.
Physical Exam:
  Pink edematous plaques (wheals) with no surface changes such as scales or crust.
  May exhibit dermatographism.
  Angioedema of lips, eyelids tongue, hands, and feet may be present.
  Anaphylaxis can occur and may present as dyspnea, wheezing, abdominal pain, dizziness, and hypotension.
  Typical Locations: Can occur anywhere.
  Distinguish from bug bites by duration <24 hours and absence of central crust or punctum.
  (see Chapter 16)

(continued)

Table 42-1. Differential diagnosis of skin diseases involving multiple body regions. (Continued)

Disease	Epidemiology, History, and Physical Examination
Drug exanthem 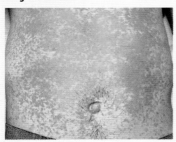	Epidemiology: 　Common. 　F > M. 　Age: Any age, but increased prevalence in older adults. History: 　Asymptomatic or pruritic. Rarely painful. 　Symptoms, onset, and duration variable, depending on offending agent. History of recent changes or adjustments to medications typically within 2 weeks. Hepatitis, acute kidney injury and eosinophilia can occur with more severe drug eruptions with internal involvement, also referred to drug-induced hypersensitivity syndrome. 　Risk factors: Elderly, concomitant viral infections, especially HIV (trimethoprim-sulfamethoxazole), and EBV/CMV (amoxicillin or ampicillin). 　Antibiotics, anticonvulsants, and NSAIDs most common cause. Physical Exam: 　Symmetric eruptions, often starting on the trunk and pressure-bearing areas and may generalize. Wide variation in morphologies including scarlatiniform (erythema), morbilliform (pink macules and papules), urticaria-like, and petechial. Morbilliform most common. May resolve with desquamation. 　Facial involvement with swelling, especially ears, mucosal involvement, purpura, and pain, rather than pruritus, may signify more severe drug rashes with systemic involvement. Blisters may be a sign of SJS/TEN. 　Typical Locations: Starts on trunk and spreads to extremities. 　Can be difficult to distinguish from viral exanthem. Recently initiated new medication would favor drug exanthem. 　(see Chapter 17)
Stevens-Johnson, Syndrome (SJS)/Toxic Epidermal Necrolysis (TEN) 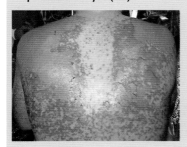	Epidemiology: 　Rare. 　F > M. 　Age: Any age, but usually adults. 　Increased risk in older patients and those with HIV/AIDS. 　High mortality. History: 　Prodrome of nonspecific symptoms such as fever, malaise, headache, cough, fever, sore throat with mucosal irritation followed by development of cutaneous eruption, which can be painful. 　Most common offending agents: allopurinol, carbamazepine, lamotrigine, NSAIDs, phenobarbital and sulfonamide, taken within 4 weeks of rash. Physical Exam: 　Erythematous, purpuric, dusky, targetoid macules and patches that expand and coalesce. 　Lesions develop necrotic centers and flaccid bullae with a positive Nikolsky sign. Typically start on trunk and then spread to extremities and face. 　Mucous membrane involvement common and can precede or follow skin involvement. 　Typical Locations: Trunk and face with frequent mucosal involvement. 　Distinguish from drug exanthem by systemic symptoms, skin pain, dusky nature of lesions, development of blisters, and frequent mucosal involvement. 　(see Chapter 18)

(continued)

Table 42-1. Differential diagnosis of skin diseases involving multiple body regions. (Continued)

Disease	Epidemiology, History, and Physical Examination
Autoimmune Bullous Diseases	

Bullous pemphigoid

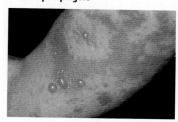

Epidemiology:
Uncommon.
M = F.
Age: 60–80 years of age.
History:
Pruritus with or without blisters.
Can be medication induced.
Physical Exam:
Urticarial plaques +/- tense bullae. Mucous membranes involved in <20%.
Typical Locations: Trunk and proximal flexural extremities.
Distinguish from eczematous dermatoses such as atopic dermatitis and allergic contact dermatitis by older age at presentation, widespread nature, possible mucosal involvement and the presence of bullae. Distinguish from urticaria by duration of lesions >24 hours.
(see Chapter 19)

Pemphigus vulgaris

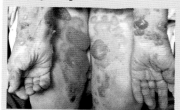

Epidemiology:
Rare.
M = F.
Age: 40–60 years of age.
High mortality prior to advent of corticosteroids.
History:
Painful blisters and erosions on mucosal surfaces (most commonly oral cavity) and skin. Usually no pruritus.
Patients may complain of pharyngitis and/or dysphagia due to other areas of mucosal involvement.
Physical Exam:
Painful, flaccid bullae with a positive Nikolsky sign and crusted erosions with a wet base
Mucosal lesions may involve the oral cavity, pharynx, larynx, genitals, esophagus or conjunctiva.
Typical Locations: Oral cavity. Head, upper trunk, and intertriginous areas.
Distinguish from aphthous ulcers by persistent, recalcitrant, and more widespread nature as well as cutaneous or other mucosal site involvement. Distinguish from SJS/TEN by chronicity.
(see Chapter 19)

Dermatitis herpetiformis (DH)

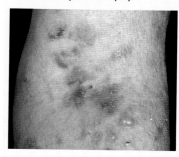

Epidemiology:
Uncommon.
M > F.
Age: Any age, but most common 20–60 years of age.
History:
Severe episodic pruritus.
Almost all patients have an associated gluten-sensitive enteropathy (celiac disease) although it may not be symptomatic.
DH is also associated with several other cell-mediated autoimmune diseases including type I diabetes mellitus, vitiligo, alopecia areata, autoimmune thyroid disease, and pernicious anemia.
Physical Exam:
Grouped, pink, crusted papules and erosions. Vesicles rarely seen due to excoriation.
Typical Locations: Extensor extremities, including elbows and knees, as well as buttocks, scalp, and neck in a symmetric distribution.
Distinguish from widespread dermatitis by morphology of grouped eroded papules and involvement of classic areas (e.g., post-auricular scalp, elbows, knees and buttocks).
Gastrointestinal symptoms can also be a clue.
(see Chapter 19)

(continued)

Table 42-1. Differential diagnosis of skin diseases involving multiple body regions. (Continued)

Disease	Epidemiology, History, and Physical Examination
Connective Tissues Disease	
Acute cutaneous lupus erythematosus (ACLE) 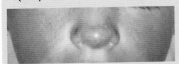	**Epidemiology:** Uncommon. F > M. Age: Any age, but most commonly 30–40 years of age. **History:** Always associated with systemic lupus erythematosus (SLE). Pruritus or burning. Exacerbated by sun exposure. Associated with hair loss, arthritis, fatigue, oral ulcers, and other systemic findings consistent with SLE. **Physical Exam:** Pink to red edematous papules, plaques, and patchy erythema with variable scale. Typical Locations: Photosensitive distribution involving the forehead, malar cheeks (also known as butterfly rash), bridge of the nose, neck, upper chest, and dorsal hands. Classically sparing nasolabial/melolabial folds and skin overlying the joints of the hand. Distinguished from dermatomyositis by typically sparing the nasolabial/melolabial folds and dorsal joints of the hands, areas which are classically involved in dermatomyositis. (see Chapter 15).
Dermatomyositis 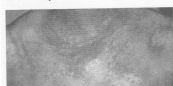	**Epidemiology:** Rare. F > M. Age: Bimodal; peaks at ages 5–10 and 50 years of age. Associated with malignancy in older adults (>60 years of age) and male sex. **History:** Typically very pruritic, but may be asymptomatic. Chronic course. Associated with photosensitivity, scalp pruritus/burning, and symmetric proximal muscle weakness. Associated with malignancy in approximately 20% of adult cases. **Physical Exam:** Pink-violet patches on scalp, periocular region (heliotrope rash), upper chest (V-sign), upper back/shoulders/upper arms (shawl sign), overlying joints, especially elbows, knees, and joints of the hands (Gottron's sign), and thighs (holster sign). Can have centrofacial erythema that classically involves the melolabial folds. Flat-topped violaceous papules overlying knuckles and interphalangeal joints (Gottron's papules). Periungual erythema and ragged cuticles with cuticular overgrowth. Typical locations dependent on manifestation. Distinguished from acute cutaneous lupus erythematosus (ACLE) in SLE by involvement of nasolabial/melolabial folds and skin overlying joints, which are classically spared in ACLE. (see Chapter 15).

(continued)

Table 42-1. Differential diagnosis of skin diseases involving multiple body regions. (Continued)

Disease	Epidemiology, History, and Physical Examination
Pigment Disorders	

Vitiligo

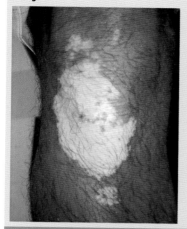

Epidemiology:
  Common.
  M = F.
  Age: Typically 10–30 years of age.
  If new onset > 50 years of age, consider melanoma-associated leukoderma and perform full-body skin exam to evaluate for melanoma.
History:
  Asymptomatic. Chronic course.
  Personal or family history of autoimmune disease.
Physical Exam:
  Well-demarcated depigmented, stark white macules and patches in symmetric distribution Accentuate with Wood's lamp.
  Typical Locations: Dorsal hands, ventral wrists, extensor forearms, genitals, and face, favoring the perioral and periocular regions.
  Distinguish from pityriasis alba by well-demarcated nature and depigmentation on Wood's lamp.
  (see Chapter 23).

Neoplastic

Mycosis fungoides (cutaneous T-cell lymphoma)

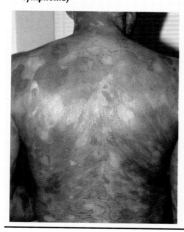

Epidemiology:
  Uncommon.
  M > F.
  Age: Usually in middle-aged adults.
History:
  Asymptomatic to severe pruritus.
  Onset over months to years with chronic course.
  Very slow or absent disease progression.
Physical Exam:
  Well-defined eczematous or psoriasiform patches and plaques that may progress to thicker plaques, nodules, tumors or erythroderma with lymphadenopathy).
  Typical Locations: Sun-protected sites, especially the buttocks, asymmetrically distributed.
  Distinguish from eczematous dermatoses such as atopic dermatitis by involvement of "bathing suit distribution", older age at onset, and no prior history of dermatitis. Requires a biopsy for diagnosis.

F, females; M, males; HSV, herpes simplex virus; NSAID, nonsteroidal anti-inflammatory drug.

Index

Note: Page numbers followed by *f* and *t* indicate figures and tables.